MALIGNANT MELANOMA

MALIGNANT MELANOMA

Irving M. Ariel

M.D., F.A.C.S., M.S. (SURGERY), M.S. (RADIOLOGY)

Professor of Clinical Surgery

New York Medical College
New York, New York

State University of New York at Stony Brook
Stony Brook, New York

Attending Surgeon

Long Island Jewish Hospital
New Hyde Park, New York

Cabrini Medical Center
New York, New York

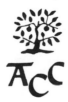

APPLETON–CENTURY–CROFTS/New York

81 82 83 84 85 / 10 9 8 7 6 5 4 3 2 1

Prentice-Hall International, Inc., London
Prentice-Hall of Australia, Pty. Ltd., Sydney
Prentice-Hall of India Private Limited, New Delhi
Prentice-Hall of Japan, Inc., Tokyo
Prentice-Hall of Southeast Asia (Pte.) Ltd., Singapore
Whitehall Books Ltd., Wellington, New Zealand

Library of Congress Cataloging in Publication Data
Main entry under title:

Malignant melanoma.

Bibliography.
Includes index.
1. Melanoma. I. Ariel, Irving M. [DNLM:
1. Melanoma. QZ 200 M2495]
RC280.S5M35   616.99′4   81–485
ISBN 0–8385–6114–4   AACR1

Cover design: Gloria Moyer
Text design: Alan Gold

PRINTED IN THE UNITED STATES OF AMERICA

Dedicated to the Memory of
Dr. George T. Pack (1898–1969)
for his outstanding contributions to clinical cancer,
particularly malignant melanoma

and

Harold S. Brady (1909–1976)
for his dedicated devotion to medical research and education.

CONTRIBUTORS

Rajendra M. Agrawal, M.D.
Chief Resident in Surgery
New York Infirmary
New York, New York

Irving M. Ariel, M.D., F.A.C.S.,
    M.S. (SURGERY), M.S. (RADIOLOGY)
Professor of Clinical Surgery
  New York Medical College
  New York, New York
  State University of New York at Stony
    Brook
  Stony Brook, New York
Attending Surgeon
  Long Island Jewish Hospital
  New Hyde Park, New York
  Cabrini Medical Center
  New York, New York

Myron Arlen, M.D., F.A.C.S.
Clinical Associate Professor of Surgery
Downstate Medical Center;
Chief of Surgical Oncology
Brookdale Hospital Medical Center
New York, New York

Philip W. Banda, Ph.D.
Department of Dermatology
University of California
San Francisco, California

Graeme L. Beardmore, M.B., B.S.,
    D.D.M., F.A.C.D.
Honorary Research Fellow
Queensland Melanoma Project
Princess Alexandra Hospital
Brisbane, Queensland, Australia

William H. Beierwaltes, A.B., M.D.
Professor, Physician-In-Charge
Department of Internal Medicine
Division of Nuclear Medicine
Ann Arbor, Michigan

Alexander Breslow, M.D.
Head of the Surgical Pathology Division
Professor of Pathology
George Washington University Medical
  Center
Washington, D.C.

Arthur S. Caron, M.D., F.A.C.S.
Clinical Assistant Surgeon of Breast
  Service
Memorial Sloan Kettering Cancer
  Center;
Attending Surgeon
Doctors Hospital
New York, New York

John Conley, M.D.
Professor of Clinical Otolaryngology
  (Emeritus)
Columbia Presbyterian Medical Center;
Chief, Head and Neck Surgery
St. Vincent's Hospital and Pack Medical
  Foundation
New York, New York

Neville C. Davis, M.D., HON. D.S.,
    F.R.C.S., F.R.A.C.S., F.A.C.S.
Co-ordinator, Queensland Melanoma
  Project
Princess Alexandra Hospital
Brisbane, Queensland, Australia

Laurence Desjardins, M.D.
Fellow in Ophthalmic Oncology
Edward S. Harkness Eye Institute of
    Columbia Presbyterian Medical
    Center
Department of Ophthalmology of the
    Columbia University of Physicians
    and Surgeons of New York City,
    New York, New York

John M. Edwards, M.S., F.R.C.S.,
    F.A.C.N.M.
Consultant Surgeon and Senior Lecturer
St. Thomas' Hospital
London, England

Mary Anne Fitzmaurice, M.S.
Department of Microbiology
Pacific Northwest Research Foundation
Seattle, Washington

Glenn W. Geelhoed, M.D.
Associate Professor of Surgery
George Washington University
    Medical Center
Washington, D.C.

Satinder T. Gill, M.D.
Chief of Nuclear Medicine Service
Veterans Administration Medical Center
Martinsburg, West Virginia

Stephen L. Gumport, M.D., F.A.C.S.
Professor of Surgery
Consultant, Division of Oncology
Department of Surgery
New York University Medical Center
New York, New York

Ronald C. Hamaker, M.D.
Assistant Professor
Department of Otorhinolaryngology
Indiana University School of Medicine
Indianapolis, Indiana

Matthew N. Harris, M.D., F.A.C.S.
Professor of Surgery
New York University School of
    Medicine;
Director, Division of Oncology
Department of Surgery
New York University Medical Center
New York, New York

Ariel Hollinshead, Ph.D.
Professor of Medicine
George Washington University College of
    Medicine
Washington, D.C.

John Holt, B.Sc., Ph.D.
Lecturer in Numerial Analysis
Department of Mathematics
University of Queensland
Brisbane, Queensland, Australia

Ira S. Jones, M.D.
Clinical Professor of Ophthalmology
Columbia University College
    of Physicians and Surgeons;
Attending Surgeon
Edward S. Harkness Eye Institute
    of the Presbyterian Hospital
New York, New York

John H. Little, M.B., B.S., D.P.H.,
    D.C.P., F.R.C.Path., F.R.C.P.A.
Director of Pathology
Princess Alexandra Hospital
Brisbane, Queensland, Australia

G. Roderick McLeod, M.B., B.S.,
    F.R.C.S.(Edin), F.R.C.S., F.R.A.C.S.
Senior Research Fellow
Queensland Melanoma Project
Princess Alexandra Hospital
Brisbane, Queensland, Australia

Ruben Oropeza, M.D., F.A.C.S.
Assistant Professor in Surgery
Columbia University;
Assistant Clinical Professor in Surgery
Mount Sinai Medical School
New York, New York

Redmond L. Quinn, M.B., B.S., B.Sc.,
M.C.Path., F.R.C.P.A.
Anatomical Pathologist
Princess Alexandra Hospital
Brisbane, Queensland, Australia

Vernon Riley, D.Sc.
Chairman, Department of Microbiology
Pacific Northwest Research Foundation;
Member, Fred Hutchinson Cancer
    Research Center;
Professor (Adjunct)
Department of Rehabilitation Medicine
University of Washington School of
    Medicine
Seattle, Washington

Joseph Scherrer, M.A.
Research Associate
Department of Surgery
Brookdale Hospital Medical Center
New York, New York

Darrel H. Spackman, Ph.D.
Department of Microbiology
Pacific Northwest Research Foundation;
Research Scientist
Fred Hutchinson Cancer Research
    Center;
Associate Professor (Adjunct)
Department of Rehabilitation Medicine
University of Washington School of
    Medicine
Seattle, Washington

Marianne Wolff, A.B., M.D.
Associate Professor of Clinical Surgical
    Pathology
College of Physicians and Surgeons
Columbia University;
Associate Attending Surgical Pathologist
Presbyterian Hospital of the City
    of New York
New York, New York

CONTENTS

Part One
GENERAL CONSIDERATIONS

Part Two
MALIGNANT MELANOMAS
OF SPECIFIC ANATOMIC SITES

PREFACE

The magnificent melanocyte and the malefi-
cent melanoma are discussed in this volume.
The melanocyte present throughout most of
the animal kingdom is a truly remarkable cell.
Its protective function varies from instan-
taneous camouflage, as in the chameleon, to
inherited pigmentary characteristics developed as part of the evolutionary development
of a given species, to its production of protective pigmentary changes for protection as occurs by tanning in the human after exposure to
solar radiation.

Although the number of melanocytes are
more or less equal for the different races, the
genetic transfer of the amount of pigmentary
granules produced by these melanocytes has
resulted in different skin coloration varying
from the Caucasian to the Negro. The social
implications of this melanocyte function are
universally evident.

The melanocytes arise from the precursor
melanoblast during embryonic development
within the neural crest and migrate throughout the body (skin, mucous membrane, nervous system, eye, and other locations). All except those of the retinal pigment can undergo
malignant transformation and form a malignant melanoma. The skin is the most frequent
site. The actual number of melanocytes in a
given individual or in different locations in the
same individual does not seem to influence
the formation of a melanoma. The amount of
pigment produced, the eumelanins, do influence the development of malignancy.
Darker-pigmented individuals have a much
lower incidence of malignant melanoma
(Chapter 2).

Just as the term *cancer* is meaningless inasmuch as certain lesions called *cancer* can be
cured by conservative measures (basal cell carcinoma) whereas others spell a death sentence
with the diagnosis, so the term melanoma is
losing its sting as certain subdivisions of the
generic term have different meanings. The
clinician is deeply indebted to certain
pathologists and dermatologists for their
painstaking researches describing malignant
melanoma as a multifaceted disease with
subclassifications requiring different forms of
treatment and having different prognoses.
Some of these evolutionary changes in the
natural history of melanoma have been
published in the excellent book by W. E.
Clark, Jr., Leonard I. Goldman, and Michael J.
Mastrangelo, and also one by Alfred W. Kopf.

This volume focuses upon the diagnosis,
treatment techniques, and accomplishments
in curing malignant melanoma. Many of the
chapters express the clinical story of patients
with malignant melanoma treated by surgeons
at the Pack Medical Group during the years
between 1935 and 1972.

Although the classification of levels of invasion (Clark et al.) or thickness of the lesion
(Breslow—Chapter 6) were not available during the study, the cases were classified as
superficial or invasive. We do not consider
level I as a metastasizing melanoma and it is
not included in the presentation. Level III
(Clark's classification) is somewhat am-
biguous. Great strides have been made in staging, but strict adherence to mechanistic
parameters may be too simplistic as the formation growth and spread of melanoma involve
many metabolic interactions which include
genetic, chronologic, sexual, hormonal, and
immunologic factors. Considerations of the
histologic, immunologic and other markers
are necessary to define better the clinical conduct of a patient with malignant melanoma.

The vast majority of our patients during
1935 to 1972 suffered from infiltrating melanomas suggesting a late stage of involvement.
The clinical climate is different now since
earlier diagnoses are being made due to lay
education and professional awareness.

This volume commences with general considerations discussing the role of the ubiqui-

tous mole and the iniquitous melanoma; discussions regarding the suggestive causes of melanoma; the universality, incidence, and epidemiology of malignant melanoma. Then Chapter 4 deals with the pathology of melanoma, written by a great student and authority on melanoma, Dr. Marianne Wolff. Drs. Myron Arlen, Ariel Hollinshead, and Joseph Scherrer in Chapter 8 discuss the strides rapidly being made in investigating how melanoma is influenced by the immune system of the host.

Besides the histologic characteristics of different melanomas with the identification of the juvenile melanoma (Spitz nevus) and the B.K. mole, certain biochemical markers illustrating metabolic pathways are discussed by Doctors Vernon Riley and Phillip Banda (Chapter 9).

Principles of clinical evaluation, prognostic indices, routes of lymphatic spread, and the dynamics of lymphatic spread are also discussed. The role of chemotherapy, endolymphatic isotope therapy, and the accomplishments of treating melanoma as a community disease in a location with the highest incidence of melanoma—Queensland, Australia—are presented.

Once a diagnosis of melanoma is established, definitive treatment often depends on the anatomic setting; in fact, melanoma in different locations will be referred to doctors of different specialties. The second section of the volume is presented according to the specific anatomic sites. Melanoma of the head and neck, including mucous membranes, are presented by Doctors Hamaker and Conley, largely from the Pack Medical Group series. Melanoma of the eye and orbit, an important site from the standpoint of etiology, therapy, and immunology, is discussed by Drs. Ira Jones and Laurence Desjardins, authorities in this field. The delay of 10 to 25 years for metastases to present in the liver after enucleation of an eye melanoma evokes speculation regarding the immune mechanisms involved.

In later chapters, the trunk is divided into those melanomas arising from the thorax and those from the skin of the abdomen, because of the lymphatic vessels which are at risk.

Subungual melanomas are treated in a separate chapter stressing the clinical picture and treatment policies of this unique site for melanoma formation.

Melanomas arising at various rare sites are presented for the sake of completeness, such as those arising from the gastrointestinal tract, genitalia, and central nervous system.

The volume closes with a chapter describing the diagnosis of a pulmonary mass in a patient treated previously for melanoma and the conduct of treating such a patient.

There is an ebb and flow in the growth of melanoma and reaction of the host as evidenced by increased pigmentation and size (growth), redness (inflammation), interspacing white areas (host-reaction-destroying melanoma). There is an increased incidence of melanoma but a decrease in deaths as earlier diagnoses are made and adequate therapy instituted.

The authors paradoxically hope that the techniques herein described may soon become obsolete and that preventive early conservative treatment be instituted before the full malignancy of the lesion develops, preferably by instituting immune techniques in preventing and/or treating melanoma. In the meantime this volume offers techniques and accomplishments in treating the patient with infiltrating melanoma today. Further study is needed to define the best treatment for patients with superficial melanomas, level II (Clark), or less than 0.75 mm thickness (Breslow).

ACKNOWLEDGEMENTS

It is a dutiful pleasure to acknowledge with appreciation our indebtedness to the many authorities and their notable contributions which have made this book possible.

The superior medical illustrations contribute greatly to the value of the text. I express my gratitude to each of the medical illustrators and to our own medical photographer, Mr. Harry Weissfisch, for his cooperation in supplying excellent illustrations. I join with the other authors in acknowledging the generous cooperation of the many journals and publishers who freely permitted the use of graphic and statistical material. Specific acknowledgements are given throughout the text.

Our research assistants, Mrs. Brenda Lewy, Mrs. Ingegard Angerer, and Mr. Robert Ariel, have been most assiduous and competent in the assemblage of statistical and referential data for reporting.

Mrs. Pamela Bartle, our editorial associate, tirelessly typed complicated and sometimes unintelligible tapes into rough manuscripts from which the final copy was derived.

The following individuals or foundations have made contributions which were utilized for the vast task of assembling the raw data into reportable manuscripts with the final assemblage of the complicated and complex variables into this coordinated text:

The Pack Medical Foundation
The Foundation for Clinical Research
The Harold S. Brady Cancer Research Fund
The Marilyn Fixman Memorial Cancer Research Fund
The Benjamin Schwartz Foundation
The Janet K. Hetherington Fund
The Arnold and Muriel Rosen Cancer Fund
Mr. Philip Bornstein
The Hudson Chapter of the Pack Medical Foundation, with special thanks to Mr. Rudolph J. DeAngelo.

The author is deeply indebted to the above for their support, without which this volume could not have been produced.

Finally, we are most indebted to Appleton-Century-Crofts and especially to Mr. Robert E. McGrath and Ms. Holly Reid for their patience and industry in the multitude of editorial tasks in the preparation and production of this book.

MALIGNANT MELANOMA

PART ONE

GENERAL CONSIDERATIONS

CHAPTER ONE

A HISTORICAL INTRODUCTION

Is The Beauty Mark a Mark of Beauty or a Potentially Dangerous Cancer?

IRVING M. ARIEL

The expression "black is beautiful" has become common in recent times, applying primarily to the black race. From the standpoint of melanoma, the expression "black is beautiful" becomes pertinent since this form of cancer rarely occurs in the black population. It almost always is found among Caucasians. In fact, if a Negro develops melanoma, it will be at Caucasoid sites—the nonpigmented areas such as the palms, soles, and mucous membranes.

Caucasians often consider a small pigmented lesion to be a sign of beauty. The average Caucasian has approximately 15 to 20 "birthmarks" on the skin, whereas in the Negro these lesions are not found in the pigmented portion of the body but may be found in the nonpigmented areas (palms and soles). Asiatics frequently have tiny birthmarks located in the lumbar region at birth, called "Mongolian spots," which disappear within a few years.

In the evolution of human relationships pigmented lesions have had a bizarre history. The following is an abridged translation from the article *La Française et son grain*, published in Arts Loisirs, August, 1966, Paris, France.[2]

The interest that women have demonstrated toward beauty marks dates back to antiquity. The ancient Gauls exploited them to heighten the value and desirability of their white skin for the purpose of seduction during the Roman occupation. Very quickly, the term *Gallia*, which designated the newly conquered province, became synonymous with the color of milk. With the arrival of Christianity, freckles were seen as a moral indicator: If they were deeply pigmented or raised, theologians welcomed them as a sign from above and recommended that the women expose them clearly in order to protect their virtue. Those marks, however, that might awaken lust had to be concealed under a coarse fabric.

At the end of the Middle Ages, the doctrine was revised. It no longer mattered what the beauty mark was used for, now their presence could bring death. It was no longer the theoretical fires of hell but the real fires of the Inquisition that were promised to the woman whose pigmentation showed a bit too much fantasy. The judges recognized these as the marks of the Devil, and the women were tried for sorcery and often ended on the stake. Exorcists spent entire nights bent over the body of the suspect in an effort to receive clarification from above of the true state of the suspect.

THE SIGNATURE OF THE DEVIL

In the southwest of France, if the women had beauty marks near their mouths, on their breasts, or on their inner thigh it was because the demons of the Basque countries had read Brantôme and Aretin, and had learned which were the erogenous zones and they lingered there amorously before digging in their claws. Victims would complain to their confessors that Lucifer's sex organs were covered with fish scales that lay flat as he entered them but would stand out and up and sting as he would leave them. Satan was coiled like a serpent, his semen was glacial and his breath fiery.

In Lorraine, Satan was prudish. He made love covertly while hidden behind a cloud of smoke.

3

Very often he did not consummate the marriage but contented himself by acting out a parody of baptism. This is why, explain the Exorcists, so many women of this province have beauty marks on their foreheads or their shoulders and always at a respectful distance from the throat or the sex organs.

In the North, Lucifer exhibited himself as a methodical and imaginative lover. "He places marks in shameful places as a sign that one has had an affair with him" explains Marie De Sains. That is, as a sign that one has committed sodomy, or on the heart area as a sign of love, or the lower back as a sign of lust, or on the hands as a sign that one has committed something abominable.

The more beauty marks present, the more highly placed is their possessor in the society of hell and, by consequence, dangerous to Christianity. Jacques Fontaine, Henry IV's doctor, assured us that "a good accountant of beauty marks is worth more in the defense of a kingdom than half a dozen choice regiments." The frightening outcome, notes J. Suyeux, is that in 150 years more than 200,000 witches betrayed by their pigmented skin lesions were reduced to ashes.

A MARK ON THE NOSE

With the Renaissance a mysterious connection between the universe and the body was claimed, and astrologers compared beauty marks to the constellations (Fig. 1-1). This new divining science would for a century eclipse that of wrinkles and palmistry. Before taking any step, such as beginning an affair, one would consult one's reader of beauty marks. A person with a beauty mark on the top of his ear is a thief and a gambler and is capable of killing his mother and father for his own benefit. A woman whose nose is adorned on the top and on the left side with a jet black mark will be quarrelsome and will have two husbands. By contrast a good, honest and fertile wife has a beauty mark on her knee, while a loyal associate has a beauty mark above the right eyebrow. Trips, pleasures, financial and literary adventures were organized by those read into beauty marks as the gypsies would interpret a crytal ball. The Cabalists and members of certain secret societies were recruited on the basis of their beauty marks.

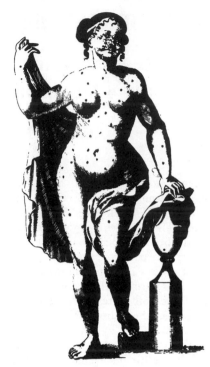

FIGURE 1–1. The distribution of "beauty marks" were interpreted to represent different constellations. Fortune telling on the destiny of the bearer was performed by "experts" in this field as is palmistry today.

WHEN LOVE IS BASED ON BEAUTY MARKS

The age of enlightenment marked the return to saner esthetic traditions. Under Louis XVI, women no longer had to fear the Inquisitors or the interpreters of the divine, nor did they have to hide their beauty marks. On the contrary, they became respectable. Women now darkened them with charcoal, enlarged them, applied false ones or decorated them with small pieces of fabric. At first, they were demurely placed near the temples and behind the ear. Gradually their size and number grew in proportion to the ever-diminishing shadow of the Devil. In the era of the Encyclopedia, no one any longer doubted their personal safety, and the epidermis of flirts was covered with endless designs (moudres pour bal). Some showed signs of the zodiac, while others, inspired by the plates of Buffon, reproduced exotic animals (Fig. 1–2). In less than 100 years, beauty marks became most fashionable.

At Court, the beauty marks had their own language. Some invited flirtation or discouraged gestures that were too suggestive. One gave the green light, while others signified that its wearer's heart was taken. Certain ones were removed to show changing sentiments. The Duchesse of New Castle had her silversmith fashion half a dozen about 4 to 5 millimeters long, depicting a coach drawn by four horses, which could be seen lounging on her cheeks at the outset of some new adventure and descending slowly toward her throat as the fish was hooked, not resuming its original position until the victory was complete. With sensual women, discreet moles made of velvet were placed inside certain anatomical areas, which were of particular interest in love play and served to intensify the at-

traction and heighten erotic sensitivity. Natural or not, these "favorable moles" had definitely lost all religious or magical significance and became instead, instruments of voluptuousness.

THE GOLDEN AGE OF THE BEAUTY MARK

At the festival of white skin, they became the indispensable complement to rice powder, and were placed everywhere; on the face, the breasts, the arms, the legs (Fig. 1–3), on the veils of women of the world and on the stockings of women of the streets.

In 1908, all of France was singing one of Vincent Solto's first songs, "He was counting her beauty marks just as he would count his rosary beads, kiss them and if you find that pleasing, only with the tip of the lips count them again." Monologues, plays, reviews, postcards celebrated their glory. A military vaudeville show received

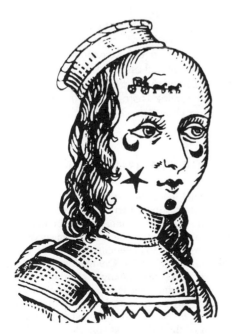

FIGURE 1–2. The beauty marks became more numerous, developed different shapes, and at times depicted her amorous state.

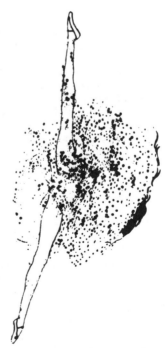

FIGURE 1–3. A dance depicting the "Festival of the White Flesh." Here the "beauty mark" is king.

rave reviews by recounting in an obscene tone the adventures of a gad-about who seduced, by virtue of his beautiful mole, his colonel's mistresses.

WHERE SHOULD ONE PLACE THEM?

For the first time, the beauty mark was not the appendage of a social minority. By fantastic notorious publicity, the obsession of beauty marks gained more territory. J. Suyeur discovered a popular novel wherein the heroine bewitched men by means of three small black marks situated, one at the corner of her mouth, another one at her throat and the third one on her derriere. All males became victims of the passion they inspired. One of her lovers killed her, believing these marks were the sole reason for his love, and proceeded to perform a bizarre operation. With the point of his knife, around each beauty mark he cut a circle of flesh and removed them. After a fifty-year eclipse, the beauty mark is making a comeback. Historians are studying its influence during the evolution of mankind. Ethnologists are asking themselves why so many Africans show such an interest in beauty marks when they discover them on a Caucasian's body. To their eyes does it not indicate the beginning of a cutaneous kinship? A racial kinship? The germ of black skin? A forerunner of black skin? In addition to wearing it as a means to accentuate the beauty, the proud Marquise also often wore it to hide the marks of smallpox, the common disease of the 18th century, and the "waterloo" of women (Fig. 1–4). In this same period, on special occasions beauty marks were held in lorgnette fashion, completely covering the face, and the masks were adorned with beauty marks or patches (Fig. 1–5).

Moles during the 18th century were a sign of beauty, of sexuality, and were expressed by various poets in their writings (Fig. 1–6). An ancestor of the late Dr. George T. Pack (a surgeon who has contributed tremendously to the study of malignant melanoma) whose name was Dr. Richardson Pack, of Oxford, England, wrote a poem published in a book entitled, *Miscellanies in Prose and Verse*, published by E. Curll of London, England in 1727. In this collection is an ode to "Dear

Molly Spring'' whereby he praises her moles as sensuous and beautiful:

> Not far from the Hide* lives a Damsel,
>   so Fair,
> I'd Give Her my Heart for one Lock of
>   her Hair.
> Her Cheeks are like Roses that Blush in
>   their Prime;
> Her Lips sweet as Cherries just Gathered
>   in Time.
> To Gaze on her Eyes might an Hermit
>   inflame;
> And Who Looks *on her Moles* but thinks
>   o' That same?
> Her Waist is as Taper as Mercury's Rod,
> And the Treasures below were a Prize for
>   a God.

MOLES AND THE OLD TESTAMENT

According to Rosner's translation of Preuss' Biblical and Talmudic medical; moles were described as being familial, but it was debated whether they could be used to identity a corpse because some believed the mole changes after death; others questioned this.[3]

A hairy mole on the face makes a woman disfigured; if located on the genitalia of a child might be mistaken for pubic hair. The son of the priest, Zaddek, recognized his sister by a mole on her shoulder when they were both in prison.

MOLES OF THE DALAI LAMA

The regional location or disposition of moles on the skin of the upper part of the trunk played a significant role in the incarnation of the fourteenth Dalai Lama.[1,4] The Dalai Lamas of Tibet were regarded as a single spirit occupying a succession of bodies. In 1933, when the thirteenth Dalai Lama became critically ill, he prophetically hinted about the place of his rebirth. After his death his body sat in state facing south but later the monks noted that his face had turned in the direction of the sunrise; at this the State Oracle flung a khata (white scarf) toward the east, in-

* A celebrated wood in Suffolk.

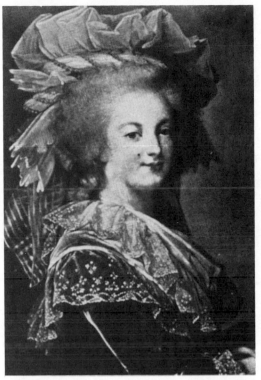

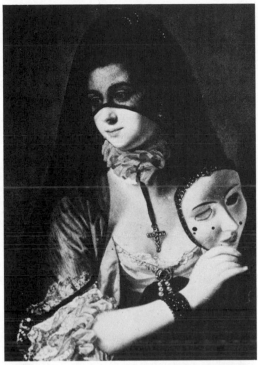

FIGURE 1-4. A famous portrait of Marie An-
toinette (by Elizabeth Louise Vigée-Lebrun) shows
the distinguishing beauty mark.

FIGURE 1-5. The aristocratic woman attended a
social affair with a mask held lorgnette-fashion on
which were painted the beauty marks. (The Fair
One Unmasked by Henry Robert Moreland.)

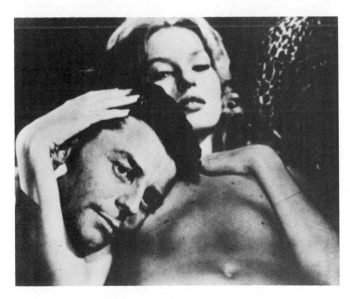

FIGURE 1-6. A French movie, "Les
Liaisons Dangereuses," shows the
heroine Annette Stroyberg bearing 45
beauty marks over her body, a sign
of a sensuous lover. (Courtesy Arts
Loisirs.)

dicating the direction of search for the new Dalai Lama. Dzaza Kungsangtse, the commander-in-chief of the Tibetan army, in his search eastward in the Chinese province of Chinghai, came to a monastery with golden towers which the great thirteenth had described. According to Heinrich Harrer, in his book, *Seven Years in Tibet*, a two-year-old boy ran from a hut and clutched the raiments of a disguised priest in the party crying out, "Sera lama." The disguised priest was said actually to come from the Sera monastery. On the child's body were found the marks or stigmata that the incarnation of Chenrezi, the fourteenth Dalai Lama, should bear—prominent ears and moles in the proper location on his upper trunk; this finding and regional distribution were consonant with the ancient ritualistic qualification.

The concept of black spots being a sign of beauty has survived through the years. They are so considered to this day by many women, either as naturally occurring pigmented lesions or as artificial beauty marks blackened with a cosmetic pencil. Beauty is often conceded to be a dangerous attribute, and this can readily apply to the paradoxical aberration of moles and to the fact that some of these moles may be precursors of dangerous cancers or actually consist of a form of cancer, "malignant melanoma."

REFERENCES

1. Harrier H: Seven Years in Tibet, Graves R (trans). London, Rupert Hart Davis, 1953
2. La française et son grain. Arts-Loisirs, Vol 40, July 1966, pp 6–8
3. Julius Preuss' Biblical and Talmudic Medicine, Rosner F (trans). New York, Sanhedrin Press, 1978, pp 200–201
4. Urtega O, Pack GT: On the antiquity of melanoma. Cancer, 19:607–610, 1966

CHAPTER TWO

THEORIES REGARDING THE ETIOLOGY OF MALIGNANT MELANOMA *

IRVING M. ARIEL

We do not know the exact cause of malignant melanoma. The factors that produce a melanoma de novo or cause a preexisting mole to undergo malignant transformation are undetermined. Certain circumstantial features indicate factors that may be causative agents. (Environmental conditions such as ultraviolet radiation may be melanogenic or comelanogenic.) Others may make the patient susceptible to the development of malignant melanoma (inheritance, complexion etc.). These shall be presented in the hope that the physician may be alerted to such features.

PLACENTAL TRANSMISSION OF MELANOMA

In a number of instances a mother suffering from disseminated melanoma was responsible for the dissemination of that melanoma through the placenta to the child, the offspring then born bearing malignant melanoma.

Holland[46] reported a case of placental transmission of melanoma with microscopic evidence of melanoma in the mother, fetus, and placenta. Gottron and Gertler[42] reported a case of a mother with proven melanoma whose child developed melanoma at age 5 months and died. Dargeon et al.[27] also reported a

---

* An expanded version of an article, Theories regarding the cause of malignant melanoma, published in *Surgery, Gynecology and Obstetrics*, June 1980, Vol. 150, 907–917, reprinted with permission of publisher.

mother with melanoma whose child died of melanoma at the age of 11 months, proven at autopsy. The mother died on the fourth postpartum day with a perforated metastatic melanoma of the small intestine. Byrd and McGaffity reported a melanoma involving the placenta but not the fetus. Reynolds[84] reported a 29-year-old mother with disseminated melanoma including the placenta; at the time of the report the child was 10 months old and did not reveal any melanoma.

Experimentally, Retig and colleagues[83] inoculated the Cloudman S-91 melanoma into the tail arteries of pregnant mice. Disseminated melanoma was found in the mothers, and eight blood samples of newborn offspring showed circulating melanoma cells, but none of the offspring developed melanoma, and the placenta failed to reveal any evidence of melanoma.

INHERITED TENDENCIES FOR DEVELOPING MELANOMA IN ANIMALS

Melanomas have existed within the animal kingdom for millions of years. Virchow, at the turn of the century, recorded an instance of a white stallion whose melanoma of the anal region was transmitted to all his white dependents, but those who had pigment did not get the melanoma (after Feldman) (Fig. 2–1A,B).[34]

The classic study of Myron Gordon on hybrid fish conclusively demonstrates this

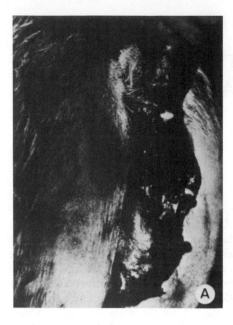

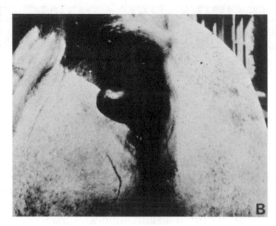

FIGURE 2–1A and B.   Perianal melanoma in gray
Percheron horse.

relationship.[39,40] He and co-workers crossed
two species, the Mexican platyfish (*Platypoe-
cilus maculatus*), and the swordtail (*Zipho-
phorus helerii*). They observed that the
pigmentation of the hybrid depended upon the
presence of two types of pigmented cells,
the macromelanofors and the micromelanofors, and determined that the distribution of
these melanofors was controlled by five genes,
all dominant and sex-linked. In both species,
none of the animals developed melanomas
when mated among themselves, but a constant number of hybrid offspring developed
malignant melanomas that caused death. They
observed that the macromelanofors were the
offending cells: those who had inherited the
macromelanofors developed the melanomas,
whereas those who were amelanotic, or inherited only micromelanofors, did not.

Melanomas have been described in many
species of lower animal life including the
Drosophila, Exolotols (salamanders), mice,
swine, and pine snakes.

Moulton, in a book devoted to tumors in
domestic animals, calls attention to the fact
that melanomas are rather common in the
dog. The incidence is highest between 7 and
14 years of age and very rare in younger dogs.
Scottish terriers, Boston terriers, Airedales,
and cocker spaniels have a higher incidence of
melanoma than most others. In general, the
incidence is higher in dogs with a greater skin
pigmentation, in contrast with the incidence
of melanoma in horses with grey or white
skin. Interestingly, the Dalmatian coach dog,
which has black or brown spots of pigmentation in a white overall skin area, has never
been reported to have suffered a malignant
melanoma.

There appears to be no sex predilection. The
melanomas are usually solitary, and the most
common site for dogs in the United States
is the oral cavity. But in Great Britain,
squamous cell cancers are found more frequently than melanomas. They grow as they
do in the human being, with a 10%–20% local
recurrence after local excision, and spread by
means of the lymphatics and blood stream,
producing death.

Both benign nevi and malignant melanomas
occur in 80% of grey horses but are rare in
horses of other colors. They are also found in
grey, white, and brown mules and donkeys.
The cause is believed to be a disturbance in

metabolism after middle age with a whitening due to cessation of manufacture or absorption of melanin in the hair routes, with the deposition of either new melanoblasts or increased activity of those existing. There is a steady increase in incidence of melanoma in horses over six years of age. Some believe that all horses would develop malignant melanoma if they lived long enough. The most common sites for melanoma in the horse are the perineum lateral to the anus and the underside of the origin of the tail. Melanomas have also been found in the skin of the head (particularly at the base of the ear), on the neck, eyelids, scrotum, udder, and limbs. This tumor when malignant is usually slow-growing, but may metastasize and cause death, as it does in humans.

Melanomas have also been described in the ox, pig, sheep, chicken, cat, and goat. They have also been described in young calves and pigs. The relatively high incidence reported in Angora goats in South Africa is believed due to the fact that these animals are permitted to live long because of the mohair production. Melanomas occur most often in the aged females, and most commonly in the perineum and less often in the ears, horn, stumps, and other body sites. They metastasize and cause death.[97]

HEREDITARY ASPECTS OF HUMAN MALIGNANT MELANOMA

Norris, in 1820, was apparently the first to report an inherited malignant melanoma in a human, which he believed to be of fungus origin.[72] The literature remained rather dormant on the subject until 1952 when Cawley reported the genetic aspects of malignant melanoma occurring in three members of one family: father aged 60, melanoma of the forearm, son aged 24, melanoma of the abdomen, and daughter aged 31, who developed a melanoma of the leg during pregnancy.[19]

The hereditary nature of malignant melanoma was frequently commented upon in relation to the familial occurrence of ocular melanoma.

Miller and Pack[66] have listed three criteria on which to base a conclusion that the melanomas are indeed due to a familial tendency. This is important because of the possibility of melanomas developing coincidentally, regardless of a family tendency: (a) the tumor must be of the same histogenetic type, i.e. melanoma; (b) the tumor must originate in the same type of organ, the skin, eye, oral, anal, and genital mucous membranes; and (c) the tumor would more naturally occur in siblings at approximately the same age, or in successive generations at progressively earlier ages (Fig. 2–2).

Greene and Fraumeni, in reviewing the literature, call attention to the fact that there have been 34 reports of familial cutaneous malignant melanoma existing in 155 kindreds, and 490 cases, an average of three melanomas per family.[43] The largest kindred had 15 individuals.[19] They further call attention to the fact that almost 40% of the familial tumors developed in a parent and one or more children. The exact incidence of familial malignant melanoma is difficult to determine, because the possibility exists that other factors may play a role, such as exposure to sunlight, which has resulted in a higher incidence of familial melanoma in southern climates. Of 377 hereditary melanomas, Greene and Fraumeni state that, when sex was specified, 179 (47.5%) were male and 198 (52.5%) were female. In these data are two sets of twins, one monozygous and one dizygous. They state that in 217 cases where age information was available, the mean age was 41.9 plus/minus 16.2, and that there was no significant difference between males (41.5 years) and females (42.3 years). All reported cases were of Caucasian background, and the lightly pigmented Celts and those from northern Europe seemed to be more susceptible to both the familial type of melanoma as well as the sporadic melanoma.

The increasing number of reported familial melanomas focuses the need for evaluating the causative factors.

The conclusion regarding the genetic aspects of familial malignant melanoma is summarized by Anderson, Smith, and McBride:

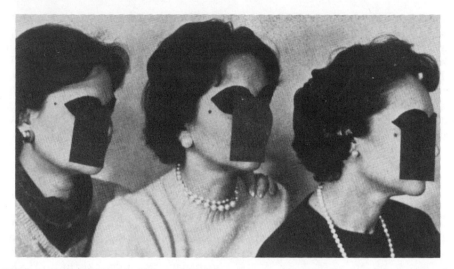

FIGURE 2–2.   Congenital benign nevi in three sisters: note approximate similarity in regional location. (From Miller TR, Pack GT: The familial aspect of malignant melanoma. Arch Dermatol 86:35–39, 1962. Copyright, 1962, American Medical Association. Reproduced by permission.)

This report focuses attention on familial malignant melanoma and some of its clinical characteristics by documenting its occurrence in 22 kindreds, including one in which this malignant neoplasm has developed in a total of 15 individuals. The data convincingly demonstrate a genetic basis for the occurrence of this tumor in these kindreds. Furthermore, the tumor is apparently inherited through the autosomal and not the sex chromosomes. The mode of inheritance involves dominance although the pattern is not always that of a regular dominant. A change in terminology is proposed from "familial" to "hereditary malignant melanoma." Hereditary malignant melanoma is also characterized by the victims' significantly early age at first diagnosis and an increased frequency of multiple primary lesions. The findings have important bearing on early detection of this malignant neoplasm in the relatives of patients.[3]

An example of a genetically related melanoma reported by Miller and Pack is herein presented:

A 16-year-old white girl was first seen in September, 1951, at which time a fungating, black, bleeding skin lesion was seen on the left lower leg above the ankle. The transition from a congenital mole had apparently occurred within the past 3 months. She was pregnant at the time of examination. A 3-dimensional wide excision of the malignant melanoma was done in September, 1951. Three months later, in December, 1951, she gave birth to an 8-pound girl (Fig. 2–3).

Twenty-six years after her surgery, the patient developed metastases to the leg, groin, and brain, and died.

This patient's maternal grandfather died at the age of 42 years of a malignant melanoma originating on the lower leg, and her maternal uncle also died of melanoma. . . The patient's female infant had a black congenital nevus situated in the skin of the left lower leg in the identical location of her mother's melanoma. This junctional nevus was excised when the child was 5 years old.

The child remains well to date.

Miller and Pack reported nine instances of familial melanoma to 1962. Since then eight additional cases considered to be familial melanomas have been seen at the Pack Medical Group.

Do familial melanomas arise from preexisting moles? Most reported series attribute between 50% and 85% of melanomas to preexisting moles. Pack believed that all melano-

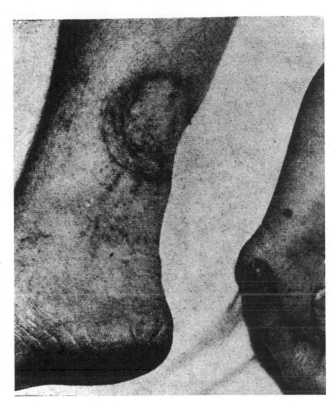

FIGURE 2-3. Mother at age 16 had resection of melanoma of ankle, which developed during pregnancy, and her infant daughter with a large junction nevus at the same site. (From Miller TR, Pack GT: The familial aspect of malignant melanoma. Arch Dermatol 86:35–39, 1962. Copyright, 1962, American Medical Association. Reproduced by permission.)

mas arise from preexisting nevi, many of which are invisible to the naked eye.[73] Greene and Fraumeni reported a 67% incidence of preexisting moles in patients with familial melanomas. St. Arneault et al. reported malignant melanoma in twins (of triplets) each of whom had a nevus on the left chest for a prolonged period before melanoma transformation occurred.[93]

An important contribution was made by Reimer, Clark, Greene, et al in 1978 when they described an atypical nevus labelled the B.K. mole (after the first two families investigated).[82] The characteristics of the B.K. mole are different from the usual benign nevus, which generally appears soon after birth but does not develop beyond the age of 25 years or so. The clinical characteristics of the B.K. nevus are summarized by Reimer. Histologically they are the same as a compound nevus plus: (1) atypical melanocytic hypoplasia; (2) lymphatic infiltration of dermis; (3)

fibroses; (4) neurovenal formation; (5) melanocytes are large, with rare mitoses; abundant cytoplasm filled with melanin in a charcoal-like fashion.

Greene and Fraumeni call attention to two individuals from families that were prone to produce melanomas to demonstrate the B.K. moles transferring into superficial spreading melanomas. They further state that the B.K. mole syndrome has tended to segregate into autosomal-dominant patterns within these families. They add that these moles tend to appear far more susceptible to neoplastic change than the usual acquired melanocytic nevi, as evidenced by the earlier age at which the melanomas may develop and the tendency towards producing multiple primaries. Despite their increased susceptibility, it seems that they require some external stimulus, the nature of which is not known but may include ultraviolet irradiation or changes in hormonal balance,[73] oncogenic viruses, or carcinogenic chemicals to induce the malignant changes. It appears that a substantial fraction of melanoma-prone families have an underlying syndrome of multiple atypical nevi that provide a cutaneous marker for identifying family members with a high risk of melanoma. In such cases, thorough periodic skin examinations and early removal of suspicious lesions may be life-saving.

Another factor to consider in patients with a familial tendency or a sporadic melanoma may be hormonal influences. For example, women usually have a better prognosis than men, and it has been stated that parous women fare better than nulliparous women.[45] Instances have been described of melanomas exacerbating during pregnancy, (Fig. 2–4)[78] and there have been several cases on record where the melanoma presumably disappeared after pregnancy. It has recently been claimed that oral contraceptives have contributed to the formation of melanoma.[12] Hormonal studies between those with sporadic melanomas and those with familial melanomas are sketchy and the data rather problematic.

The detection of estrogen receptors in melanoma cells lends support to the hormonal influence on the life history of the malignant melanoma.[36] The influence of environmental factors seems even more convincing. Sunlight is considered a cocarcinogen for melanoma. Patients with xeroderma pigmentosa, a genetic disease associated with defective DNA repair induced by ultraviolet light, have a tendency to develop skin cancers including malignant melanoma (Fig. 2–5).[24] Spontaneous regression of melanomas in siblings has been reported.[58] Greene and Fraumeni state that patients with familial melanoma have no greater susceptibility to ultraviolet light than normal persons. It appears that in hereditary malignant melanoma the melanocytes are genetically susceptible to the harmful effects of the ultraviolet radiation and that this susceptibility is further increased for those atypical melanocytes that exist in the B.K. mole syndrome.

Neurocutaneous melanosis with its high incidence of cutaneous melanomas is another entity due to a genetic disorder associated with

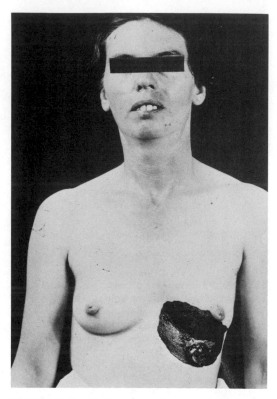

FIGURE 2–4.   Malignant melanoma of the breast which expanded rapidly during her pregnancy.

an autosomal recessive disorder (Fig. 2–6).[81]

Studies on albinism show that certain genes regulate cell metabolism, including melanin synthesis and the metabolism of the various ingredients including tyrosinase.[37]

Although it is well known that patients with albinism are highly susceptible to skin cancer, only about eight cases of cutaneous malignant melanomas have been reported in the albino to date (Fig. 2–7).[106] The mechanism of the genetic influence is too complex for this volume, and the reader is referred to Greene and Fraumeni.[43]

The early and proper treatment of patients with familial malignant melanoma may be life-saving. Where there are two or more cases of malignant melanoma in a family, the melanomas should be treated exactly as if they were sporadic melanomas. Careful review is

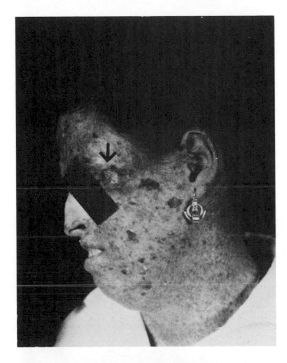

FIGURE 2–5. Melanoma in a patient with xeroderma pigmentosa.

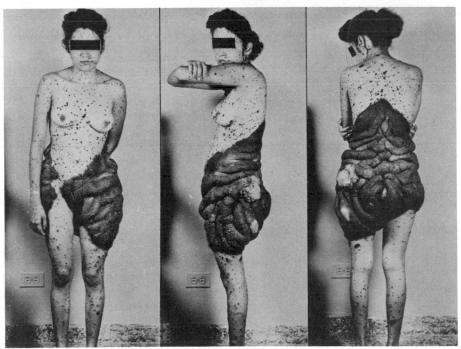

FIGURE 2–6. Melanoma developed in a patient with a huge bathing trunk nevus associated
with neurofibromatoses (Von Recklinghausen's disease).

necessary by someone deeply interested in the study of melanoma of the entire family, and any suspicious-looking lesion should be locally and conservatively excised. Other forms of therapy such as escoratics or electrodissection should be emphatically avoided. Other members of the family should be examined, with particular attention to areas where the melanomas occur most frequently. Such families should be warned against exposure to sun and advised to wear protective clothing or use sunscreens such as para-aminobenzoic acid. Sunlamps should be avoided. Such families should also be warned against undue exposure to petrochemicals, as these have been responsible for the induction of melanomas in susceptible animals experimentally, although the data are not conclusive for humans. Careful scrutiny is indicated for

susceptible families during periods of pigment metabolism stress, especially during adolescence and pregnancy.

The value of such a program is implied by the report of Reimer, who discovered and treated six patients with superficial spreading melanoma who were unaware they had such a disease and in whom the prognosis seems excellent, in that no metastases existed. The question of hormonal manipulation in these families is an enigmatic one and pertains especially to patients taking corticosteroids, oral contraceptives, or sex hormones.

There have been reports of nongenetic transmission of malignant melanoma within given families. Several cases of melanomas in husband and wife,[85] and one example of a melanoma in a genetically unrelated stepbrother have been reported, suggesting some nongenetic but rather environmental (viral) factor.[8]

BENIGN MOLES AND MALIGNANT MELANOMAS

In the preceding section describing the inherited tendencies for developing malignant melanoma, an entity was described in which the B.K. nevus was responsible for the so-called B.K. syndrome, in which certain inherited nevi with specific characteristics were more prone to the development of malignant melanomas. This section will discuss the theories pertaining to the development of malignant melanomas in benign nevi.

In approximately 75% of the patients questioned, the nevus was present for a variable period before it underwent malignant transformation.

The first report of a benign mole undergoing malignant transformation is attributed to Laennec in 1806. Sir James Paget in 1864 remarked that the occurrence of cancer in or under pigmented moles was a well-known phenomenon.[79] Later, Traub noticed that malignant melanomas arose from benign junctional nevi.[98] Becker, however, believed that most melanomas originate from isolated

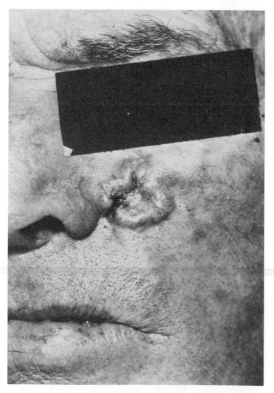

FIGURE 2–7. Malignant melanoma of the face of an albino.

melanocytes at the epidermal-dermal junction of normal skin and only rarely from preexisting nevus cells, and after careful study, was able to find neval tissue in only 23% of the specimens of melanoma he studied.[9] He further believed that melanomas may arise from lentigo malignum.

Pack and Davis[74] believed that nearly all melanomas arise from preexisting nevi, some of which may be invisible to the naked eye. Allen has demonstrated quite conclusively that melanomas arise from nevi with junctional activity.[1,2] Pack et al.[75] determined that approximately 15 nevi exist in the average Caucasian, and the incidence of melanoma is so rare that the likelihood of a benign nevus undergoing malignant melanoma transformation would be approximately one per million. One could, therefore, not remove all nevi prophylactically, and the determination of which nevi may be removed prophylactically depends upon many parameters, both clinical and histologic.

Histologically, only junction or compound nevi can undergo malignant transformation, whereas the intradermal nevus, for all practical purposes, never does. The blue nevus of Jahdasson (Fig. 2–8) has rarely undergone malignant changes, and Hutchinson's freckle may undergo malignant changes, with a rather low degree of malignancy.[35]

Very few nevi exist in the newborn. The large bathing trunk nevus or garment nevus is usually congenital and frequently is a precursor for a malignant melanoma (Fig. 2–9). There is no unanimity of opinion as to whether sporadic congenital nevi should be removed, but care must be taken both from an oncologic as well as a cosmetic standpoint to develop a surgical plan for removing them.

Most nevi appear during the early days of life; it is believed that they seldom undergo malignant transformation. Nevi that appear later in life are more suspicious. Dubreuilh termed them "precancerous circumscribed melanosis."[29] Becker, in 1945, emphasized the danger of delayed nevi, which he called "malignant lentigo."

Veronesi et al.[100] have observed that a pa-

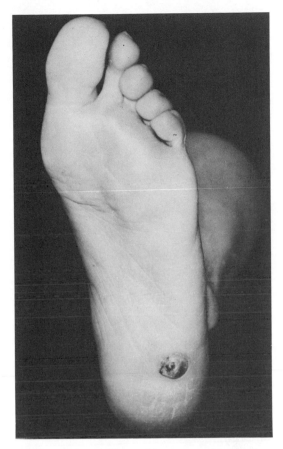

FIGURE 2–8. **Malignant blue nevus of Jadassohn, which produced metastases in the lymph nodes of the groin.**

tient who has or had a malignant melanoma is 900 times more likely to have a second primary than an individual in the general population. The risk is age and sex-dependent.

Billroth[15] is credited with being the first to describe multiple primary melanomas in the same patient, and since then over 2,000 such cases have been reported.[67]

Some claim a higher incidence of noncutaneous cancer in patients who had melanoma.[1,2,90] Bellet et al found an 8.2% prevalence for such an occurrence to be no greater than would be expected from chance alone.[11]

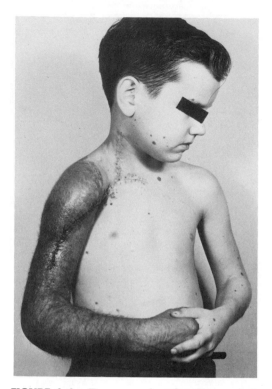 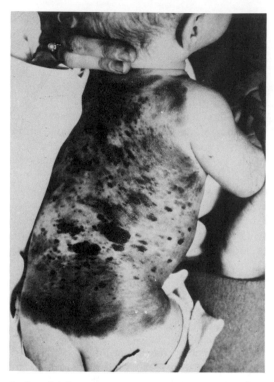

FIGURE 2–9. Two examples of malignant melanoma developing in giant congenital nevi. The boy on the left had a wide excision and neck dissection for metastases to the neck. The baby on the right had multiple melanomas scattered about her giant nevus. She died at 16 years of age, cerebellar metastases.

Pack et al. have studied the distribution of benign nevi as well as the distribution of malignant melanoma as seen at the Pack Medical Group, and noted a high incidence of junction and compound nevi on the palms of the hands, soles of the feet, and genitalia. These doctors have recommended that these are potentially malignant and should be excised prophylactically (Fig. 2–10). Wilson and Anderson reviewed this subject and came to the conclusion that the incidence of malignancy in these regions was approximately 0.18%, which argues against routine excision.[105]

Malignant change is indicated by changes in size or color (increased or decreased pigmentation), ulceration, pruritis, bleeding, irregularity of the margin, or satellitosis.

FACTORS INFLUENCING BENIGN NEVI TRANSFORMATION

TRAUMA

While trauma is frequently claimed by patients to have induced malignant changes, the possibility of this occurring is most unlikely. Constant irritation, such as pressure from a belt, collar, suspenders, brassiere, a tight shoe, or the repeated trauma from shaving or scratching, have been implicated by patients. However, no definite proof exists, and studies of location of melanomas do not support such hypotheses. It is more likely, in fact, that ulceration and bleeding has been caused by an irritation upon a lesion that has previously gone through transformation.

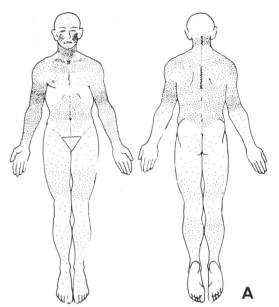
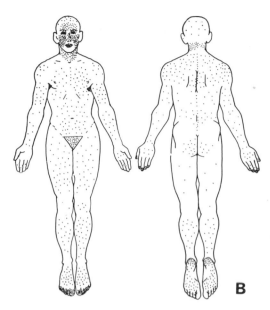

FIGURE 2–10. Distribution of moles and melanomas. A. Regional distribution of nevi found on general examination, based on 1,000 adult patients. Each dot represents five nevi. B. Regional distribution of malignant melanomas, based on 1,225 patients. Each dot represents one malignant melanoma. Internal malignant melanomas not shown above: Eyes, 64; oral cavity, 18; nasal cavity, 8; inner ear, 2; lung, 1; esophagus, 1; anorectal region, 19.

All irritations, such as electrolysis, irradiation, cauterization with pastes or electrocautery, or any escarotics, must be avoided. There is a possibility that infection is a factor in the induction of subungual melanomas.

There are numerous reports where a claim is made that trauma was a causative factor.[14,44,89] It is possible that persistent and continuous trauma does play a role in certain instances of melanoma of the sole of the foot, but sufficient examples exist where a similar degree of trauma occurs in certain populations with no melanoma formation, and other examples of melanoma developing where there was no history of trauma.[65]

Ewing[32,33] states that the traumatic stimulation of cutaneous nerves may be a factor in initiating the metamorphosis of a specific cell of sensory nerve terminal into melanoma. In discussing the role of trauma to nevi, one must include the iatragenic trauma often induced by physicians who incompletely remove nevi, shave nevi, apply irritating and caustic substances to nevi, and or otherwise traumatize the nevus. Although it is difficult to state that the offending agent was the causative factor in the production of the melanoma, it is a fact that a constant irritation was produced and that cells were left behind with a potential for malignant changes, and emphatically argues against such procedures.

HORMONAL INFLUENCES

The pigmentary system of the human undergoes constant changes. At the time of puberty many unnoticed or invisible nevi become prominent. During pregnancy, the areola undergoes deeper pigmentation with enlargement and increased pigmentation of many nevi. A nevus removed from a pregnant woman often shows considerable activity. The fact that malignant melanoma is so extremely infrequent in the preadolescent child focuses upon the hormonal influence on pigmentary metabolism in general, and on the life history of the nevus in particular. One instance was observed by us of a metastasized prepubertal melanoma with hormonal imbalance and precocious puberty due to a masculizing tumor of the adrenal gland in a 5-year-old Negro boy. In support of the possible effect of hormonal influence, malignant melanoma has never been described in a castrated male.[76]

Efforts to control malignant melanoma dissemination by hormonal manipulation such as bilateral adrenalectomy, hypophysectomy, castration, or estrogen administration, were all without effect in our experience with 80 patients.

The influence of pregnancy on melanoma formation is disputed. Although moles do become larger, no known factors conclusively prove that pregnancy induced the transformation of a mole to a melanoma. The effect of pregnancy on the behavior of an existing melanoma is also uncertain; most authors claim there is no statistical proof that pregnancy, per se, adversely affects the prognosis of the melanoma, although some believe that it does. Several cases have been reported of increase in the growth of a melanoma during pregnancy, and partial or complete regression with the delivery of the baby.[2,18,96]

Stewart reports the opposite finding: tumors recurring weeks after the patient delivered her babies on three separate occasions.[95]

The influence of menopause on the course of a melanoma is also unclear. White quotes a number of patients who noted the onset of the disease, or increased growth, or the presence of metastases, associated with the onset of menopause.[104] He cites one patient who had survived seven years without evidence of recurring tumor, who died with widespread metastases two months after she had missed her first period. This problem remains very enigmatic.

SUNLIGHT AND MALIGNANT MELANOMA

McGovern, in 1952, first suggested that solar radiation played a role in the oncogenesis of melanomas.[63] This theory has gained wide acceptance, but warrants further elucidation because of its extreme importance.

It is a fact that sunlight produces the usual skin cancers (squamous and basal cell carcinomas). In experimental animals (especially the hairless mouse) ultraviolet light has been conclusively demonstrated to be a carcinogen. Presumptive evidence exists that sunlight may also be a carcinogen, or cocarcinogen, in the etiology of malignant melanomas. Evidence supporting this viewpoint is as follows:

1. In those parts of the world where light-skinned Caucasians receive large amounts of solar radiation (Australia and Israel), the incidence of malignant melanoma is highest,[28] especially in regions of the skin exposed to the sun. Regions that are generally protected from exposure to sunlight, such as the breasts in women, or the portion of the trunk in men and women covered by clothing, have a lower incidence of melanomas.

2. This observation may not be limited to different countries. In countries with many latitudes malignant melanoma is greatest in those who reside closest to the equator. Thus, Magnus[60] found that the incidence of melanoma in the southern part of Norway was almost three times that in the northern part. Movshovitz and Modan[71] found that the incidence of melanoma was highest in native-born Israelis, indicating that the period of exposure played a role.[71]

3. Individuals with deep pigmentation, such as Negroes or dark Caucasians, have a much lower incidence of malignant melanoma, demonstrating the protective effect of the melanin pigment (Table 2–1). The pigmentation of the Negro population is not due to an increased number of melanocytes, which is actually equal to the number of melanocytes in the white population, but rather to the elaboration of greater amounts of pigment present in the layers more superficial to the site of the melanocytes (Fig. 2–11).

4. Approximately 11% of the population are of dark complexion, whereas in our series of 3,305 melanoma patients reported from the Pack Medical Foundation in New York, approximately 85% of the patients were of light

TABLE 2-1. Comparative Frequency of Nevi in Various Racial Groups

Group	Number of Individuals	Number of Nevi	Average Number
Negroes	208	376	2
Bantus of South Africa	133	375	3
Indians of Bombay	124	983	9
Filipinos	103	2,641	26
Japanese	103	1,752	16
Chinese	102	3,019	30
Mestizo Indians	98	2,552	26
Maya Guarani Indians	95	258	3
Maoris of New Zealand	88	234	3

extraction. (This, however, is biased in that many of the patients came from different parts of the country.)

5. Patients with xeroderma pigmentosa, where the sunlight induces numerous cutaneous tumors, such as keratoses, basal and squamous cell carcinomas, and other lesions, develop malignant melanomas more frequently than do others. Moore and Iverson (1954) found that 3% of 360 patients with xeroderma pigmentosa developed malignant melanoma, and at the National Institutes of Health, of 15 patients with xeroderma pigmentosa, seven (47%) developed malignant melanoma.[68]

6. Metastasizing melanoma was induced in animals, such as hairless mice, exposed to artificial ultraviolet light in combination with a topically applied carcinogen (dimethyl benzanthracene).[31]

7. Measurements supporting the ultraviolet light theory were performed by Scotto, Fears, and Gorie using a "sunburning ultraviolet meter," which measures the effectiveness of ultraviolet light in inducing erythema of the skin.[88] In repeated recordings in ten widely spread geographic areas of the United States, the incidence of all skin cancers, including basal and squamous cell carcinomas and malignant melanomas, increased with the increased exposure to ultraviolet light.

8. An interesting theory was promulgated by Lee and Merrill in 1970, who raised questions about the actual role of sunlight in inducing melanoma.[56] They postulated a "solar circulating factor" as an etiologic cause to explain the incidence of malignant melanoma of unexposed areas. They believe that this factor is circulated via the blood to different sites, exciting the melanocyte to undergo malignant transformation.

9. If exposure to ultraviolet light is indeed a factor, two current practices warrant evaluation. One is that the fluoro-carbon gases used as propellants for sprays deplete the ozone layer, which filters out much of the carcinogenic ultraviolet light that reaches the surface of the earth. Recent legislation has outlawed their use. Furthermore, the use of commercial supersonic aircraft, flying at high altitudes unprotected by the ozone layer, has been estimated to have resulted in at least 8,000 more skin cancers a year in the white population, and in about 300 more deaths from skin cancer including melanoma.[17] It is estimated that the ozone shield has been reduced by 5%. These factors strongly suggest the use of sunscreens, and public education may be rewarding.

10. Fitzpatrick postulates that nonexposed parts of the body may still receive injurious amounts of ultraviolet irradiation.[37]

11. Houghton, Munster, and Viola have presented data suggesting that the incidence of melanoma increases during periods of maximum sunspot activity.[48] They show that the incidence for malignant melanoma in Connecticut has risen from 1.1 per 100,000 individuals in 1935 to 6.2 per 100,000 in 1975.

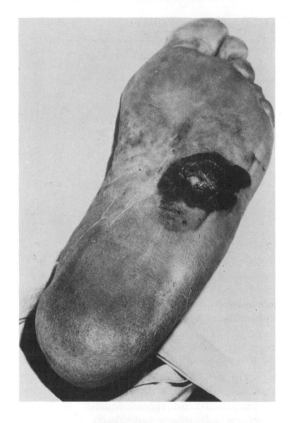

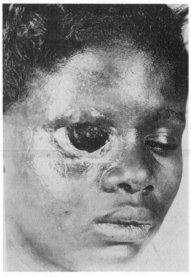

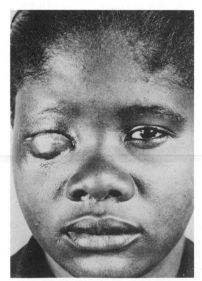

FIGURE 2–11.   Melanoma of foot (upper) and eye (lower) in Negroes.

Superimposed on the steady rise in incidence are 3 to 5 year periods in which the rate of increase in incidence rises. These periods have a cycle of 8 to 11 years and follow times of maximum sunspot activity. A similar cyclic activity was observed in New York and may be related to reduction of the ozone layer.

A recent survey on the linkage of solar ultraviolet radiation to skin cancer, performed under the auspices of the Federal Aviation Administration for the High Altitude Pollution Program by P. Cutchis,[26] casts doubt on the carcinogenic activity of ultraviolet radiation in malignant melanoma (Figs. 2-12 and 2-13). His conclusions can be summarized as follows:

1. Ultraviolet radiation is a dominant factor in the induction of squamous and basal cell carcinomas.

2. A very large number of inexplicable anomalies of various kinds are found in the worldwide incidence data, which are inconsistent with the hypothesis of solar ultraviolet radiation being a significant factor in the induction of malignant melanoma, leading to the conclusion that the primary cause(s) for this class of tumor must be sought elsewhere.

3. There is no clear evidence of a latitude gradient for the incidence of melanoma.

4. For most geographical regions the malignant melanoma sex ratio is less than unity, a finding that is inconsistent with the solar ultraviolet radiation hypothesis for malignant melanoma.

5. The incidence of malignant melanoma in males in Norway is 20 times higher than for Zaragoza, Spain. Since Norway is much further from the equator than Spain, this finding contradicts the lifetime solar ultraviolet dose hypothesis. Residents of all Mediterranean countries of Europe show a very low malignant melanoma mortality rate, while residents of all Scandinavian countries and Finland suffer a high mortality rate.

6. Age-specific incidence cures for malignant melanoma differ fundamentally from those of other skin cancers. In recent years the risk for other skin cancers increases almost exponentially with age, while the risk of malignant melanoma is essentially the same for adults between approximately 40 to 65 years of age. These data suggest that the malignant melanoma incidence is not a significant function of a lifetime dose nor, in all likelihood, the number of acute ultraviolet doses received.

7. There has been a worldwide increase in the incidence of other skin cancers and malignant melanoma in almost all countries with a predominantly white population. Exceptions can be found. Squamous cell carcinoma incidence decreased in Finland from approximately 6 per 100,000 in 1960 to 3.5 in 1973, whereas malignant melanoma increased from 2 to 3.5 in the same period. In Australia, mortality from malignant melanoma doubled from 1950 to 1964, but mortality from other skin cancers decreased by 50% during the same period. These are examples in which time variations of incidence run in opposite directions over a long period and constitute anomalies for solar radiation hypotheses linking solar radiation with malignant melanoma.

8. Malignant melanoma mortality exceeds other skin cancer mortality for both males and females and has increased with time, whereas other skin cancer mortalities have decreased with time. There is evidence in some countries of latitude gradient for malignant melanoma mortality. Since malignant melanoma also occurs in younger age groups, it poses a far more serious problem. Other skin cancers favor the most exposed anatomic sites (head, neck, and hands) whereas malignant melanoma favors the relatively unexposed anatomic sites (trunk and lower limbs). The lower limb is more favored in females. However, this finding is consistent with the solar radiation hypothesis.

9. Malignant melanoma is particularly found in members of professional and managerial classes, whereas other skin cancers are particularly found in some of the skilled and nonskilled workers more exposed to ultraviolet radiation.

10. Recent evidence in Finland, Norway, Denmark, and Poland suggest that urbanization is a factor in the etiology of malignant melanoma.

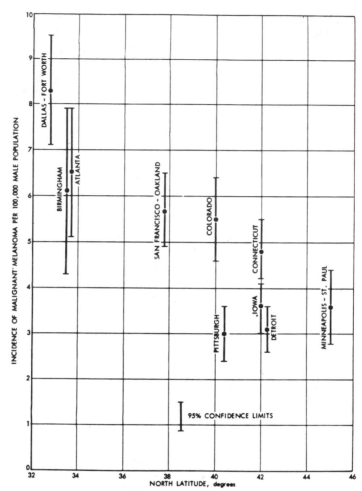

FIGURE 2-12A. Incidence of malignant melanoma for U.S. white male population in ten areas for the period 1969-1971. (From Cutchis P: On the Linkage of Solar Ultra Violet Radiation to Skin Cancer. Institute of Defense Analysis Paper P-1342, 1978. With permission of author and publisher.)

11. The etiology of malignant melanoma is in a chaotic state, and the acute ultraviolet dose hypothesis for malignant melanoma is in need of further investigation. Sunburn data for various populations and melanoma cases by anatomic site will be essential.

It is essential to question the ultraviolet radiation theory as a melanogen or co-melanogen; if the theory is valid, prophylaxis can be practiced; if not valid, it deters further investigation regarding the exact cause(s) of malignant melanoma.

VIRUS AND ITS RELATIONSHIP TO MALIGNANT MELANOMA

Viruslike particles have been found in 15 of 26 melanoma biopsies (58%) by P. G. Parsons of Brisbane, Australia [80] Similar findings have

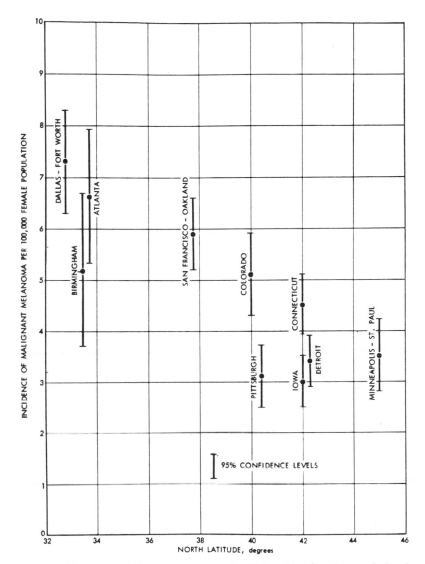

FIGURE 2-12B. Incidence of malignant melanoma for U.S. white female population in ten areas for the period 1969-1971. (From Cutchis P: On the Linkage of Solar Ultra Violet Radiation to Skin Cancer. Institute of Defense Analysis Paper P-1342, 1978. With permission of author and publisher.)

been made by others[6,16] but the exact nature remains undefined.

Findings of antimelanoma antibodies suppose some infectious factor.[61] A recent finding by Goldsmith that melanoma could develop from subcellular fractions is noteworthy.[38b]

DIET AND ITS RELATIONSHIP TO MALIGNANT MELANOMA

Can "what we eat" cause skin melanomas? There is now controversy over whether diet plays a role in the etiology of malignant

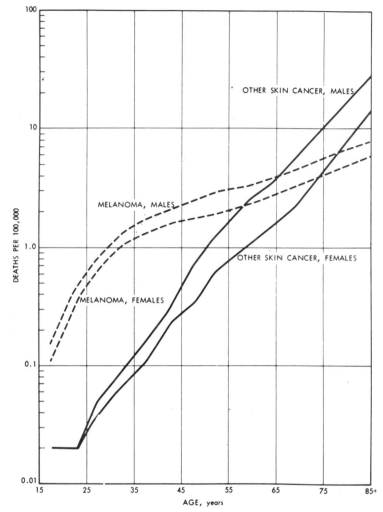

FIGURE 2-13. **U.S. white mortality rates for malignant melanoma and other skin cancer, 1950-1969.** (From Cutchis P: On the Linkage of Solar Ultra Violet Radiation to Skin Cancer. Institute of Defense Analysis Paper P-1342, 1978. With permission of author and publisher.)

melanoma. Of 500 consecutive patients who came to a plastic surgeon's office in Los Angeles, 54% forced polyunsaturated foods into their diet, and 60% of this group had had at least one skin lesion removed because of suspected malignancy, while only 8% who made no special effort to eat polyunsaturated foods reported removal of precancerous or cancerous lesions from their skin at any time in the past.[59]

Mackie reported five malignant melanomas in the lower limb of patients who had changed from butter to polyunsaturated margarine. Four of these patients were female, and Mackie believes that it is a common observaton that cutaneous reaction to oral chemicals tends to affect the legs first, probably because the sluggish circulation of the legs allows a longer period of cellular exposure to the chemicals.

LEVODOPA THERAPY AND MALIGNANT MELANOMA

There has been some concern regarding the role of Levodopa in the induction or stimulation of cutaneous malignant melanoma. Concern began when it was noted that six patients who developed melanoma had taken Levodopa. Three patients who had received the drug had a history of melanoma and allegedly showed recurrences or increased growth after taking the drug.

In a study by Sober and Wick, from the Harvard Medical School, a prospective query of 1,099 patients of the Melanoma Clinical Cooperative Group at the time of the presentation of the primary melanoma showed only one patient who had been taking Levodopa.[92] They concluded that Levodopa, if a factor in the induction of melanoma, plays a most inconspicuous role in the rapid rise in incidence observed for this tumor over the past decade.

MELANOMA AND THE APUD CELL CONCEPT

The existence within derivatives of the primitive gut of a miscellaneous collection of cells of common neural crest ancestry, with common cytochemical properties, are termed APUD cells. The acronym APUD refers to a few of the numerous capabilities of these cells, namely, amine precursor uptake and decarboxylation leading to amine and polypeptide synthesis. The concept offers a unified explanation of multiple endocrine syndromes, the secretion of peptide hormones. The endocrine tumors of this system are labelled APUDomas. The secretions of the APUD system are polypeptid hormones or hormone-like substances such as seratonin, gastrin, glucogen, secretin, ACTH, or calcytonin. Melanocytes belong to this system but have not yet been shown to produce hormone or hormone-like structures, although Horai et al. have reported a malignant melanoma of the intestine that did produce seratonin.[47] Absence of pigmentation vitiligo occurs in some patients who have a strong immunity against malignant melanoma, which indicates the hormonal relationship.

IS MALIGNANT MELANOMA A SINGLE FORM OF CANCER OR DIFFERENT CANCERS?

There is a possibility that the term malignant melanoma refers to different cancers, with different etiologies, different natural histories, and different prognoses (Table 2-2). The different results from different institutions may be explained by a preponderance of different types of melanomas (Table 2-3).

A committee of pathologists in Australia in 1966 divided the lesions into three types. (1) Hutchinson's melanotic freckle or premalignant melanosis. (2) Superficial spreading melanoma (pagetoid melanoma) is a macular spreading lesion, smaller (2 to 3 cm in diameter), more circumscribed and more uniform in color and margins. It occurs in covered skin and mucous membrane, conjunctiva as well as exposed parts of the body. Eventually a nodule occurs (vertical growth) within one to seven years. (3) Nodular melanoma commences without any antecedent spreading pigmented macule and invades from the very beginning. Dubreuilh described these: *d'emblée sur une peau Seine.*

Histologically and clinically the three lesions behave differently. Hutchinson's senile freckle consists of a linear proliferation in the basal level of the epidermis, seldom forming clusters until dermal invasion occurs. Both the primary lesion and surrounding skin usually show marked solar degeneration.

Premalignant melanoses show proliferation of melanocytes with cluster formation in the basal layer and pagetoid invasion of the epidermis before infiltrating into the dermis. Solar degeneration is seen in exposed regions but not as marked as in Hutchinson's freckle.

Nodular melanoma shows invasion from the beginning with a minimum of changes in the surrounding tissue.

Further investigation may elucidate the similarities, biologic interrelationships, and differences between these types of malignant melanomas.

TABLE 2-2. Primary Melanoma of Skin (in White Persons)

Type of Melanoma	Median Age, yr	Specific Sites*	Rate of Development	Appearance
Lentigo-maligna melanoma	70	Face, neck and hands	Slow: 5–20 yr	Predominantly flat spot 2–20 cm in size, with *irregular* borders and with raised portions throughout.
Superficial spreading melanoma	56	Face, neck, upper trunk, and lower legs (in females)	Moderately slow:1–7 yr	The brown or black color is notched; or speckled; blue, white, and red; or both
Nodular	49		Rapid: months	Isolated, small (3.0 cm) nodule with *smooth* borders; color uniform blue-black

* All three types occur either on the exposed parts of the face, neck, and hands or on the relatively exposed areas of the chest, back, and legs. Only a few lesions are seen on covered areas such as the breasts of females, bathing trunk areas of males, and bathing suit areas of females.
Source: National Academy of Sciences, 1976

TABLE 2-3. Percentage of Type of Melanoma by Institution *

Institution	No. of Cases	Lentigo-Maligna Melanoma, %	Superficial Spreading Melanoma, %	Nodular Melanoma, %	Indeterminate, %	Unknown, %
Massachusetts General Hospital	228	3.5	70.6	17.9	5.2	2.6
San Francisco Hospital	136	1.4	65.4	17.6	5.8	9.5
New York University Hospital	389	3.8	73.7	13.3	8.7	0.2
Temple University Hospital	320	7.8	62.8	14.3	12.5	2.5
All	1073	4.6	68.7	15.1	8.7	2.6

* Personal communication with T.B. Fitzpatrick, Harvard Medical School, August 1977.

REFERENCES

1. Allen AC: A re-orientation on the histogenesis and clinical significance of cutaneous melanomas and nevi. Cancer 2:28, 1949
2. Allen EP: Malignant melanoma: spontaneous regression after pregnancy. Br Med J 1:647, 1955
3. Anderson DE, Smith JL, McBride CM: Hereditary aspects of malignant melanoma. JAMA 200:741–746, 1967
4. Attie JL, Khafil RA: Melanotic Tumors: Biology, Pathology, and Clinical Features. Springfield, Ill, Charles C Thomas, 1964
5. Australian Committee for Terminology and Classification of Melanoma. Report Med J Aust 1:123, 1967
6. Balda BR, et al.: Oncornavirus-like particles in human skin cancers. Proc Natl Acad Sci (USA) 72:3697–3700, 1975
7. Batten GH: Cancer incidence in Hawaii, 1968–1972. In Waterhouse J, Muir C, Correa P, Powell J, (eds): Cancer Incidence in Five Continents, Lyon (IARC Sci Publ no 15), 1976
8. Bauman L: Melanoma in relatives. JAMA 218:1300–1301, 1971
9. Becker SW: Pitfalls in the diagnosis and treatment of melanoma. Arch Dermatol Syphilol 69:11, 1954
10. Becker SW: Black lesions of the skin. Calif Med 88:228, 1958
11. Bellet RE, Vaisman I, Mastrangelo MJ, Lustbader E: Multiple primary malignancies in patients with cutaneous melanoma. Cancer 4:1974–1981, 1977
12. Beral V, Ramcharan S, Faris R: Malignant melanoma and oral contraceptive use among women in California. Br J Cancer 36:804–809, 1978
13. Beierwaltes WH, Knarpp CT: Lack of selective uptake of radioactive iodine, phosphorus and copper by melanomas in mouse and man. J Lab Clin Med 38:786, 1951
14. Bickel WH, Meyerdung HW, Broders AC: Melano-epithelioma of extremities. Surg Gynecol Obstet 76:570, 1943
15. Billroth T: Die Allgemeine Chirurgische Pathologie und Therapie. Berlin, G Reimer, 1889, p 908
16. Birkmayer GL, Balda BR, Miller F: Oncornaviral information in human melanoma. Eur J Cancer 10:419–424, 1974
17. Booker HS: Environmental Impact of Stratospheric Flight: Biological and Climatic Effects of Aircraft Emissions in the Stratosphere. Natl Acad Sci, 1975, pp 177–227
18. Breslow A: Thickness, cross-sectional areas and depth of invasion in the prognosis of cutaneous melanoma. Ann Surg 172:902–908, 1970
19. Cawley EP: Genetic aspects of malignant melanoma. AMA Arch Dermatol 65:440–450, 1952
20. Clark WH Jr: A classification of malignant melanoma in man correlated with histogenesis and biologic behaviour. Advanc Biol Skin 8:621, 1967
21. Clark WH Jr, From L, Bernardino EA, Mihm MC: The histogenesis and biologic behaviour of primary human malignant melanoma of the skin. Cancer Res 29:705, 1969
22. Clark WH Jr, Goldman LI, Mastrangelo MJ: Human Malignant Melanoma. New York, Grune & Stratton, 1979
23. Clark WH Jr, Reimer RR, Green MH, et al: Origin of familial malignant melanomas from heritable melanocytic lesions—the B.K. mole syndrome. Arch Dermatol 114:732–738, 1978
24. Cleaver JE, Bootsma D: Xeroderma pigmentosum—biochemical and genetic characteristics. Annu Rev Genet 9:19–38, 1975
25. Cole WH, Roberts S, Watne A, et al.: The Dissemination of Cancer Cells. Bull NY Acad Med 34:163, 1958
26. Cutchis P: On the Linkage of Solar Ultra Violet Radiation to Skin Cancer. Institute of Defense Analysis Paper P-1342, 1978
27. Dargeon HW, Eversole JW, DelDuca V: Malignant melanoma in an infant. Cancer 3:299, 1950
28. Davis NC: Cutaneous melanoma, the Queensland experience. Current Probl Surgery 13:1–63, 1976
29. Dubreuilh MW: De la melanose circonscrite précancéreuse. Ann Derm Syph 3:129 and 205, 1912
30. Engell HC: Cancer cells in the blood—a five to nine year follow-up study. Ann Surg 149:457, 1959
31. Epstein JH, Epstein WL: A study of tumor types produced by ultraviolet light in hairless and hairy mice. J Invest Dermatol 41:463–473, 1963
32. Ewing J: Problems of melanoma. Br Med J 2:852, 1930
33. Ewing J: Neoplastic Diseases. Philadelphia, WB Saunders Co, 1940
34. Feldman WH: Neoplasms of Domesticated Animals. Philadelphia, WB Saunders Co, 1932, pp 247–268
35. Fisher ER: Malignant blue nevus. Arch Dermatol 74:227–231, 1956.

36. Fisher RI, Neifeld JP, Lippman ME: Oestrogen receptors in human malignant melanoma. Lancet 2:337–338, 1976

37. Fitzpatrick TB, Quevedo WC Jr: Albinism. In Stanbury JB, Wyngaarden JB, Frederickson DS (eds): The Metabolic Basis of Inherited Disease (ed 2). New York, McGraw-Hill, 1966, pp 324–340

38a. Friesen SR: Surgical Endocrinology: Clinical Syndromes. Philadelphia, JP Lippincott & Co, 1978

38b. Goldsmith HS, Stettiner L: Melanoma development from subcellular fractions. Surg Gynecol Obstet 149:491, 1979

39. Gordon M: Hereditary basis for melanosis in hybrid fishes. Am J Cancer 15:1495–1523, 1931

40. Gordon M: The production of spontaneous melanotic neoplasms in fishes. Am J Cancer 30:362–375, 1937

41. Gordon M: Effects of five primary genes on the site of melanomas in fishes and the influence of two color genes on their pigmentation. The Biology of Melanomas, NY Acad. Sci. New York, 1948, pp 216–250

42. Gottron H, Gertler W: Zur frage des Ubertutts von melanogen von der mutter auf den saugling uber die wittermilch. Arch Dermatol Syphilol 181:91, 1940

43. Greene MH, Fraumeni JF Jr: The hereditary variant of malignant melanoma. In Clark WH Jr, et al (eds). Human Malignant Melanoma. New York, Grune & Stratton, 1979, pp 139–166

44. Hall JR, Phillips C, White RR: Melanoma: study of 222 cases. Surg Gynecol Obstet 95: 184, 1952

45. Hersey P, Morgan G, Stone DE, et al: Previous pregnancy as a protective factor against death from melanoma. Lancet 1:451–454, 1977

46. Holland E: A case of transplacental metastasis of malignant melanoma from mother to fetus. J Obstet Gynecol Br Emp 56: 529, 1949

47. Horai T, Nicholson H, Haltori S, Taleichi R: Malignant melanoma producing seratonin. Cancer 43:294–298, 1979

48. Houghton A, Munster EW, Viola MV: Increased incidence of malignant melanoma after peaks of sunspot activity. Lancet, April 8, 1978, p 759

49. Hutchinson J: Senile freckles. Arch Surg 3: 319, 1892

50. Hutchinson J: Lentigo-melanosis. A further report. Arch Surg 5:252, 1894

51. Katzenellenbogen I, Sandbank M: Malignant melanomas in twins. Arch Dermatol 94:331–332, Sept. 1966

52. Kopf AW, Bart RS, Rodriguez-Sains RS: Malignant melanoma: a review. J Derm Surg Oncol, pp 41–121, 1977

53. Kraus MM, Ariel IM, Bekar AJ: Primary malignant melanoma of the small intestine and the APUD cell concept. J Surg Oncol 10:283–288, 1978

54. Lee JAH: The current rapid increase in incidence and mortality from malignant melanoma in developed societies. Epidemiology of Melanoma, Pigment Cell, vol 2, pp 414–420, Karger, Basel, 1976

55. Lee JAH, Hill GB: Marriage and fatal malignant melanoma in females. Amer J Epidemiol 91:1, 1970

56. Lee JAH, Merrill JM: Sunlight and the aetiology of malignant melanoma; a synthesis. Med J Aust 2:846–851, 1970

57. Lewison B: Spontaneous regression of malignant melanoma. Brit Med J 1:458, 1955

58. Lynch HT, Frichot BC, Lynch JF: Familial atypical multiple mole-melanoma syndrome. J Med Genet 15:352–356, 1978

59. Mackie BS: Malignant melanoma and diet. Med J Aust, May 18, 1974

60. Magnus K: Epidemiology of malignant melanoma of the skin in Norway with special reference to the effect of solar radiation. Excerpta Medica International Congress Series no 375, Biological Characterization of Human Tumours, Copenhagen, May 13–16, 1975, Excerpta Medica, Amsterdam, ISBN 90 219 03067

61. Mastrangelo MJ, Bellet R, Berd D: Immunology and immunotherapy of human cutaneous malignant melanoma. In Clark WH Jr, et al (eds): Human Malignant Melanoma. New York, Grune & Stratton, 1979, pp 355–419

62. Matthews FS: Melanosarcoma of shoulder and nodes about the shoulder; well after incomplete operation. Ann Surg 62:114, 1915

63. McGovern VJ: Melanoblastoma. Med J Aust 1:159, 1952

64. McGovern VJ: The classification of melanoma and its relationship with prognosis. Pathology 2:85, 1970

65. McNeer G: The clinical behavior and management of malignant melanoma. JAMA 176:1–4, 1961

66. Miller TR, Pack GT: The familial aspect of malignant melanoma. Arch Dermatol 86:35–39, 1962

67. Moertel CG: Multiple primary malignant neo-

plasms. New York, Springer–Verlag, 1966, p 1

68. Moore C, Iverson PC: Xeroderma pigmentosum, showing common skin cancers plus melanocarcinoma controlled by surgery. Cancer 7: 377–382, 1954

69. Moschella SL: A report of malignant melanoma of the skin in sisters. Arch Dermatol 84:1024–1025, (Dec) 1961

70. Moulton JE: Tumors in Domestic Animals. Univ of Calif Press, 1961, pp 56–62

71. Movshovitz M, Modan B: Role of sun exposure in the etiology of malignant melanoma: epidemiologic inference. J Natl Ca Inst 51:777–779, 1973

72. Norris W: A case of fungoid disease. Edinb Med Surg J 16:562–565, 1820

73. Pack GT: A clinical study of pigmented nevi and melanomas. In Miner RW, Gordon M (eds): The Biology of Melanomas, vol 4. New York, NY Acad Sci, 1948, pp 52–70

74. Pack GT, Davis J: The pigmented mole. Postgrad Med 27:370–382, 1960

75. Pack GT, Lenson N, Gerber DM: Regional distribution of moles and melanomas. AMA Arch Surg 65:862–870, 1952

76. Pack GT, Livingston EM: Treatment of Cancer and Allied Diseases, ed 1. New York, Hocber, 1940

77. Pack GT, Miller TR: Metastatic melanoma with indeterminate primary site. JAMA 176: 55–57, April 8, 1961

78. Pack GT, Scharnagel IM: The prognosis for malignant melanoma in the pregnant woman. Cancer 4:324–334, 1951

79. Paget J: Report of a clinical lecture on cases of tumours under moles. Med Times & Gazette 1:58, 1864

80. Parsons PG, Klucis E, Gross P, Oncornavirus-like particles in malignant melanoma and control biopsies. Int J Cancer 18:757–763, 1976

81. Reed WB, Becker SW, Becker SW Jr, et al: Giant pigmented nevi, melanoma and leptomeningeal melanocytosis. Arch Dermatol 91:100–119, 1965

82. Reimer RR, Clark WH Jr, Greene MH, et al: Precursor lesions in familial melanoma—a new genetic pre-neoplastic syndrome. JAMA 239:744–746, 1978

83. Retig AB, Sabesin SM, Hume R, et al: The experimental transmission of malignant melanoma cells through the placenta. Surg Gynecol Obstet 114:485–489, 1962

84. Reynolds AG: Placental metastasis from malignant melanoma. Obstet Gynecol 6:204, 1955

85. Robertson MG: Malignant melanoma in husband and wife. JAMA 217:1553, 1971

86. Salamon T, Schnyder UW, Storck HA: A contribution to the question of heredity of malignant melanomas. Dermatologica 126:65–75, 1963

87. Schoch EP Jr: Familial malignant melanoma: a pedigree and cytogenetic study. Arch Dermatol 88:445–456, Oct. 1963

88. Scotto J, Fears TR, Gori GB: Measurement of ultra violet radiation in the United States and comparisons with skin cancer data. Natl Ca Inst of Health, DHEW no. (N.I.H.) 76–1039, 1976

89. Sequeira JH, Vint FW: Malignant melanoma in Africans. Brit J Dermatol 46:361–367, 1934

90. Shafir R: Malignant melanoma and subsequent other malignancies. J Dermatol Surg Oncol 4:7, July 1978

91. Smith FE, Henley WS, Knox JN: Familial melanoma. Arch Intern Med 117:820–823, June 1966

92. Sober AJ, Wick MM: Levodopa therapy and malignant melanoma. JAMA 240:6, Aug 11, 1978, P 554

93. St. Arneault G, Nagel G, Kirkpatrick D, et al: Melanoma in twins—cutaneous melanoma in identical twins from a set of triplets. Cancer 25:672–677, 1970

94. Stewart DE, Hay LJ, Vargo RL: Malignant melanomas. Int Abst Surg 97:209, 1953

95. Stewart H: Case of malignant melanoma and pregnancy. Brit Med J 1:647, 1955

96. Sumner WC: Spontaneous regression of melanoma: report of a case. Cancer 6:1040, 1953

97. Thomas AD: Skin Cancer in the Angora Goat in South Africa. 15th Dir Vet Serv S Afr, Pt 2: 661 761, 1929

98. Traub EF: The pigmented, hairy and warty nevi and their relation to malignancy. South Med J 40:1000–1005, 1947

99. Turkington RW: Familial factor in malignant melanoma, JAMA 192:77–82, April 12, 1965

100. Veronesi U, Cascinelli N, Bufalino R: Evaluation of the risk of multiple primaries in malignant cutaneous melanoma. Tumori 62: 127–130, 1979

101. von Greifelt A: Malignes melanom: Beziehungen zu Schwangerschaft, Pubertat, Kindheit: Familiare maligne Melanome. *Arztliche Vocherschrift* 7:676–679 July 18, 1952

102. Wallace DC, Beardmore GL, Exton LA: Familial malignant melanoma. Ann Surg 177: 15–20, 1973

103. Waterhouse J, Muir C, Correa P, Powell J (eds): Cancer Incidence in Five Continents, vol 3, Lyon (IARC Scientific Publications no 15), 1976

104. White LP: Studies on melanoma: sex and survival in human melanoma. New Eng J Med 260:789, 1959

105. Wilson FC, Anderson PC: A dissenting view on the prophylactic removal of plantar and palmar nevi. Cancer 14:102–104, 1961

106. Witkop CJ Jr: Albinism. In Harris H, Hirschhorn K (eds). Advances in Human Genetics, vol 2. New York, Plenum Press, 1971, pp 61–142

CHAPTER THREE

ANTIQUITY, INCIDENCE, AND EPIDEMIOLOGY OF MOLES AND MALIGNANT MELANOMA

IRVING M. ARIEL

ANTIQUITY OF MALIGNANT MELANOMA

Information concerning the antiquity of malignant melanoma in the human has been obtained from pre-Colombian Inca mummies of Peru, from seven mummies from Chancay and two mummies from Chongos, Ica, Peru. These were estimated to be 2,400 years old, which age was determined by the use of radiocarbon 14. The diffuse metastases to bones, particularly of the skull and extremities, were particularly startling (Figs. 3–1, 3–2, 3–3). This is consonant with modern findings whereby 49% of patients dying from melanoma and subjected to autopsy revealed metastases to the bone, as determined by Selby, Sherman, and Pack in 1956.[25] In the mummies' skin were recognizable hair follicles and rounded melanotic masses, which seemed to be common melanoma satellites. The histopathological sections of the bones of the mummies showed decalcifying fluid (formic acid and sodium citrate) to have dissolved the melanin, leaving osseous trabeculations empty (Fig. 3–4). The incidence of melanoma in the Inca mummies is paradoxical in view of the infrequency of melanoma in dark-skinned individuals. Metastases of melanoma to bone have been found in Neanderthal man and in the mummy of a Pharoah, according to Urtega and Pack.[26]

Urtega and Pack state that the legendary rumor that melanoma (or as it was previously called, the "black cancer" or "black death") was mentioned in the Egyptian papyri is apocryphal. They believe that the Edwin Smith papyrus dating from the 17th century B.C. deals largely with wounds and that the term "tumor" applies to "swelling" rather than to tumor as we know it. In none of the translations of the Ebers papyrus written about 1500 B.C. is there any description of a melanoma.

INCIDENCE AND EPIDEMIOLOGY OF MALIGNANT MELANOMA

Malignant melanoma is increasing throughout the world in rather astounding proportions (Figs. 3–5, 3–6, 3–7). In 1974 the National Cancer Survey of 7 million people in the United States from ten geographic areas, randomized from a socioeconomic and racial standpoint, revealed the following:[24]

1. The age-adjusted annual incidence of melanoma for the United States is 4.2 per 100,000 population (males 4.3; females 4.1).
2. Negroes have a much lower age-adjusted annual incidence (0.8 per 100,000) than whites (4.5 per 100,000).
3. The highest annual incidence (7.1 per 100,000) is in the south (Dallas–Fort Worth), and the lowest (2.7 per 100,000) is in the north (Detroit).

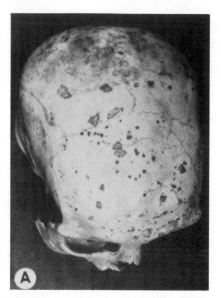 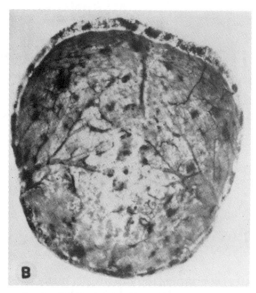

FIGURE 3–1.   Skulls of pre-Colombian mummies from Peru; estimated to be over 2,400 years old, showing evidence of metastatic melanoma. A. External view. B. Internal calvarium. (Reproduced through the courtesy of Urtega O, Pack GT: On the antiquity of melanoma. Cancer 19:607, 1966. With permission of the American Cancer Society, Inc.)

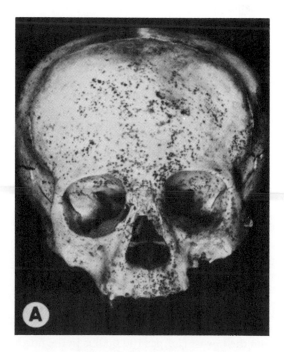 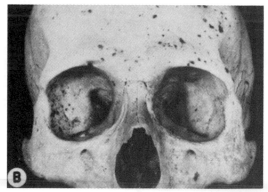

FIGURE 3–2A and B.   Metastatic melanoma to two skulls of pre-Colombian Inca mummies. (Reproduced through the courtesy of Urtega O, Pack GT: On the antiquity of melanoma. Cancer 19:607, 1966. With permission of the American Cancer Society, Inc.)

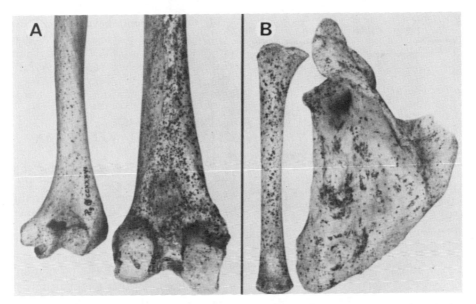

FIGURE 3-3. Metastatic melanoma in the femur (A) and humerus and scapula (B) of pre-Colombian mummies. (Reproduced through the courtesy of Urtega O, Pack GT: On the antiquity of melanoma. Cancer 19:607, 1966. With permission of the American Cancer Society, Inc.)

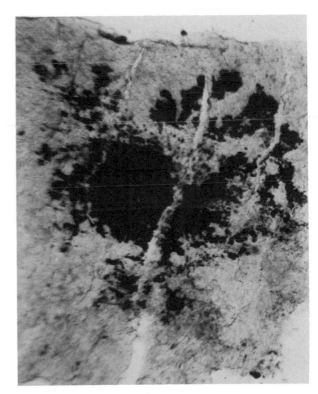

FIGURE 3-4. Demonstrates the site of dissolved melanin from the decalcifying fluid (formic acid and sodium citrate). (Courtesy, Doctor O. Urtega.)

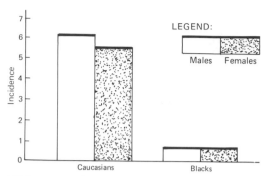

FIGURE 3–5. Overall incidence in the United States per 100,000 per year. (Reprinted from Sober & Fitzpatrick, CA vol 29(5), September/October 1979, with permission.)

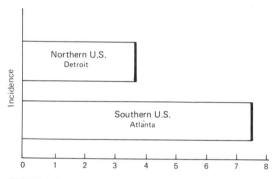

FIGURE 3–6. Latitude dependency—crude incidence rates per 100,000 Caucasions per year during 1969–1971. (Reprinted from Sober & Fitzpatrick, CA vol 29(5), September/October 1979, with permission.)

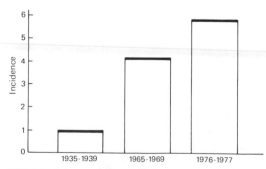

FIGURE 3–7. Increasing incidence as shown by the Connecticut registry per 100,000 per year. (Reprinted from Sober & Fitzpatrick, CA vol 29(5), September/October 1979, with permission.)

4. Older patients have a higher annual incidence (at age 5 it is 0.1 per 100,000; at age 85 it is 16.4 per 100,000). The total number of cases is greatest in the 40–49-year-old age group.

INCIDENCE OF MALIGNANT MELANOMA

While earlier diagnosis and improved medical measures are improving the overall survival rates, the growing mortality from melanoma is due largely to the increase in population, increase in expected years of life, and the absolute increase in the numbers of melanoma (Figs. 3–8, 3–9, 3–10, 3–11).

The United States has a population of over 210 million, of which approximately 9,000 individuals develop malignant melanoma, 300,000 develop other skin cancers, and approximately 600,000 develop cancers of all other organs exclusive of the skin each year. Thus, approximately one of three new cancers of man is a cancer of the skin, and one of 100 is a malignant melanoma.

The increased incidence of melanoma among the white races can be noted throughout the world. In Queensland it has quadrupled in 30 years.[1,2] In Norway,[16] Britian,[14] the United States,[12] and Canada,[9] the incidence has doubled since World War II. This marked increase in incidence has not been observed among other skin cancers. In fact, in some countries, the mortality from other skin cancers exclusive of melanoma has declined.

Elwood and Lee[9] have evaluated recent data regarding the changing incidence and epidemiology throughout the world. Table 3–1 presents a summary of the changes in age standardized rates in different countries. In this chart, the last column gives the percentage increase per year as a simple way to describe the trend. The data are not comparable between different studies because of certain differences in the study, particularly the different time periods evaluated. Nevertheless, certain facts stand out strongly. One is the rise of about 3% to 9% per year in the mortality, so that the

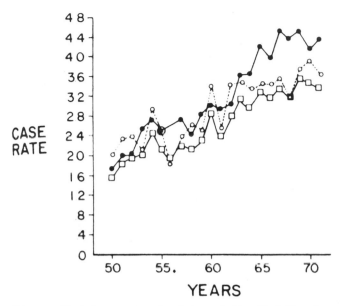

FIGURE 3-8. The age-adjusted case rates of melanoma in New York State from 1950 to 1971. (The squares represent the total case rate per year, the open circles are the rates in females, the dark circles the rates in males.)

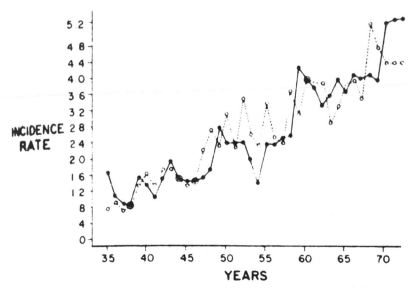

FIGURE 3-9. The age-adjusted melanoma incidence rate per 100,000 population in Connecticut, from 1935 to 1972. (The open circles represent the incidence in females per year, the dark circles the incidence in males.)

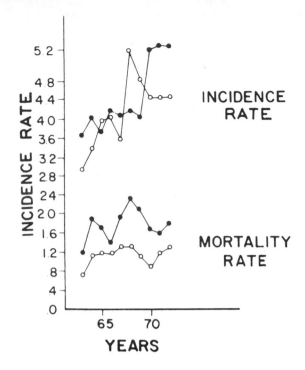

FIGURE 3-10. A comparison of the age-adjusted melanoma incidence rates per 100,000 population and the age-adjusted melanoma mortality rates per 100,000 population—in Connecticut from 1967 to 1972. (The open circles are female rates, the dark circles are male rates.)

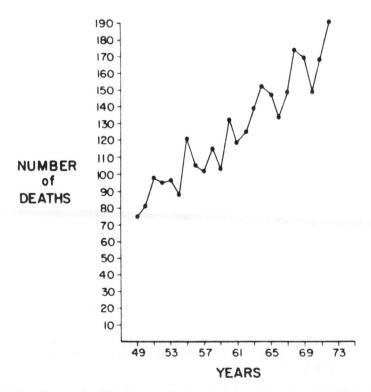

FIGURE 3-11. The number of melanoma deaths per year in New York City from 1949 to 1972.

TABLE 3-1. Increases in Incidence and Mortality from Malignant Melanoma from Different Countries

Reference		Country	Sex	First Period of Observation		Second Period of Observation		Total % Increase	No. of Years	Annual % Increase
				Time	Rate per 10^6	Time	Rate per 10^6			
1	Incidence	New York State	M	1941–1943	12.2	1967	33.7	175	25	7.0
			F	1941–1943	17.7	1967	29.3	65	25	2.6
2	Incidence	Norway	M	1955	17.9	1970	63.0	254	15	17.6
			F	1955	25.5	1970	68.4	195	15	13.0
2	Mortality	Norway	M	1956–1960	15.9	1966–1970	26.8	69	10	6.9
			F	1956–1960	13.3	1966–1970	18.1	36	10	3.6
3	Mortality	Canada	M	1951–1955	7.1	1966–1970	13.7	93	15	6.2
			F	1951–1955	5.9	1966–1970	12.2	107	15	7.1
4	Mortality	USA	Both	1950	9.3	1967	16.0	72	16	4.5
4	Mortality	UK	Both	1950	5.1	1967	10.2	100	16	6.3
5	Mortality	Australia	M	1931–1940	9.8	1961–1970	36.0	267	30	8.9
			F	1931–1940	7.6	1961–1970	24.9	227	30	7.8
6	Mortality	Denmark	M	1956–1960	15.9	1966–1969	23.7	49	10	4.9
			F	1956–1960	16.1	1966–1969	21.3	32	10	3.2
6	Mortality	Sweden	M	1956–1960	16.5	1966–1968	21.4	30	9	3.3
			F	1956–1960	10.6	1966–1968	14.8	40	9	4.4
6	Incidence	Connecticut	M	1935–1939	13.7	1965–1969	48.1	250	30	8.3
			F	1935–1939	10.5	1965–1969	47.7	354	30	11.8

Courtesy of the World Health Organization

death rate has doubled in the past 15 years. They bring out the fact that in Canada the rate of increase is greater than that of any other tumor except for lung cancer in males. These rates are real, and not due to better reporting or other factors in evaluation. If there were a common factor, all tumor rates would rise; however, such is not the case, for the increase in incidence and mortality is greater among younger people than those over 65 years of age.

The fact that people born in more recent years have both a higher incidence rate and a higher death rate from malignant melanoma, at all ages, than those born earlier is intriguing. There is thus an unhealthy generation gap. Lee and Carter[14] have suggested that people born between 1900 and 1920 in England and Wales were the first group to experience higher rates. Elwood and Lee further point out that the increase varies with different anatomic regions. There has been a slight increase in melanomas of the head and neck; the most striking increases have been the lower limb in females, the trunk in men, and the upper limb in both sexes. It has been hypothecated that this variation in site is due to greater exposure to sunlight of the anatomic regions that have the highest increase. The increase in the lower extremities of women applies only to the legs and not to the upper thigh or foot, particularly in the 15- to 34-year-old age group.

The data from England suggests that some factor causing melanoma was inactive in those born before 1903 and was most fully active in those born after 1923. The exact nature of this factor or factors remains enigmatic.

The Relationship of Race and Complexion to the Incidence of Moles and Melanomas. Inasmuch as the effects of external exposure to melanogenic factors (for example, sunlight) may play a role it is pertinent to evaluate the susceptibility of individuals with different pigmentary features as being more or less susceptible to these outside factors. The genetic effects in certain families being prone to develop melanomas have been described (see Chapter 2). This section will evaluate the role of inherited pigmentation patterns by different individuals and their susceptibility to the development of malignant melanomas.

The development of melanomas in albinos demonstrates that the melanocyte from which the melanomas arise, which is present in the albino patient but its pigment production is prevented by metabolic factors, may develop the apigmented melanoma. Similarly, patients with xeroderma pigmentosa present a hypersensitivity to ultraviolet radiation in association with melanin deficiency. These patients may develop both basal cell and squamous cell carcinomas as well as melanomas at early ages. Studies of different races from different parts of the world reveal that as a rule the darker the complexion of the individual the more resistant he is to develop melanoma. Negroes are most resistant except where they are not pigmented (palms, soles, and mucous membrane).

EPIDEMIOLOGY OF MALIGNANT MELANOMA

Epidemiologic evaluation of melanomas offers possible examples of factors that either cause or contribute to the cause of melanomas, and also certain features that may indicate a special susceptibility to the development of malignant melanomas. The profession owes a great debt of gratitude to Eleanor MacDonald[17] of the M. D. Anderson Hospital and also to Dr. J. A. Lee[14] who were amongst the first in the United States to institute such epidemiologic studies, contributing noteworthy results regarding the natural history of melanoma based on epidemiologic data. Many of the following statements are based on their studies.[17]

Malignant melanoma accounts for less than 2% of all cancers. One-tenth of the melanomas occur in the eyes, and almost all of the rest arise in the skin. Two of three occur in preexisting moles, and one-sixth in a recognizable congenital nevus.

The number of reported cases increases in a

nearly stepwise fashion as the equator is approached. In El Paso, the incidence was three times the mortality rate, which is the usual figure throughout the world except in New Zealand and Australia. The ratio of incidence to mortality was 4:1 in San Antonio, 5:1 in Corpus Christi, 6:1 in Laredo, and 7:1 in Harlingen (Texas). MacDonald states that this great difference in improving survival rates with increased incidence suggests that the lesions in the lower latitudes are being detected earlier or are probably less aggressive than those reported from cancer centers, or represent different criteria in the diagnosis of melanoma.

A study by the World Health Organization revealed great differences in different countries and different ethnic groups. The study consisted of 69 population groups in 23 countries in five continents; ten were in the different regions and ethnic groups in Texas. It soon became apparent that there were different types of melanoma with varying degrees of seriousness, which necessitated a uniform series of classifications. A landmark regarding this feature was the meeting of pathologists in 1972 in Sydney, Australia. McGovern, Mihm, Clark, and others presented a uniform classification by which to judge not only the incidence of melanoma and its epidemiology, but to compare different types within the same or different groups. As the studies progressed, it became evident that there was a relationship between sunlight and melanoma, as first suggested by McGovern in 1952.[18] Evidence from Australia supports this theory, and the studies in Texas by MacDonald revealed that in the subtropical regions except El Paso, the location of most of the lesions (lower leg, arm, face in women; face, arm, shoulders, and back in men) suggests that sun exposure plays a part in the genesis of melanoma.

El Paso had a significantly lower rate for melanoma than Laredo, Harlingen, or Corpus Christi (Table 3–2). MacDonald believes the reason is that El Paso lies in an area of desert-like aridity with nearly total sunshine; the population tends to wear protective clothing to conserve body moisture, and remains indoors during the heat of the day. In other regions of Texas where the sun shines a smaller proportion of the time, the humidity and high temperature are conducive to less clothing and more outdoor exposure, with a higher rate of skin cancer including melanoma. She further calls attention to the fact that in Texas, melanoma is a disease of whites rather than Latins, among whom it is rare and occurs slightly more frequently in women than in men. In similar studies performed by Davies et al., for whites in Uganda, evaluating the same latitude from the equator, the rates were almost identical as in Texas.[6]

A similar situation exists in Australia. Godfrey Scott has examined the ancestry of the modern Australian population in order to determine any relation of ethnic background to the likelihood of hosting a malignant melanoma.[21] He states that studies of the distribution of blood groups supports the hypothesis that the modern Celt, who in Australia has the highest incidence of melanoma in the world, has a different ethnic background from the inhabitants of other parts of the British Isles. There is a higher frequency of B and AB genes in Scotland, Wales, and Northern Ireland, the lowest frequencies occurring in Lancashire, East Anglia, and Sussex. The Celts also have a higher frequency of group O and a significantly lower frequency of the Rh negative gene than other parts of Britain. He further states, "There is clear evidence that the present-day Irish, Welsh, and Scots have linguistic and cultural traits that can be directly related to the European Celts. They have ethnic characteristics that can be directly related to the ancient aboriginal inhabitants and through them to the race of Neolithic man spread over Europe after the passing of the Ice Age."

He points out that Australia is somewhat cooler than the other land masses of the Southern Hemisphere and considerably cooler than the same latitudes in the large continental area of the Northern Hemisphere. Because of the insular nature of Australia, an atmospheric movement transports cooler air from higher southern latitudes into the sub-

TABLE 3-2. Malignant Melanoma of the Skin Average Annual Age-Adjusted Incidence Rates per 100,000 (1970 Standard) Six Regions in Texas (56 Counties)—1944-1966*

	Harlingen	Laredo	Corpus Christi	San Antonio	Houston	El Paso	All Regions
Males							
W–62–66	6.6(19)	10.5(9)	7.0(41)	8.2(123)	7.3(154)	4.5(14)	7.4(360)
44–66	5.0(58)	5.6(18)	6.3(144)	5.5(325)	5.6(405)	3.7(40)	5.5(990)
NW–62–66			0.0	.6(1)	.5(3)		.6(5)
44–66			0.0	.3(2)	.4(8)		.4(11)
SS–62–66	3.1(12)	1.3(2)	3.5(8)	1.3(7)	1.6(3)	1.8(3)	2.1(35)
44–66	.9(15)	.7(5)	2.4(19)	1.3(29)	.7(4)	2.1(13)	1.3(85)
W+SS–62–66	4.6(31)	4.5(11)	5.9(49)	6.1(130)	6.9(157)	3.4(17)	5.9(395)
44–66	2.6(73)	2.2(23)	5.0(163)	4.3(354)	5.3(409)	3.0(53)	4.3(1075)
Females							
W–62–66	7.6(22)	5.8(5)	6.8(42)	7.9(134)	9.0(219)	3.0(11)	8.0(433)
44–66	5.3(61)	4.9(15)	6.6(156)	5.7(371)	5.6(463)	4.3(53)	5.7(1119)
NW–62–66			2.6(1)	0.0	1.0(4)		.8(5)
44–66			.9(1)	.5(3)	.8(12)		.8(17)
SS–62–66	2.5(8)	2.3(4)	1.6(5)	1.5(10)	.9(1)	1.3(4)	1.8(32)
44–66	1.3(16)	2.0(14)	2.3(20)	1.2(27)	1.7(9)	2.2(20)	1.6(106)
W+SS–62–66	4.3(30)	3.4(9)	5.2(47)	5.9(144)	8.5(220)	2.3(15)	6.2(465)
44–66	2.8(77)	2.9(29)	5.3(176)	4.3(398)	5.4(472)	3.3(73)	4.5(1225)
Latitude	26	27–28	27–28	29–30	30	31–32	26–32

* W–White excluding SS; NW–Nonwhite; SS–Spanish surnamed; W+SS–White including SS.
Reproduced through the courtesy of MacDonald EJ.

tropical region. He considers this an important factor in encouraging solar exposure; the moderate air temperature is conducive to spending long hours exposed to the sun. Seldom does the heat become so extreme that the farmer or the sports enthusiast feels the need to seek shelter. With the exception of Christmas Day, the siesta is unknown in Australia. The greater part of Australia has more than 3,000 hours of sunshine per year (the east coast of New South Wales and Queensland enjoy from 2,500 to 3,000 hours), in contrast to the British Isles, with a maximum of 1,750 hours. Numerous books extol the benefits of sunlight and emphasize the fact that sunlight filtered through glass will not form vitamin D. The finding of the 1920's that sunlight has both preventive and curative effects on rickets and other disorders of calcium metabolism provided scientific support for widely held beliefs in the healthful nature of solar radiation. A large majority of Australians equated a good suntan with general good health. Several commented in a derogatory fashion on the pallor that is the hallmark of certain groups in the community—the prisoner, the weakling, and the overprotected child.

Prior to 1902, bathing in the sea was virtually unknown in Australia. In fact, bathing in public was prohibited by law between the hours of 6 a.m. and 8 p.m. These laws were more relevant to the maintenance of standards of modesty than to the prevention of skin cancer. Swimming, surfing, and board riding developed rapidly as accepted recreational activities and an added impetus was given by such events as the introduction of the one-piece bathing costume by Annette Kellerman, the success of many Australian swimmers in international competition, and the introduction of swimming as a school sport in the twenties. The Second World War added additional stimulus to the suntan cult with the wearing of shorts and no shirt. In this respect the data and conclusions are the same as those of MacDonald for Texas.

Since 1948, when large-scale immigration began, the proportion of the Australian population claiming Celtic or Anglo-Saxon origin has decreased. At present, only about one out of ten has been born elsewhere than in the British Isles or Australia. Perhaps in the future the new genetic material, changes in lifestyle in respect to recreational habits, and the growth of commerce and industry should lead to a decrease of Australians exposed to solar radiation. Less and less emphasis is being placed upon "the healthy suntanned appearance" both in Australia and in America, and it is hoped that these factors will lead to a decrease in the incidence of skin cancer, including melanoma.

Beardmore has recorded a real and significant increase in the number of deaths from melanoma in Australia since 1931. Those states closer to the equator have the highest death rate. Melanomas occur in lighter-complexioned people, and have never been reported in a Queensland aboriginal.

There is great variation in the incidence of melanoma in different countries and different regions of the same country. Norway and Sweden, at higher latitudes than England or Canada, have much higher rates than most regions of the latter two countries. Saskatchewan, which is higher in latitude than California or Connecticut, has skin cancer rates as high as the latter two states. Melanoma among women constitutes 3.8% of the total cancers of native born Israelis and 4.0% of total cancers among females in New Zealand. It constitutes more than 2.0% of total cancers among white women in Hawaii, San Antonio and Houston, Texas, and Norway.

Among Latins (both male and female), Cali, Colombia has the highest proportion of melanomas to total cancers. Among Latin males, Harlingen and Houston, Texas have nearly as high a proportion of melanomas to total cancers as Cali, Colombia.

A study throughout the world revealed that melanoma is more frequent in females than in males, with females enjoying a better prognosis.

The Negro population has a higher incidence of melanoma on the feet, whether they are African or American, Indians or Indonesians.

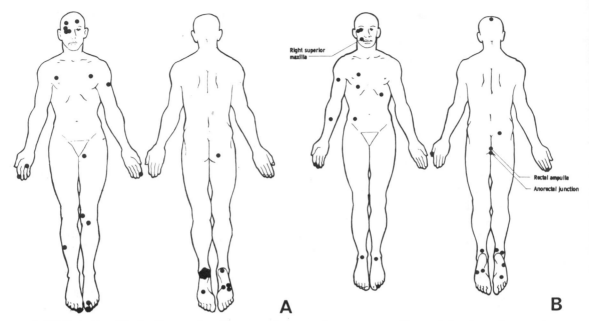

FIGURE 3–12. The incidence of malignant melanoma in the Indians compared with a scattergram of the American Negro's incidence of malignant melanoma. A. Indians of Bombay. B. American Negroes.

Since rural people often go without shoes, it is believed that trauma to the bare foot may be a factor. Lewis indicated that the incidence of melanoma was correlated with the prevalence of black spots on the soles of the feet.[15] Very few American Negroes go barefooted, but the concentration of pigmented areas on the soles appears to persist and may result in melanomas (Figs. 3–12, 3–13, and 3–14).

MacDonald found the annual incidence amongst Negroes in Texas to be 1.28 per 100,000, and 1.2 per 100,000 among Latin Americans and Anglo-Americans. Although the incidence is roughly similar, there is a great difference in site distribution between Negroes on the one hand and Latin Americans and Anglo-Americans on the other. In Texan Negroes, the foot was the most common site. Among Latin Americans the incidence of melanoma in the head and neck, the trunk, the upper extremities, and the lower extremities was similar. In Texan Anglo-Americans the head and neck was the principal site.

The death rate for males in Australia from malignant melanoma is three times that in England and Wales. The white male death rate in Massachusetts is 14 per million, as it is in New York, but it is 17 in California and 22 in Texas.

The increased susceptibility of Swedes and Norwegians is noteworthy (the Registrar General's Statistical Review 1965). The incidence in England and Wales for the years 1962–1965 was 1.4 per 100,000 for men and 2.4 for women, while in Sweden during the same period the incidence was 3.9 per 100,000 for men and 4.2 for women, although the Scandinavian countries are of much higher latitude.

Further epidemiologic studies may shed light on the reasons for the increased incidence of melanomas, whether they be intrinsic, extrinsic, or both.

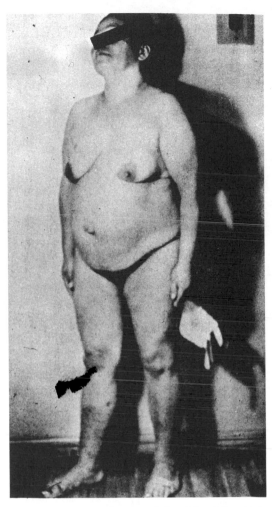

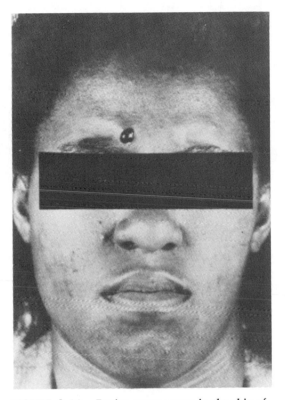

FIGURE 3-14. Benign neuro nevus in the skin of a Negro. It had the clinical appearance of a melanoma but because the patient was a full-blooded Negro, it was clinically diagnosed as benign.

FIGURE 3-13. Melanoma of the skin of the thigh of an Indian woman from the Peruvian Andes.

REFERENCES

1. Beardmore GC: The epidemiology of malignant melanoma in Australia. In Melanoma and Skin Cancer, Proceedings of the International Cancer Conference, Sydney, VCN Blight by Government Printer, 1972, pp 40-64
2. Beardmore GC: The epidemiology of malignant melanoma in Australia. In McCarthy WH (ed): Melanomas and Skin Cancer. Sydney, VCN Blight by Government Printer, 1972, pp 39-64
3. Burbank F: Patterns in cancer mortality in the United States: 1950-1967. Natl Ca Inst Mimeograph 33:370-396, 1971
4. Cutler SJ, Young JL: Third National Cancer Survey: Incidence Data. N.C.I. Monograph 41, DHEW # NIH 75-787, March, 1975
5. Cutler SJ Myers MH, Green SB: Trends and survival rates of patients with cancer. New Engl J Med 293:122-124, 1975
6. Davies JNP, Myer R, Tank R, Thurston P: Cancer of the integumentary tissues in Uganda Africans; the basis for prevention. J Natl Ca Inst 41:31-51, 1968
7. Doll R, Muir C, Waterhouse J: Cancer Incidence in Five Continents, vol 2, Springer-Verlag, 1970

8. Elmes BGT, Baldwin RBT: Malignant disease in Nigeria; an analysis of 1,000 tumours. Ann Trop Med 41:321–328, 1947

9. Elwood JM, Lee JAH: Data on the epidemiology of malignant melanoma. In Clark W Jr, et al., (eds) Human Malignant Melanoma, New York, Grune & Stratton, 1979, pp 261–272

10. Hewer TF: Malignant melanoma in coloured races: The role of trauma in its causation. J Pathol Bacteriol 41:473–477, 1935

11. Kopf AW, Bart RS, Rodriguez-Sains RJ: Malignant melanoma: a review. J Dermatol Surg Oncol 3:41–44, 1977

12. Lee JA: Current evidence about the causes of melanoma. In Ariel IM (ed), Prog Clin Cancer. 6:151–161, 1975

13. Lee JA, Eisenberg HJ: A comparison between England and Wales and Sweden and the incidence and mortality of malignant skin tumors. Brit J Cancer 26:59–65, 1972

14. Lee JA, Carter AP: Secular trends in mortality from malignant melanoma. J Natl Ca Inst 45:91–100, 1970

15. Lewis ME, Kiryabwire WM: Aspects of behavior and natural history of malignant melanoma in Uganda. Cancer 21:876–887, 1968

16. Magnus K: Incidence of malignant melanoma of the skin in Norway from 1955–1970. Cancer 32:1275–1280, 1973

17. MacDonald EJ: Epidemiology of melanoma. In Ariel IM (ed): Prog Clin Cancer, 6:139, 1975

18. McGovern VJ: Melanoblastoma. Med J Aust 1:159, 1952

19. Pack GT, Davis J, Oppenheim A: The relation of race and complexion to the incidence of moles and melanomas. Ann NY Acad Sci 100 (II):719–742, 1963

20. Paymaster JZ: Epidemiologic study of cancer in Western India. In Ariel IM (ed): Prog Clin Cancer. 3:107–124, 1967

21. Scott G: Some sociologic observations on skin cancer in Australia. In Melanoma and Skin Cancer, Proceedings of the International Cancer Conference, Sydney, VCN Blight by Government Printer, 1972, pp 16–37.

22. Scotto J, Kopf AW, Urbach F: Non-melanoma skin cancer among Caucasians in four areas of the United States. Cancer 34:1333–1338, 1974

23. Sequeira JH, and Vint FW: Malignant melanoma in Africans. Brit J Dermatol 46:361–367, 1934

24. Third National Cancer Survey—Advanced Three Year Report: 1969–1971 Incidence (excluding carcinoma in situ). Biometric Branch, NCI, DHEW #NIH 74-637, 1974

25. Selby HH, Sherman C, Pack G: A roentgen study of bone metastases from melanoma. Radiology, 67:224–228, 1956

26. Urtega O, Pack G: On the an... noma. Cancer, 19:607–610, 1966

CHAPTER FOUR

THE PATHOLOGY OF CUTANEOUS MELANOCYTIC LESIONS

MARIANNE WOLFF

In this section we will discuss the common melanocytic lesions of the skin, with differential diagnostic criteria, areas of controversy, approach to diagnostic and therapeutic aspects, and natural history of the various conditions.

Because of space limitations, melanocytic lesions of the eye, of the nervous system, and of mucous membranes will not be included. Furthermore, as details of gross presentation of various lesions will be thoroughly discussed and illustrated in chapters on clinical aspects, and regimens of therapy in chapters on treatment, no attempt will be made to deal with them exhaustively in this chapter.

PATHOLOGY

In order to depict the pathology of malignant melanoma of the skin, it is essential to consider the normal skin, the embryologic derivation of pigment cells, as well as a number of benign lesions that may be mistaken, clinically or pathologically, for malignant melanoma.

The epidermis of the skin, it will be remembered, takes its embryological origin from the ectoderm, while the melanocytes, which inhabit the basal layer, migrate to their ultimate position from the neural crest, which is a specialized area of the ectoderm. Normally, melanocytes are fairly regularly spaced along the basal layer, occurring one every 8, 10, or 12 basal cells.[12] Usually they are not conspicuous on routine staining, except for a characteristic halo (constant artifact), which separates a melanocyte from the adjacent epidermal cells. With the use of special staining techniques for the pigment-producing apparatus within melanocytes, they can be demonstrated more distinctly. It will be seen that melanocytes are dendritic, i.e. they have an irregular shape, with long tapering extensions, reminiscent of other cells of neural crest derivation. Pigment extends into the dendritic processes and, as has been proved experimentally, can be transferred from one cell to another, as well as to the basal cells of the epidermis.[39]

BENIGN MELANOCYTIC LESIONS

Junctional nevi. These lesions are said to occur most commonly in the palms and soles, but may be found anywhere. In children the cells in the junctional nests often assume a spindle shape. Under certain conditions (e.g. pregnancy or in the presence of malignant melanoma elsewhere) junctional foci become "activated," i.e. their nuclei assume characteristics of greater immaturity, such as prominence of nucleoli, larger nuclei, or even mitotic activity. Such "activated junctional nevi" may pose a problem of differential diagnosis from malignant melanoma.

In this entity there is a proliferation of melanocytes, occurring in clusters at the base of the rete ridges, and confined to the interface between epidermis and dermis, called the "junction." These clusters are surrounded by a clear space or halo, so that they appear to be

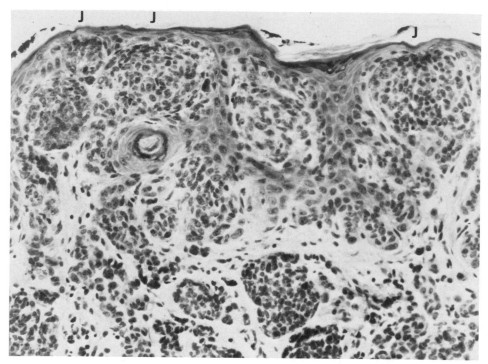

FIGURE 4-1. Compound nevus, characterized by several nests of melanocytes in a junctional position (J), as well as nests of typical intradermal nevus cells in lower part of field. HPS × 224

about to "drop off" into the dermis. (German: *Abtropfung*) Junctional nevi are pigmented clinically and microscopically; they are flat and impalpable clinically. This is the lesion that develops in young children, when they first acquire the pigmented lesions that all of us possess in varying numbers.

Compound nevus. This consists of a combination of junctional and intradermal nevus (Fig. 4-1).

Intradermal nevus. This is probably the most common type of melanocytic lesion, and may occur anywhere. It is grossly elevated, sometimes dome-shaped, often hair-bearing and consists microscopically of numerous aggregates of small, polygonal cells within the dermis. These are generally only lightly pigmented, if at all. They are frequently admixed with a few multinucleated nevus cells.

Such nests of cells may extend quite deeply into the dermis, and often concentrate about dermal appendages, such as hair follicles.

One of the variants seen in intradermal nevi is the so-called "neuronevus." This is not at all uncommon, and is said to occur most frequently in older patients; however, we have seen this change in nevi of patients in the third decade. Microscopically the superficial dermis contains ordinary nevus cells. However, in the deeper portion of the dermal lesion one finds wavy, fibrillary structures bearing a strong resemblance to Schwann cells in neurofibromas. In addition one may at times encounter small circular structures, having a whorled internal appearance, reminiscent of Meissner's tactile corpuscles, which are normally found in the upper dermis (Fig. 4-2A,B). As Schwann cells and sensory nerve endings are embryologically derived from the neural crest, the association of nevus cells with these struc-

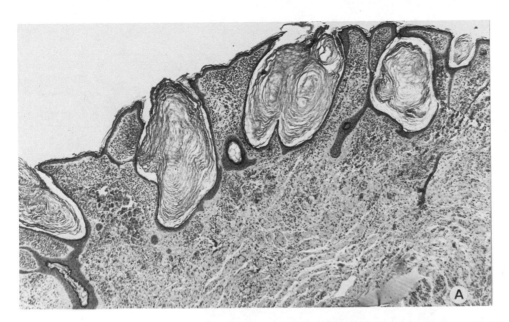

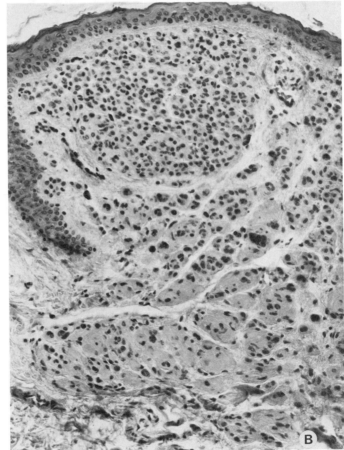

FIGURE 4-2A. Neuronevus. Typical nevus cells occupy the upper dermis, while the lower dermis is occupied by rounded cellular aggregates, which contain more cytoplasm than do nevus cells, and which, architecturally, form structures resembling Meissner's tactile corpuscles. The surface of this particular lesion is papillary and hyperkeratotic, and is reminiscent of seborrheic keratosis. Hematoxylin, phloxin, and safran × 38
B. Detail of same lesion. Note the presence of several multinucleated nevus cells in center of field; these are not unusual in intradermal nevi, but have no premalignant significance. Hematoxylin, phloxin and safran × 160

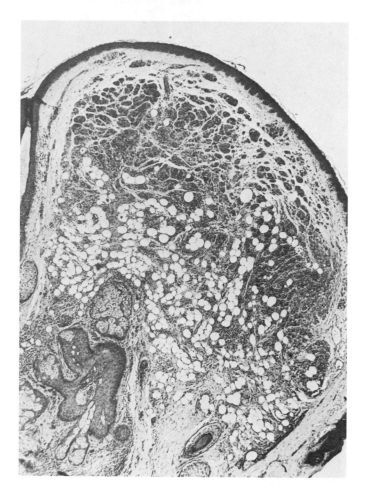

FIGURE 4-3. Dome-shaped lesion, typical of intradermal nevus. The unusual feature of this lesion is the presence of fat cells intermingled with intradermal nevus cells. Hematoxylin, phloxin, and safran × 38

tures is not too surprising, when it is remembered that melanocytes also originate from the neural crest. Whether the neuroid elements represent maturation, dedifferentiation, or metaplasia from nevus cells is not understood. A dual origin of the intradermal components from Schwann cells as well as from melanocytes has also been postulated. A much rarer event, which is even harder to explain, is the finding of fat cells admixed with nevus cells in the dermis (Fig. 4-3). This peculiar combination was explained by Masson as reflecting a malformative error during development of the skin, perhaps a type of hamartoma. (Normally there is no fat in the

dermis and adipose tissue comes from the mesoderm, rather than the neuroectoderm).

Another theory for the occurrence of fat in a dermal nevus is that fat cells grow in, following the disappearance of nevus cells due to atrophy.[29]

At times one may observe a small rounded focus of mature bone within the intradermal portion of a benign nevus; (Fig 4-4) such an osteoma cutis has no prognostic significance. It may be related to a remote inflammatory lesion, such as folliculitis.[29]

Blue nevus. These lesions may occur anywhere, but have a number of favorite lo-

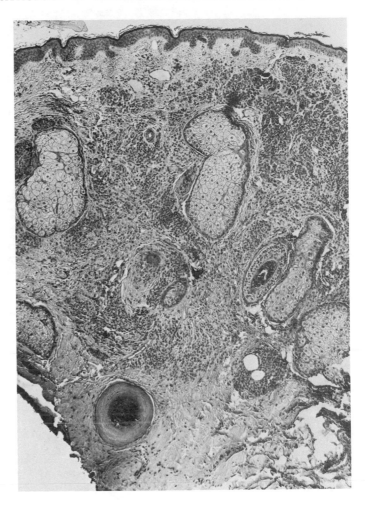

FIGURE 4-4. Intradermal nevus, associated with a rounded focus of compact bone (osteoma cutis), located in lower left portion of the field. HPS × 63

cations, such as the base of the spine ("Mongolian spot"), buttocks, extremities, and face. They often reach a very large size, and present grossly as blue or bluish black lesions; the brownish-black melanin pigment is located fairly deep in the dermis, and the light reflected from the lesion has to pass through a certain depth of normal dermis, from which all but blue light is absorbed. Histologically a pure blue nevus consists of elongated (dendritic), heavily pigmented cells, associated with variable amounts of collagen (Fig. 4-5A, B). These lesions are often almost flat or even slightly depressed because of the contractility of the associated collagen. At times this kind

of growth is associated with an ordinary intradermal nevus or, less commonly, with junctional nests.

A rare variant of blue nevus is the "cellular blue nevus." In this lesion there is abundant proliferation of spindle cells, which may or may not be pigmented, which grow in typical epithelial-like packets, with minimal accompanying fibrous tissue. This cellular proliferation may extend very deeply into the tissue, and may be difficult to extirpate adequately, hence the propensity for local recurrences. However, cytologically the cells are rather uniform (Fig. 4-5C) and mitotic figures extremely sparse or entirely absent. Thus these

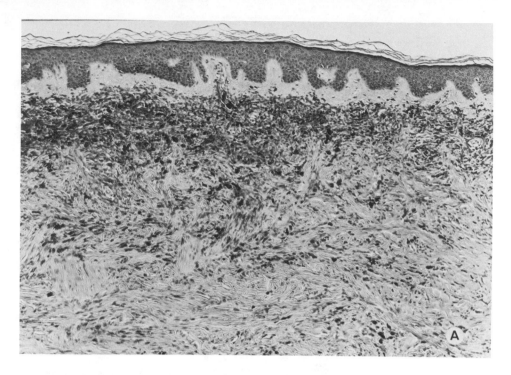

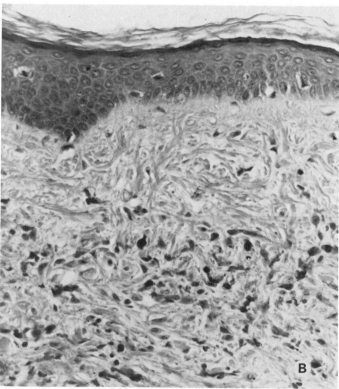

FIGURE 4-5A. Blue nevus. The pigmented cells are elongated and are dispersed by numerous fibroblasts. Note the uninvolved zone in the upper (papillary) dermis. HPS × 80. B. Detail of same case. HPS × 240.

lesions should not be considered malignant. They bear some resemblance, histologically, to pigmented neurofibromas, with which they share a common ancestry, as both have their origins from the neural crest.

There is, however, a rare malignant tumor composed of a densely cellular, spindle-shaped cell population with or without pigmentation, in which the cells have all morphological attributes of malignancy, including a high rate of mitotic activity. These tumors are in actuality a variant of malignant melanoma, although they do not have a demonstrable epidermal junctional component. They involve regional lymph nodes, by direct local extension or possibly by embolic metastasis. In one reported case the patient succumbed to disseminated visceral metastases.[41] Such lesions are known as "malignant blue nevi."

Congenital nevi. These are often very large, hairy, unsightly, and a problem in management. Their importance lies not only in their cosmetic consideration but also in the fact that there is a significant incidence of the subsequent development of malignant melanomas from these lesions. Histologically they are compound nevi, indistinguishable from those described previously except for their unusually large size.

Halo nevi. This is an unusual variant, so-called because of its gross appearance. A central pigmented lesion is surrounded by a depigmented halo. This phenomenon is believed to be due to depigmentation in an area that was previously occupied by pigmented nevus cells, which have since been destroyed by lymphocytes. Depigmentation of the basal

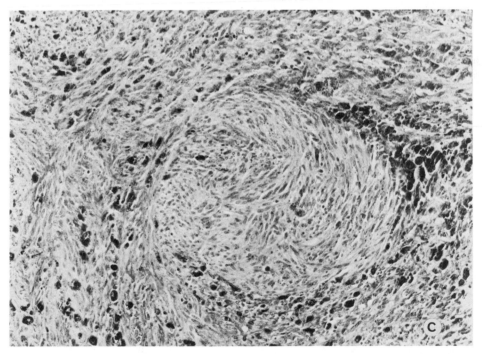

FIGURE 4–5C. Cellular blue nevus. These benign, spindle-shaped cells, some of which are pigmented, are not separated by fibroblasts or collagen. H&E × 160

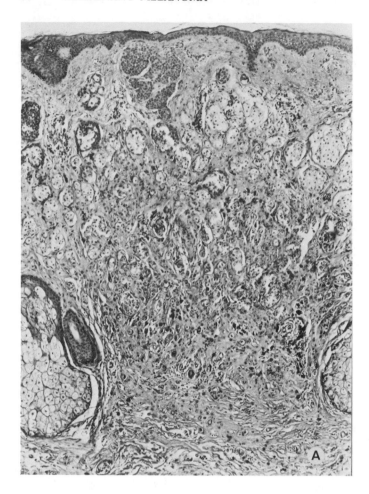

FIGURE 4-6A. Balloon cell nevus. In addition to nests of typical intradermal nevus cells (top, to left of center) numerous groups of cells have abundant pale cytoplasm. H&E × 63

layer occurs in this same area. The lesion most usually occurs on the skin of the back of young people in the first and second decades.[29]

Balloon cell nevus. This is a variant of intradermal nevus, in which the cytoplasm of benign nevus cells becomes voluminous and pale, although pigment can still be observed (Fig. 4-6A,B). The phenomenon of ballooning is explained ultrastructurally by extensive degeneration of melanosomes, with vacuolization of the cytoplasm of these cells.[24,37]

Balloon cells are often seen side by side with ordinary intradermal nevus cells. The lesion is benign.

Other unusual nevi. Pathologists may occasionally encounter rare variants of benign nevocytic lesions; for example, the epithelioid cell nevus (Fig. 4-7) and the spindle cell nevus (Fig. 4-8).

JUVENILE MELANOMA

This designation applies to a pathological entity, rather than to an age group, making the name a misnomer. McGovern states that he has encountered typical juvenile melanoma up to the age of 65.[31] Grossly, the lesion is often well-delimited, reddish, and polypoid (Fig. 4-9).

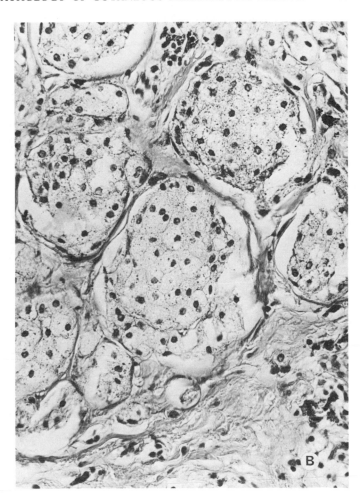

FIGURE 4–6B. Detail of same lesion. Note that the pale cells contain finely dispersed melanin pigment granules. The cells of sebaceous gland origin, to which balloon cells bear some resemblance, have a finely vacuolated cytoplasm that contains lipid, but never melanin. H&E × 285

The typical lesion consists microscopically of a variable number of rounded aggregates of spindle-shaped cells, located in the region of the epidermal-dermal junction, along the edges of rete ridges or between them (Fig. 4–10A). Not infrequently a few cells have abundant eosinophilic cytoplasm and may be multinucleated. These bear a superficial resemblance to malignant cells of skeletal muscle origin and have been dubbed "rhabdomyoid" (Fig. 4–10B). There is also an intradermal component, consisting of more polygonal epithelioid cells. Occasional single cells may be seen migrating through the epidermis. The cells have fairly prominent nucleoli, occasional mitotic figures and sparse melanin pigment. Often there is prominent dilatation of blood vessels (Fig. 4–11), which explains the reddish color clinically evident in these lesions, as well as the frequent preoperative impression that these are tumors of blood vessels. There is frequently a conspicuous chronic inflammatory cell infiltrate in the dermis, beneath the lesion.

In a melanocytic lesion, featuring prominent nucleoli, mitotic activity, epidermal involvement, and typical giant cells, it is of the utmost importance to distinguish a juvenile "melanoma" from a true malignant melanoma, and this may be quite difficult. It is a

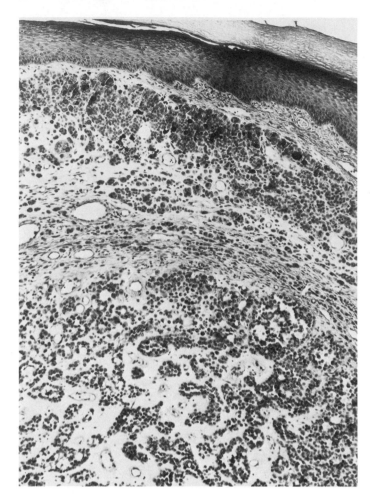

FIGURE 4–7. Epithelioid cell nevus, a somewhat unusual variant of intradermal nevus, characterized by epithelial cell nests that tend to form alveolar structures. This was interpreted as benign, but atypical. HPS × 69

wise rule not to diagnose malignant melanoma in a child unless *all* criteria of malignancy have been met and the diagnosis of juvenile melanoma excluded. Features helpful in leading to a diagnosis of benign juvenile melanoma include: clusters of spindle-shaped cells near the dermal epidermal junction, presence of rhabdomyoid cells, and telangiectases.

True melanomas do occur in the pediatric age group, but with the utmost rarity (Fig. 4–12). The distinction between benign juvenile melanoma ("Spitz lesion") and true malignant melanoma is one of the most difficult problems in the entire pathology of melanocytic lesions.

Ephelis. This is the common "freckle" and is characterized histologically by increased pigmentation in the basal layer of the epidermis, without other changes.

Lentigo. In addition to basal cell pigmentation, there is lengthening and club-shaped widening of rete ridges (Fig. 4–13). The epidermis itself is somewhat atypical, such as is seen in solar keratosis. Lentigines are also commonly seen in sun-exposed areas.

Other pigmented lesions to be included in the clinical differential diagnosis. Not infrequently, biopsies of pigmented lesions are taken, in order to rule out the possibility of

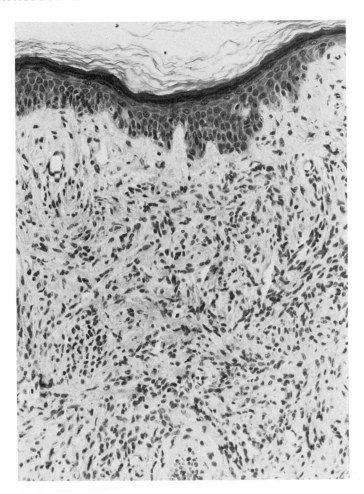

FIGURE 4-8. Another variant of intradermal ncvus, this one composed almost exclusively of spindle cells. HPS × 176

malignant melanoma. Histologically the distinction between melanoma and such lesions as seborrheic keratoses (Fig. 4-14), pigmented basal cell epitheliomas, or foreign body reaction to graphite presents no real problem.

MALIGNANT MELANOMA

Anatomic Distribution. Excluding primary melanomas of the eye, the central nervous system, the mucous membranes, and the autonomic nervous system, the most common site for the occurrence of melanomas is the lower extremities, for both sexes. Other frequently involved areas are the head and neck region, back (especially in males), chest and abdomen and upper extremities, the relative order of frequency depending on the series under investigation, and the geographical origin of the material. In Queensland, Australia for example, the trunk is a slightly more frequent site of involvement than are the lower extremities for both sexes; in males 47% of a series of 523 malignant melanomas occurred on the trunk, while in females 38.6% of 644 melanomas arose in the lower extremites.[17] At our own institution the lower extremities are the most common sites involved in female patients, followed by head and neck, abdomen, upper extremities, chest and abdomen and back, while in males in-

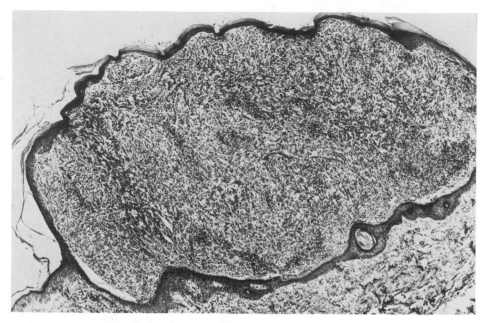

FIGURE 4-9. Juvenile "melanoma." This elevated, dome-shaped lesion appears to be surrounded by an epidermal collar. It is composed of closely packed cells, many of which are spindle-shaped. HPS × 94

volvement of the chest slightly exceeded that on the back, followed by head and neck and upper limbs, the lower limbs representing the lowest incidence of the five areas analyzed.[15] The figures from Connecticut fairly well duplicate the local experience, in that in male patients melanomas tend to occur on the trunk most frequently, and in females the lesions develop most commonly in the lower limbs. The other sites show slight change in the order of involvement, when compared with the figures at CPMC.[18]*

Although the technique of biopsy falls within the province of the surgeon, certain principles should be set forth, to be assured of adequate diagnostic tissue and to maximize the patient's chances for recovery.

If the lesion in question is small, i.e. less than 1 cm in major dimension, it can be excised with a margin of normal skin surrounding it. The depth of excision should include

* Columbia Presbyterian Medical Center

some subcutaneous fat so that the level of extension in depth can be evaluated. Shave biopsies of pigmented lesions suspected of being melanoma are to be avoided, because of the inability to judge the depth and also because of the possible but unproven role of irritation of the lesion by this trauma.

Larger lesions, and pedunculated lesions should be sampled with an incisional biopsy. This should include some normal skin at the margin, and subcutaneous tissue, if possible. The surgeon should try to obtain viable and representative tissue, i.e. to incise well into the lesion, but in areas not involved by hemorrhage and necrosis. The reason for including normal skin at the edge of the biopsy is for evaluation of the transition between normal skin and invasive melanoma, to look for junctional nests, or a preinvasive phase of melanoma. The former is important for establishing the diagnosis in some melanotic lesions and for evaluating whether a given lesion is

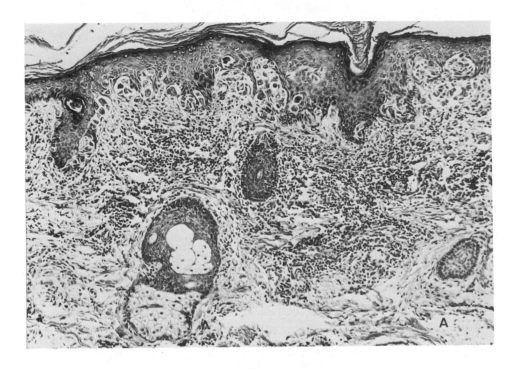

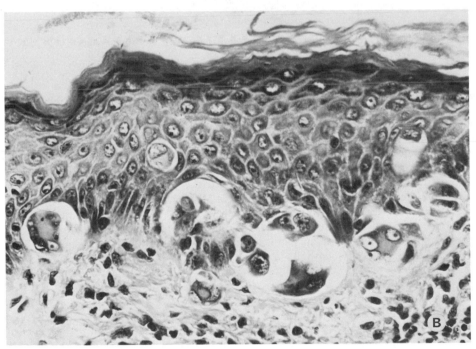

FIGURE 4–10A. Another juvenile "melanoma" in which there is a prominent junctional component, some of the cells being spindle-shaped. Others are large, with abundant cytoplasm. HPS × 94. B. Detail of same case, showing large, bizarre multinucleated cells that have strongly acidophilic cytoplasm and have been referred to as "rhabdomyoid cells." HPS × 375

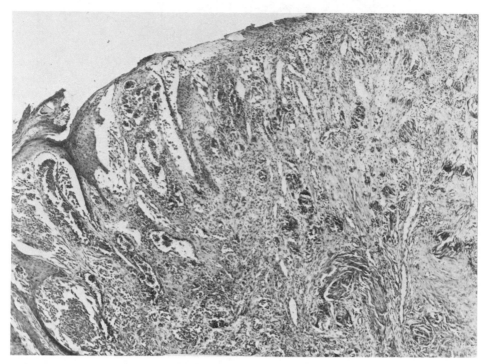

FIGURE 4–11. Superficially ulcerated polypoid lesion, composed of spindle-shaped cells, in which telangiectases are a conspicuous feature. H&E × 38

primary or metastatic. The latter is important in assigning a prognosis to a given lesion, in light of the modern classification of malignant melanoma (q.v.). Objections have been raised to the practice of performing incisional biopsies on lesions suspected of being malignant melanomas, on the grounds that such a procedure might mobilize tumor cells and cause spread of disease. However, repeated studies of this problem have failed to substantiate any danger to the patient from having had an incisional biopsy, followed in a few days by a definitive surgical procedure.[19,27]

The role of frozen section in the diagnosis of malignant melanoma. Whereas the vast majority of malignant melanomas are diagnosed by frozen section in major centers in Australia[17,31] the interpretation requires a considerable degree of experience, exposure, and expertise on the part of the pathologist. In most

American laboratories, including our institution, we prefer to section well-fixed paraffinized tissue; a similar viewpoint was recently expressed by Ackerman.[2] When dealing with excisional biopsies we paint all surgically created margins with India ink[16] in order to evaluate the proximity of the lesion to the margin. By permitting adequate fixation we believe we can better discern fine details of cellular morphology, as well as more precisely estimate architectural relationships.

CLASSIFICATION

The modern assessment and treatment of malignant melanoma is based upon a classification devised in 1967 by Clark[10] and almost simultaneously by McGovern in Australia.[32] This classification has been quite generally followed by pathologists, oncologists, and

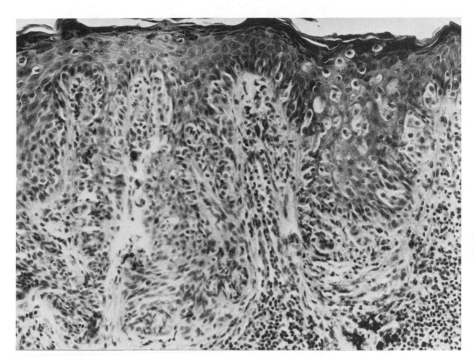

FIGURE 4-12. Lesion from the back of a 17-year-old boy, illustrating a prominent junctional element, some spindle-shaped cells, and the presence of occasional intraepidermal cells (upper right of field). A prominent inflammatory cell infiltrate is noted beneath the lesion in lower right of field. Occasional mitoses were found in the lesion and this was interpreted as a true malignant melanoma. HPS × 160

surgeons, and is not only useful in assigning a prognosis to a given case, but is an example of the multidisciplinary approach, in which all specialists adhere to the same criteria and terminology, with only minor modifications.

I. MALIGNANT MELANOMA ARISING IN HUTCHINSON'S FRECKLE. SYNONYM: LENTIGO MALIGNA MELANOMA

In this, the most favorable of the three main types of malignant melanoma, a focus of invasive melanoma develops in a preexisting, usually long-standing intra-epidermal lesion, known as Hutchinson's freckle, or lentigo maligna. These lesions affect persons over 50 years of age. They are usually quite large, irregularly pigmented, and occur virtually exclusively in sun-exposed areas, most commonly in the malar region of the face.

The frequency with which invasive melanoma complicates lentigo maligna has not been determined. In order to establish this, a prospective study on a large number of patients with biopsy-proven, but not otherwise treated lentigo maligna would have to be carried out, and these patients followed for the remainder of their lives.

Grossly, lentigo maligna is a flat tan or brownish patch having irregular outlines. When invasive melanoma develops in one of these lesions the clinical aspect will include one or more zones of deeper brown or blue-black pigmentation and elevation from the surface, perhaps with some surface hyperkeratosis.[35] Microscopically, lentigo maligna is characterized by the presence of an increased number of melanocytes, so that instead of one melanocyte for every 10 or 12 basal cells they

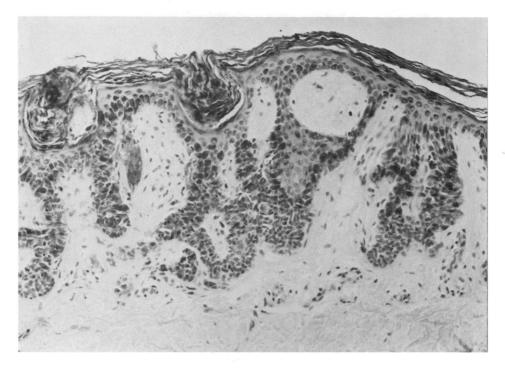

FIGURE 4-13. Senile lentigo. This lesion is pigmented because of increased pigment in the basal cells. Note also the elongation of rete pegs, many of which are club-shaped. HPS × 160

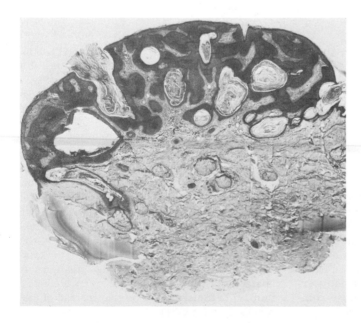

FIGURE 4-14. Seborrheic keratosis. The proliferating basal cells often contain pigment, and there are numerous keratin horn cysts within the lesion, which appears to be everywhere superficial. HPS × 16

become more closely spaced, i.e. every 3 or 4 basal cells. In addition melanocytes are larger, more hyperchromatic and thus more prominent than in normal skin (Fig. 4–15). When the lesion progresses to lentigo maligna melanoma, melanocytes form an almost continuous band at the basal layer, the cell nuclei become even larger and more bizarre in configuration, and most importantly there is evidence of separation of melanoma cells from the epidermis, with invasion of the dermis (Fig. 4–16A,B). The intradermal portion shows cells with large nuclei, prominent nucleoli, amphophilic cytoplasm, usually containing melanin pigment granules, and mitotic activity can often be demonstrated. The depth of invasion in these lesions is generally not very deep, and occurs late in the course of the disease. The dermis invariably shows the changes of severe sun-damage, i.e. solar elastosis. The prognosis for these lesions is by far the best of the three groups. It is difficult to know how wide a margin of skin to excise in treating these lesions. Should the entire intraepidermal lesion be removed in order to prevent the development of one or more additional foci of invasive melanoma? Since Hutchinson's freckles are generally quite sizable, this would entail an extensive procedure.

Levels of Invasion. This schema developed by Clark et al.[11] divides the skin into five levels, for purposes of staging melanoma (Fig. 4–17A): level I = intraepidermal (in situ, preinvasive); level II = invasion into papillary layer of dermis; level III = invasion to junction of papillary and reticular dermis, with indentation of the reticular layer; level IV = invasion into reticular layer of dermis (Fig 4–17B); level V = invasion into subcutaneous fat.

An alternative scheme of expressing the degree of invasiveness of melanomas has been proposed by Breslow,[8] and is predicated upon the thickness of the melanoma in mm; although Breslow claims that his scheme correlates more closely with prognosis, the five levels delineated above have been more generally adopted (Chap. 6).

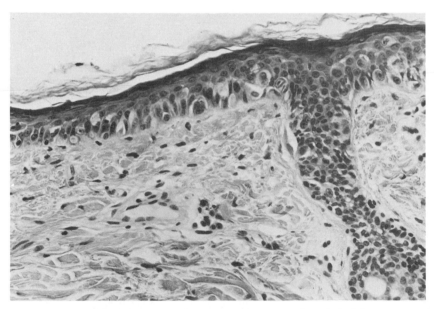

FIGURE 4–15. Lentigo maligna, showing melanocytes to be more numerous and anaplastic than in normal skin. Note the presence of abnormal melanocytes along hair follicle, as well as surface epidermis. HPS × 208

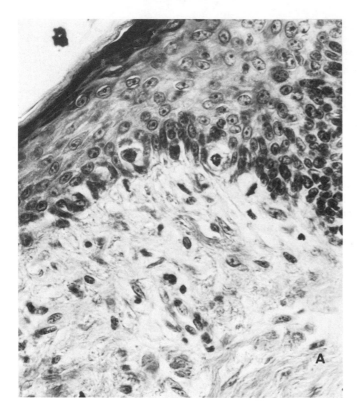

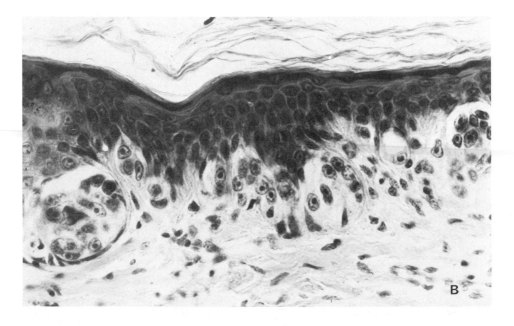

FIGURE 4-16A. Lentigo maligna. Note two mitoses to right of center, upper portion of photograph. HPS × 375. B. Same case, showing nests of malignant melanocytes at epidermal junction. HPS × 375

II. Superficial Spreading Melanoma (Page-toid Melanoma)

This is the second class of malignant melanoma, which is preceded by an intraepidermal or in-situ stage, or a "premalignant melanosis." Superficial spreading melanoma is the most common of the three types. It occurs either on sun-exposed skin or on skin that is usually covered by clothing. The basic in situ lesion is smaller than lentigo maligna, but when invasive melanoma supervenes the lesion grows more rapidly than does the invasive component in a lentigo maligna melanoma. Grossly, the preinvasive lesion is flat, variable in color, with a fairly discrete but irregularly shaped outline. Indentations or notches often occur in these lesions. The superimposed invasive lesion is an elevated nodule, often with a verrucous surface, showing loss of normal skin markings.[36] The coloration of superficial spreading melanomas shows great variability, and often includes a variegated assortment of pink, red, blue, black, tan, and white (Fig. 4-18). The white areas are ascribed to areas of depigmentation, which correspond to areas of regression microscopically.

The histological appearance of superficial spreading lesions is characterized by involvement of the full thickness of the epidermis by malignant melanocytic cells, usually containing melanin pigment, and showing large nucleoli and mitotic activity (Fig. 4-19A). Not infrequently such cells can be seen in the exfoliated keratotic layer at the surface (Fig. 4-19B). In addition there are frequently prominent junctional nests of malignant cells and, in the invasive phase, cells of the melanocytic series are seen to invade the dermis. The depth of invasion is graded according to the schema (v.s.), level I-V. Dermal changes of solar elastosis are usually far less pronounced than is the case for lentigo maligna melanoma. Underlying the invasive portion there is usually a band-like infiltrate of lymphocytic cells (Fig. 4-19C). Such cells are always seen beneath the white areas observed grossly, where the malignant pigmented epithelial cells have disappeared and presumably been destroyed by "killer" lymphocytes (Fig. 4-20).

III. Nodular Melanoma

This type is sometimes referred to as "melanoma without adjacent intraepidermal component." It is the most ominous of the three varieties of malignant melanoma, in that it grows more rapidly, invades more deeply, and is more likely to metastasize, via the blood stream and/or via lymphatics.

Grossly, the lesion is elevated, convex, or even pedunculated (Fig. 4-21), and is frequently deeply pigmented, with a black or dark blue color (Fig. 4-22). It has been described as resembling a blueberry.

Microscopically typical melanoma cells occur at the junction of rete ridges and dermis, as well as invading well into the dermis. Involvement of the epidermis is seen only directly overlying the invasive tumor, i.e. there is absence of what was called "lateral junctional spread" 20 years ago.[27] Even though the terminology was different then, the conclusion reached was identical, i.e. that melanomas without any adjacent intraepidermal component have a far worse biological behavior than those with lateral junctional spread.

It is the nodular melanomas that are sometimes amelanotic, and that often ulcerate the overlying epidermis, so that evidence of junctional change may be difficult to demonstrate. In such a case the diagnosis rests on a thorough familiarity with the appearance of melanoma cells, as well as the exclusion of other possibilities. A dopa stain on fresh tissue might serve to demonstrate melanin that could not be discerned on routine stain, while a short Fontana stain on fixed tissue (Fig. 4-23) blackens pigment that might be only faintly visible on routine stains. If the facilities of an electron microscope are available it may be possible to demonstrate melanosomes in the cells (Fig. 4-24).

Not infrequently malignant melanoma of any of the types, but mostly in the case of nodular melanoma, is accompanied by a pronounced overgrowth of squamous epithelium in the vicinity, resulting in pseudoepitheliomatous hyperplasia (Fig. 4-25). It is understandable, under such circumstances, that a nonpigmented lesion might be misdiagnosed as squamous cell carcinoma. One of

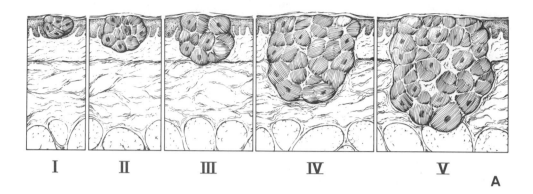

I   II   III   IV   V

A

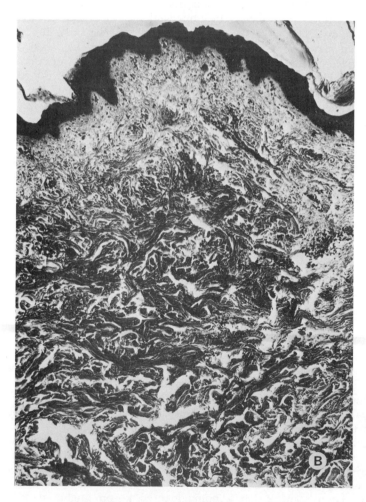

B

FIGURE 4–17A. Schematic diagram to demonstrate levels of invasion in melanomas (after WH Clark, Jr). B. This deliberately overstained section clearly illustrates the contrast between papillary and reticular dermis. The former consists of fine collagen fibers, loosely woven, while the latter consists of heavy thick collagen bundles. It is the boundary between papillary and reticular dermis that presents the main difficulty to pathologists in assigning a level of invasion. HPS × 69

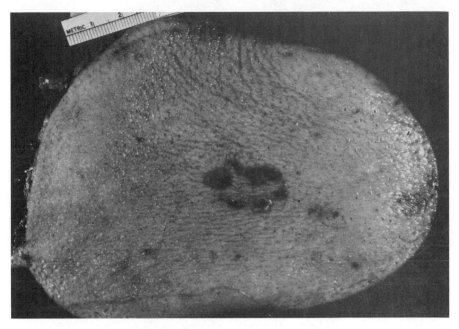

FIGURE 4–18. Gross photograph of a superficial spreading malignant melanoma, showing multiple shades, irregular outline, area of depigmentation, and the elevated, nodular focus in lower portion of the lesion.

the melanin stains would be helpful in indicating the nature of the malignant cells.

When first seen nodular melanomas have usually invaded at least to level III or deeper. The mitotic rate is higher than seen in the two previous categories of malignant melanoma; lymphatic or blood vessel invasion can frequently be demonstrated in these lesions (Fig. 4–26), and the incidence of lymph node and hematogenous metastases from these tumors is very high. Perineural invasion may also be encountered in the primary lesion.

Nodular melanomas are unassociated with solar changes in the underlying dermis, and frequently occur in zones of the body not directly exposed to the sun. There is often a history of sun exposure of other parts of the skin in such patients, leading to the theory of a humoral factor released from sun-exposed skin, which incites a malignant melanoma in skin of another area.[7,28]

DESMOPLASTIC MELANOMA

This is a rare variant of melanoma, which was first described by Conley, Orr, and Lattes in 1971.[14] These lesions are bulky, infiltrative, and aggressive, and are characterized microscopically by invasive bundles of spindle-shaped cells, some of which are fibroblasts but many of which are spindle-shaped melanoma cells (Fig. 4–27). Most such lesions have been reported in the region of the head and neck. All have been associated with more typical superficial melanomas, either concurrently or lesions previously removed from the area in question. Thus desmoplastic melanoma represents invasive spindle-cell melanoma with a prolific fibroblastic response and collagen deposition (Fig. 4–28). The importance of this entity is in being able to distinguish it from various mesenchymal neoplasms that also consist of spindle-shaped cells. A silver stain

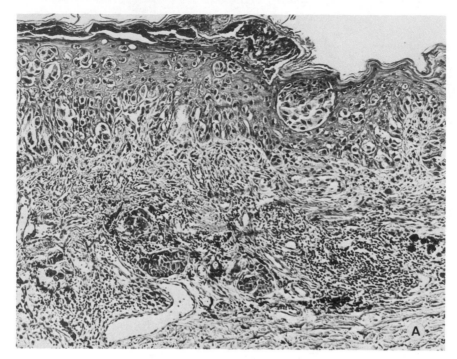

FIGURE 4–19A. Superficial spreading melanoma, showing nests of malignant melanocytes in all layers of the epidermis, and invading dermis down to reticular layer. Note presence of widely patent lymphatic channels within dermis. H&E × 94.

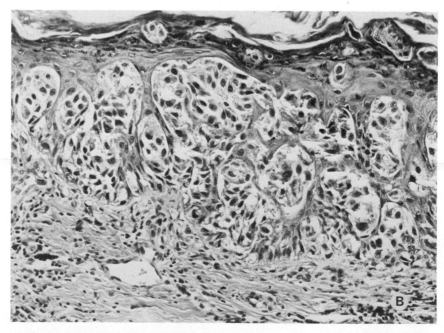

FIGURE 4–19B. Higher magnification of same lesion. Note melanoma cells that have migrated into stratum corneum (extreme right upper corner) H&E × 192

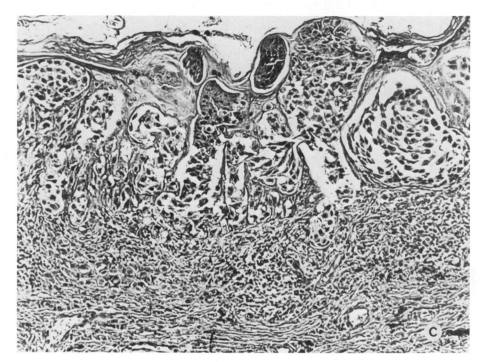

FIGURE 4–19C. Note band of lymphocytic infiltrate beneath the lesion. H&E × 160

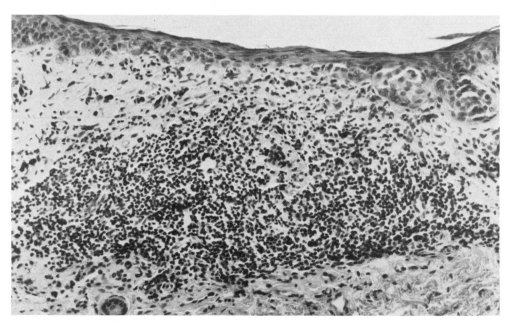

FIGURE 4–20. Melanocytes present only at the junction. The papillary dermis shows fibrosis and a heavy concentration of lymphocytes, along with pigmented macrophages. This section was taken from an area of depigmentation and is thought to represent regression of an invasive focus. HPS × 160

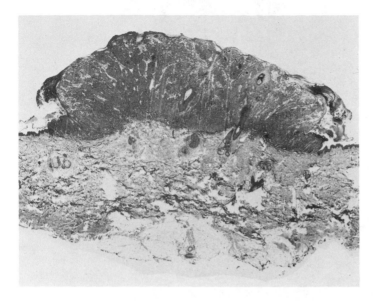

FIGURE 4–21. Low-power micro-photograph of a polypoid nodular melanoma. HPS × 8

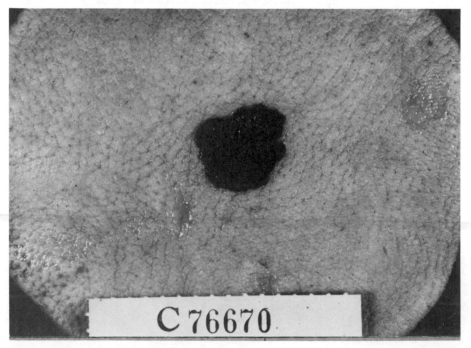

FIGURE 4–22. Gross photograph of nodular melanoma. Note fairly sharp circumscription, deep pigmentation, and absence of satellite lesions.

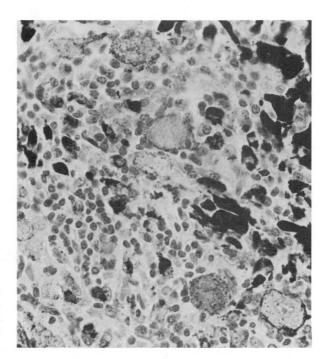

FIGURE 4-23. Typical melanin granule stain. In the more lightly stained cells, the delicate character of melanin pigment granules and the sparing of nuclei will be apparent. Short Fontana × 375

will often help to delineate the nest-like epithelial type of reticulin distribution (Fig. 4-29). The demonstration of a superficial melanoma overlying the lesion is pathognomonic, but often only a history of such a lesion having been removed is obtainable. This must be substantiated by reviewing the previous pathological preparations. Desmoplastic melanomas are rarely pigmented; occasionally evidence of pigment-forming organelles can be demonstrated ultrastructurally.

PRIMARY VERSUS METASTATIC MELANOMAS

It has been generally affirmed that when a malignant lesion has arisen at a particular site, there will be evidence of junctional change in the immediate vicinity of the lesion; in contrast a metastatic melanoma will be unassociated with overlying junctional changes. As a rule metastatic melanoma will be deposited in and grow in the subcutis or dermis, the overlying epidermis being unbroken.

These basic rules are unfortunately not always fulfilled. For example, a rapidly growing ulcerated melanoma may have undergone extensive necrosis, with destruction of all evidence of junctional changes, before it arrives for pathological evaluation. A metastatic lesion could fortuitously be deposited and grow in an area of skin in which there happens to be a pigmented lesion with a junctional component. Furthermore, locally recurrent melanomas may have junctional changes in the overlying epidermis. This is explained on the basis of a "field effect" surrounding the original cutaneous lesion.

THE SPREAD OF MALIGNANT MELANOMA

In addition to superficial intraepidermal (horizontal) spread by melanoma cells with the possible formation of satellite lesions, and

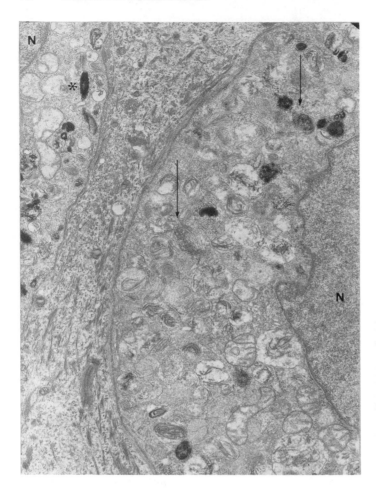

FIGURE 4–24. Electron micrograph of two intraepidermal melanoma cells, showing a varying degree of melanosomal maturation. N = nuclei of melanoma cells; arrows indicate poorly cross-linked filaments in abnormal melanosomes, while * indicates a normal, fully melanized melanosome in a melanoma cell. Original magnification × **9000** (Courtesy Dr. David N. Silvers)

penetration into the depth of the skin (vertical spread), melanoma cells can gain access to lymphatic channels and metastasize to regional lymph nodes; they can also invade vein walls and give rise to hematogenous metastases. These can be found in virtually any organ: bowel, lungs, liver, brain (including meninges) and bone are common sites. Submucosal metastases to the gastrointestinal tract can give rise to massive hemorrhage, obstruction, or even intussusception. Polypoid mucosal metastases to the gallbladder are well known to radiologists. Certain viscera that are rare targets for metastases by most other tumors are notoriously involved in cases of widespread malignant melanoma; these target organs include spleen and heart (any layer).

Thus it is apparent that even if a patient with melanoma has been demonstrated to be free of lymph node metastases, there remains a significant possibility of hematogenous metastases. However, since we know of no foolproof method of preventing or curing hematogenous metastases it is felt that regional lymphadenectomy has a definite place in the management of malignant melanoma (v.i.) Another type of presentation of malignant melanoma, in an advanced stage of the disease, is called "in-transit metastases." In this condition the primary skin lesion has been excised and a lymphadenectomy of the draining lymph nodes performed. A few weeks or months later the patient may develop multiple visible and palpable nodules in the skin of the extremity, which are probably originating in cells located in lymphatic vessels. The explanation for this phenomenon is that tumor cells had become detached from the primary lesion prior to or during surgery; since the draining nodes were removed at the time of the procedure the in-transit cells, which proceeded to grow, were trapped within lymphatics.

It is for this type of recurrent melanoma that isolated perfusion of an extremity, using such chemotherapeutic agents as phenylalanine mustard, has been utilized. Because of this ominous complication, some have advocated delaying lymphadenectomy for 3 to 6 weeks in order to permit in-transit tumor cells to reach the draining lymph nodes; others have recommended en bloc removal of the primary lesion, with a strip of intervening skin and subcutis and the regional node dissection, in an attempt to obviate the in-transit metastases.

Do melanomas arise from benign nevi? This is a practical and pertinent question, as the average person has 10 to 30 pigmented nevi[44] yet the chances that one of these will become malignant are 1 per 72,000.[17] It is thus impractical to remove all nevi prophylactically. However, patients with xeroderma pigmentosum have a very high incidence of

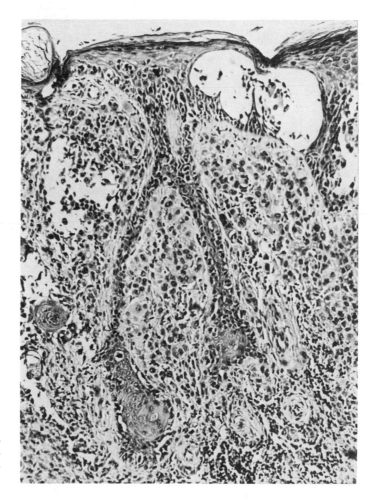

FIGURE 4–25. Pseudo-epitheliomatous hyperplasia (wishbone-shaped area) in a malignant melanoma. H&E × 120

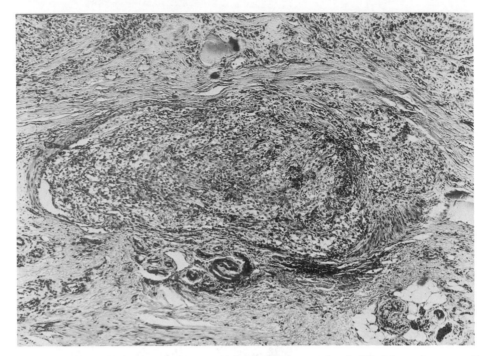

FIGURE 4–26. Vein (Occupying center of field) almost completely filled by melanoma cells. HPS × 69

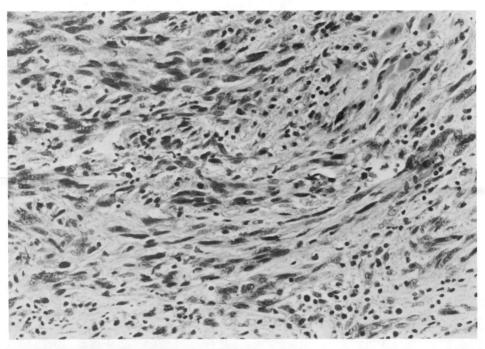

FIGURE 4–27. Desmoplastic melanoma. Bundles of plump spindle-shaped cells are admixed with fibroblasts and lymphocytes. H&E × 240

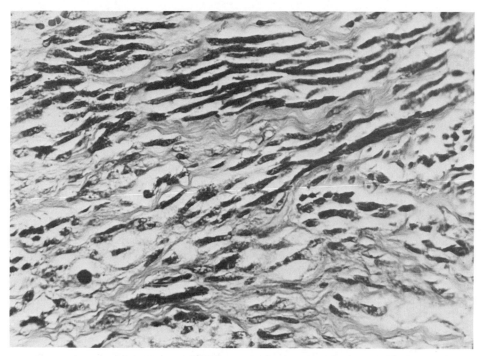

FIGURE 4-28. High-power view of a desmoplastic melanoma with dense collagen bundles between nests of spindle-shaped cells. Tumor cells have extremely hyperchromatic, somewhat wavy nuclei, with a suggestion of palisading, vaguely reminiscent of Schwann cell tumors. HPS × 375

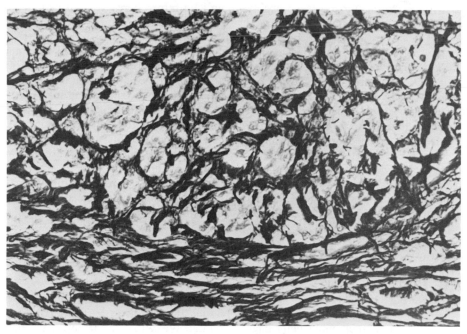

FIGURE 4-29. Desmoplastic melanoma. Reticulin stain brings out epithelial nests in upper portions of field, indicating this is not a mesenchymal tumor. Laidlaw × 240

developing malignant melanoma. In addition, congenital nevi, which are large, hairy, and usually of the compound type, have a predisposition for malignant alteration,[40] and such lesions should be removed, if feasible. Other nevi that ought to be surgically excised are those in which a change has occurred (in size, pigmentation, integrity of the surface, appearance of satellites); those which are exposed to constant mechanical trauma by clothing; sizable (> 0.5 cm), black, presumably junctional nevi; lesions in which the diagnosis is not certain; lesions posing cosmetic problems; and finally those causing a high degree of apprehension in the patient.

Perhaps one reason why there has been a widespread belief that most malignant melanomas arise from benign nevi is that in the deeper portions of many invasive melanomas the cells appear smaller and the nuclei less anaplastic than in the superficial portions. The modern interpretation of this finding is that the deeply situated cells represent maturation of melanoma cells rather than preexisting benign nevus cells. Their presence is associated with a better prognosis—probably because of their low rate of mitotic activity.[33]

In a study of 209 patients with melanoma Clark found that 9.6% had evidence of undoubtedly benign nevus cells associated with their malignant melanoma.[11] From the point of view of duration of lesions, the majority had known of the presence of their lesions for a very few years (average 6.6 years).[11] In the series of Lane et al.[27] more than 50% of the patients gave a history of having had a pigmented lesion in the area where a melanoma subsequently developed. As this was a clinical observation, the figure undoubtedly included the intraepidermal phase of melanoma, i.e. lentigo maligna and superficial spreading (preinvasive) melanosis.

GENERAL HISTOLOGICAL ASPECTS OF MALIGNANT MELANOMA

Whatever the subtype, melanoma cells have certain properties in common, by which they can be recognized even in the absence of pigment production.

Melanoma cells are usually large, polygonal, or spindle-shaped with an amphophilic, grayish cytoplasm and large nuclei, which often have very prominent nucleoli (Fig. 4–30). The nucleoli may be acidophilic and sometimes are so large that they resemble inclusion bodies. Not infrequently melanoma cells have bilobed nuclei, and the finding of a large cell with a bilobed nucleus having prominent acidophilic nucleoli can be strikingly similar to a Reed–Sternberg cell of Hodgkin's disease.[45] Melanoma cells grow in clusters but do not cohere to each other in the manner of the pavement cells of squamous cell carcinoma. This lack of cohesiveness serves to explain the phenomenon of an alveolar pattern in some melanomas, in which the cells of a solid cluster pull apart, the central cells drop out, and the peripheral ring of cells remains. Mitoses can almost always be demonstrated in malignant melanomas, in considerable numbers.

Pigment production by melanoma cells can occur in an irregular manner. Not uncommonly one may see pigmented cells in the deep portions of a melanoma (Fig. 4–31). It will be remembered that in benign nevi (excluding blue nevi for the moment) pigment is seen superficially but is absent in the deeper dermal nevus cells, which are older and more mature. This production of pigment in deeply situated cells can be helpful towards arriving at a diagnosis in some doubtful cases.

Many, if not most malignant melanomas are underlain by a zone of chronic inflammatory cell infiltration. This is cited by some as indicative of the malignant nature of the lesion. However, inflammatory cells are also present in the vicinity of "juvenile melanomas," and thus should not give rise to erroneous diagnoses of malignant melanoma.

THE ROLE OF REGIONAL LYMPH NODE DISSECTION

This has become one of the most controversial issues in the entire area of malignant melanoma. We will not attempt an exhaustive debate of the problem, but will simply highlight some arguments and state our stance in this matter.

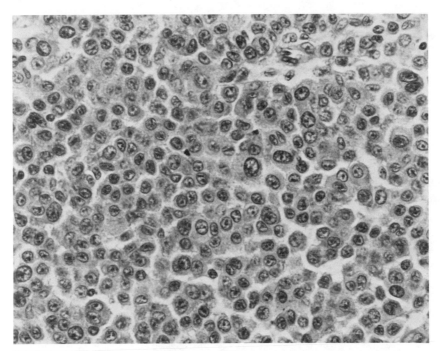

FIGURE 4-30. Focus of amelanotic melanoma showing typical appearance of cells, polygonal in shape with pleomorphic nuclei and prominent nucleoli. Note lack of cohesiveness between cells. HPS × 375

Opponents of lymphadenectomy cite the value of lymph nodes as an immunologic barrier and that their extirpation removes a line of defense from the patient. Further they state that not every cell that reaches a lymph node will stay there or even survive, and that the mere demonstration of melanoma cells in lymph nodes does not necessarily bode ill for the patient. With the advent of the generally accepted system of levels of invasion in malignant melanoma, the current approach is to carry out elective regional lymph node dissections for patients whose melanomas reach level III or beyond. This is based on statistical studies, which point out the rarity of lymph node metastases in lesions invading to levels more superficial than III.

In this institution we have seen widespread lymph node metastases, ultimately causing the patient's death, originally considered to be level I but later proved to be level II. Thus, even though metastases occur with great rarity, the potential for metastases exists as soon as the melanoma has reached the dermis; this was also the conclusion of Mehnert and Heard.[34] Some of us believe that if the patient can tolerate the procedure medically he deserves a prophylactic lymphadenectomy. In the exceptional case in which the primary is in a location where lymphadenectomy is not feasible, such as the very middle of the back, which would entail four lymphadenectomies, such a procedure is not recommended. Usually, however, the primary can be lateralized to one side or the other.

The value of prophylactic lymphadenectomy, i.e. removal of draining lymph nodes while they are clinically uninvolved, was convincingly demonstrated by Lane et al.,[27] even though some patients had microscopic metastases (Fig. 4-32). This conclusion has since been confirmed by a number of other investigators.[1,13,22,23,25] These authors all found that a regional lymph node dissection per-

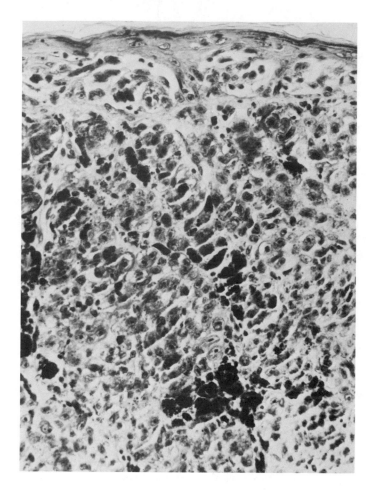

FIGURE 4-31. Lentigo maligna melanoma. Invasive melanoma has supervened. Note pigment production in deep portion of the lesion, as well as prominent nucleoli in nuclei of melanoma cells. H&E × 240

formed in continuity (Fig. 4-33) or discontinuously in patients with melanoma, even though lymph nodes were not clinically palpable, was followed by a significantly greater survival rate than if node dissection were not carried at all or if nodes were already palpable. In the latter situation very few patients survived five years.

INDETERMINATE LESIONS

With all the available descriptions, criteria, and increasing understanding of melanocytic lesions, there still remain instances in which the diagnosis of malignancy is in doubt. With a well-taken, well-fixed, and properly oriented biopsy this should not happen too frequently. Often level-sections through the paraffin block can solve the problem in one direction or the other. In this institution we find it helpful to seek the opinion of other members of the staff, who have had considerable experience with melanocytic lesions. If the particular case is totally irresolvable, it is recommended to the surgeon to carry out a wide local excision, in order to totally extirpate the local lesion with its adjacent skin.

What constitutes a wide local excision? Empirically it has been found that a radius of 5 cm all about the margin of a malignant melanoma seems to prevent local recurrences, and thus this has been widely adopted. Recently, however, a margin of 6 cm, where anatomically feasible, has been recommended.[4] Naturally, wide local excision entails skin grafting.

MULTIPLE PRIMARY MELANOMAS

The incidence of the occurrence of more than one primary malignant melanoma varies, according to the criteria applied. Multiple primary melanomas are not exceptional; they may be seen concurrently or metachronously. The incidence of more than one primary melanoma in various reported series ranges from 1.3%[38] to 3.8%[6] and even 3.9%.[9] Although most reported cases concern patients with two primary malignant melanomas, Beardmore and Davis reported a case with six

independent melanomas,[6] while Kahn and Donaldson reported a patient with at least 49 primary lesions.[26] In most instances the second lesion arose within five years of the first, but occasionally the interval was much longer. It is of note that the second primary lesions were detected at an earlier stage, due undoubtedly to the suspicion of both patient and physician, leading to earlier biopsy and diagnosis.

HEREDITARY FACTORS OPERATIVE IN MALIGNANT MELANOMAS

The occurrence of malignant melanomas in several members of a family is a rare but well-recognized event. It is well known that malig

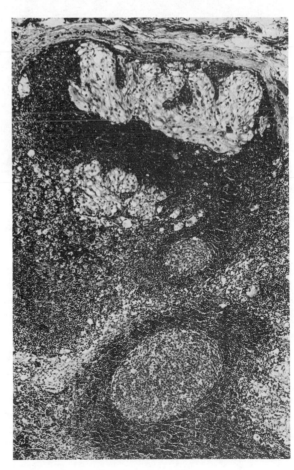

FIGURE 4-32. Metastatic melanoma (pale areas) in one out of 33 regional lymph nodes resected prophylactically. HPS × 64

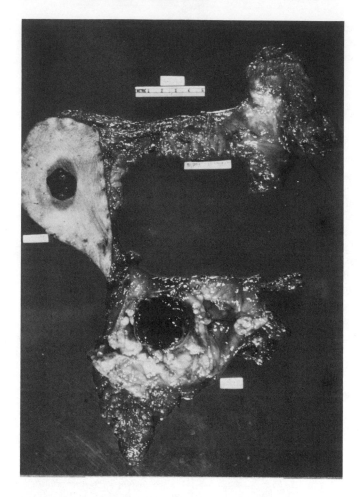

FIGURE 4–33. Gross photograph of widely excised nodular melanoma of shoulder, in continuity with supraclavicular and axillary lymphadenectomy. In this case nodes were palpable, and the lymphadenectomy was "therapeutic" rather than "prophylactic."

nant melanoma occurs preferentially in fair-skinned blonde or red-haired individuals, and particularly in those of Celtic origin. It appears that in families in which several members have malignant melanoma, there is a greater tendency for individual patients to have more than one melanoma, and for the patients to be younger than is true for sporadic cases of melanoma. In a study of first-degree relatives of patients with melanoma, it was found that the liability for developing malignant melanoma was 11%.[46] The exact manner of inheritance did not follow simple Mendelian rules but was interpreted as being polygenic. In reviewing a total of 74 kindred with malignant melanoma[3] it was observed that in

familial cases the survival is significantly longer than in sporadic cases. This may indicate that familial cases have a different degree of biological potential or that patients and their families are more alert to the disease, and present more promptly for medical attention, after signs and symptoms first appear.

THE EFFECT OF PREGNANCY ON MALIGNANT MELANOMA

It is well known that there is increased melanocytic activity during pregnancy, as exemplified by the darkening of the nipples, occurrence of chloasma, darkening of the linea alba, etc. It is also a well-known clinical and pathological manifestation that new nevi appear during pregnancy and that already existing nevi become darkened. Pathologically one observes "activation" of junctional zones, i.e. actively growing, young melanocytes (without the features of frank malignancy), which undoubtedly produce the additional pigment that is visible clinically. As for the fate of established melanomas during pregnancy, reports have arrived at conflicting conclusions. A recent study[43] found that pregnant patients were more likely to have lymph node metastases; to develop local changes at the site of the lesion such as ulceration, bleeding, and itching; and to have shorter survival rates if lymph node metastases were present than a comparable group of nonpregnant patients.

Conversely there have been reported cases in which spontaneous regression of malignant melanoma occurred during pregnancy[31] and McGovern feels that pregnancy probably exerts no effects on pigmentary lesions of the skin.

METASTATIC MELANOMA WITHOUT A KNOWN PRIMARY (See also Chapter 7)

The discovery of metastatic melanoma in lymph nodes or other viscera without a known primary melanoma is a puzzling, though not an exceptional situation. In a recent review of almost 2,500 patients with melanoma, 4% did not have a known primary.[5] The following circumstances could explain such a situation: (1) The patient had a lesion at some time in the past, which was removed; if it was sent for pathological examination it may have been incorrectly interpreted or the patient may not have been told of the result. More likely the lesion was fulgurated, no pathological examination was ever performed, and no scar remained. In either of these circumstances the patient did not remember the episode. (2) A melanoma was present, and underwent spontaneous regression (q.v.). (3) A primary melanoma is present in a site that the physician did not examine adequately, e.g. scalp or mucous membranes, such as nasal cavity, oral cavity, anorectal or urogenital regions, or even esophagus. (4) The primary has arisen in the lymph node itself, from nests of nevus cells. These nests are found in the capsule or in fibrous trabeculae of the node (Fig. 4–34). Such nests are found incidentally in nodes that are examined for the presence of metastases during the course of pathological staging in cancer operations. The exact manner in which nevus cells reach the nodes is not known, but it is thought to be the result of displaced tissues, probably an error of embryological development. An alternate theory is that they represent a form of benign metastasis.[30] A statistical estimate of the magnitude of this problem was recently published from Memorial Hospital.[42] It was found that 0.33% of mastectomy specimens and 3.0% of node dissections for malignant melanoma contained some nodes in which nests of benign nevus cells were present. It was argued that the anatomical distribution of nodes so involved, the relatively better prognosis in patients who had node dissections without a demonstrable primary, and the fact that the disease remains confined to lymph nodes, would all be consistent with an origin in the nodes themselves.

SPONTANEOUS REGRESSION OF MALIGNANT MELANOMA

Of all malignant neoplasms, malignant melanoma is surpassed only by renal cell carcinomas and neuroblastomas in its propensity to undergo spontaneous regression.[20] This known potential of malignant melanomas obviously raises doubt regarding any statistics dealing with results of various modes of therapy.

Grossly, a lesion undergoing regressive changes shows a lightening of the degree of pigmentation, which often eventuates in vitiligo, i.e. the end stage has a paler color than does the surrounding normal skin.

Microscopically one sees large numbers of lymphocytes and plasma cells in the dermis, along with considerable numbers of melanin-containing macrophages (melanophores). (Fig.

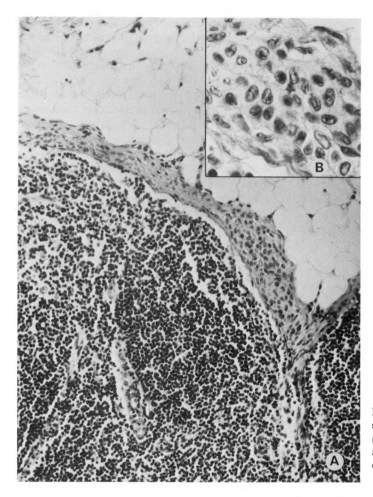

FIGURE 4-34A. Nevus cells (grey-staining) in capsule of a lymph node. (HPS × 160). B. Detail of same area, showing benign appearing cells confined to the capsule. (HPS × 580)

4-21) No viable malignant cells are in evidence. Melanocytes along the basal layer are normal or decreased in number. There is increased vascularity in the dermis and ultimately a cicatrix will be formed. The explanation for these events is that some immunological stimulus has evoked the activation of cytotoxic lymphoid cells, which destroy malignant melanocytes, and that the melanin pigment released is phagocytosed by macrophages. Features of regression or partial regression are not uncommon in malignant melanomas; they do not necessarily imply that the patient is cured, for the primary lesion may regress while its metastases may continue to grow and eventually cause the patient's death.

Due to the gratifying clinical results in some cases of spontaneous regression of melanomas, many modalities of immunotherapy have been administered. Perhaps the best known is the use of BCG, injected into the melanoma itself; this is usually reserved for cases of recurrent melanoma, as illustrated in Figure 4-35.

THE ROLE OF TRAUMA

Although anecdotal reports exist implicating trauma in the etiology of malignant melanoma, it is more likely that trauma has drawn attention to an already existing melanoma or perhaps that constant trauma to a benign pigmented lesion causes ulceration and bleeding, which would raise the clinical suspicion of malignant melanoma. We do not believe that trauma can convert a benign nevus to a malignant melanoma. We agree with Davis[17] that once a melanoma exists, trauma can play a significant role in disseminating tumor cells. Here one should include shave biopsies and various forms of electrocautery, curettage, or removal of suspicious lesions by means of a high-frequency current, because it has been the experience in this institution and others that patients whose melanomas were subjected to thermal, electrical, or mechanical manipulation had a far worse prognosis than those who, after a careful biopsy, underwent wide excision, with or without regional lymphadenectomy.

THE ROLE OF SUNLIGHT

It is now generally acknowledged that sunlight plays an etiological role in the genesis of malignant melanoma. Briefly summarized the evidence includes geographic incidence, anatomic distribution, as well as individual habits related to sun exposure. In order to explain the remarkable increase in the incidence of melanomas in various parts of the world, it has been postulated that there has been a change in the physical quality of the offending solar rays, rather than solely a purely quantitative increment.[15] Using a statistical approach coupled with physicochemical investigations Fears et al.[21] postulate that more short-wavelength ultraviolet light is reaching the surface of the earth, as the ozone layer is gradually becoming depleted, due to technological advances in the 20th century.

OVERALL PROGNOSTIC ATTRIBUTES OF MALIGNANT MELANOMA

A number of simple clinical-pathological features that are correlated with a favorable

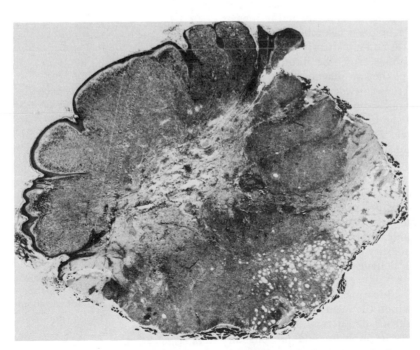

FIGURE 4–35. Re-excision of locally recurrent melanoma, which had been injected with BCG. Upper part of dermis is infiltrated by melanoma cells. Deeper dermis and subcutaneous fat are occupied by noncaseating granulomata, secondary to BCG. HPS × 6.5

prognosis deserve mention. Several of these were established in a previous study conducted in this laboratory[27] and have been amply reconfirmed by others.

1. Primary tumors smaller than 2 cm in greatest diameter have a better prognosis than larger lesions.

2. Melanomas in females have an overall better prognosis than those in males.

3. Invasive melanomas arising from preexisting intra-epidermal lesions (i.e. those with "lateral junctional spread") have a better prognosis than those beginning d'emblée (nodular melanomas).

4. Within each classification—lentigo maligna, superficial spreading, and nodular-melanoma—the deeper the level of invasion the greater the likelihood of lymph node metastases, and the poorer is the ultimate prognosis.

5. Lesions located on the extremities have a good prognosis, while those on the trunk (which usually occur in males) have a particularly poor prognosis. Subungual lesions as a group are particularly favorable—they are on the extremities and are also situated at a considerable distance from the draining lymph nodes. Perhaps they are diagnosed early by virtue of their accessible location.

6. The overall survival rates for Queensland Australia are significantly better than those of all other series. This is undoubtedly related to a vigorous education campaign directed at the laity as well as the medical profession in a region having the highest incidence of malignant melanoma of any population in the world. As a result, patients present for and receive treatment at a stage of their disease that is amenable to cure in a high percentage of cases. The majority of their lesions are small, superficial, and have not yet reached lymph nodes.

A similar educational campaign in this country, in which the incidence of this tumor is rising, might serve to alert patients and their physicians to the problem and prevent unnecessary delays in treating the lesion aggressively.

ACKNOWLEDGMENTS

The author wishes to thank Ms. Ida Nathan for the photographic work and Ms. B. John for preparing the manuscript. The case illustrated in Figures 4–4 through 4–6A and B was kindly provided by Dr. B. A. Ackerman.

REFERENCES

1. Abu-Dalu J: Prophylactic regional lymph node excision in malignant melanoma. Harefuah 80:128, 1971
2. Ackerman AB: Malignant melanoma: clinical and histological diagnosis, by Vincent J McGovern (book review). Hum Pathol 8:356, 1977
3. Anderson DE: Clinical characteristics of the genetic variety of cutaneous melanoma in man. Cancer 28:721, 1971
4. Arons MS: The surgical treatment of cutaneous melanoma. Yale J Biol Med, 48:417, 1975
5. Baab GH, McBride CM: Malignant melanoma. The patient with an unknown site of primary origin. Arch Surg 110:896, 1975
6. Beardmore GL, Davis NC: Multiple primary cutaneous melanomas. Arch Dermatol 111:603, 1975
7. Black HS, Lo WB: Formation of a carcinogen in human skin, irradicated with ultraviolet light. Nature 234:306, 1971
8. Breslow A: Tumor thickness, level of invasion and node dissection in stage I cutaneous melanoma. Ann Surg 182:572, 1975
9. Cascinelli N, Fontana V, Cataldo I, et al.: Multiple primary melanoma. Tumori 61:481, 1975
10. Clark WH Jr: A Classification of malignant melanoma in man, correlated with histogenesis and biologic behavior. In Montagna W: Advances in Biology of Skin. The Pigmentary System. New York, Pergamon Press, 1967, pp 621–647
11. Clark WH Jr, From L, Bernardino EA, et al.: The histogenesis and biologic behavior of primary human malignant melanomas of the skin. Cancer Res 29:705, 1969
12. Cochran AJ: Incidence of melanocytes in normal human skin. J Invest Dermatol 55:65, 1970
13. Cochran AJ: Malignant melanoma. A review of 10 years' experience in Glasgow, Scotland. Cancer 23:1190, 1969
14. Conley J, Lattes R, Orr W: Desmoplastic malignant melanoma (a rare variant of spindle cell melanoma). Cancer 28: 914, 1971

15. Cosman B, Heddle SB, Crikelair GF: The increasing incidence of melanoma. Plast Reconstr Surg, 57:50, 1976
16. Crikelair GF, Lattes R: A useful method to determine the adequacy of surgical resection of skin lesions. Trans IV Int Cong Plast Reconstr Surg Rome, 1967, pp 117–121
17. Davis NC: Cutaneous melanoma: the Queensland experience. Current Problems in Surgery XII, #5. Year Book Medical Publishers, Chicago, May, 1976
18. Eisenberg H: Cancer in Connecticut. Incidence and rates. 1935–1962. Cited in Cosman B, Heddle SG, Crikelair GF: The Increasing Incidence of Melanoma. Plast Reconstr Surg 57:50, 1976
19. Epstein E, Bragg K, Linden G: Biopsy and prognosis in malignant melanoma. JAMA 208:1369, 1969
20. Everson TC, Cole WW: Spontaneous Regression of Cancer. Philadelphia, WB Saunders, 1966, pp 164–220
21. Fears TR, Scotto J, Schneiderman MA: Skin cancer, melanoma and sunlight. Am J Public Health. 66:461, 1976
22. Goldsmith HS, Shah JP, Kim DH: Prognostic significance of lymph node dissection in the treatment of malignant melanoma. Cancer 26:606, 1970
23. Gumport SL, Harris MN: Results of regional lymph node dissection for melanoma. Ann Surg 179:105, 1974
24. Hashimoto K, Bale G: An electron microscopic study of balloon cell nevus. Cancer 30:530, 1972
25. Holmes EC, Clark WH Jr, Morton DL, et al.: Regional lymph node metastases and the level of invasion of primary melanoma. Cancer 37:199, 1976
26. Kahn LB, Donaldson RC: Multiple primary melanoma. Cancer 25:1162, 1970
27. Lane N, Lattes R, Malm J: Clinicopathological considerations in a series of 117 malignant melanomas of the skin of adults. Cancer 11:1025, 1958
28. Lee JAH, Merill JM: Sunlight and the oetiology of malignant melanoma: a synthesis. Med J Aust 2:846, 1970
29. Lund HZ, Kraus JM: Melanotic Tumors of the Skin. Atlas of Tumor Pathology, section 1, fasc 3, Armed Forces Institute of Pathology, Washington DC
30. McCarthy SW, Palmer AA, et al.: Naevus cells in lymph nodes. Pathology 6:351, 1974

31. McGovern VJ: Malignant Melanoma: Clinical and Histological Diagnosis. John Wiley & Sons, New York, 1976
32. McGovern VJ, Caldwell RA, Duncan CA, et al.: Moles and malignant melanoma—terminology and classification. Med J Aust 1:123, 1967
33. McGovern VJ, Mihm MC, Bailly C, et al.: The classification of malignant melanoma and its histologic reporting. Cancer 32:1446, 1973
34. Mehnert JH, Heard JL: Staging of malignant melanoma by depth of invasion. Am J Surg 10:168, 1965
35. Mihm MC, Clark WH, From L: The clinical diagnosis, classification and histogenetic concepts of the early stages of cutaneous malignant melanomas. N Eng J Med 284:1078, 1971
36. Mihm MC, Fitzpatrick TB, Lane Brown MM, et al.: Early detection of primary cutaneous malignant melanoma. A color atlas. N Engl J Med 289:989, 1973
37. Okun MR, Dunnellan B, and Edelstein L: An ultrastructural study of balloon cell nevus. Cancer 34:615, 1974
38. Olsen G: The Malignant Melanoma of the Skin. The Finsen Institute and Radium Center, Copenhagen, 1966
39. Peterson NC, Bodenham DC, Lloyd OC: Malignant melanoma of the skin. Br J Plast Surg 15:49, 1962
40. Reed WB, Becker SW, Becker SW Jr, et al.: Giant pigmented nevi, melanoma and leptomeningeal melanocytosis. Arch Dermatol 91:100, 1965
41. Reiss RF, Gray GF: Malignant blue nevus. Occurrence with aggressive behavior. NY State J Med 1749, Sept 1975
42. Ridolfi RL, Rosen PP, Thaler H: Nevus cell aggregates associated with lymph nodes: estimated frequency and clinical significance. Cancer 39: 164, 1977
43. Shiu MM, Schottenfeld D, Maclean B, et al.: Adverse effect of pregnancy on melanoma. A reappraisal. Cancer 37:181, 1976
44. Stegmeier OC, Becker SW Jr: Incidence of melanocytic nevi in young adults. J Invest Dermatol 34: 125, 1960
45. Strom SB, Park JK, Rappaport H: Observation of cells resembling Sternberg–Reed cells in conditions other than Hodgkin's disease. Cancer 26:176, 1970
46. Wallace DC, Exton LA, McLeod GRC: Genetic factor in malignant melanoma. Cancer 27:1262, 1971

CHAPTER FIVE

MOLES AND MALIGNANT MELANOMAS OF THE PREADOLESCENT CHILD

IRVING M. ARIEL

This chapter discusses diagnosis and treatment of solitary pigmented lesions in prepubertal children. Such congenital lesions as the Mongolian spot or the facial nevus of Ota, often arising on the backs or faces of Oriental people (see Fig. 5–1), or longitudinal pigmentations seen subungually often in Asiatic or Negro patients, are not discussed in detail.

INTRADERMAL NEVUS

This, the common mole, accounts for approximately 75% of all nevi seen in the adult, but occurs infrequently in the infant. Such nevi are usually raised, papular, sometimes nodular. They are most often found on the skin; rarely involve the eye or mucuous membrane. Most of the large, hairy congenital nevi, or the hugh bathing trunk nevi or garment nevi, are of the intradermal type, but areas of junctional changes are usually found throughout. They are composed of atypical melanoblasts, usually located in the dermis. The average young adult has about 20 pigmented moles, which become evident as the infant grows to childhood (Fig. 5–2).

JUNCTION NEVUS

Allen[4,4a] demonstrated that 98% of 50 nevi in children possessed junctional activity, whereas only 12% of 400 intradermal nevi in adults presented junctional activity. The nevi of the child gradually migrate downward from the epidermal–dermal junction into the dermis and at certain stages are located both within the junction and/or within the intradermal location. Ackerman[1] demonstrated excessive junction activity in 100 of 156 moles in children.

This important subcategory possesses the potentiality for undergoing malignant changes.[2] Most malignant melanomas are believed to develop either de novo or from preexisting junction or compound nevi (Fig. 5–3). The incidence of malignant transformation is actually extremely small—about one in a million moles. Van Scott et al.[113] and Wilson and Anderson[119] believe that junction nevi of the palms and soles show such a slow rate of malignant transformation that their removal routinely as a prophylactic measure is not advisable. The tumors are usually smooth and hairless, flat macular, sometimes slightly raised, varying from light to dark brown, occasionally black. They have a superficial look, and are usually relatively small, varying from 2 mm to $1\frac{1}{2}$ cm. Most become manifest near puberty or in early adult life. In a study performed by Pack and Davis[92] on the relative incidence of junction nevi with intradermal nevi, it was discovered that a large preponderance of nevi on the palms, soles, genitalia, and mucocutaneous junctions were of the junctional variety.

Clinical diagnosis becomes difficult and one would consider in the differential, hematomas angiomas, histiocytomas, granuloma pyogenicum, and others.

Junction nevi may mature in various manners. They may regress, remain stationary, or evolve into intradermal nevi or compound nevi. Rarely, they may undergo malignant transformation and form a full-fledged malignant melanoma.[6] Allen and Spitz[4] believe that approximately 90% of all melanomas arise

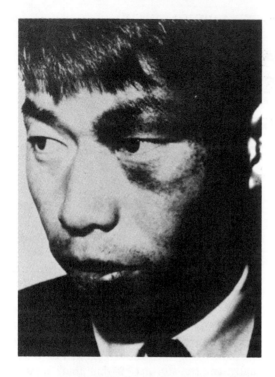

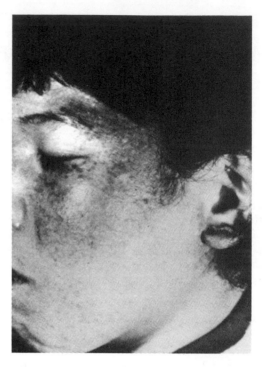

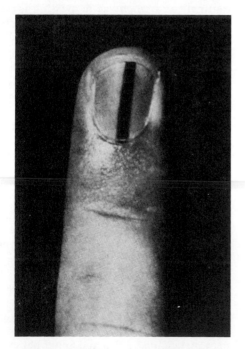

FIGURE 5-1. Congenital prepubertal lesions that do not require treatment. Top: Facial discoloration often seen in Orientals—the nevus of Ota. It most frequently disappears spontaneously. This is a rare example of the discoloration persisting into adult life in a Japanese male. Bottom: Subungual linear pigmented lesion seen shortly after birth, usually in Orientals, which disappear spontaneously.

from junctional nevi, and at times there is a prolonged period between the demonstration of a unction nevus and its malignant counterpart, malignant melanoma. It is extremely unlikely for the ubiquitous mole to become malignant.

COMPOUND NEVUS

Approximately 98% of dermal nevi in adolescence are compound nevi, according to Allen and Spitz,[5] whereas only 12% in adults are

FIGURE 5-2. Scattergram illustrating five nevi in 203 newborn babies. These 203 white children, when they become adults, can be expected to have 15 × 203 = 3,645 nevi. These are not "acquired" nevi, but invisible nevi that become apparent later in life. (Courtesy Dr. Jeff Davis)

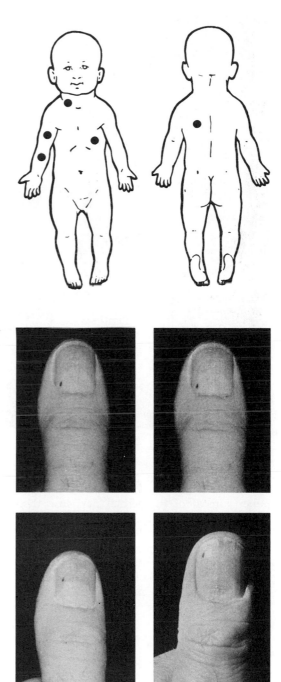

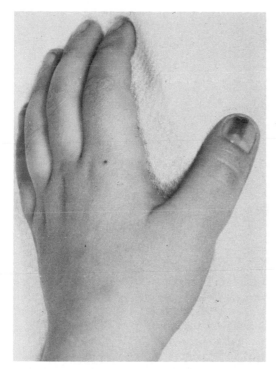

FIGURE 5-3. Above: Subungual junction nevus in a child, treated by local conservative excision. A mistaken diagnosis of malignant melanoma would result in amputation of the thumb. We have never observed a subungual malignant melanoma in a prepubertal child. Right: Subungual hemangioma. A differential diagnosis from melanoma is demonstrated by the distal propagation of the lesion, which retains a constant size.

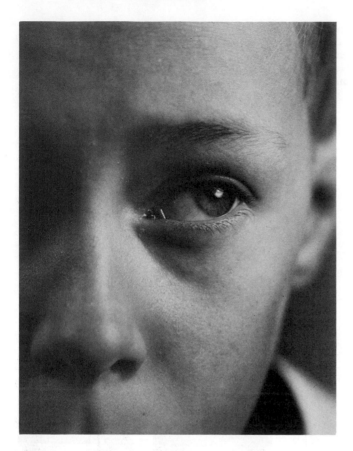

FIGURE 5-4. A pigmented compound melanoma (Spitz nevus) in the inner canthus of a young child. A conservative local excision resulted in a cure.

compound (Fig. 5-4). The reason is that after puberty most of the dermal nevi lose their junctional components. It is impossible to distinguish these clinically; they can only be diagnosed microscopically (Fig. 5-5). Extremely few develop into melanomas. Allen and Spitz found 3.9% of their 362 melanomas analyzed to originate in a compound nevus.

BLUE NEVUS (JADASSOHN-TIÈCHE)

The blue nevus, (Jadassohn-Tièche nevus) is deeply pigmented, varying from a deep blue to almost jet black, and clinically presents a frightening appearance (Fig. 5-6). These tumors are benign, arising from cells in the dermis. When white light is transmitted through the epidermis to the dermal pigment, the dermal pigment absorbs almost all the red light and reflects the blue, which is then scattered back to the observer's eye, creating the appearance of bluish-black color (Tyndel effect). Very rarely have they been reported as undergoing malignant changes. Of Lerman et al.'s 12 cases of malignant melanomas in children, two arose from a Jadassohn nevus[73]. Although they do have a clinically characteristic appearance, the diagnosis should not rest strictly on clinical evaluation, but the nevi should be conservatively excised with a small portion of surrounding skin, and subjected to

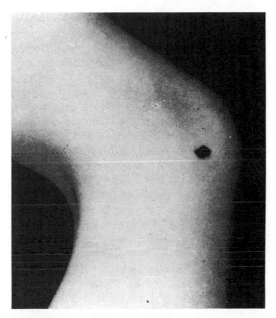

FIGURE 5-5. Juvenile melanoma of the leg in a child who had multiple nevi over the body. The nevus was locally excised.

histologic analysis. In almost every instance they will be found to be benign.

THE MONGOLIAN SPOT

The Mongolian spot is a solitary nonelevated, nonindurated, smooth, brownish-black, pigmented lesion, varying in size from 2 to 10 cm and located in the lumbosacral region of infants, often of Mongolian races, but occasionally in Caucasian races. It is usually present at birth, in contrast to Jadassohn's blue nevus, gradually fades away after the first few months of life, and disappears usually by one year of age. It is seldom, if ever, seen after puberty. It is said to occur in 100% of Japanese babies, 95% in Negroes, 90% in Chinese, Malayancsc, Koreans, Eskimos, and American Indians. They are observed in only 1% to 5% of Caucasian babies. The spots rarely occur in other locations. Treatment is never indicated.

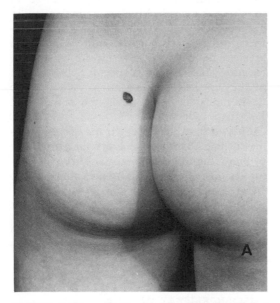

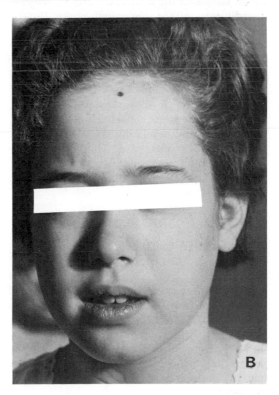

FIGURE 5-6A and B. Blue (Jadassohn-Tièche) nevus involving the buttock and forehead in young prepubertal children.

THE NEVUS OF OTA

The nevus of Ota is rare, usually benign, although there have been three reports where they developed into malignant melanomas. This nevus commonly occurs in Japanese, Koreans, and Chinese, but it is occasionally seen in Caucasians and Negroes. It was first described by Ota[87a] in 1939, who attached the appellation *fusco caeruleus maxillofacialis* because of its unusual and striking pigmentation, which involves the periorbital skin. It usually occurs in combination with pigmentation of the eyeball; however, either the skin or the ocular manifestations may occur independently. The pigmentation appears at birth, or shortly thereafter, and is characterized by grey to brown, through blue–black color area, located, as a rule, unilaterally on the face, involving the eyelids, the circumorbital melar, preauricular region, cheeks, forehead, hairline area of the scalp, and occasionally the tip or the ala of the nose. It usually follows the distribution of the trigeminal nerve. Rarely, this pigmentation occurs bilaterally. With orbital involvement, the sclera is usually affected or the conjunctiva, iris, choroid, and the optic disc may be involved. The nevus of Ota is considered as an aberrant or misplaced Mongolian spot. It always disappears.

In the Japanese, the incidence is less than 1 to 1,000 of the population, and some of the cases are quite aggressive. There is no treatment for this lesion, and they tend, at times, to disappear, but not to the extent that the Mongolian spot does.

THE CONGENITAL NEVUS

The average nevus is an acquired one, but some children are born with a congenital nevus. Pack and Davis[92] observed them to be present in 2.5% of newborn babies; they may be either "small" or extremely large (Fig. 5–7). The so-called "small" ones are usually larger than the average acquired nevus, and are usually more than 1.5 cm in their greatest diameter.

The larger ones may involve huge areas of the body and have earned the appellation of "bathing trunk nevus" because they involve that portion of the skin usually covered by a bathing suit, or a "garment nevus," indicating the extremely extensive size, which portion would ordinarily be covered by a garment and almost give the appearance of a garment-like covering of the skin (Figs. 5–8 and 5–9).

Ainsworth, Fulberg, Reed, and Clark, in the volume *Human Malignant Melanoma*, edited by Clark, et al., Grune and Stratton, 1979, pp 167–208, call attention to the histologic variation which these larger nevi can show as a function of time. They cite specimens from a child at 5 weeks, 7 months, and 13 months. Several experienced pathologists seriously considered the diagnosis of malignant melanoma in the 5-week specimen. In the 7-month specimen the histology was disturbing; no consultant pathologist made a diagnosis of melanoma; and at age 13 months, the histology was that of "a classical congenital melanocytic nevus with reasonably mature intraepidermal components." They accordingly recommended exceeding caution in making a diagnosis of malignant melanoma in a congenital melanocytic nevus when examined during the early period of life. These nevi present developmentally bizarre histologic features, some of which suggest Schwann cell origin, or they may resemble cellular blue nevi, malignant blue nevi, and spindle-cell malignant melanoma.[29]

Ainsworth et al. state: "It may be impossible at times to properly classify such lesions or to know the biologic potential of the disturbing lesions. We have the impression that the slowly evolving, deep nodular growths are probably a source of overdiagnosis of malignant melanoma."

INCIDENCE OF MALIGNANT MELANOMA DEVELOPING FROM CONGENITAL NEVI

The incidence of malignant melanoma developing in the smaller congenital nevi is an

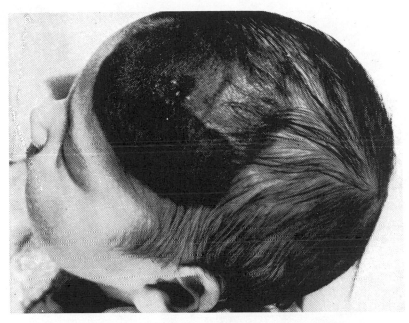

FIGURE 5-7. Massive melanotic nevus of the scalp in a young infant. This tumor may undergo malignant changes. Excision and skin grafting will be done at approximagely six years of age.

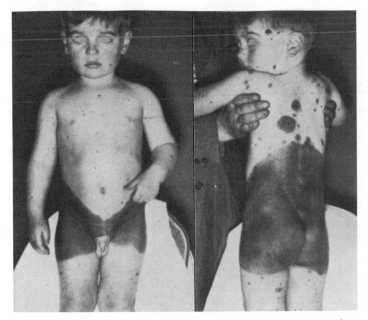

FIGURE 5-8. Bathing trunk nevus present since birth. Note the numerous other nevi scattered about the face, trunk, and extremities.

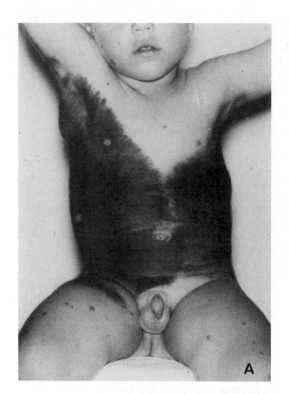

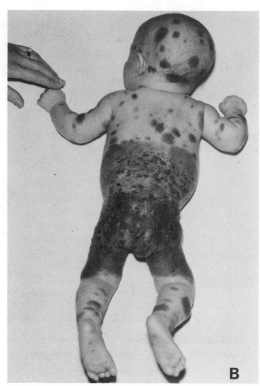

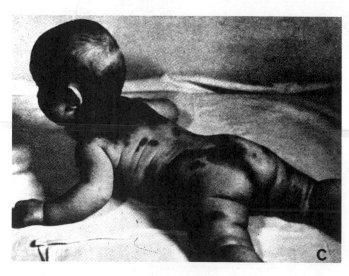

FIGURE 5-9A, B, and C. Three examples of bathing trunk (garment) nevi in infants. The incidence of melanomas developing in such lesions is high.

enigmatic variable with no absolute proof that the incidence is higher than that in the ordinary acquired junctional or compound nevus.

If located in an area of constant trauma, if they increase in size, or if they are very deeply pigmented, we recommend conservative excision.

The true incidence of malignant melanomas developing on the giant congenital nevi varies from 15% to 42%. Although the precise incidence is unknown, it is pertinent that approximately 40% of all malignant melanomas seen in the preadolescent child has arisen from a giant congenital nevus (Fig. 5-10), and the prognosis is uniformly very poor.

The treatment of a giant nevi is a most complex problem requiring the services of a dermatologist, surgical oncologist, and plastic surgeon. We have treated some by wide excision with split-thickness skin graft with semi-satisfactory results. At times segmental resection through the center portion of the tumor with primary closure at yearly intervals have been found semi-satisfactory. Although there is a theoretical risk in cutting into a tumor, we have never encountered such a case that developed into a malignant melanoma.

JUVENILE MELANOMAS (THE SPITZ NEVUS)

At one time it was believed that malignant melanomas never occurred before puberty. Previously, the pathologist often requested the age of the patient before making his diagnosis. If the child's age was before puberty, the diagnosis would usually be benign nevus; if after puberty, as malignant melanoma. It was

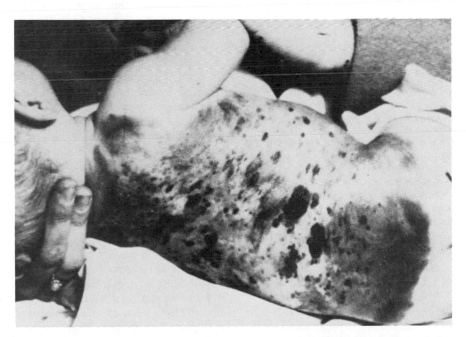

FIGURE 5-10.   At five months of age, 19 juvenile melanomas were excised. Cerebral melanomatous metastases were found at craniotomy when the patient was 16 years of age. The patient died two months later. Between infancy and the age of 16 there was no demonstrable clinical evidence of new or recurrent melanomas of the skin.

believed that puberty acted as a boundary, that the endocrine environment before puberty prevented malignant transformation of certain nevi into true melanomas, whereas as soon as puberty occurred the hormonal environment so altered that the growth potential of certain nevi would permit some of them to undergo malignant transformation into true metastasizing malignant melanomas. The occasional occurrence of showers of nevi, and sometimes enlargement of preexistent nevi at the time of adolescence, seemed to favor this concept. The hormonal alterations associated with pregnancy, such as increased pigmentation of the areola and sometimes generalized increase in pigmentation as well as increase in size and depth of pigmentation of nevi, also seemed to favor the concept that an altered environmental state influenced the growth and depth of pigmentation of certain pigmented sites and nevi.

In 1948, Pack made the following statement:

> There is one important type of pigmented nevus which bears such a close resemblance to malignant melanoma that it is not possible clinically to distinguish between the two. This nevus may be found in children from age one to the time of puberty. Usually they are rather darkly pigmented, blueish, blue-black, or dark brown in color, smooth and well demarcated. When this tumor is excised in infancy or childhood and submitted to pathologists for diagnosis, they are frequently unable to state whether the neoplasm is benign or malignant inasmuch as the histologic criteria, exclusive of the permeation of vessels, are practically identical with the malignant variety of melanoma as encountered in adults.[89]

He coined the term ''prepubertal melanoma'' for this lesion, and argued that surgical removal of all dark, deeply pigmented nevi in childhood be conservatively performed.

Attention had been previously directed to this oncologic enigma in the prepubertal child. Darier and Civatte, in 1910, described a pigmented lesion of the nose of an eight-year-old child, concluded histologically to be malignant, but clinically benign.[32] Darier continued his studies on the question of malig-

nancy in pigmented lesions of children with mixed conclusions.[31]

Woringer (1939) described a pinkish, slightly raised, lesion of the hand of an eight-year-old girl, whose histology revealed unusual neval cells.[121] He considered it benign even though it contained some mitosis, and believed the cells were atypical because of the growth potential of the tumor, giving the histologic characteristics of malignant melanoma. He later accepted Spitz's term, juvenile melanoma.

Webster, Stevenson, and Stout (1944) described pink elevated lesions in children that had the microscopic appearance of malignancy, but which very rarely metastasized.[114]

In 1948, Spitz[108] presented her classic paper describing the benign juvenile melanoma as a distinct entity with characteristic histologic features. The clinical and pathologic, as well as the prognostic, features of this entity were further elaborated by the husband-and-wife team Spitz and Allen, to whom the profession is indebted for their contribution of great clarity to this rather confusing oncologic situation. Instead of prepubertal melanoma, as designated by Pack, they call the lesion ''juvenile melanoma.'' Kopf[69] favors the term ''benign juvenile melanoma'' to emphasize the benign nature of the tumor, and to segregate the entity from the malignant metastasizing neoplasm. A few other synonyms are: spindle cell and epithelioid cell nevus; spindle cell, epithelioid cell, and round cell juvenile cell melanoma; pseudomelanoma; nevus with large cells.[28]

A committee of Australian pathologists in 1967 recommended the term ''Spitz nevus.'' Weedon and Little's paper, ''Spindle and epithelioid cell nevi in children and adults: A review of 211 cases of Spitz nevus,[115] credits Sophie Spitz with originally describing the entity and separating it from other pigmented lesions. Their term avoids the connotation of malignancy of the term ''melanoma.''

Kopf states: ''It is a wise rule not to diagnose malignant melanoma in a child unless *all* criteria of malignancy have been met and the diagnosis of juvenile melanoma excluded.'' He further states: ''True melanomas do occur in the pediatric age group, but with the utmost rarity. The distinction between juvenile 'melanoma' ('Spitz lesion') and true malignant melanoma is one of the most difficult problems in the entire field of pathology of melanocytic lesions.''

ETIOLOGY

There is no known etiologic factor.[33] Heredity does not seem to play a role, in most instances, although Kopf and Andrade (1966) reported several instances of familial relationships.[69]

The so-called giant nevus cell nevi appearing on the trunk, or garment nevi contain areas of juvenile melanoma as well as certain regions that may later become malignant melanomas.

INCIDENCE

The true incidence of juvenile melanoma is unknown as most reports are from surgically excised specimens for which indications for their removal existed. Kopf[69] accumulated reports from various authors of 4,556 nevi excised in children, 71 (1.6%) were the benign juvenile melanomas. In 100 patients reviewed by Spitz, she encountered eight instances of juvenile melanoma. The high incidence reflected her great interest in this entity.

Weedon and Little reported 211 cases from the Queensland project in Australia. From that locality, they estimate the incidence to be 1.4 cases per 100,000 population, compared to an incidence in the same area of melanoma of 25.4 per 100,000.

The Spitz nevus occurs in adults as well and the prepubertal child. Of Allen's 308 patients, 19% were adolescent or adults, the remainder were prepubertal. A report by Coskey and Mehregan[27] showed that 26% of Spindle cell nevi were from patients 18 years and older. In Weedon and Little's series, 30% were from patients over the age of 20 years, which may be a false representation regarding age incidence, as only the complicated cases were sent to the pathologists skilled in pathology of melanotic lesions.

CLINICAL FEATURES

A typical benign juvenile melanoma is a papillar, pinkish lesion usually occurring on the cheek of a child. Although the color may vary from a tan to a deep brown color, so many are of a pinkish hue that a melanomatous lesion is often not considered a possibility. The correct diagnosis is seldom made on a clinical basis, at least in the past. As more cases are reported and greater familiarity is obtained with this form of tumor, it will undoubtedly be suspected or properly diagnosed clinically in the future.[38,39]

Of 27 lesions reported by Kernen and Ackerman, none were clinically diagnosed.[68] In the series by Kopf and Andrade, approximately one-third of their 43 lesions were clinically considered as being juvenile melanoma.

Although juvenile melanoma may occur anywhere in the body, the most frequent site is the face, seconded by the trunk, and to a lesser extent the lower extremities.

Kopf calls attention to some element of telangiectasia superficially located over the lesion, a finding frequently overlooked.

The juvenile melanoma usually vary in shape, increase in size (the average size is 7 to 10 millimeters), and then remain stationary. If traumatized they may break down and bleed. The patient may experience pruritis and may complain of pain. Lesions diagnosed in adulthood may arise de novo or may have existed since childhood.

TREATMENT OF BENIGN JUVENILE MELANOMAS

Inasmuch as these lesions are benign, the treatment should consist of a conservative elliptical excision with a small margin of normal skin (Fig. 5–11).

A number of reports exist where recurrences developed after incomplete excision, or where the lesion was shaved off leaving the base behind. In these instances the recurrences were also benign; none developed malignancy. Jakubowicz[65] reported eight recurrences in fifty cases, of which two acted locally ag-

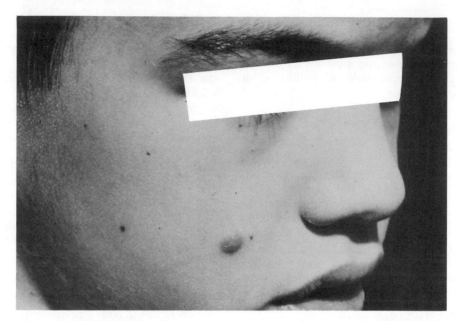

FIGURE 5-11. A juvenile melanoma (Spitz nevus) of the cheek of a young boy; treated by conservative surgical excision. Its pink color served to obscure the true diagnosis. (Courtesy, Dr. Alfred W. Kopf)

gressively. In a series reported by Kopf, there were four recurrences of benign juvenile melanomas. Allen, in 1963, emphasized the fact that these recurrences did not represent an ominous clinical entity, as he had never seen any metastases develop from a recurrence of a true juvenile malanoma.[3]

PROGNOSIS

The eventual outcome of an untreated benign juvenile melanoma varies. There are several reports of the tumor remaining stationary for a period after which the lesion became flattened, and in one instance remained as a reddened macular area.[121]

The four courses that juvenile melanoma may follow are:

1. It may remain unchanged until adulthood and remain in adulthood. The incidence of juvenile melanomas in adults is increasing as more pathologists are aware of this entity. From 15% to 40% of all juvenile melanomas have been reported in adults, the oldest being 65 years of age.

2. It may undergo involution, as do the ordinary nevus cell nevi with fibrosis and spontaneous disappearance.[69]

3. It may change into an ordinary intradermal nevus. The findings of cells characteristic of juvenile melanoma coexisting with ordinary neval cells have led to this hypothesis.

4. The possibility exists that it may undergo malignant transformation, which is extremely rare, if, in fact, it does exist.

THE QUESTION OF MALIGNANT TRANSFORMATION OF BENIGN JUVENILE MELANOMAS INTO METASTASIZING MALIGNANT MELANOMAS

The best assumption at this time is that these lesions are benign and have only the same potential of forming malignant melanomas as do the usual compound nevi, which is extremely rare. There have been some authors, as Attie and Khafif,[7] who believe that benign juvenile melanomas do have an increased potential of becoming malignant, especially after adulthood, due probably to Allen and Spitz's findings[5] that cells characteristic of juvenile melanoma were found in 5.9% of their 362 cases of malignant melanoma. Kernen and Ackerman failed to find any relationship between juvenile melanoma and malignant melanoma. In fact, they believe that those few lesions, reported since 1948, that have been called juvenile melanomas and metastasized were diagnosed in error.

Another possibility has been suggested that juvenile melanomas and malignant melanomas coexist in the same lesion and the malignant melanomas' produced the metastases (Delacreatz,[34] Duverne and Prunieras,[40,41] Montgomery[84]). Further histologic evaluation is necessary (Fig. 5–12).

Kopf, after correspondence with Allen and complete review of the subject, published the following conclusions:

. . . . we conclude that the consensus of most authors is that juvenile melanoma act as benign lesions in nearly all instances. The rare exceptions reported need critical review to determine if they indeed are indisputable examples of malignant transformation.

INDICATIONS FOR EXCISING BENIGN LESIONS IN THE PREPUBERTAL CHILD

Despite the fact that puberty is not an absolute boundary segregating the preadolescent child (thought previously to be completely immune to developing malignant melanoma) from the postpuberty child, we have observed a number of cases of malignant melanomas that occurred in adolescents just after puberty with rapid growth, and, at times, dissemination of the tumors during this early age. The following criteria are presented to assist in determining which nevi should be removed in the young child. Inasmuch as malignant melanomas are so extremely rare in childhood, it is

wise to wait until a child is six to eight years of age, at which time he can cooperate in the excision and not fight the procedure, which should be done under local block anesthesia and not general anesthesia. The younger child will resist local anesthesia, and general anesthesia is not indicated unless under very rare circumstances, where it is mandatory that the excision be performed because of fear that the child has one of the rare malignant melanomas.

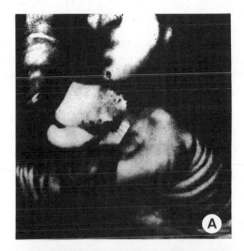

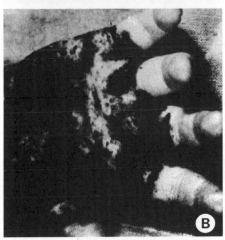

FIGURE 5–12A. Malignant melanoma of the second toe, which metastasized to the lymph nodes of the groin, occuring in a prepubertal boy. B. Malignant melanoma of the palm with metastases to the axillary lymph nodes in an 11-month-old girl.

Indications for Removal of Nevi

1. Juvenile melanomas that usually have a pinkish hue should be locally excised, especially if there is deepening in pigmentation or increase in size.

2. Any nevus subjected to repeated trauma, such as irritation from shaving, a brassiere or garter belt, belt, etc.

3. Any nevus showing any evidence of change, including increase in size, contour, increased pigmentation, pruritis, inflammation about the nevus, and very rarely, bleeding. Such changes would be an indication for excision at any age.

4. Nevi of the genitalia, mucous membrane, palms of the hands, soles of the feet, and subungual nevi. Incidence of junction or compound nevi is highest in these regions.

5. All very deeply pigmented lesions that vary in color from a deep blue to black. Occasionally such a lesion may be a Jadassohn-type nevus, but the deeply pigmented lesions are best removed prophylactically. This is especially true in a child with light complexion, with blond or red hair.

6. If the parent had a melanoma in the location where the child presents a nevus, such nevi should be removed before puberty. As there is a significant incidence of familial relationship, a more critical evaluation should be given children whose siblings or parents have suffered from a malignant melanoma.

7. Hair growing from a nevus has often been considered as prima-facia evidence that no melanoma exists. Although this is usually true, there are so many exceptions that the presence of hair in a nevus should not deter the physician from removing the nevus under the assumption that such nevi are never, or never become malignant. If a patient has a hairy nevus and the hairs fall out spontaneously, advise excision of such a nevus (Fig. 5–13).

8. Extensive nevi covering large skin areas (the bathing suit or garment-type nevus). Treatment of these huge nevi is difficult and should always be surgical. Treatment can vary from excising suspicious areas that are darker in color, more nodular, or bleeding, to efforts at fractional resection with skin graft at different surgical sessions. The donor site may be lacking; a satisfactory procedure in certain instances has been to resect a segment of the nevus, which would permit primary closure, and after a period of six to nine months repeat the procedure. The deformity is so horrendous and the potentiality for melanoma so great, that this would be one exception where surgical treatment can be started early in life. Malignant transformation arises in 10% to 30% of such patients.

9. Prepubertal children with neurocutaneous nevi and central nervous system melanomas. Malignant changes in the central nervous system and skin can occur.

10. Pigmented lesions in patients with xeroderma pigmentosa (Fig. 5–14). The incidence of melanoma is higher in this group of patients.

11. Repeat follow-up in any child who has had nevi removed for various considerations, with careful surveying under bright light for any suspicious-looking nevi.[35] Careful instruction should be given to parents to look for signs and symptoms that might warrant excision of additional nevi at a later date. Congenital nevi should be critically observed.

The definitive treatment of nevi consists of:

1. Surgical excision, using local anesthesia, leaving a full margin of normal skin. (A radical excision is never indicated at the first surgical approach.)

2. Nevi are radioresistant and any form of radiation therapy is never employed.

3. Small lesions should not be partially biopsied, but a conservative excision of the entire lesion should be accomplished, both in depth and in border.

4. Electrodessication or cryotherapy is not indicated and may be hazardous because (a) biopsies cannot be obtained; (b) electrodessication may be superficial, leaving neval cells at the base, and such cells after the irritation of electrodessication may grow more rapidly than normally; (c) a good cosmetic result is the rule after local excision.

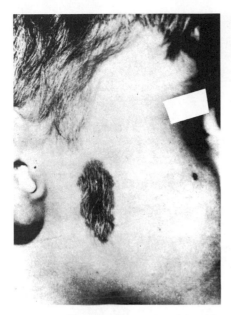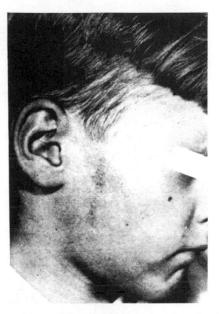

FIGURE 5–13. **Left. Hairy nevus involving the face of a young lad; it was treated by local surgical** excision. **Right. Appearance one year after local excision and primary closure.**

5. All patients should be followed for the possibility of residual pigmentation at the site of the neval removal, and if the pathologist calls the excised nevus a malignant melanoma, it should be reexamined by a pathologist skilled in the histopathology of pigmented lesions to confirm the diagnosis before embarking upon the radical treatment necessary to cure a malignant melanoma.

MALIGNANT MELANOMA IN CHILDREN

Malignant melanoma in the prepubertal child is extremely rare.[30] Less than 100 cases have been reported to date. Allen, in 1977, had personally seen 52 instances of malignant melanoma in the preadolescent, some of which had been reported by others (personal communication). Skov-Jensen et al., in 1966, reviewed the literature and reported 43 acceptable cases, including two of his own previously unreported.[107] Since then there have

been five case reports by Oldhoff and Koudstaal.[87] Lerman et al., in 1970, reported 12 cases from Memorial Hospital in New York. The only cases of malignant melanoma that are unequivocably acceptable by these authors are those that have "documented metastatic disease." The reason for this is that (1) there is great rarity of malignant melanoma in childhood, and (2) "the admitted difficulty in separating some cases from juvenile melanoma."

It is essential that the pathologist be well-versed in this area, in view of the extreme difficulty in determining malignant melanoma pathologically as well as the seriousness of the diagnosis (radicalness of treatment and prognosis).

Before the classic studies in 1948 by Spitz, it was believed that the histologic appearance of childhood melanoma was indistinguishable histologically from melanoma in the adult. The clinical behavior of these two lesions was believed to be different in that melanoma in the child never metastasized, in contrast to its

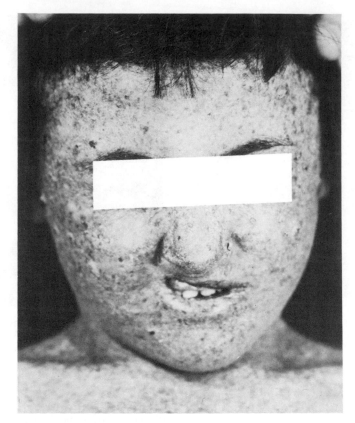

FIGURE 5–14.   Malignant melanoma of the inner canthus, left eye, in a patient with xeroderma pigmentosa.

behavior in the adult. Allen and Spitz originally suggested that two-thirds of juvenile melanomas could be correctly diagnosed histologically. McWheaten and Woolner believe that all can be correctly diagnosed. The difficulty is emphasized by Truax et al.[112] who studied the slides of 247 preadolescent patients claimed to have had malignant melanomas who were long-term survivors. They list 62 cases that were incorrectly diagnosed: 34 (55%) had cellular compound or blue nevi; 7 (11%) had the epithelioid or spindle-cell nevi.

A patient in Lerman's review demonstrates the complexity of diagnosis. A biopsy of a bathing trunk nevus in a one-year-old child revealed a compound nevus with focal atypia "at a borderline level of interpretation," and at eight years of age an excised femoral node revealed it to be partially replaced by focally pigmented nevus cells of a generally benign appearance distributed in subcapsular and interstitial sinuses and in the peripheral and hilar capsule of the lymph node. The patient was without evidence of disease one year later. Benign nevus cells in a lymph node have been reported, including one case of a patient with malignant melanoma[67] and one patient with a cellular blue nevus.[102]

ETIOLOGY

One exciting case was reported by Poore et al. in 1954,[96a] and rereported by Lerman et al.,[95] of a disseminating malignant melanoma occurring in the left buccal mucous membrane. This occurred in a five-year-old Negro child who also suffered from an adrenal-cortical tumor that caused precocious development. It was believed that this hormonal environment aged the child prematurely, creating a situation more conducive to the development of the malignant melanoma than in the average child of this age. The boy died two years and ten months after onset of melanoma.

Approximately 12 instances of spread of a melanoma from a mother with widespread melanoma to the unborn fetus have been reported (see Chapter 2). The placenta has contained melanoma either exclusively or concomitantly with metastases to the fetus in seven instances. One case is on record of an infant being born bearing malignant melanoma metastatic to the skin, liver, and brain and arising from a bathing trunk nevus. Could the hormonal environment of the mother explain the development of the malignant melanoma in the fetus, as suggested by Sweet and Connerty?[110]

Malignant melanoma in the child can arise in giant hypertrophic nevi, the so-called nevus pigmentosus giganticus. Ten of the 41 cases recorded in the literature, and two of the cases reported by Lerman et al., had such an origin. Both of Lerman's patients died within 15 months of widespread metastases. All the patients reported in the literature of malignant melanoma arising from the congenital giant nevus died of widespread metastases, with the exception of one case reported by Oldhoff and Koudstaal. Lerman states that the extremely poor prognosis is in part due to the difficulty and subsequent delay in recognizing the signs of malignant changes in these large pigmented lesions. Reed et al.[99] have quoted other melanomas existing with giant nevi, although these were never verified, and were only considered clinically suspicious of being malignant melanoma. The incidence of melanomas arising from giant nevi has been estimated from 2% to 13% by Reed et al.

Two of the cases reported from Memorial Hospital arose from Jadassohn's nevi.

The sex distribution is more or less similar (five boys and seven girls) in the Memorial Hospital series. The ages ranged from 10 months to 14 years, although none of the patients had any signs of postpubertal development, except for one case referred to above who had an adrenal-cortical carcinoma with precocious virulism. Only one Negro was encountered in the series reported by Lerman et al., all the others were Caucasian.

SITE OF ORIGIN

Malignant melanomas in the child may arise anywhere in the body, those reported by Lerman arose from the scalp, forehead, mouth, neck, back, arm, hand, sole of the foot (two cases). Two cases arose from blue nevi (Jadassohn's nevus), one was in the groin, and one was in the urethral-bulbar soft tissues of the orbit. There was a minimum of six months delay before the diagnosis.[73] The pathology is discussed in Chapter 4, but as with melanomas of the adult, the deeper or thicker the melanoma the poorer the prognosis.

PACK MEDICAL GROUP EXPERIENCE

In 1951, Pack and Scharnagel[93] reported on 1,050 melanomas and noted that there were never any metastases or fatalities in a child from malignant melanoma.

Since then, five metastasizing melanomas in children were observed among 3,305 patients with melanomas. All were surgically treated by wide resection and simultaneous regional lymph node resection, four died within three years after treatment. In each the diagnosis was not originally suspected and from one to two years elapsed from the onset of the melanoma until adequate therapy was instituted. Two developed in a giant nevus; one in a patient with xeroderma pigmentosa; one apparently de novo; and one who survived was a ten-year-old boy with melanoma of the arm, which arose from a preexisting mole. His case report is appended.

A ten-year-old boy had a brown mole on his left shoulder for one year, which changed to a dark blue/brown coloration and was treated by electrodessication. Two months later it recurred as a blue/black lesion. It was biopsied and reported as malignant melanoma at the University of Pennsylvania Hospital, which diagnosis was confirmed at the Pack Medical Group. Ten months later, the patient developed a metastasis to his left axilla. This was treated by a radical axillary dissection and 15 years later the patient is well, without any evidence of metastasis. This is an example of a malignant melanoma which produced metastasis in a pre-adolescent boy, or it could be an example of a metastasizing juvenile melanoma. The pathology report from the Memorial Hospital was metastatic melanoma, spindle type, with numerous lymph nodes invaded by the melanoma.

MELANOTIC PROGONOMA

Medenis, Slaughter, and Barber[83] reported one instance in a five-month-old girl which involved the right upper alveolar ridge when the child was three months old. No recurrence was found 18 months later. They state that 25 previous cases of melanotic progonoma were found during the first year of life. The site of predilection was the maxilla in 18 cases, and the mandible in five cases. In one case, tumor was found in the shoulder, and in another in the epididymis. This tumor is usually benign, although local recurrences occur after incomplete surgical resection. It must be separated from the true malignant melanoma.

TREATMENT AND PROGNOSIS OF MALIGNANT MELANOMA IN CHILDREN

The best treatment is wide surgical resection preferably with closure by skin graft. The treatment should be the same as that for an adult, and the surgeon must be bold in his treatment to effect a cure, because these

cancers in children are as malignant as they are in adults.[137] They are usually infiltrating. However, elective node dissection when no nodes are palpable is debatable.

Inasmuch as the mortality rate of patients with stage II melanomas of the child is very slightly better than the 19% cure rate reported from Memorial Hospital, Lerman and colleagues state: ". . . . we feel that these patients should have the benefit of an elective dissection to try to improve the survival rate."

Skov-Jensen et al. noted[107] a 24% three-year survival of patients with localized or with metastases to the lymph nodes from malignant melanoma in childhood. Other instances of fatal melanoma in children are recorded.[36]

Sylven[111] reported in 1949 eleven cases of prepubertal melanoma with 100% cures, which would suggest that he was reporting some benign juvenile melanoma.

The five-year survival rate in children culled from the literature in 1966 by Skov-Jensen et al. was 17%. The five-year survival of the Memorial Hospital group was 33%. Four of those patients were alive at the time of their report—one at five years; one at six years; and two at 20 years. Eight of their patients died, all within 18 months; two arose in patients with xeroderma pigmentosa; and two arose from congenital giant nevi.

SUMMARY AND CONCLUSIONS

1. The benign juvenile melanoma, which has specific histologic characteristics, is a distinct entity that exists not only in the preadolescent child but also in adults. It has a characteristic clinical appearance and definite histologic criteria by which to establish its diagnosis. The treatment is a conservative local excision, with an excellent prognosis. Whether the benign juvenile melanoma ever undergoes malignant transformation is not known.

2. Various benign nevi afflict the preadolescent child, each of which has a distinct clinical and histologic nature, a few of which may

undergo malignant transformation. The junction nevus and the compound nevus are believed to be the benign tumors from which malignant melanomas may arise. The fact that the nevus is ubiquitous and malignant melanoma very rare indicates that approximately one in a million nevi will undergo malignant transformation.

3. Criteria are suggested so as to determine which benign nevi should be surgically excised primarily those in young patients with a particular genetic background such as a family history of malignancy, or light complexion with blue eyes; and nevi that are subject to irritation from external factors.

4. Any nevus that undergoes change in the size, shape, color, or consistency should immediately be surgically excised and histologically evaluated.

5. Approximately 100 metastasizing malignant melanomas have been reported in the preadolescent child. The behavior is essentially similar to that of a malignant melanoma in the adult. The overall five-year survival for stage II malignant melanomas of the preadolescent child is approximately 25%.

6. Most authors do not accept stage I melanoma in children as absolutely being the metastasizing type because of confusion in differentiating the juvenile melanoma of Spitz from the true metastasing malignant melanoma.

REFERENCES

1. Ackerman LV: Malignant melanoma of the skin. Am J Clin Pathol 18:602, 1948
2. Allen AC: A reorientation on the histogenesis and clinical significance of cutaneous nevi and melanomas. Cancer 2:28 (Jan) 1949
3. Allen AC: Juvenile melanomas. Ann NY Acad Sci 100:29, 1963
4. Allen AC: Juvenile melanomas of children and adults and melanocarcinomas of children. Arch Dermatol 82:325, 1960
4a. Allen AC, Spitz S: Histogenesis and clinicopathologial correlation of nevi and malignant melanomas. Arch Dermatol 69:150, 1954
5. Allen AC, Spitz S: Malignant melanoma. A clinicopathological analysis of the criteria for diagnosis and prognosis. Cancer 6:1 (Jan), 1953
6. Andrews GC: Diseases of the Skin, ed 2, Philadelphia, WB Saunders, 1938, p. 666
7. Attie JN, Khafif, RA: Melanotic Tumors. Springfield, Ill, Charles B Thompson, 1964
8. Bandiera DC: Nevo giante pigmentado com transformaco maligna. Rev Brasil Cirug 54:120, 1967
9. Battin J, Vital C, Alberty J, et al: La mélanose neurocutanée. Arch Fr Pediatr 25:277, 1968
10. Becker WS: Origin and nature of pigmented nevi (Schwannomas). Arch Dermatol Syphilol 30:779 (Dec), 1934
11. Beerman H, Lane RAG, Shaffer B: Pigmented nevi and malignant melanoma of the skin. Am J Med Sci 229:444, 1955
12. Bezecny R: Beitragzur Frage de blaven Naevus. Arch f Dermat u Syph 164:314, 1931
13. Booher, RJ, Pack GT: Malignant melanoma of the hands and feet. Surgery 108:121, 1957
14. Booher RJ: Recognition and treatment of melanoma. Surg Clin North Am 49:389, 1969
15. Boyd W: A Textbook of Pathology, ed 4, Philadelphia, Lea and Febiger, 1943, p. 313
16. Brodsky L, Baren M, Kahn S, et al: Metastatic malignant melanoma from mother to fetus. Cancer 18:1040, 1965
17. Cahalane SF, Meenan FOC: Benign juvenile melanoma: A clinical and pathological survey. Irish J Med Sci 2:489, 1969
18. Cancer Registry of Norway: Survival of Cancer Patients. Oslo, The Norwegian Cancer Society, 1975
19. Cavell B: Transplacental metastasis of malignant melanoma. Acta Pediatr (Suppl) 146:37, 1963
20. Cawley EP, Rathbun D, Wheeler CE: Infra-red spectroscopic studies of pigmented tumors. Arch Dermatol Syphilol 70:748 (Apr), 1954
21. Cheah JS, Ting SK: Fetal malignant melanoma in a prepubertal Chinese boy. Singapore Med J 10:174, 1969
22. Clark WH Jr, Trom L, Bernadino EA, Mihm MC: The histogenesis and biologic behavior of primary human malignant melanomas of the skin. Cancer Res 29:705, 1969
23. Coe HE: Malignant pigmented mole in an infant. Northwest Med 24:181, 1925
24. Coffey RJ, Berkely WT: Prepubertal malignant melanoma: Report of a case. JAMA 147:846, 1951
25. Conu A, Nicholescu H, Popescu GL: Malig-

nant melanoma developing in intrauterine life. Romanian Med Review 2:41, 1971

26. Conway H: Bathing trunk nevus. Surgery 6:585, 1939

27. Cosky RJ, Mehregan A: Spindle cell nevi in adults and children. Arch Dermatol 108: 535–536, 1973

28. Dabska M: Melanoma juvenile. Nowotwory 6:103, 1956

29. Dailly R, Forthhomme J, Samson M, et al.: Mélanose neuro-cutanée à l'évolution tumorale. Presse Med 73:2867, 1965

30. Dargeon, HW, Eversole JW, Del Duca V: Malignant melanoma in an infant. Cancer 3:299, 1950

31. Darrier J: Des naevocarcinomes. Bull Assoc Fr Étude Cancer 6:145, 1913

32. Darrier J, Civatte A: Naevus ou naevo-carcinome chez un nourisson. Bull Soc Fr Dermatol Syphiligr 21:61, 1910

33. Degos R: Naevus cellulaire prépubertaire. In Noirclerc AP: Dermatologie, Flammarion, Paris, 1958, pp 760a and 760b

34. Delacreatz J: Mélanome juvénile (mélanome de Spitz) à l'évolution maligne. Dermatologica 139:79, 1969

35. Delacreatz J, Jaeger H: Sur deux cas de mélanomes juvéniles (de Spitz). Oncologica 10:80, 1957

36. Derrick JR, Thompson JA: Fatal malignant melanoma in a Negro child. Pediatrics 21:222, 1958

37. Dobson L: Prepubertal malignant melanomas. Am J Surg 80:1128, 1955

38. Dupperat B: Le mélanome juvénile. Bull Soc Fr Dermatol Syphiligr 62:500, 1955

39. Dupperat B, Dufourmentel C: Étude de mélanome juvénile d'àprès 40 cas personnels. Minerva Dermatol 34:190, 1959

40. Duverne J, Prunieras M: Trois cas de mélanome juvénile. Bull Soc Fr Dermatol Syphiligr 63:259, 1956a

41. Duverne J, Prunieras M: Trois cas de mélanome juvénile. Lyon Med 88:442, 1956b

42. Echevarria R, Ackerman LV: Spindle and epithelioid cell nevi in the adult—clinico-pathologic report of 26 cases. Cancer 20:175, 1967

43. Eeg Larsen T, Grude T, Iversen OH, Magnus K: Histological classification of malignant melanoma in relationship to prognosis and cytogenesis. In Proc VI Int Symp Biol Character Human Tumors. Copenhagen, 1975, Excerpta Medica, Int Congr Ser No 375: 260–273

44. End Result in Cancer. Report No. 5 DHEW Pub 77-992 (NIH) 1976, pp 223–227

45. Ellsworth RM: Juvenile melanoma of the urea. Trans Am Acad Opthalmol 64:148, 1960

46. Epstein E, Poragg K, Linden G: Biopsy and prognosis of malignant melanoma. JAMA 208:1369, 1969

47. Fish J, Smith EB, Canby JP: Malignant melanoma in childhood. Surgery 59:309, 1966

48. Forbuscited in Lund HZ, Kraux JM: Melanotic tumors of the skin. In Atlas of Tumor Pathology, Section 1, Washington DC: AFIP, 1962

49. Fox H, Emery JL, Goodbody RA, Yates PO: Neuro-cutaneous melanosis. Arch Dis Child 39:508, 1964

50. Freedman WL, McMahon FJ: Placental metastasis. Obstet Gynecol 16:550, 1960

51. Fuste R, Morales LM: Degeneracion maligna de un nevi pigmentario giante de la espalda. Rev Med Cuba 55:307, 1944

52. Gartmann H: Das Sug Juvenile Melanom. Münch Med Wuchenschr 104:587, 1962

53. Gartmann H: Benignes Juveniles Melanom. In Braun-Falco O, Petzoldt D (eds): Fortschritte der Prakitschen Dermatologie und Venerologie. Vol 7, Berlin, Springer-Verlag, 1973, pp 66–72

54. Gartmann H, Thurm K: Juveniles Melanom der Augenbindehaut. Dermatol Wochenschr 142:805, 1960

55. Giertsen JC: Malignant melanoma with metastases in a six-year-old boy. Acta pathol Microbiol Scand 60:173, 1964

56. Greeley PW, Curtin JW: Giant pigmented nevi. GP 34:132, 1966

57. Greeley PW, Middleton AG, Curtin JW: Incidence of malignancy in giant pigmented nevi. Plast Reconstr Surg 36:26, 1965

58. Groothuis FBG: Melanomata juvenilia. Dermatologica (Basel) 119:61, 1959

59. Gross PR, Carter DM: Malignant melanoma arising in a giant cerebriform nevus. Arch Dermatol 96:536, 1967

60. Grupper C, Tubiana R: Mélanome juvénile de Spitz ou pseudo mélanome. Bull Soc Fr Dermatol Syphiligr 62:300, 1955

61. Hendrix RX: Juvenile melanomas, benign and malignant. Arch Pathol 58:363, 1954

62. Hoagland PW, Hughes CW: Melanocarcinoma of childhood. Arch Surg 81:957, 1960

63. Hoffman HJ, Freeman A: Primary malignant leptomeningeal melanoma in association with giant hairy nevi. J Neurosurg 26:62, 1967

64. Holland E: A case of transplacental metastasis of malignant melanoma from mother to foetus. J Obstet Gynaecol Br Emp 56:529, 1949

65. Jakubowicz K: Uber Die Zugehorigkeit Des Sogenannten Juvenilen Melanomas Zur Gruppe de Antiven Nevuszellnaevus. Hautarzl 16:411, 1965

66. Jernstrom P, Aponte GE: Juvenile melanoma of the tongue. Am J Clin Pathol 26:1341, 1956

67. Johnson WT, and Helwig EB: Benign nevus cells in the capsule of lymph nodes. Cancer 23:247–253, 1969

68. Kernen JA, Ackerman LV: Spindle cell nevi and epithelioid cell nevi (so-called juvenile melanomas) in children and adults. Cancer 13:612, 1960

69. Kopf AW, Andrade R: Benign juvenile melanoma. In Year Book of Dermatology, 1965–1966, Chicago, Year Book of Med Pub, 1966

70. Koudstaal J, Oldhoff J, Panders AK, Hardonk MJ: Malanotic neuroctodermal tumor of infancy. Cancer 22:151, 1968

71. Lane N, Lattes R, Malm J: Clinicopathological correlations in a series of 117 malignant melanomas of the skin in adults. Cancer 11:1025, 1958

72. Lee JAH, Carter AP: Secular trends in mortality from malignant melanoma. J Natl Cancer Inst 45:91–97, 1970

73. Lerman RI, Murray D, O'Hara JM et al.: Malignant melanoma of childhood. Cancer 25:436, 1970

74. Lockwood K, Stancke B, and Clemmesen J: Survival rates for melanomas of the skin. In, S. Cutler (ed): Int Symp on End Results of Cancer Therapy, Nat Cancer Inst Monogr 15:185–195, 1964

75. Lyall D: Malignant melanoma in infancy, JAMA 202:1153, 1967

76. Magnus K: Incidence of malignant melanoma of the skin in Norway, 1955–1970. Cancer 32:1275–1286, 1973

77. Masters PL: Malignant melanoma in a child. Med J Aust 7:620, 1963

78. McGovern VJ, Brown MM Lane: The Nature of Melanoma. Springfield Ill, Charles C Thomas, 1969

79. McGovern VJ, Goulston E: Malignant moles in childhood. Med J Aust 1:181, 1963

80. McLeod RG: Factors influencing prognosis in malignant melanoma. In Melanoma and Skin Cancer. New South Wales, VCN Blight, Government Printer, 1972, pp 367–373

81. McWhorter HE, Woolner LB: Pigmented nevi juvenile melanomas and malignant melanomas in children. Cancer 7:564, 1954

82. McWhorter HE, Figi FA, Woolner LB: Treatment of juvenile melanomas and malignant melanomas in children. JAMA 156:695, 1954

83. Medenis R, Slaughter DP, Barber TK: Melanotic progonoma in childhood. Pediatrics 29:600, 1962

84. Montgomery H: Die Histopathologische Untercheidung der Pigment Naevi, Juvenilen Mclanome und Melanomalignome. Hautarzt 9:52, 1958

85. Morris LL, Danta G: Malignant cerebral melanoma complicating giant pigmented nevus: a case report. J Neurol Neurosurg Psychiatry 31:628, 1968

86. Myhre E: Malignant melanomas in children. Acta Pathol Microbiol Scand 59:184, 1963

87. Oldhoff J, Koudstaal J: Congenital papillomatous malignant melanoma of the skin. Cancer 21:1193, 1968

87a. Ota M: Nippon No Igaku. Tokyo, Mimpusha, 1946

88. Pack GT: The Pigmented Mole and the Malignant Melanoma. Am Cancer Soc, 1962

89. Pack GT: Prepubertal melanoma of skin. Surg Gynecol Obstet 86:374, 1948

90. Pack GT, Anglem TJ: Tumors of the soft tissues in infancy and childhood. J Pediatr 15:372, 1939

91. Pack GT, Davis J: Moles. NY State J Med 56:22, 1956

92. Pack GT, Davis J: Nevus giganticus pigmentosus with malignant transformation. Surgery 49:347, 1961

93. Pack GT, Scharnagel IM: Prognosis for malignant melanoma in the pregnant woman. Cancer 4:324, 1951

94. Penman HG, Stringer HC: Malignant transformation in giant congenital pigmented nevus. Arch Dermatol 103:428, 1971

95. Pers M: Naevus Pigmentosus Giganticus. Ugeskr Laeger 125:613, 1963

96. Pontius EE, Dziabis M.: Malignant melanoma in children. J Indiana Med Assoc 54:478, 1961

96a. Poore JB, Mermann AC, Yu JS: Adrenalcortical carcinoma and melanocarcinoma in a 5-year-old Negro child. Cancer 7:1235–1241, 1954

97. Potter JF, Schoeneman M: Metastases of maternal cancer to the placenta and fetus. Cancer 25:380, 1970

98. Recent trends in survival of cancer patients. DHEW Pub No (NIH) 52, 1974; 75–767.

99. Reed WB, Becker JW Jr, Whiting I, Nickel WR: Giant pigmented nevi melanoma and leptomeningeal melanocytosis. Arch Dermatol 91:100, 1965

100. Retik AB, Sebastian SM, Roxane H, et al.: The experimental transmission of melanoma cells through the placenta. Surg Gynecol Obstet 114:485, 1962

101. Reynolds AG: Placental metastasis from malignant melanoma. Obstet Gynecol 6:205, 1955

102. Rodriguez HA, Ackerman LV: Cellular blue nevus. Cancer 4:9–38, 1951

103. Saksela E, Rintala A: Misdiagnosis of prepubertal malignant melanoma. Cancer 22:1308, 1968

104. Samuels SL: Juvenile melanoma of the iris. Trans Am Acad Ophthalmol Otolaryngol 67:718, 1963

105. Schultz RC: Fatal malignant melanoma in children with giant nevi. Plast Reconstr Surg 27:551, 1961

106. Shaw MH: Malignant melanoma arising from a giant hairy nevus. Br J Plast Surg 15:426, 1962

107. Skov-Jensen T, Hastrup J, Lambrethsen E: Malignant melanoma in children. Cancer 19:620, 1966

108. Spitz S: Melanomas in childhood. Am J Pathol 24:591, 1948

109. Stegmaier O: Natural regression of the melanocytic nevus. J Invest Dermatol 32:413: 1959

110. Sweet LK, Connerty HV: Congenital Melanoma—A report of a case in which antenatal metastasis occurred. Am J Dis Child 62:1029, 1951

111. Sylven B: Malignant melanoma of the skin. Acta Radiol (Stockh) 32:33, 1949

112. Truax KF, Page HG: Prepubertal malignant melanoma. Ann Surg 137:255, 1953

113. Van Scott EJ, Reinertson RP, McCall PB: Prevalence, histologic types and significance of palmer and plantar nevi. Cancer 10:363–367, 1953

114. Webster JP, Stevenson, TW, Stout AP: The surgical treatment of malignant melanomas of the skin. Surg Clin North Am 24:319, 1944

115. Weedon D, Little JH: Spindle and epithelioid cell nevi in children and adults—a review of 211 cases of the Spitz nevus. Cancer 40:217–225, 1977

116. Wells GC, Farthing GJ: Juvenile melanoma: a histochemical study. Br J Dermatol 78:380, 1966

117. White LP: Studies on melanoma. N Engl J Med 260: 789–797, 1959

118. Williams WF: Melanoma with fatal metastasis in a five-year-old girl. Cancer 7:163, 1954

119. Wilson MC Jr, Anderson PC: A dissenting view of the prophylactic removal of plantar and palmar nevi. Cancer 14:102–104, 1961.

120. Winkelmann RK: Juvenile melanoma. Cancer 14:1001, 1961

121. Woringer F: A propos d'un naevus actromique de la joue chez une fillette de 8 ans. Bull Soc Fr Dermatol Syphiligr 46:550, 1939

122. Woringer F: Le mélanome juvenile de Spitz. Sem Hop Paris 32:1723, 1956

123. Woringer F: L'évolution d'une tumeur de Spitz. Bull Soc Fr Dermatol Syphiligr 70:246, 1963

124. Woringer F, Alt J: A propos des mélanomes malins prépubertaires. Congress Derm Syph Lgue Fr Lausanne. IX:152, 1956

125. Yagawa K, and Nakamura K: An autopsy case of the widely metastasized juvenile malignant melanoma arising from "naevus pigmentosus." Gan. 45:278, 1954.

126. Zwaveling A, Westbrsek DL, Vande Heul RA, Blok AP: Maligne Melanoon Bijkinderen. Ned Tijdschr Geneeskd 110:754, 1966

CHAPTER SIX

TUMOR THICKNESS AS A GUIDE TO TREATMENT IN CUTANEOUS MELANOMA

ALEXANDER BRESLOW[†] AND

GLENN W. GEELHOED

Evaluation of prognosis in cutaneous melanoma is important to the surgeon, to the medical oncologist, and, of course, to the patient. Many factors are believed to influence the clinical course of melanoma (Table 6–1), but this chapter will be concerned only with the level of invasion and with maximal tumor thickness.

LEVEL OF INVASION

The idea that prognosis in melanoma might be related to the ability of melanoma cells to invade the dermis and subcutaneous fat was first suggested by Allen and Spitz.[1] They found that superficial lesions had a better prognosis than did deeply infiltrating tumors, but the term "superficial" was not defined in a useful way. Menhert and Heard[26] proposed a more precise system with an in-situ level and invasive levels involving the papillary dermis, the reticular dermis, and the subcutaneous fat. Mortality increased with increasing level of invasion. This was modified by Clark et al.[8] who subdivided the invasion of the papillary dermis into a deep group in which melanoma cells accumulate at the junction of the reticular and papillary dermis (level III), and a superficial group in which they do not (level II). The mortality for patients with level II to V lesions was 8, 35, 46, and 52%, and similar progressions were found by other observers.[3,17,23] More recently McGovern[25] and

† Deceased.

Elias et al.[10] found no difference in survival between levels III and IV at ten years.

There are several problems with the use of this method. The first is that the differentiation between levels III and IV depends on the identification of the junction between the papillary and reticular dermis.

In some parts of the body this is simple, but in many the interface is vague and the distinction is difficult or impossible. A second problem is the definition of a level IV lesion. It is not enough to find a few melanoma cells in the reticular dermis. "Isolated intrusion of cells between the collagen bundles of the upper reticular dermis at the base of level III tumors is not considered sufficient for classification as a level IV lesion. There should be distinct invasion well into the reticular dermis."[8] This is vague and makes the separation of level III and level IV melanomas extremely subjective.

TUMOR THICKNESS

Because of this subjectiveness in the interpretation of the level of invasion, an attempt was made to develop a more objective measure of prognosis in cutaneous melanoma. It was thought that tumor volume might be such a factor and that the maximal cross-sectional area, the product of maximal surface diameter and maximal thickness, would be proportional to tumor volume. Maximal thickness is measured with an ocular micrometer, and is the distance from the deepest point of invasion to the top of the granular cell layer of the overlying epidermis. Measurement is made at

TABLE 6-1. Prognostic Variables in Cutaneous Melanoma

1. Clinical history	9. Satellitosis
2. Sex	10. Mitotic rate
3. Age	11. Level of invasion
4. Anatomic site	12. Size of tumor
5. Ulceration	a. Volume
6. Amelanosis	b. Diameter
7. Histologic type	c. Thickness
8. Inflammatory reaction	

Adapted from Geelhoed GW, Breslow A, McCune WS. Am Surg 43:77-85, 1977.

right angle to the surface of the skin surrounding the tumor. If the lesion is ulcerated, the ulcer base serves as the point of reference. Invasion is defined as the presence of melanocytes in the dermis, surrounded by collagen and/or inflammatory cells. Melanocytes in junctional nests are not considered invasive even though they may extend deeply into the papillary dermis due to epidermal hyperplasia. If residual benign melanocytes from an antecedent intradermal nevus are found in the bottom of the melanoma, they are not used in measurement. Finally, if deep nests of melanoma appear to arise from junctional nests of adjacent skin appendages, they are not used in measurement. Rarely one finds a lesion in which a column of melanocytes extends at a right angle into the deep dermis from the lower border of the tumor. This should not be measured, since its contour strongly suggests that it represents tumor arising from an appendage, and this can often be demonstrated by serial section.

TUMOR THICKNESS AND INCIDENCE OF METASTASES

For reasons that will be discussed later, the correlation between the maximal cross-sectional area and the metastatic rate was poor. By contrast, however, the correlation between maximal tumor thickness and the rate of metastasis was excellent.[3] This study was extended prospectively with similar results[4] (Table 6-2), and was then confirmed by others.[15,31] Tumors ≤ 0.75 mm thick were found to have a metastatic rate of about 1% (Table 6-3). The correlation of maximal thickness and the rate of metastasis in this study[4] of melanomas from all body sites was very close, but nonlinear, with a correlation coefficient of 0.931 (P=0.022). In a separate study, we recently found an almost linear relation between thickness and mortality in a group of 248 melanomas of the extremities (χ^2 = 13.33 P = 0.0002).[5] The lack of linearity in the first study may be a reflection of variation in prognosis at different body sites.

Simultaneous analysis of the thickness and the level of invasion[4,15,31] reveals a marked variation between them, as much as tenfold. Because thickness correlates so well with mortality, it could be anticipated that the level would not be as good a measure of prognosis. Wanebo et al.[31] found maximal tumor thickness to be superior to the level in predicting mortality. For thick lesions, the level consistently underestimated the mortality, but for thin lesions both methods were comparable. The basic question is whether these two methods are measuring the same prognostic factor by different means or are measuring different factors. If they are measuring different factors, the level of invasion, though less accurate, might still add significant prognostic information after tumor thickness has been measured. A 1.5 mm thick level IV melanoma might be more lethal than a 1.5 mm thick level III tumor. To test this, data presented by Wanebo et al.[31] were combined with our own for extremity melanomas. When the metasta-

TABLE 6-2. The Rate of Metastasis as a Function
of Thickness

Thickness (mm)	Number	% Metastasis
0–0.75	54	0
0.76–1.50	27	33
1.51–2.25	19	32
2.26–3.00	13	69
>3.00	25	84

TABLE 6-3. Published Metastatic Rates for Melanomas
≤0.75 mm Thick

Author	Number of Cases	Metastasized	
		No.	Percent
Gromet et al.[12]	98	2	2
Balch et al.[2]	17	0	0
Breslow and Macht[6]	62	0	0
Total	177	2	1.1

tic rates of combined level III and IV tumors 1 to 1.9 mm thick and 2 to 2.9 mm thick are compared, the rate for the thicker group was 53% and that for the thinner, 26% (P = 0.01). When the two groups are subdivided by level, there is no significant difference in the metastatic rates (P>0.40). Once thickness is measured, it seems that little is added by determining the level.

CORRELATION OF LEVEL OF INVASION AND TUMOR THICKNESS

This was also the conclusion of a study of extremity melanomas,[5] which by multiple logistic regression analysis found that 95% of the available prognostic information was recovered when thickness was measured first, leaving only 5% to be recovered by determining the level. When the level was measured first, it provided only 40% of the prognostic information, leaving 60% for thickness. Similarly, another study,[2] using the same statistical analysis, reached similar conclusions (Table 6-4). Maximal tumor thickness was found to be an independent variable and "the single most important determinant for stage I disease." By contrast the level of invasion was found to be "a dependent variable whose only predictive value lay in its rough correlation with tumor thickness." The poor correlation between the level of invasion and survival and the failure of the determination of invasive level to be useful in prognosis is not difficult to understand. There is a marked variation in the thickness of the skin in different parts of the body. Assuming a melanoma to be a flat level III lesion, a tumor on the eyelid will be much thinner than one of the sole of the foot; also, if one is raised and the other is flat, the variation will be even greater. In addition the lethal nature of a melanoma is not due to the ability of its cells to infiltrate the reticular dermis, but to their ability to invade blood and lymphatic vessels. Though the most vascular part of the skin is the papillary dermis, level II melanomas rarely metastasize. By contrast the rate of metastasis is quite high for level IV tumors, though the

TABLE 6–4. Multiple Logistic Regression Analysis of Level and Thickness in Cutaneous Melanoma

Percent of Prognostic Information			
Breslow et al.[5]		Balch et al.[2]	
LEVEL	THICKNESS	LEVEL	THICKNESS
1st	2nd	1st	2nd
40%	60%	50%	50%
95%	5%	100%	0%
THICKNESS	LEVEL	THICKNESS	LEVEL
1st	2nd	1st	2nd

reticular dermis has relatively few vessels. There may be a simple explanation for this enigma. As tumors invade the dermis they enlarge; once their diameter exceeds the maximal distance that oxygen can diffuse in tissue, the tumor must stimulate the formation of new blood vessels, which increases the chance of metastasis. If this hypothesis is correct, the failure of the maximal cross-sectional area to correlate closely with the metastatic rate, alluded to earlier in this chapter, may be due to the inclusion of large thin tumors in this study. The correlation between the maximal cross-sectional area of the segment of the tumor greater than 0.75 mm thick would probably have resulted in a closer correlation, but was not measured. I would not expect the results to have been better than that achieved by only measuring thickness.

Shape of Melanoma. The cross-sectional shape of the melanoma is determined by the ability of the tumor cells to invade the dermal connective tissue, the ratio of the mitotic rate to the tumor cell death rate, and the ability of the tumor to extend laterally at the junction of the dermis and epidermis, possibly a manifestation of a field change at the time of tumor induction rather than a result of direct extension of the tumor. These variables explain the shape of the four major subgroups of melanoma: the lentigo maligna, the superficial spreading, the nodular and the polypoid

tumors. Lentigo maligna melanomas and superficial spreading tumors both extend laterally, are quite variable in thickness, but differ in their rate of growth. The nodular and the polypoid tumors are almost always thick tumors, reflecting their rapid growth rate, but differ in that the nodular type infiltrates the reticular dermis early in its development while the polypoid type, though highly malignant, seems to be unable to invade the reticular dermis and is often confined to the superficial papillary dermis. If the level of invasion were a dominant prognostic variable, the polypoid tumors should have a low, not a high malignant potential, and this contradiction has led some to consider them as unclassified as to the level of invasion.[22]

Melanoma Morphology. It is generally believed that the morphology of the tumor provides us with important prognostic information with the lentigo maligna the least malignant, the nodular and polypoid the most malignant and the superficial spreading in an intermediate position. Though this is true when they are considered as groups, for individual cases of similar thickness[31] or similar level[16] there is no significant difference between nodular and superficial spreading tumors. This is probably also true for lentigo maligna melanomas, but the incidence of thick tumors is so low in this group that one cannot be certain.

MITOTIC RATE AND PROGNOSIS

The mitotic rate has been found to be of value in assessing the prognosis of melanoma by some[9,20,23,26,32] but this was not confirmed by others.[18] A recent study[28] compared mitotic counts per square millimeter in the area of greatest mitotic activity, level of invasion, tumor thickness, and prognostic index (mitotic count × thickness) in a group of 146 melanomas treated only by excision. If adjunctive treatment had been used for patients with tumors of levels III-IV the total error rate (the percent that developed subsequent metastases whose lesions were level II and those who did not develop metastases whose lesions were levels III–V) was 40%. With a dividing line at 2 mm the error rate for thickness was 29%, at 4 mitoses/mm^2, 21%, and only 14% for prognostic index with a division at 12 mitoses/mm. If this is confirmed, and if there is reasonably good agreement on mitotic counts between different pathologists examining the same slides, this will certainly be the preferred method for evaluating prognosis. It must be remembered that the identification of the area of greatest mitotic activity is a subjective assessment and that a group of pathologists at an international workshop were unable to reach agreement on many slides simply evaluated as to low, intermediate, and high mitotic activity. (Results of W.H.O. Workshop, Milan, November) 1977; personal oral communication from N. Cascinelli, MD).

TUMOR THICKNESS AND TREATMENT POLICIES

In treating a tumor he believes is a stage I cutaneous melanoma, the surgeon is faced with two problems: how much apparently normal skin should be removed from around the tumor and whether to perform an elective node dissection. The scientific literature concerning the optimal size of the resection margin in melanoma is scanty. Suggested margins ranged from 2 to 15 cm with little or no data to support any decision the most frequent recommendation is a 5 cm margin; this has almost become surgical dogma. It has been attributed to Handley,[13,14] and if this is true, the evidence in favor of a 5 cm margin is no better than that for any other margin. It consists of a postmortem study of the lymphatic distribution of tumor surrounding metastatic cutaneous lesions, which as far as I know has no proven relationship to that for primary tumors. The best paper dealing with this problem that I am aware of is that of Olsen[27] who, in a study of 302 melanomas, found no relationship between the incidence of local recurrence and the size of the resection margin in the range from less than 1 cm to more than 5 cm. She divided local recurrences into those that contain areas of junctional activity, (23% of her series) essentially newly formed melanomas, and those that do not have junctional activity and are believed to be due to local lymphatic spread of the tumor. Since we have already seen that the rate of distant dissemination is closely correlated with maximal tumor thickness, it seems likely that the incidence of local recurrence might be related to tumor thickness. This was found to be true for tumors less than 0.75 mm thick.[6] In a series of 62 thin tumors the in vitro resection margins ranged from 0.1 to 5.5 cm with 32% no more than 1 cm and none metastasized or recurred locally in the five or more years following excision. For such tumors the optimal size of the resection margin depends on the anatomic site of the tumor, and skin grafts should be required only in a minority of cases for optimal cosmetic results. A recent study of 799 stage I and II cases from the W.H.O. Melanoma Group Registry found no correlation between the local recurrence rate and the size of the resection margin for tumors no thicker than 2 mm (N. Cascinelli, MD, personal oral communication). There was a negative correlation for thicker tumors, but this was not statistically significant. By contrast, the correlation between thickness and the incidence of local recurrence was close (r = 0.98, P < 0.005). Since the size of the resection margin did not influence the mortality rate for the 593 stage I patients, a randomized clinical trial is planned that will compare 1 cm margins with margins of at least 3 cm. It is reasonable to include stage II cases in the aforementioned study, since there is no evidence that nodal metastases can cause recurrences in scars.

For the measurement of tumor thickness to have a bearing on the primary treatment of melanoma, the surgeon must decide on biopsy before planning the extent of the resection margins and lymphadenectomy. The use of frozen sections, though employed frequently in parts of Europe and in Australia, has not achieved universal acceptance and, if used, would necessitate new criteria for the measurement of tumor thickness. In such a situation (which should occur infrequently) a preferable course would be a minimally traumatic incisional biopsy through the area that appears to be the thickest part of the tumor followed by complete excision in 24 to 48 hours. There is no convincing evidence that this approach decreases the rate of survival.[11a,19,21] It is reassuring that surgeons were able to select the thickest part of the tumor by visual inspection in 92% of a series of 42 cases at the National Cancer Institute (S. A. Rosenberg, MD, personal oral communication 1977).

ELECTIVE NODE DISSECTION

As for the role of elective node dissection in the treatment of cutaneous melanoma, the literature prior to 1977, including part of my 1975 paper,[4] is difficult if not impossible to evaluate. Because of the likelihood of bias in patient selection, retrospective studies cannot be used to compare different methods of treatment. For example, on the basis of a retrospective study, Hansen and McCarten[15] concluded that elective node dissection appeared to double survival for patients with tumors at least 1.5 mm thick while having no effect on the survival of patients with thinner tumors. We confirmed these findings[4] in a similar retrospective study, but realized that a properly executed prospectively randomized study was required to answer this question. Such a study, carried out by the W.H.O. Melanoma Group,[30] revealed no significant difference in five-year survival between those treated with immediate node dissection and those followed at monthly intervals and dissected only upon the discovery of nodal enlargement. In a similar study Sim et al.[29] were unable to demonstrate improved survival with elective node dissection. Re-examination of our data (Table 6–5) revealed that our surgeons tended to select for elective node dissection those patients whose tumors had a readily predictable lymphatic drainage, i.e. melanomas of the extremities while avoiding dissections for patients with axial tumors. Extremity tumors have a significantly better prognosis than axial tumors; to make matters worse, none of our patients with far advanced level V tumors were treated by elective node dissection. Inadvertently, our surgeons had selected for node dissection the patients with the best prognosis.

By measuring thickness of the melanomas in the W.H.O. study we hoped to find a subgroup that would have benefited from elective node dissection.[5] Though there was no significant difference for any subgroup at five years, there was a suggestion for the 3 to 4.5 mm subgroup with a 19% improvement in survival for the immediate node dissected patients (P–0.12). At eight years these curves have come closer together, but there now appears to be a marginal difference in favor of node dissection for tumors > 4.5 mm. thick, although the numbers are small. If the tumor is too thin, node dissection is not needed, and if it is too thick, it will not improve survival because of subclinical dissemination beyond the regional nodes. There may well be a suitable intermediate range in which elective node dissection will prove to be beneficial. That this range may be somewhere beyond 3.0 mm shows how good the prognosis is in extremity melanoma, especially in a patient population that proved to be 81% female. This brings us to a frequently voiced criticism of the W.H.O. study: the patient population was at very low risk because there were too few men and the tumors were all in the extremities. Since the risk was so low, these cri-

TABLE 6-5.   Elective Lymph Node Dissection

Site	Number	% Dissected
Axial	32	28
Extremity	24	50
Level V	9	0

tics claim that it is difficult to demonstrate a benefit from node dissection. This criticism can be tested by comparing mortality rates in the W.H.O. study with those of a comparable study[31] in which there were more males. Thickness for thickness there is no significant difference in survival between the two groups (Table 6-6), but the W.H.O. group had more than 2.3 times the percentage of tumors thicker than 3 mm than did the other group. This does not appear to have been a population at exceptionally low risk.

PROBLEMS IN MEASURING TUMOR THICKNESS

There are four problems in measuring maximal tumor thickness. The first is sampling. If one does not study the entire lesion one cannot be certain one has found the area of maximal thickness. The entire lesion should be step-sectioned, at 1 to 2 mm intervals. This is especially true for thin tumors. With the thicker tumors it is often possible to identify the area of maximum thickness on gross examination. In a study at the National Cancer Institute, the thickest part of the tumor was identified by the surgeon by gross examination in 41 of 45 cases (S. A. Rosenberg, MD, personal communication, 1977).

The second is error in sectioning and embedding the tissue. The angle must be 90 degrees to the skin surface to measure the true thickness of the tumor. Tangential sections or embedding errors increase the apparent thickness, with a 41% increase at 45 degrees but only an 8% increase at 22.5 degrees. With care one should be able to keep the error of the angle to much less than 22.5 degrees.

The third problem is that of tumor regression. A tumor may grow until it is 0.75 mm thick or a thicker lesion may become that thin by undergoing spontaneous regression. Unfortunately, such a tumor may metastasize before it regresses, and regression is much less likely to occur at metastatic sites. There is no way to evaluate the prognosis of regressed tumors. Gromet et al.[15] found an incidence of metastasis of 5 of 23 cases of regressed tumors less than 0.76 mm thick as compared to only 2 of 98 thin tumors without evidence of regression. Such tumors are easily identified by the presence of dense, fibrous tissue and large dilated blood vessels not seen in the normal dermis, or unusually large mononuclear inflammatory infiltrates with relatively few melanoma cells.

The final problem is that of variation in histologic technique. It has been suggested that this may alter the apparent thickness of the tumor. This does not appear to be a practical problem. The slides of the 248 melano-

TABLE 6-6.   Melanomas of Extremities

Wanebo et al.[31] M:F = 0.41		Breslow et al.[5] M:F = 0.23	
Thickness (mm)	Mortality (%)	Thickness (mm)	Mortality (%)
1.1–1.5	16	1.25	22
1.6–2.0	18	1.75	24
2.1–3.0	38	2.50	27
>3.0	46	>3.0	41

mas of the extremities referred to before[5] were prepared by many technicians in 17 laboratories from Lima to Moscow and from Oslo to Naples. If variation in histologic technique had altered apparent thickness, we would not have found such a close correlation between thickness and mortality ($\chi^2 = 13.33$ P = 0.0002). Most of the errors in histologic technique result in slides of very poor quality and are easily avoided.

ACKNOWLEDGMENT

This work was partly supported by funds provided in part by the International Cancer Research Data Bank Programme of the National Cancer Institute, National Institutes of Health (US), under Contract No. No1-CO-65341 (International Cancer Research Technology Transfer - ICRETT) with the International Union Against Cancer.

REFERENCES

1. Allen A, Spitz S: Malignant melanoma—a clinicopathology analysis of the criteria for diagnosis and prognosis. Cancer 6:1–45, 1953
2. Balch CM, Murad TM, Soong S et al.: A multifactorial analysis of melanoma: Prognostic histopathological features comparing Clark's and Breslow's staging methods. Ann Surg, in press
3. Breslow A: Thickness, cross-sectional areas and depth of invasion in the prognosis of cutaneous melanoma. Ann Surg 172:902–903, 1970
4. Breslow A: Tumor thickness, level of invasion and node dissection in stage I cutaneous melanoma. Ann Surg 182:572–575, 1975
5. Breslow A, Cascinelli N, van der Esch EP, Morabito A: Stage I melanoma of the limbs: Assessment of prognosis by levels of invasion and maximum thickness. Tumori, 64:273–284, 1978
6. Breslow A, Macht SD: Optimal size of resection margin for thin cutaneous melanoma. Surg Gynecol Obstet 145:691–692, 1977
7. Breslow A, Macht SD: Evaluation of prognosis in stage I cutaneous melanoma. Plastic Reconstr Surg 61:342–346, 1978
8. Clark WH Jr, From L, Bernadino EA, Mihm MC: The histogenesis and biologic behavior of primary human malignant melanomas of the skin. Cancer Res 29:705–726, 1969
9. Cochran AJ: Histology and prognosis in malignant melanoma. J Pathol 97:459–468, 1969
10. Elias EG, Didolkar MS, Goel IP, et al.: A clinicopathologic study of prognostic factors in cutaneous malignant melanoma. Surg Gynecol Obstet 144:327–334, 1977
11a. Epstein E, Bragg K, Linden G: Biopsy and prognosis of malignant melanoma. JAMA 208:1369, 1969
11b. Greelhoed GW, Breslow A, McCune WS: Malignant melanoma: Correlation of long-term follow-up with clinical staging, level of invasion, and thickness of the primary tumor. Am Surg 43:77–85, 1977
12. Gromet M, Epstein WL, Blois MS: The regressing thin malignant melanoma: a distinctive lesion with metastatic potential. Cancer 42:2282–2292, 1978
13. Handley WS: The pathology of melanotic growths in relation to thin operative treatment. Lancet 1:996, 1907
14. Handley WS: The pathology of melanotic growths in relation to thin operative treatment. Lancet 1:927, 1907
15. Hansen MG, McCarten AB: Tumor thickness and lymphocytic infiltration in malignant melanoma of the head and neck. Am J Surg, 128:557–561, 1972
16. Hermanek P, Hornstein OP, Tonak J, Weidner F: Malignant melanoma depth of invasion and histologic typing. Beitr Pathol Bd 157:269–282, 1976
17. Huvos AG, Mime V, Donnellan MJ, et al.: Prognostic factors in cutaneous melanomas of the head and neck. Am J Path 71:33–48, 1973
18. Huvos AG, Shah JP, Mike V: Prognostic factors in cutaneous malignant melanoma: A comparative study of long-term and short-term survivors. Hum Pathol 5:347–357, 1974
19. Jones NM, Jones Williams W, Roberts MM, Davies K: Malignant melanoma of the skin; Prognostic value of clinical features and the role of treatment in 111 cases. Br J Cancer 22:437, 1968
20. Jourdain JC: Étude de critères cliniques et histiologiques du prognostic des mélanomes malins primaires. Ann Dermatol Syphil (Paris). 101:171–178, 1974
21. Knutson CO, Hori JM, Spratt JS: Melanoma. Curr Probl Surg, December, 1971, pp 1–55
22. Little JH: Histology and prognosis in cutaneous malignant melanomas. In McCarthy WH (ed):

Melanoma and Skin Cancer. Sydney Australia, VCN Blight, Government Printer, 1972, pp 107–119

23. McGovern VJ: The classification of melanoma and its relationship with prognosis. Pathology 2:85–98, 1970

24. McGovern VJ: Melanoma: Growth patterns, multiplicity and regression. In McCarthy WH (ed): Melanoma and Skin Cancer. Sydney Australia, VCN Blight, Government Printer, 1972, pp 95–106

25. McGovern VJ: Malignant Melanoma, Clinical and Histologic Diagnosis. John Wiley & Sons, New York, 1976, p 125

26. Menhert JH, Heard JL: Staging of malignant melanomas by depth of invasion. Am J Surg, 110:168–176, 1965

27. Olsen G: The malignant melanoma of the skin, Acta Chir Scand [Suppl] 365:140, 1966

28. Schmoeckel C, Braun-Falco O: Prognostic in-dex in malignant melanoma. Arch Dermatol 114:871–873, 1978

29. Sim FH, Taylor WF, Ivins JC, et al.: A prospective randomized study of the efficacy of routine elective lymph-adenectomy in management of malignant melanoma. Cancer 41:948, 1978

30. Veronesi U, Adamus J, Bandiera DC, et al.: In-efficacy of immediate node dissection in stage I melanoma of the limbs. N Engl J Med 297: 627–629, 1977

31. Wanebo IIJ, Fortner JG, Woodruff J, et al.: Selection of the optimum surgical treatment of stage I melanoma by depth of microinvasion: use of the combined microstage technique (Clark-Breslow). Ann Surg 182:302–313, 1975

32. Williams WJ, Davies K, Jones WM, et al.: Malignant melanoma of the skin: prognostic value of histology in 89 cases. Br J Cancer 22:452–460, 1968

CHAPTER SEVEN

BIOLOGIC REGRESSION WITH DISAPPEARANCE OF MALIGNANT MELANOMA

(Results of Treating Metastases to Lymph Nodes with No Known Primary)

IRVING M. ARIEL

A middle-aged patient presents himself with a large mass in the lymph nodes of the axilla or groin that proves to be a metastatic melanoma. What is the nature of this metastasis without a known primary? What should be done regarding "adequate" therapy, and what is the prognosis for such a patient?

Spontaneous regression with eventual disappearance of cancer, although rare, does occur. The classic study of Everson and Cole,[16] who culled 176 instances of spontaneous regression of cancer from the world literature, of which 20 were metastatic melanoma, focused upon this phenomenon. Although the melanoma incidence of all cases surveyed was less than 1%, it represented 11% of all spontaneous regressions, exceeded by hypernephroma (18%) and neuroblastoma (16%). In order to consider spontaneous regression of a cancer as a possibility, they proposed the following criteria:

Spontaneous regression could only be considered if there were (1) histologic confirmation of the primary or metastatic tumor plus (2) partial or complete disappearance of the malignant tumor in the absence of all treatment or in the presence of therapy which is inadequate to exert a significant influence on the neoplastic disease.

THE NATURE OF OCCULT PRIMARY MELANOMA

The exact nature of occult or regressed primary melanoma in the presence of metas-tases is difficult to ascertain. Several possibilities must be evaluated. (1) An occult primary exists but has not been discovered. This would not be true in the case of long-term survivors (5–25 years) after treatment of the metastases to lymph nodes. (2) There has been actual regression with disappearance of the primary site, akin to the surgical removal of the tumor. The cells that had metastasized to regional lymph nodes while the tumor was in existence became clinically manifest at a later date. The site where the primary tumor existed may reveal areas of leukoderma, melanophages, or chronic inflammatory infiltrates, including large numbers of lymphocytes and fibroses (Figs. 7–1 and 7–2). There is a possibility that the desmoplastic spindle-cell melanoma described by Conley et al.[12] may represent one phase of the host's reaction to the presence of the malignant tumor which, theoretically, could go on to complete destruction of the tumor with only the fibrotic reaction remaining.

Everson and Cole postulated certain factors that could contribute to spontaneous regression, namely: (1) endocrine influences such as pregnancy and menopause; (2) complete resection of the tumor, which was thought to be only partially excised; (3) unusual sensitivity of certain tumors to irradiation or other therapy; (4) destruction of some tumors by fever and/or acute infection; (5) unusual allergic reaction; (6) some mechanism causing interference with the nutrition of the tumor during incomplete resection; (7) removal of a

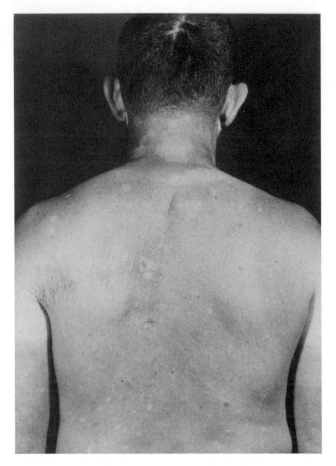

FIGURE 7-1. Patient with leukoderma, halo nevi, and metastatic melanoma of the posterior thoracic wall, treated by wide surgical resection and radical axillary dissection. Patient remained well for over ten years.

carcinogenic agent; (8) incorrect original diagnosis. They stress the fact that the histology must always be confirmed by expert pathologists before spontaneous regression can be accepted as a diagnosis.

McGovern[26] believes that cutaneous melanomas have a tendency to disappear spontaneously, and describes 54 (12.2%) of 437 primary cutaneous melanomas that demonstrated evidence of regressive features characterized by dense lymphocytic infiltrate similar to that found around nevi that disappear spontaneously (Fig. 7-3). All the melanomas that he claimed regressed were the superficial spreading type. He records that the clinical patterns of the process can be recognized as follows: (1) inflammatory nodules with or without pigmentation; (2)

scarring of the tumor; (3) several foci of malignancy simulating multicentricity; (4) a pigmented lesion with a deep pigmented halo; (5) a pigmented scar with surviving malignant cells; (6) a pigmented scar without surviving tumor cells; (7) metastatic melanoma with no demonstrable cutaneous primary.

In support of this concept, the study of Gromet, Epstein, and Blois[19] demonstrates that although certain of the melanomas may be very thin with limited invasion of the host tissue, metastases can occur. They postulate that these tumors may have been thicker and infiltrated more deeply, but that host reaction has partially destroyed the tumors, so that they are now thin with limited invasion but with a high potential for producing metastases (as existed before partial destruction of the

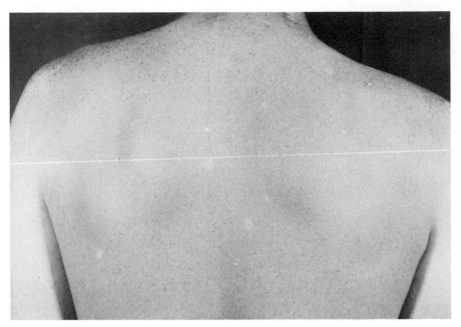

FIGURE 7-2. Young male with multiple halo nevi and foci of leukoderma. He suffered from metastatic melanoma to the left axillary lymph node. It is believed that one (or more) of the leukoderma may have been the site of the primary melanoma, which involuted spontaneously.

tumor had occurred as a result of host defenses).

An interesting case report by Pack[29] is that of a 32-year-old female who had several melanotic nodules removed from her leg. One year later, after being bitten by a dog, she received a course of 14 rabies vaccine injections. Five and one half years later, two additional nodules appeared, were excised, and the patient remained cured for the succeeding ten years of observation. Because of this unusual biologic behavior of the melanoma Pack believed the course of rabies vaccines may have altered the biologic determinism. Subsequently, at the Pack Medical Group, we treated many patients with a course, and sometimes two full courses, of rabies vaccine with no demonstrable benefit.

Another most interesting instance of spontaneous regression is that reported by Sumner[35] in a 30-year-old female whose subcutaneous nodules of the trunk and metastases to the groin disappeared after pregnancy, and she has remained well for over 11 years. Because of this unusual event, Sumner and Foraker[36] later injected a plasma infusate into a 28-year-old male with metastases to the scalp and buttocks, as well as the axillary lymph nodes. The metastases disappeared and the patient remained well for over five years. The author has tried a similar experiment on other patients with metastatic melanoma and no demonstrable benefit was observed, indicating the unpredictable behavior of many aspects of malignant melanoma.

In Wallace's series, spontaneous regressions of four female patients were associated with pregnancy. This constituted one-third of all the females with spontaneous regression. One such patient seen by Pack Medical Group surgeons had a tremendous growth of malignant melanoma during her first pregnancy. The melanoma was treated surgically and she developed cutaneous metastases, which disappeared after her second pregnancy.

In eight of Wallace's patients (36%) no fac-

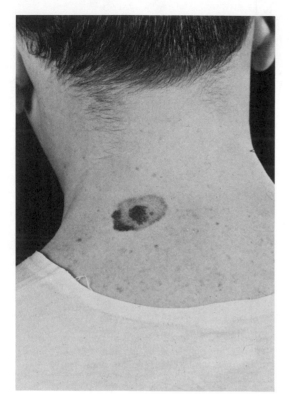

FIGURE 7–3. A pigmented superficial melanoma undergoing depigmentation. This could conceivably become entirely depigmented in time.

tors could be found to account for the spontaneous disappearance of the malignant melanoma. In three of these cases, subsequent tests suggested some immune mechanism was responsible.

HORMONE RELATIONSHIP TO REGRESSION

The theory that hormonal influences cause regression is based upon the following considerations: (1) Certain other tumors, such as the breast and the prostate, do respond to endocrine manipulation. (2) Malignant melanoma is extremely rare before puberty. (3) The fact that there is a better prognosis for females for most melanomas suggests some beneficial endocrine climate. (4) There have been a number of reports of spontaneous regression of melanoma associated with pregnancy. In three cases metastases developed and grew during

pregnancy and regressed after childbirth; in a fourth case, metastases developed during the first pregnancy, regressed during the second pregnancy, and reappeared during the third pregnancy. Although it was once believed that pregnancy exerts a detrimental influence upon the melanoma, studies have demonstrated no significant difference in longevity (Wallace).

We have attempted many forms of endocrine manipulation varying from hypophysectomy, adrenolectomy, orchiectomy, oophorectomy, plus many forms of endocrine administration, each of which has proved to be a failure. In assessing the possible influence of endocrine factors, one must bear in mind the considerable variations in the biologic history of malignant melanomas. One case comes to mind of a young man who had a melanoma that appeared on his ankle, gradually spread to his knee, and then throughout the skin of his thigh. At this point I recommended that he have a bilateral orchiectomy. The patient wisely refused. I followed him for the next ten years, at which time melanoma developed throughout the leg, but never went beyond the inguinal ligament, produced no dysfunction, and the patient continued working on his job without any loss of time.

IMMUNOLOGIC FACTORS AND SPONTANEOUS REGRESSION

Support for the immunological factors in producing spontaneous regression is demonstrable by the life cycle of malignant melanoma. There is constant competition between the growth impulse of the cancer and the body's attempt to retain or destroy the tumor. This is manifested by altered coloration, and irregular boundaries due to partial to complete destruction of different parts of the melanoma. It is stressed that the defense is local, in that the primary melanoma may show areas of partial regression to complete regression, whereas the metastases will continue to grow without any hindrance.

After primary treatment, certain melanomas, especially those of eyes and some of the extremities, may remain quiescent for over 25 years. This was the case with a patient of mine for 27 years after treatment of her primary melanoma, after which the melanoma metastasized, and the patient died within a short period. What happened to the cancer cells during the long period of quiescence, and what immunological mechanisms subsequently permitted such precipitous growth, remains an enigma.

The existence of cytotoxic melanocytoxic lymphocytes in the serum of some patients seems to substantiate further the role of immunology in the life history of melanoma. In view of these host reactions, Robert Madden has rightly suggested the term spontaneous regression be changed to biologic regression.

OTHER EXPLANATIONS

There is the possibility that primary melanoma may originate in the lymph nodes. This was suggested by Ewing, who in 1933 described nevus cells in axillary lymph nodes: ". . . in the septa of the lymph node itself, not metastatic, because there was no lesion of the skin." Pigmented melanocytes are found in approximately 5% of axillary and groin lymph nodes (Lectures to Cornell Medical School Students, P 108, 1934).

In addition, one must be aware of noncellular pigment within the lymph nodes. In patients with a primary melanoma of the extremity, a pigmented lymph node must show melanoma cells and not just the pigment to be considered metastatic melanoma. The primary site may be in one of the viscera, such as the gastrointestinal tract, the central nervous system, or the genitourinary tract.

Practically all of the regressions occurred in either cutaneous or in metastases to lymph nodes. In about six cases, it was claimed that pulmonary metastases subsided based on roentgenological evidence, but the data are too indefinite to be accepted with conviction.

Hepatomeglia due to metastases have been reported in three cases, but in most instances the data are insufficient, except in a case reported by Bulkley, which demonstrated histologic diagnosis of an hepatic metastasis; a biopsy taken 12 years later revealed it to be negative, demonstrating an absolute case of spontaneous regression in the liver.

INCIDENCE OF OCCULT PRIMARY MELANOMA

The exact incidence of spontaneously regressed tumors is not known (Table 7–1). Inasmuch as certain patients may have their tumors regress without producing metastases to lymph nodes, no knowledge of their previous presence exists. Bodurtha, in a collected series, records 29 cases of regression.[4] The series does not include 39 cases recorded by Milton,[27] and records only one case reported from the Pack Medical Foundation, whereas 118 cases were observed there, of which 29 were recorded originally by Pack, Gerber, and Scharnagel in 1952.[30] These cases represent 3.6% of the 3305 patients with

TABLE 7-1. Incidence of Occult Primary Melanoma

Author	No. of Patients with Melanoma	No. of Patients with Occult Primary	Percent of Occult Primaries
Brownstein and Helwig (1972) (Armed Forces Institute of Pathology)	1000 patients with metastases	150	15.0
Einhorn et al. (1974)	426 patients with metastases	64	15.0
Das Gupta et al. (1963)	992	37	3.7
Baab and McBride (1975)	2446		4.0
Milton et al. (1967)		39	
Pack Medical Group	3305	118	3.6
Smith and Stehlin.	461	40	8.7

melanoma surveyed by the Pack Medical Group.

Das Gupta, Bowden, and Berg[14] reported 37 spontaneous regressions of 992 patients with melanoma (3.7%) in a 1963 review of patients at Memorial Hospital, New York City.

Bodurtha estimates a representative value of spontaneous regression of metastatic melanoma can be obtained where it is described as an incidental finding. By this method, he estimated one case of regression of metastases per 400 patients.

CLINICAL FEATURES

There is usually an increased incidence in males (4.6 to 1 in Milton's series—32 men and 7 women; in Beardmore's series[3] the ratio was 2:1 in favor of males). In the 28 recorded cases summarized by Bodurtha, there were 16 males and 12 females; the patients' mean age was 48 years for males and 42 years for females. Bodurtha believes that the younger mean age for the females, and the fact that 10 of 12 females whose melanoma spontaneously regressed were under 55 years of age, suggest that some endocrine factor may be responsible.

In Milton's series the mean age was 45.5 years, the youngest being 18 years and the oldest 78 years at the time of diagnosis.

The 39 patients are divided into two groups. Eighteen patients (13 men and 5 women) were true occult primaries inasmuch as no history of a primary melanoma was obtained. In 21 patients (19 men and 2 women), a history was obtained that suggests that a primary tumor may have been present but spontaneously disappeared.

The sites of metastases described by Milton are: 9 to the cervical lymph nodes; 10 to the axillary lymph nodes, 11 to the inguinal lymph nodes; and 9 indeterminate in that they presented multiple subcutaneous nodules that represented either tumors in transit or blood-born metastases; one patient presented with generalized metastases in addition to subcutaneous satellites.

In the Pack Medical Group series (See Table 7-2), of the 118 patients with occult primaries, in 98 the primary was truly occult, but in 20 there was a history of spontaneous regression. (One patient who presented with metastases to his cervical region described a dried-up black lesion on his neck, which he scraped off about two years before the appearance of the metastases in the cervical region.)

Of these patients, 21 had metastases to the cervical region; 30 to the axilla; 24 to the inguinal region; 6 to the axilla and cervical region, and 37 had miscellaneous extra nodal deposits.

Of the 118 patients, 56 were females and 62 were males. The average age was 45 years; 43 for females and 47 for males.

TREATMENT OF OCCULT OR SPONTANEOUSLY REGRESSED MELANOMAS

If a careful search has been made for a primary lesion, including other metastases (because of the vagaries of metastases), then the metastases should be handled as if the primary tumor had been successfully treated (Fig. 7-4).

If evidence of visceral metastases or multiple metastases, to several lymph node lesions are uncovered, only palliative therapy should be instituted. If careful survey does not record other metastases, a radical lymph node dissection is the indicated procedure. Resecting only the involved node is contraindicated because of the strong probability that the other regional nodes are invaded by the melanomas. This is emphasized by Milton, who recorded multiple node involvement in the resected specimen of 16 patients treated by radical resections. The prognosis for patients with multiple skin nodules and/or visceral involvement is poor, and Milton calls attention to the fact that 9 patients with occult metastases, with systemic and no nodal metastases, all died within 12 months. At the Pack Medical Group, the 37 patients with extra nodal metastases treated only by palliation survived 9 months.

SURVIVAL

In the series of 118 patients with occult metastases, or with primaries that had spon-

TABLE 7-2. Incidence and Survival of Metastases from an Occult Primary Melanoma Treated at the Pack Medical Group

Location	Number of Patients	Number of 10-Year Survivors	Percent of 10-Year Survivors
Cervical lymph nodes	21	0	0
Axillary lymph nodes	30	12	40
Axillary and cervical lymph nodes	6	1	17
Groin lymph nodes	24	8	33
Extranodal metastases including metastases to viscera	37	0	0
Total	118	21	

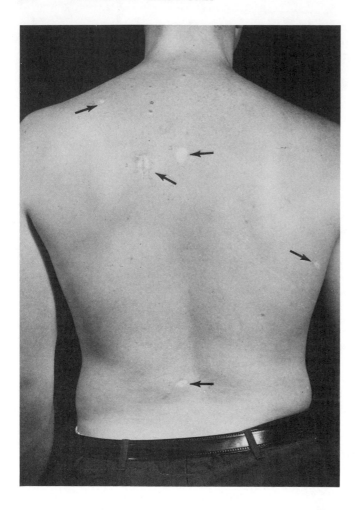

FIGURE 7–4. Spontaneous disappearance of junctional nevi. The leukoderma also occurred around the scar where a malignant melanoma was treated by excisional biopsy. This one region was treated by tridimensional resection.

taneously regressed with no clinical evidence of their existence, were 75 who had metastases to one group of lymph nodes and were subjected to resection of that group of lymph nodes. The overall 10-year survival rate equalled 26.7% (20 of 75). None of the 21 patients subjected to cervical neck dissection survived, reported by Conley and Hamaker (see Chapter 17). Of 30 with axillary lymph node involvement, 12% survived for ten years (40%), and 8 of 24 patients with metastases to the lymph nodes of the groin survived a minimum of ten years (33%). These values are similar to those for stage II melanomas of patients with metastases to the axilla from known primaries of the upper extremities (26% of 272 patients), and for stage II melanomas of the lower extremities (24% of 263 patients). These data suggest that an immune factor that influenced the primary melanoma may have prolonged survival.

Booher[6] stated that when the metastasis was confined to one regional node, the rate was 41.7% (10 of 24 patients) and when the metastases involved one lymph node basin, the results demonstrated a 29.7% survival rate for treating metastases with an unknown primary melanoma.

In the series of 29 patients undergoing spontaneous regression reported by Bodurtha, 19 survived over five years (75%). Six of these 19 long-term survivors have died of recurrent metastatic melanoma. He states that spontaneous regression, although indicative of an improved prognosis, is therefore not synonymous with cure.

Six of nine patients of the Smith and Stehlin series[33] developed metastases and died in less than 5 years. In Milton's series, 17 of the 32 men and 2 of the 7 women have died, giving a survival rate of 51%.

One male in Milton's series had multiple small-bowel metastases, but lived free of evidence of his disease for over five years. The outcome of this case is not stated. Milton notes that several other patients showed temporary regression or retrogression for up to 18 months, but the disease finally proved fatal.

These figures justify an adequate surgical attack upon melanoma metastatic locally to one group of lymph nodes in patients whose primary tumor is occult.

This is especially true for metastases to axillary and groin nodes. Since no cures were obtained for the 21 patients with metastases to the cervical nodes, the performance of a radical neck dissection does not seem warranted. If more than one group of nodes are invaded, or if extranodal metastases exist, surgical extirpation seems futile.

SUMMARY AND CONCLUSIONS

1. Metastatic melanoma with no known primary lesion (either a cryptic primary, or the primary melanoma has been biologically destroyed) has been observed in from 3.5% to 15% of patients in different series. One hundred eighteen instances were observed in a series of 3305 patients with melanoma seen at the Pack Medical Group, New York City.

2. An axillary dissection performed in 30 patients resulted in a 40% 10-year survival; a groin dissection performed in 24 patients yielded a 33% 10-year survival. These results are superior to those obtained for stage II melanoma with a known primary. A radical neck dissection for metastases to cervical nodes did not yield a single long-term survivor.

3. When extranodal metastases occurred, or

if several lymph node basins were involved, there were very few long-term survivors.

4. Biologic regression demonstrates the ability of the host in combatting the cancer. Careful critical evaluation of all metabolic factors may lead to biologic (hormonal, immunologic, etc.) methods of combatting malignant melanoma.

5. The existence of the phenomenon of biologic or spontaneous regression should caution against claims of "unusual cancer cures" by certain systemic treatments.

6. Attempts should be made to maintain and possibly enhance the host's natural immunity.

REFERENCES

1. Allen EP: Malignant melanoma, spontaneous regression after pregnancy. Br Med J 2:1067, 1955
2. Baker HW: Spontaneous regression of malignant melanoma. Am Surg 30:825–829, 1964
3. Beardmore GL: The epidemiology of malignant melanoma in Australia. In McCarthy WH (ed): Melanoma and Skin Cancer. Proceedings of the International Cancer Conference, Sydney, Government Printer, 1972, p 39
4. Bodurtha AJ: Spontaneous regression of malignant melanoma. In Clark WH et al. (eds): Human Malignant Melanoma, New York, Grune & Stratton, 1979, pp 227–241
5. Bodurtha AJ, Berkelhammer J, Kim YH, et al.: A clinical, histological and immunological study of a case of metastatic malignant melanoma undergoing spontaneous remission. Cancer 37:735–742, 1976
6. Booher RJ: Recognition and treatment of melanoma. Surg Clin of N Am 49:389, 1969
7. Boyd W: The Spontaneous Regression of Cancer. Charles C Thomas, Springfield Ill, 1966, pp 15–24
8. Boyd W: Spontaneous regression of cancer. J Can Radiol 8:45–49, 1957
9. Bulkley GB, Cohen MH, Banks PM, et al.: Long-term spontaneous regression of malignant melanoma with visceral metastases. Cancer 36:485–494, 1974
10. Cochran AJ, Diehl V, Stjernsward J: Regression of primary malignant melanoma associated with a good prognosis despite metastases to lymph nodes. Rev Eur Etudes Clin Biol 15:969–972, 1970

11. Conley J, Hamaker RC: Melanoma of the head and neck. Laryngoscope 87:760–764, 1977

12. Conley J, Lattes R, Orr W: Desmoplastic malignant melanoma (a rare variant of spindle cell melanoma). Cancer 28:914–986, 1971

13. Daland ME, Holmes JA: Malignant melanoma. N Engl J Med 220:651–660, 1939

14. Das Gupta T, Bowden L, Berg JW: Malignant melanoma of unknown primary origin. Surg Gynecol Obstet 117:341–345, 1963

15. Doyle JC, Bennet RC, Newing RK: Spontaneous regression of malignant melanoma. Med J Aust 2:551–552, 1973

16. Everson TC, Cole WH: Spontaneous Regression of Cancer. Philadelphia: WB Saunders, 1966, pp 1–10, 164–220

17. Foley WJ, Coon WW: Unusual clinical course in patients with malignant melanoma. Med J Aust 2:551–552, 1973

18. George PA, Fortner JG, Pack GT: Melanoma with pregnancy (a report of 115 cases). Cancer 13:854–859, 1960

19. Gromet MS, Epstein WL, and Blois MS: The regressing thin malignant melanoma, a distinctive lesion with metastatic potential. Cancer 42:2282–2292, 1978

20. Howes WE: Removal of testes in treatment of melanoma. JAMA 123:304, 1943

21. Levison VB: Spontaneous regression of a malignant melanoma. Br Med J 1:458–459, 1955

22. Malleson N: Spontaneous regression of malignant melanoma. Br Med J 1:668, 1955

23. Mastrangelo MJ, Kim YH, Bernstein RS, et al.: Clinical and histological correlation of melanoma regression after intralesional BCG therapy (a case report). J Natl Cancer Inst 52:19–24, 1974

24. Maurer LH, McIntyre OR, Rueckert F: Spontaneous regression of malignant melanoma. Am J Surg 127:397–403, 1974

25. Medical Journal of Australia editorial. Med J Aust 2:761, 1975

26. McGovern VJ: Spontaneous regression of melanoma. Pathology 7:91–99, 1975

27. Milton GW: Malignant Melanoma of the Skin and Mucous Membrane. London, Churchill, Livingstone, 1977, pp 153–156

28. Mundth ED, Guralnick EA, Raker JW: Malignant melanoma; a clinical study of 427 cases. Ann Surg 162:15, 1965

29. Pack GT: Note on the experimental use of rabies vaccine for melanomatosis. Arch Dermatol Syphilol 62:694–695, 1950

30. Pack GT, Gerber DM, Sharnagel JM: End results in the treatment of malignant melanoma. Ann Surg 136:905–911, 1952

31. Pack GT, Miller TR: Metastatic melanoma with inter-determinate primary site. Report of two instances of long-term survival. JAMA 176:55, 1961

32. Shimkin MB, Boldrey EB, Kelly KH, et al.: Effects of surgical hypophysectomy in a man with malignant melanoma. J Clin Endocrinol 12:439–453, 1952

33. Smith JL, and Stehlin JS: Spontaneous regression of primary malignant melanoma with regional metastases. Cancer 18:1399, 1965

34. Stewart FW: Experiences in spontaneous regression of neoplastic disease in man. Tex Rep Biol Med 10:239–253, 1952

35. Sumner WC: Spontaneous regression of melanoma. Cancer 6:1040–1043, 1953

36. Sumner WC, Foraker AG: Spontaneous regression of human melanoma: Clinical and experimental studies. Cancer 13:79–81, 1960

37. Wallace DC, Beardmore GL, Exton LA: Familial malignant melanoma. Ann Surg 177:15–20, 1973

38. Wallace DC, Exton LA: Genetic predisposition to development of malignant melanoma. In McCarthy WH (ed): Melanoma and Skin Cancer. Proceedings of the International Cancer Conference. Sydney, Government Printer, 1972, pp 65–81

CHAPTER EIGHT

IMMUNITY IN MALIGNANT MELANOMA

MYRON ARLEN, ARIEL HOLLINSHEAD
AND JOSEPH SCHERRER

Malignant melanoma remains a highly unpredicable and virulent tumor in spite of attempts at early detection, radical surgery, active combination chemotherapy and the use of nonspecific immunotherapy.[12] Recurrence can usually be expected in most patients where clinical nodal disease is present or penetration into Clark's dermal levels IV and V are noted histologically.[28] This virulent behavior is seen in spite of suggestions that an active host tumor relationship exists. Lesions may be noted to regress with zones of depigmentation resulting, or on rare occasions may be associated with spontaneous regression.[4] Long latent periods greater than ten years have been noted between initial therapy and recurrence; in spite of this picture of host resistance, eventual dissemination of disease is usually the rule.

Recent attempts at enhancement of the immune response in patients with clinically recurring melanoma have invariably been unsuccessful with regard to long-term survival. Radiated tumor cells have produced some questionable alterations in tumor growth.[35] The use of Bacillus, Calmette, and Guerin (BCG) administered by scarification and intradermal injection suggests that there may be a potentiating effect on cellular re-activity to both primary and recall antigens.[19] BCG, however, has failed to produce any form of consistant tumor regression, as had been hoped for initially. In some instances, tumor growth increased.[36]

TUMOR–ASSOCIATED ANTIGENS

As a clearer understanding of the mechanisms of tumor rejection has evolved, more direct approaches towards controlling this disease have been initiated. We now look for specific active immunotherapeutic effects using newly isolated cell membrane antigens as an ancillary measure in obtaining sought-after responses.[27] Initial studies now suggest that tumor control can be improved.

In animal systems, antigens isolated from tumor membrane can be shown to be tumor-specific after separation from various other membrane fraction (fetal, viral, tissue specific, transplantation antigens, etc). These antigens can demonstrate protection in inoculated animals against growth of transplanted tumor cells. In humans, the identification of probable tumor-specific antigen fractions have been possible only through the use of in vitro experiments such as delayed cutaneous hypersensitivity reactions; this has necessitated use of the term "tumor-associated antigen" (TAA), probably comparable to the tumor-specific antigen of animal models.

Early attempts at identifying and isolating antigens and the products they elicited were relatively crude. In 1956, Koysakov and Korosteleva[33] suggested a method for obtaining organ-specific and anticancer sera, removing nonspecific antibodies by selective tissue absorption. Rabbits were immunized with saline extracts from liver metastasis of tumors obtained from varying primary sites. Complement fixation tests were employed, appearing to indicate that the capacity of the tumor to react with appropriate sera depended on specific antigens adherent on the tumor itself. The presence of possible tumor antigens was further postulated by Hellstrom, who demonstrated that lymphoid cells from neuroblastoma patients inhibited formation of colonies of tumor cells in tissue culture. He demonstrated that cross-reactivity with these lymphocytes occurred with autologous tumor cells, suggesting recognition of a tumor antigen.

Southam[51] described three types of clinical experiments that appeared to bear on the question of cancer-specific antigens:

1. Homotransplantation of human cancerous cell lines in healthy volunteers yielded iso-antibodies that reacted with cancer cells but rarely reacted with normal cells.

2. Treatment of acute leukemia patients with autologous leukemia cell extracts while in hematologic remission, caused development of skin sensitivity of the immediate wheal and erythema type to intradermal injections of the same autogenous extract.

3. Comparison of growth from quantitated autotransplants of cancer cells, with and without the admixture of autologous leukocytes or plasma, demonstrated that cancer cell growth was often inhibited by the leukocytes and occasionally by the plasma.

TUMOR ANTIGENS AND MALIGNANT MELANOMAS

The question of defining tumor antigens specifically related to malignant melanoma arose in experiments described by Morton[43] in 1968, and later by Lewis[38] in 1969. Utilizing immunofluorescent techniques, antibodies to melanoma cells were identified in serum from tumor patients. The anti-melanoma antibodies were demonstrated in all patients where serum was tested against their own melanoma and in 61% of homologous serum, suggesting that most melanoma cells contained a common tumor antigen. Lewis noted evidence of two groups of antibodies in patients with malignant melanoma. One of these antibodies reacted with cytoplasmic constituants of the tumor cell and was found in all patients with melanoma; the second was apparently directed against a surface antigen unique to each tumor cell line. Savel[49] reported using in vitro lymphocyte transformation as a measure of autosensitization to

tumor extracts. In one patient with malignant melanoma, whose neoplasm had spontaneously regressed, lymphocytes responded slightly to an extract of the primary tumor. Jehn[30] (1970) found that lymphocytes obtained from seven patients with melanoma were stimulated when cultured in vitro with extracts of autologous tumor. Lymphocytes from normal persons did not respond to these tumor extracts. This suggested that previous sensitization to a melanoma antigen had occurred. The mitogenic material in the tumor fluid had the electrophoretic mobility of a beta globulin and could be separated from the bulk of melanoma pigment by starch bloc electrophoresis. Urine was also found to contain protein that was mitogenic in the presence of lymphocytes from patients with melanoma. Gel diffusion analysis using rabbit antiserum against tumor and urinary mitogen showed that these substances were antigenetically identical.

Carrel[7] described evidence for tumor-associated antigens in melanoma patients by preparing rabbit antiserum to concentrated lyophyllized urine from these patients. In essence, his preparation was similar to the mitogenic material isolated by Jehn. This antiserum reacted in double diffusion or single radial diffusion tests with concentrated urine samples from other melanoma patients, but failed to react with normal urine samples. Such experiments were felt to indicate the presence of a common antigen in the tumor, which was excreted into the patients' urine. It was not certain, however, whether these tumor-associated antigens were tissue- or tumor-specific. A possible embryonic origin was suggested since cross-reactivity occurred with three nonmelanoma urine samples. Two were from patients with neuroblastoma and one from a patient with ganglioneuroma.

Cutaneous hypersensitivity reactions toward autologous extracts of melanoma were later studied by Fass.[13] In order to clarify the possible existence of tumor antigens specifically related to the melanoma cell, crude membrane extracts were used for testing delayed skin hypersensitivity. Three patients with localized melanoma gave positive skin reactions and five with metastatic disease gave negative skin reactions. This suggested the reaction to be specific for identifying an immune system that had been in previous contact with melanoma but that failed as dissemination of tumor occurred. Stewart[53] evaluated the nature of this delayed hypersensitivity reaction towards extracts of malignant tumor. The reactivity did not appear to arise in nuclear material or from bacterial toxins but appeared to represent a reaction toward a fraction of the tumor cell membrane. A correlation was noted between delayed cutaneous hypersensitivity reactions towards extracts of malignant tumors and stromal infiltrate by lymphocytes. This was felt to represent a cell-mediated defense mechanism (although not an effective one) against growth and spread of tumor. In culture it has been noted that sensitized allogenic lymphocytes (originating from genetically different individuals within the same species) aggregate around tumor cells and later may produce cell destruction (Rosenau[48]), but that in general, cytotoxicity more likely represents nonspecific lymphocyte reactivity enhanced by stimulation with agents such as PPD or BCG, followed by a second step involving specific immunologic recognition (Helm and Pearlman[22]).

Hellstrom, in studying the effect of lymphocytes on target tissue cells in microcytotoxicity assay,* found that when a high ratio of lymphocytes to target tumor cells were used, no difference could be found in the cytotoxic effect from patients with growing melanoma or from patients who had become tumor-free following therapy.[21] When titrations were employed with various lymphocyte doses per chamber well it became apparent that patients with advanced melanomas were less reactive than were patients with a small tumor load. At this time, the coating of lymphocytes by blocking substances secreted off the tumor membrane was not fully appreciated.

---

* An assay where cultured tumor cells are incubated separately with serum and lymphocytes in an attempt to determine whether cytotoxicity from cellular or humoral factors exists.

The effect that tumor antigens have had on producing delayed cutaneous hypersensitivity appears for the most part related to lymphocyte response to tumor membrane protein. Eight patients with varying stages of malignant melanoma were tested by DeGast (1970).[10] Three patients with localized tumor gave positive skin reactions; those with metastatic disease gave negative reactions. One might interpret this as an indication of a weakened immune system in the presence of metastatic disease, so that the skin response becomes anergic. In 25 patients studied by Arlen and Hollinshead, the hypersensitivity reaction was positive, regardless of the stage of disease encountered. In each case allogeneic purified tumor-associated antigen (TAA) from melanoma membrane was utilized for skin testing. Only as the patient reached the end stages of the disease did the failure to respond become evident. In some instances, patients with clinical stage 1 disease have also appeared unresponsive to skin testing. This may be due to a tumor burden so minimal that the immune system has failed to recognize it. It may also represent an inherent defect in the antigen employed for skin testing that the host is to recognize. Stewart found that about one-fourth of patients with carcinomas and sarcomas gave delayed cutaneous skin reactions in response to intradermal innoculation of autologous tumor cell extracts. Herberman and Oren[23,24] did skin tests with membrane extracts of leukemia and lymphoma cells and obtained positive responses in 72% of patients.

Factors Contributing to Skin Reactivity. Various factors appear to contribute to skin reactivity and probably involve:

1. The purity of the antigen being tested
2. Circulating blocking antibodies
3. Coating of T-cells by blocking factors
4. Inhibitory antigens removed along with the tumor-associated antigen used in the skin testing

In 19 Ugandan patients with melanoma that Ziegler[58] evaluated, he found no gross impairment of humoral or cellular host-immune mechanisms, regardless of the extent of disease. This seems to fit more in line with present concepts that loss of host immunity occurs late in the course of disease and only after metastasis has appeared. A similar conclusion was arrived at by Stein et al.,[52] in a group of 225 breast carcinoma cases that included 104 operable, 44 locally advanced inoperable, and 44 with demonstrable metastatic dissemination. Parameters of immune reactivity included PPD (purified protein derivitive), DNCB (dinitrochlorobenzene), PHA transformation (phytohemagglutinin), E-rosette formation, and lymphocyte counts. Immune competence was not affected by metastatic involvement of regional nodes nor in patients with occult metastatic dissemination (as determined in retrospect). Since tumor dissemination preceded impairment of general immunoincompetence, it emerged as the cause, rather than the result of immunosuppression.

IDENTIFICATION OF TUMOR-ASSOCIATED ANTIGEN

Purification of antigenic material initially alluded to in the studies of Lewis, Jehn, and other investigators has been recently accomplished by Hollinshead.[25,26] Two separate skin reactive antigens were found in separate fractions obtained from Sephadex G-200 filtration. Gradient polyacrylamide gel electrophoresis produced further purification of the fractions (Fig. 8-1). Sephadex fraction II PAGE region (A) produced positive delayed skin hypersensitivity reactions in 43/49 (88%) of early systemic and occular melanomas as compared with 1/32 (3%) in other types of cancer. Fraction III region (B) contained more broadly reactive antigens, giving positive skin reactions in 9/21 (43%) of patients with early melanoma and 13/18 (72%) with advanced stages of melanoma. It also produced positive skin tests responses in patients with breast cancer 5/6, although negative tests were seen in a variety of other cancer types. The appearance of reactivity to these separated antigens indicates that blocking or inhibitory factors may be present in unfractionated

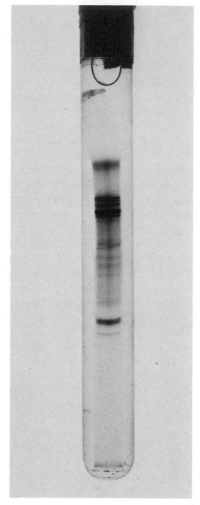

FIGURE 8-1. Fractionation of tumor antigen by gradiemt polyacrilamide gel electrophoresis from Sephadex fraction 1B.

material, which prevent the appearance of skin reactivity and which are removed during purification of the antigenic material.

ACTIVE TUMOR IMMUNOTHERAPY

In Russia, active tumor immunotherapy has existed since 1956. A current form of therapy used in treating melanoma patients (Gorodilova[18]) includes the use of polysacchride complexes extracted from melanoma membrane. A comparison of these extracts with those obtained by Hollinshead showed similarity between the glycolipoprotein of PAGE region (A) and the glycolipoprotein present in the Russian antigenic material. Further analysis using double-diffusion Agarose plates to define precipiten patterns against rabbit melanoma tumor-associated antigens (TAA) antiserum revealed that the USSR extract was serologically identical to the U.S. melanoma TAA. As a means of gaining information regarding host responses to tumor-associated antigen, various parameters in addition to skin reactivity have been considered. In-vitro lymphocyte function, T-cell, B-cell, lymphocyte migration, and colony inhibition, all provide some degree of important information.

IN VITRO MEASUREMENTS OF HOST IMMUNITY

DeGast[10] reported on in-vitro lymphocyte function in patients with different clinical stages of malignant melanoma. Lymphocytes were isolated by Isopaque-Ficoll gradient centrifugation, cultured in Eagles medium and incubated for three days with phytohemagglutinin (PHA), Hemocyanin, Diptheria toxoid and Tetanus toxoid. Reactivity of lymphocytes in patients with stage III disease was significantly lower than that of other stages of disease. Sixty-four percent of patients without lymphocyte reactivity to three test antigens showed tumor recurrence or progression within six months, against 3% of patients with lymphocyte response.

Enhancement of blastogenic response had been reported by Gerovich,[17] using specific active immunization with nonirradiated autologous and irradiated cultured allogeneic melanoma cells. Immunization with 10^6 through 8×10^7 tumor cells were carried out in draining areas of BCG scarification on day 7. Six of 11 patients had a significant increase in the blastogenic response, lasting 7—10 days.

Sequential assays for cell-mediated reactivity (CMR) serum-blocking factors, have

been performed in melanoma patients using microcytotoxicity assays and dilute agar colon inhibition tests. Currie et al.[9] found that autoimmunization of patients with an irradiated suspension of their own tumor cells resulted in the appearance of cytotoxic lymphocytes in five of 12 patients studied. Modification of the cytotoxicity assays have been described using the release of chromium-51 or Iododeoxurydine-125 from labelled tissue culture target cells (according to McCox[40] and Oldham,[45] respectively).

There have been a number of criticisms of the techniques and interpretation of results with microcytotoxicity testing. According to Herberman and Oldham, there is little question that normal human microcytotoxicity reactivity does exist; however, the reactivity of the lymphocytes from cancer patients may not be entirely directed against histologic-type tumor-associated antigens. One must carefully analyze the information obtained in evaluating the nature of the experimental model being employed. Herberman[23] suggested setting up an experiment involving a large checkerboard design with lymphocytes from several patients with different histologic types, from patients with benign disease of the same organs, and from several normal individuals tested almost an equally large array of target cells, derived from various types of cancer and normal cells.

THERAPEUTIC MODALITIES

It is felt that the use of tumor-associated antigen derived from melanoma cell membrane, when employed as a vaccine in melanoma patients who displayed delayed cutaneous hypersensitivity to test doses of antigen, will probably enhance their immunologic mechanism. This approach has been used by Stewart, Harris, and Hollinshead[54] in patients with primary bronchogenic carcinoma. They have reported results in a group of patients whose disease has been controlled for up to 42 months, using a combination of immunochemotherapy—high dose Methotrexate and innoculation with purified lung cancer antigen. The latter was prepared after separating extraneous cell surface antigen, histocompatability antigens and inhibitory or blocking antigens. The purified tumor-associated antigen was delivered in combination with complete Freund's adjuvant to allow gradual release over several months.

The value of using purified antigen is "to give the white blood cells a straight message without confusing them with messages put out by extraneous substances" found in ground-up tumor material (Hollinshead).

Sharma[50] studied the parameters for generating such cytotoxic lymphocytes against tumors; maximal cell-mediated cytoxic responses were produced in vitro using $2-4 \times 10^4$ tumor cells and 1×10^6 leukocytes after a five-day incubation period. Further increase in the number of stimulating cells usually suppressed immunization of lymphocytes. It was felt that the immunosuppression noted with larger numbers of tumor cells was due to synthesis and release of an immunosuppressor, supporting the inhibitory antigen concept described by Hollinshead. Cell-free extracts and tissue culture supernatants of certain murine tumor cells have been reported to be immunosuppressive in vitro again, suggesting liberation of a blocking factor into the serum.

The concept of immune enhancement as a means of controlling melanoma not amenable to surgical resection, appears clinically well founded at the present time. In addition to evidence supporting host recognition of melanoma antigen, evaluation of cases demonstrating spontaneous regression of melanoma corroborated the existence of human immune mechanisms in the destruction of existing tumor. Bodurtha et al.[5] reported on a patient with biopsy-proven recurrent melanoma who was observed to manifest clinical regression of disease. Biopsy of regressed areas showed:

1. Absence of malignant melanoma cells in basal layers of epidermis with relative increase in basal layer clear cells.
2. Dermal inflammatory reactions with lymphocyte infiltrate melanophages and degenerative malignant melanocytes.
3. Dermal reactive vascular proliferation and interstitial edema progressing to repairative dermal fibrosis.

Using a microcytotoxicity assay with two established allogenic melanoma cell cultures as target cells, a statistically significant increase in lymphocyte cytotoxicity values was observed over the clinical time course of regression. No significant serum cytotoxic or serum-blocking effects were detectable. The et al. further demonstrated active phagocytosis of metastatic melanoma cells in a lymph node imprint of a patient having undergone spontaneous regression.[56]

THERAPEUTIC TRIALS

Attempts at clinical enhancement of the immune system as a means of controlling melanoma began more than seven decades ago. Fowler[16] studied the end results produced by infection and toxin (Coley), and found many instances of regression and prolonged survival. Reviewed cases dating to the turn of the century were grouped into three series:

Series A: 3 operable, 17 inoperable with recurrent infection fever, acute inflammation or transfusion reaction
Series B: Operable toxin-treated - 14 cases
Series C: Inoperable toxin-treated - 14 cases

Thirteen of the 20 infection cases and nine of the 28 toxin-treated cases remained free from further evidence of melanoma 5 to 56 years after onset. The average survival of the 28 toxin-treated cases was over three times the expected survival for this neoplasm. Occasional reports have also appeared over the last few decades associating infection with regression of disease (DePace and Pack[46]). More direct attempts at immune enhancement have been made by altering the tumor through the use of radiated tumor cells (Kremetz). Passive immunotherapy seemed promising in the 1960s. Finney[14] immunized one patient having melanoma and two sarcoma patients using homogenized tumor cells prepared in Freund's adjuvent. Increased cytotoxic antibodies were noted following serum fractionation. Cross-transfusion as a means of controlling melanoma was employed by Sumner and Foraker,[55] using blood from a donor undergoing spontaneous remission; the treated patient also demonstrated tumor regression. Nadler and Moore[44] utilized cross-transplantation of tumor as a means of inducing an antibody response. Cross-transfusion with the development of an immune serum was then used to obtain tumor regression. Kremetz et al.[34] applied this technique to patients with melanoma using cross-immunization followed by cross-transfusion with plasma and leukocytes. There was an indication of tumor regression but not one significant enough to allow the technique to be expanded in depth.

Numerous investigators continued using sensitized or nonspecifically stimulated lymphocytes with minimal results. Moore and Gerner[41] attempted to increase the ratio of lymphocytes to tumor cells in order to improve tumor kill by employing larger number of autologous or allogeneic cultured lymphocytes. Of 31 patients studied, two received over 300 gm of autologous lymphocytes and showed some significant remissions. Fisher[15] reviewed lymphocyte immunotherapy in experimental tumor systems. This study concerned the effects of sensitized autologous, allogeneic, and xenogeneic lymphocytes on small transplanted tumors, on isogeneic hosts and on the growth of cells from such tumors innoculated into appropriate syngeneic recipients. Despite the variety of therapeutic regimens, the study failed to demonstrate that the employment of such cells influenced tumor growth.

CHEMOTHERAPY

In terms of melanoma therapy, the failure of clinical immunotherapy to achieve control of disease led to a more concerted attack with combination chemotherapy.[32] In a study of 73 patients at the University of California, primary and combination drug therapy using IUPR, FUDR, BCNU, Hydroxyurea, Vincristine, etc., failed to give a satisfactory response. TMAC -Tri- methyl colchicinic acid methylethyl d-tartrate produced regression in 6 of 29 patients. In separate studies, DTIC was shown to produce a similar rate of temporary tumor regression. To date, there has been no

effective methods for controlling recurrent or metastatic tumor except when localized to an extremity. This has led to further attempts at active immunotherapy, using tumor cell vaccines.

CRUDE TUMOR PREPARATIONS

In 1960, Finney et al. reported on irradiation of metastatic tumor deposits leading to increased antitumor antibody titers by tanned red cell hemoglutination. Similar increases in antibody titers were reported by Blakemore and McKenna,[3] using fluorocarbon extracts from melanoma for attempted immunization. Kremetz et al. reported on the use of repeated intradermal injection of irradiated autologous and allogeneic tumor cells carried in tissue culture. One patient had regression of tumor lasting 3½ years. Ikonoposiv[29] immunized 13 melanoma patients with irradiated autologous cells obtained by biopsy. While high titers of cytotoxic and immunofluorescent antibodies were demonstrated, no apparent effect on the course of disease was noted.

Finely minced tumor suspension refined and concentrated to yield a supernatant fraction termed Vaccine II was employed by Jewell et al.[31] in patients with stage II and III melanoma. All responses were noted in intradermal or subcutaneous disease except for one patient with a 3 cm lesion of the frontal bone, which disappeared on transfer factor therapy. A comparison survival in 44 high-risk melanomas receiving therapy appeared two times the rate expected from a comparison of 230 patients from the Ellis Fischel Hospital.

NONSPECIFIC IMMUNOTHERAPY

In the past decade, there has been a resurgence in the use of bacterial products. Morton[42] described 40 patients with metastatic melanoma treated by surgical resection of metastasis and then BCG immunotherapy. The rational for the use of BCG was that the drug appeared to have antitumor activity mediated through nonspecific stimulation of the immune system and that, if administered into the lesion, could cause a high rate of regression. In the surgical group given BCG, it appeared that this agent might have some effect on the incidence of subsequent recurrence. In a separate group of 84 patients with stage II disease, 64% remained free of recurrence when immunotherapy followed surgical resection, compared with 36% when surgery alone was employed.[12] Of those treated by operation alone, 50% had recurrence in four months. The median time to recurrence in the group treated with surgery and BCG was ten months. Little if any effect was noted in patients having systemic disease.

ACTIVE SPECIFIC IMMUNIZATION

The effects of active specific immunization with the addition of nonirradiated autologous and irradiated cultured allogeneic melanoma cells, in cell-associated immunity, was studied by Gerovich et al.[17] Eleven patients with widespread disease who were receiving immunotherapy were studied. Immunization was carried out with $1 \times 10^6 - 8 \times 10^7$ tumor cells introduced into an area of BCG scarification. Five of the 11 patients showed signs of delayed cutaneous hypersensitivity toward autologous tumor cells at a separated test site following immunization. Currie and coworkers found the appearance of cytotoxic lymphocytes in 5 of 12 melanoma patients after immunization with an irradiated suspension of their own tumor cells. The use of BCG therapy as an adjuvent to the stimulation of the immune system has not been entirely innocuous. Some undesirable side effects have been seen, particularly after intralesional injection. Accelerated growth of tumor has been reported by Bernstein and associates[2] and by Levy et al.[37] and hepatic complications have been noted by Bordurtha.[5] A possible explanation of tumor enhancement may lie in the fact that the immunosystem is not suppressed completely, but that blocking substances elaborated by the tumor decreased lymphocyte reactivity. Stimulation, under such circumstances, may therefore enhance recognition of blocking or inhibitory substances, resulting in enhancement of tumor growth. This has been noted clinically in patients with medullary carcinoma of the breast where increased lymphocyte reactivity within the tumor appears associated with enhanced growth of the tumor and a higher incidence of lymph node metastasis.[1]

As a means of obviating some of the problems associated with intradermal and intralesional BCG, MacGregor et al.[39] have reported on the use of oral BCG in 47 patients with varying stages of melanoma. The results appeared to indicate that there may be a delay in the development of local recurrence and distant metastasis when localized disease is treated. In patients with disseminated melanoma but without intracranial metastasis the survival rate was increased from 4 to 12.7 months.

With the ability to purify tumor-associated antigen glycolipoprotein from melanoma membrane, and with evidence for the ability to demonstrate delayed cutaneous hypersensitivity in such patients, clinical trials were undertaken to study the effect of the antigen on patients with recurrent disease. Such trials are now in progress (Arlen, Hollinshead, Scherrer) and appear to demonstrate control of disease not previously seen when other forms of immunotherapy have been employed. The study of such patients was approved by the Institutional Clinical Research Committee; patients were informed of the nature of their disease and gave proper consent before trials were begun.

In the presence of an adequate skin response, all patients were challenged with 500 μg of antigen given at three locations on their forearm. Four weeks later, they were given a second dose of antigen, mixed with Freund's adjuvent to enhance and prolong the antigeneic stimulation. Fifteen patients with recurrent or extensive tumors were treated over a 12- to 24-month period; each received two to four sensitizing doses of antigen (500 μg). Five patients died from their disease, three having brain metastasis at the time that the study was initiated. Of the 11 patients who have remained alive and on maintenence therapy, six are clinically free of disease. One had pulmonary metastasis that regressed; three others showed regression of nodal disease. One patient with extensive pelvic tumor had regression of visceral seeding, which allowed later resection of a localized necrotic tumor mass.

PREPARATION OF VACCINE

Separation, identification, purification and analysis of antigenic material used in the present study was carried out by removing tumor by biopsy, washing it immediately mincing the tissue mass in physiologic saline, washing it several times and separating cells by use of 60-mesh stainless steel sieves and aspiration through wide-bore 50 ml pipettes. In this procedure, as in all that follow sterility monitored by placing a drop of appropriate material on both blood agar and thioglycolate. The dispersed single cell suspension is counted in three columns of two hemocytometers; three counts of the cells are made using white blood cell diluent, trypan blue and neutral red and viable cell count is determined. The single-cell suspension is then frozen (–70 C) and thawed, and isotonic to hypotonic saline membrane extraction is performed using a modified Davies procedure. The single-cell suspension is centrifuged for 10 minutes at 2500 rpm in an IEC low-speed refrigerated centrifuge and the supernatant retained. The pellet is suspended in 10:1 v/v and again centrifuged at 2500 rpm. This resuspension and those following are carried out twice at 0.14M NaCl and 0.07M NaCl. Supernatants are retained at each step, pooled and centrifuged in a Beckman L3–50 Ultracentrifuge at 100,000 × g. The supernatant is discarded and the pellet of membrane material is washed from the tubes and resuspended in physiological saline. Membrane protein is measured at this point by the Lowry method. The material is examined by electromicroscopy to assess the membrane pieces and the lack of nuclear material. In addition, HLA determinations of whole cells and membranes are made by the chromium release cytotoxicity method using a broadly reactive serum so that quantitation of membrane components

can be calculated prior to further study. The suspension of membrane material is then subjected to sequential low-frequency (9 kc/sec) sonification in a Raytheon model DF-101 Sonic Oscillator. Centrifugation with retention of the supernatant and resuspension of the membrane pellet is carried out for one hour at 100,000 × g after each interval sonification period; the sonification periods consist of 3 min, 4½ min, and 6 min, for respective progressive intervals. The supernatants are pooled and termed the soluble pool of membrane protein, and a Lowry protein determination is made. This soluble pool is then concentrated by Diaflo ultrafiltration (Amicon) to adjust the protein concentration of the sample to approximately 100 μg protein in per 0.1 ml, which is a concentration well suited to our further procedures. Samples with protein in excess of this concentration are diluted. The sample is then subjected to one or more methods of separation.

Sephadex G-200 columns are prepared to accomodate the amount of protein obtained. The columns are washed with 0.01M phosphate buffer for several hours and the void volume determined using Dextrane blue. The next day the soluble sonicates are separated over Sephadex gels, 2 ml fractions collected and the profile recorded at 220 and 280 mu. Fractions are pooled according to protein peaks and the pools concentrated by Diaflo ultrafiltration. In all of these steps, the materials are kept at 0 C or 40 C except for the column separation, which is conducted at room temperature, with collection of eluates at 4 C in an automatic fraction collector. Standard purified proteins are separated on identical columns for molecular weight calculations. The following day, any concentrations that were not accomplished the previous day are completed and all of the material tested by the Lowry procedure for protein content. Each fraction is either diluted or further concentrated in order to have fractions of required protein for further study. Separate equipment and separate hoods are used for handling normal tissue.

Gradient polyacrylamide (discontinuous) gel electrophoresis is used for further purification. The apparatus we employ is not available from any one company, since our methodology requires a different combination of power source and gel bath. A L:1:2 gel solution is made by mixing gel buffer, distilled water and the appropriate gel solution. This mixture is added to and mixed with an equal volume of the ammonium persulfate solution immediately before preparing the column. This final catalyzed solution is then layered with flat end 23ga needle into the gel tube as follows (gel tubes are immersed in a 1:200 dilution of Kodak Photo Flow 200 and air-dried prior to use): 10% or 12%, 7%, 4.75%, and 3.5% gel solution are layered carefully to avoid mixing. Distilled water is layered onto the 3.5% gel to the top of the tube (12 cm) to allow polymerization. This water is removed by shaking prior to use (at least 40 min must be allowed for complete polymerization. Greater reproducibility is obtained if the gels are allowed to age > 12 hours).

Prepared gels are placed in the upper chamber gronmets of a Canalco Model 122 ion bath. The upper and lower chambers of the bath are then filled with chamber buffer, insuring that air bubbles are removed from the loading section of the gels tube (upper (−) portion). A drop of tracking dye (Bromophenol Blue in NaOH at pH 8.3), is added to the upper chamber to follow the extent of migration of the leading ion front. A few grains of sucrose are added to the sample to insure that it is heavier than the chamber buffer. The chamber is then carefully loaded onto the top of the 3.5% gel by means of a Hamilton microliter glass syringe. Electrophoresis is carried out using a Buchler Model 3-1155 Voltage and current regulated power supply in the constant current mode. To each column 4ma are applied and the gels run from cathode to anode. A typical gel run takes 75 to 80 minutes.

After the run, gels are removed from their tubes by means of rimming with a finely tapered needle with injection of water between the gel and the tube wall as needed. The gels are then ready for staining or for cutting and eluting protein from appropriate regions. Some of the stains employed are Coomassie Brilliant Blue, nonspecific protein stain: Oil Red O, a lipoprotein stain, and Periodic Acid Schiff

stain, a carbohydrate stain. Accurate drawings are made and photographs are taken during every study.

To prepare material for careful analysis, soluble sonicate of appropriate samples at a level of approximately 100 pg/0.1 ml are stained as a reference for further separation. Protein migration is monitored in subsequent unstained gels by scanning at 280 nm with a Gelmain ACD–15 densitometer. Relative concentration of TAA to total soluble membrane protein is then quantitated by scanning stained gels at 610 nm on the same instrument. Unstained gels are then sliced for precise regions. Gels are eluted with sterile saline at 4 C for 50 hours, concentrated by ultra-filtration, rediluted 100-fold, and reconcentrated in order to help eliminate any toxic dialyzable substances. With these new methods, recovery of material previously separated by Sephadex is often 50% to 100%; and since even amounts of 100 μg protein are applied to each column, a fairly uniform amount of protein is recovered for testing purposes, thus assuring a more standard preparation for cross-testing and for comparisons of several tests. The bands thus obtained from the different preparation are studied for their molecular weight determination, both by migration on the polyacrylamide gels in comparison with known proteins, and by their migration of the Sephadex columns in comparison with known standard curves of elution of known proteins. Further, the molecular weights of isolated purified proteins can be calculated from measurements of their sedimentation rates in a Beckman Model E analytical ultracentrifuge when sufficient amounts are available.

BLOCKING AND INHIBITORY SUBSTANCES

The weakened delayed cutaneous hypersensitivity response noted in many patients with advanced melanoma probably represents the effect of inhibitory factors elaborated by the tumor which block the normal immune response. Cummings et al.[8] evaluated cell-mediated reactivity and serum-blocking factors in 12 patients who were treated with one or both of the clinically available imidizole carboximide derivatives, DTIC or PIC mustard. Decreased levels of serum-blocking factor were seen with six patients while cell-mediated immunity was not significantly depressed.

Considering that reappearance of tumor in patients treated with TAA was possibly related to blocking or inhibitory factors, DTIC was added to the immunotherapy protocol that we have employed. All patients received 200 mg for five days prior to receiving antigen. The imidizole carboximide has been repeated every two months and the antigen given for the third time 12 weeks after the initial injection and eight weeks following the dose containing Freund's adjuvent. It now appears that an effective dose of antigen may be achieved with as little as 200–500 μg of TAA.

Other modalities of restoring the immune response to normal in conjunction with the use of active immunization may be considered. Levamisole has been utilized experimentally in attempts to restore lymphocyte reactivity. Renoux and Renoux[47] reported reduction of metastais from Lewis lung tumor in C57B1 mice. In humans there is no information to date that indicates metastatic disease may respond to therapy. Wache[57] and others showed the Levamisole effected DNA and RNA protein synthesis in human peripheral lymphocytes stimulated with mitogens. Thymosin may prove to be another method for restoring immuncompetance. Hardy et al.[20] performed in vitro studies suggesting that this agent may influence depressed host resistance by increasing T-cell-mediated immunity.

It may by necessary in anticipation of immunotherapy to physically remove blocking or inhibitory substances of humoral or cellular origin so that immune enhancement and antigenic recognition can be accomplished. Doyle et al.[11] found that blood cell separation followed by washing was an effective way to enhance lymphocyte response. Isolation of lymphocytes in a separator was able to unblock T-lymphocytes activity, as measured by PHA transformation and rosette formation. The results were similar to the unblocking of lymphocytes in patients with cancer using proteolytic enzymes such as "Brinase." Brown[6] suggested that plasmaphoresis could have a practical role in immunotherapy.

There is little question that immunotherapy has an important role in the management of patients with malignant melanoma and other neoplastic disorders. If immune suppression resulting from substances secreted from the tumor surface can decrease host reactivity, as has been reported, then removal of such factors is essential. In the protocol employed by Arlen, Hollinshead, and Scherrer, imidizole carboximide is utilized as a possible means of reducing such factors. It may eventually prove to be advantageous to employ cell separation, plasmaphoresis and/or intravenous proteolytic enzymes to accomplish this. At present, specific stimulation with known antigenic substances freed from inhibitory material appears to be required for proper development of a cell-mediated immune response. Combined treatment employing the surgical reduction of a tumor load, followed by chemotherapy and immunotherapy, appears to be the direction best suited for the management of patients with advanced malignant melanoma.

REFERENCES

1. Arlen M, Flores L, Elguezabal A, Lerowitz B, et al.: Nodal response in medullary carcinoma of the breast. Amer J Surg 131:263–266, 1976
2. Bernstein RS, Mastrangelo MJ, Sulit H: Immunotherapy of melanoma with BCG. Natl Can Inst Monogr 39:213, 1973
3. Blakemore WS, McKenna JM: Antibodies reactive with antigens derived from He La and JIII in patients with malignancies. Surg 52:213, 1962
4. Bodurtha AJ, Berkelhammer J, Kim, YH, et al.: A clinical, histologic, and immunologic study of a case of metastatic malignant melanoma undergoing spontaneous remission. Cancer 37:735 742, 1976
5. Bodurtha A, Kim YHM, Laucius JF: Hepatic granulomas and other hepatic lesions associ-

ated with BCG immunotherapy for cancer. Amer J Clin Pathol 61:747, 1974

6. Browne O, Bell J, Holland PDJ, Thornes RD: Plasmaphoresis and immunostimulation. Lancet July 1976, p 96

7. Carrel S, Thickloss L: Evidence for a tumor associated antigen in human malignant melanoma. Nature 242:609–10, 1973

8. Cummings FJ, Heppner GH, Calebrase P: Evaluation of cell mediated reactivity and serum blocking factors in melanoma patients on chemotherapy. Med Pediatr Oncol 1:195–206, 1975

9. Currie GA, Basham C: Serum mediated inhibition of the immunological reactions of the patient to his own tumor. Br J Cancer 26:427, 1972

10. DeGast GC, The TH, Schraffordt Koops H, et al.: Humoral and cell mediated immune response in patients with malignant melanoma. Cancer 36:1289–1298, 1975

11. Doyle JS, Bell J, Deasy P, Thornes RD: Activation or unblocking in on lymphocytes. Lancet Oct. 1974, p 959

12. Eilber FR, Morton DL, Holmes EC, Sparks FC, Ramming KP: Adjuvent immunotherapy with BCG in treatment of regional lymph node metastasis from malignant melanoma. N Engl J Med 294:237–240, 1976

13. Fass L, Ziegler JL, Herbsman RB, Kiryabwire JW: Cutaneous hypersensitivity reactions to autologous extracts of malignant melanoma cells. Lancet, Vol 15, 116–118, 1970

14. Finney JW, Byers EH, Wilson RH: Studies in tumor autoimmunity. Cancer Res 20:351, 1960

15. Fisher BM, Saffer EA, Fisher ER: Experience with lymphocyte immunotherapy in experimental tumor systems. Cancer 27:771, 1971

16. Fowler GA: Enhancement of natural resistance to malignant melanoma with special reference to the beneficial effects of concurrent infections or bacterial toxin therapy. Monogr NY Cancer Research Inst, 1968

17. Gerovich FG, Gutterman JV, Mavligit GM, Hersh EM: Active specific immunization in malignant melanoma. Med Pediatr Oncol 1:277–87, 1975

18. Gorodilova VV, Hollinshead AC: Melanoma antigens that produce cell mediated immune responses in melanoma patients: Joint US–USSR Study. Science 190:391–92, 1973

19. Gutterman JV, McBride C, Freireich EJ: Active immunotherapy with BCG for recurrent malignant melanoma. Lancet 1:1208, 1973

20. Hardy MA, Freund M, Friedman N: In-vitro effect of thymosin on T-cells from immunodepressed surgical patients. Surgery 80:238–45, 1976

21. Hellstrom I, Hellstrom KE, Sjogren HO: Demonstration of cell mediated immunity to human neoplasm of various types. Int J Cancer 7:1–16, 1971

22. Helm G, Pearlman P: Cytoxic potential of stimulated human lymphocytes. J Exp Med 125:721–736, 1967

23. Herberman RB, Oldham RK: Problems associated with study of cell mediated immunity to human tumors by microcytotoxicity assays. J Nat Cancer Inst 55:749–753, 1975

24. Herberman RB, Oren ME: Delayed cutaneous hypersensitivity reactions to membrane extracts of human tumor cells. Clin Research 17:403, 1969

25. Hollinshead AC: Analysis of soluble melanoma cell membrane antigens in primary melanoma. Cancer 36:1282–1288, 1975

26. Hollinshead AC, Herberman RB, Jaffurs WJ, et al.: Soluble membrane antigens of human malignant melanoma cells. Cancer 34:1235–1243, 1974

27. Hollinshead AC, McCammon JR, Yohn DS: Immunogenicity of a soluble membrane antigen from adenovirus 12 induced tumor cells demonstrated in inbred hamsters. (PD-4). Can J Microbiol 18:1365–1369. 1972

28. Huvos AG, Shah JP Mike V: Prognostic factors in cutaneous melanoma. Hum Pathol 5:347–57, 1974.

29. Ikonopisov RL, Lewis MG, Hunter-Craig ID, et al.: Autoimmunization with irradiated tumor cells in malignant melanoma. Brit Med J 2:752–53, 1970

30. Jehn VW, Nathonson L, Schwartz RS, Skinner M: In-vitro lymphocytic stimulation by a soluble antigen from malignant melanoma. N Engl J Med 283:329–33, 1970

31. Jewell WR, Thomas JH, Starchi JM, et al.: Critical analysis of treatment of Stage II and Stage III melanoma patients with immunotherapy. Ann Surg 183:543–48, 1976

32. Johnson FD, Jacobs EM: Chemotherapy of metastatic malignant melanoma. Cancer 27:1306–12, 1971

33. Kosyakov PN, Korosteleva VS: Antigens specific for human tumors. Specific Tumor Antigens (IVAC Monograph), Munksgaard, Copenhagen, 1967

34. Krementz ET, Mansell PWA, Hormung MO, et al.: Immunotherapy of malignant disease; the

use of viable sensitized lymphocytes on transfer factor prepared from sensitized lymphocytes. Cancer 33:394, 1974

35. Krementz ET, Samuels MS, Wallace JH, Benes EN: Clinical experience in immunotherapy of cancer. Surg Gynecol Obstet 133:209, 1971

36. Laucius JF, Audley J, Bodurtha, AJ, et al.: BCG in the treatment of neoplastic disease. J Reticuloendothel Soc 16:347, 1974

37. Levy NL, Mahaley MS, Day ED: Serum mediated blocking of cell mediated antitumor immunity in a melanoma patient. Int J Cancer 10:244, 1972

38. Lewis MG, Ikonopisov RL: Tumor specific antibodies in human malignant melanoma. Brit Med J. 3:547–552. 1962

39. MacGregor AB, Falk RE, Landei S, et al.: Oral BCG immunostimulation on malignant melanoma. Surg Gynecol Obstet 141:747–54, 1975

40. McCoy JL, Herberman RB, Rosenberg EB: [51]Chromium release assay for all mediated cytotoxicity. Natl Can Inst Monogr 37:49–58, 1973

41. Moore GE, Gerner RE: Cancer immunity hypothesis and clonical trial of lymphocytotherapy for malignant diseases. Ann Surg 172:733, 1970

42. Morton DL, Eilber FR, Holmes EC: BCG immunotherapy of malignant melanoma. Ann Surg 180:635–643, 1974

43. Morton DL, Melmgren RA, Holmes EG, Ketcham A: Demonstration of antibodies against human malignant melanoma. Surgery 64:233–40, 1968

44. Nadler SH, Moore GE: Clinical immunologic study of malignant disease; response to tumor transplants and transfer of lymphocytes. Ann Surg 164:482, 1966

45. Oldham RK, Herberman RB: Evaluation of cell mediated cytotoxic reactivity against tumor associated antigens with ^{125}I-iododeoxyuridine labeled target cells. J Immunol 111:1871, 1973

46. Pack GT: Note on experimental use of rabies vaccine for melanomatosis. Arch Derm Syph 62:694, 1950

47. Renoux G, Renoux M: Levamisole inhibits and cures a solid malignant tumor and its pulmonary metastasis in mice. Nature 240:217, 1972

48. Rosenau W, Moon HD: Lysis of homologous cells by sensitized lymphocytes in tissue culture. J Nat Cancer Inst 27:471–77, 1961

49. Savel H: Effect of autologous tumor extracts on cultured human peripheral blood lymphocytes. Cancer 24:56–63, 1969

50. Sharma BS: In-vitro lymphocyte immunization to cultured human tumor cells. J Natl Can Inst 57:747–48, 1976

51. Southam CM: Evidence for clinical experiments for the existence of human cancer antigens. Specific Tumor Antigens (IVAC Monograph) 1967

52. Stein JA, Adler A, Ben Efraim S, Moar M: Immunocompetence, immunosuppression and human breast cancer. Cancer 38:1171–1187, 1976

53. Stewart THM: The presence of delayed cutaneous hypersensitivity reactions in patients toward cellular extracts of their malignant tumors. Cancer 23:1968–79, 1969

54. Stewart THM, Hollinshead AC, Harris JE: Immunochemotherapy of lung cancer. Ann NY Acad Sci, 1976

55. Sumner WC, Foraker AG: Spontaneous regression of human melanoma, clinical and experimental study. Cancer 13:79, 1960

56. The TH: Some recent developments in human tumor immunology. Neth J Med 15:279–290, 1972

57. Wache, KK: Effect of Levamisole and C reactive protein on mitogen stimulated lymphocytes in-vitro. Res Commun Chem Pathol Pharmacol 8:681, 1974

58. Ziegler JL, Lewis MG, Luyombya JMS, Kiryabwire JW: Immunologic studies in patients with malignant melanoma in Uganda. Br J Cancer 23:729–734, 1969

EXPLOITABLE PHYSIOLOGICAL CHARACTERISTICS ASSOCIATED WITH MALIGNANT MELANOMA GROWTH

VERNON RILEY, DARREL H. SPACKMAN,

MARY ANNE FITZMAURICE, AND

PHILLIP W. BANDA

Tumors are not merely aggregates of malignant cells replicating in the absence of effective host controls. They are auxiliary "organs" capable of inducing profound biochemical and physiological alterations, as well as imposing detrimental changes in the defense organs, cells, and tissues of the unwilling subjects.

The intent of this chapter is to demonstrate the effects that tumors can have upon elements of the immunological apparatus, the anatomy of vital organs, and changes in the composition of the usually highly stable amino acid pools. Also discussed is the detection of unusual metabolic products associated with tumor growth, which in themselves may have potent adverse influences on the tumor-bearing host, although they may be useful markers for the detection and monitoring of tumors.

These malignant, metabolically active "organs" are also capable of inducing anorexia, which in turn leads to cachexia, and a state of malnutrition that may contribute to a decrease in host immunocompetence, and thus to the acceleration of tumor growth.

Accumulative data are presented that establish a basis for an integration of these varied tumor influences upon host physiology, and may in turn provide clues for new therapeutic approaches to cancer control, as well as rational means for approaches to an earlier detection of malignancy, or for following changes in tumor status during or following treatment.

EXPERIMENTAL TECHNIQUES

ANIMAL CAGING AND ENVIRONMENT

Standard plastic cages, $11 \times 7 \times 5$ inches, containing about 2 cm of San-I-Cel ground corncob bedding, were employed in all experiments. For physiological or immunological studies, plastic cages are superior to metal cages in terms of general insulation, resistance to temperature changes, cold conductivity, and minimization of sound and other stress factors. Inasmuch as endocrine and various circadian effects are related to light and dark exposures, the plastic cages are also preferable over metal for controlling admittance of diffuse light to the animals. Standard 12-hour intervals of light and dark were maintained by automatic clock-controlled switches.[36] The temperature was maintained at 75 F (± 3).

All animals, including both stock and experimental groups, were protected by a special low-stress barrier system consisting of ventilated enclosed shelves provided with filtered laminar air flow that is vented outside of the building following contact with the mice and their released aerosols.[32]

TUMOR

The B-16 melanotic melanoma employed was obtained from K. Adachi of the Oregon

Regional Primate Center. Tissue culture passage was utilized to free the tumor of the LDH-virus, since this inconspicuous entity is capable of compromising host response under a variety of experimental conditions.[40] Mice were implanted subcutaneously in the hip with tumor cell suspensions in physiological saline containing between 10^5 and 10^6 cells in a 0.1 ml volume. Standard three-dimensional tumor volume measurements, reflecting tumor growth, were made with calipers.

MOUSE BLOOD SAMPLES

Cold sampling procedures were employed to minimize amino acid alterations during bleeding and processing of plasma samples for amino acid analysis.[38] Blood samples of about 0.2 ml per mouse were removed by the orbital bleeding procedure.[28]

AMINO ACID DETERMINATIONS

Analysis of free plasma and urine amino acids were carried out on a Beckman Model 120 B amino acid analyzer modified to provide accelerated, semiautomatic runs of high sensitivity.[49] Recently revised and improved methods of analysis were employed. An improved sodium citrate buffer system for basic amino acids (D. H. Spackman, unpublished data, 1969) allows the routine analysis of E-N-monomethyllysine[45] along with all other basic amino acids. Lithium citrate buffers were used for the acidic and neutral amino acids.[6,44] The latter buffer system in its modified form is essential for the satisfactory separation of asparagine and glutamine, which are of critical importance in amino acid studies of tumor-bearing subjects.[37,38]

ASSAY FOR PLASMA CORTICOSTERONE IN MICE

A microfluorimetric assay was developed in our laboratories,[47,48] based on the procedure described by Glick et al.[18] Our assay used 50 μl of plasma; thus 100 to 120 μl of plasma obtained from individual mice by the nonharmful orbital bleeding procedure[28] permitted two repetitive assays to be carried out on single animals. However, in some experiments plasma samples were pooled from five mice.

MATERIALS AND METHODS FOR DPPH CHROMATOGRAPHY

The principles of detection and the general operating conditions of the DPPH (diphenylpicrylhydrazyl) analyzer have been previously described.[2,4] The results presented below were derived in part from instrumentation described elsewhere,[5] and in part from a more recent version of the analyzer that used a 0.9 × 41.5 cm column of A-5 cation-exchange resin (Bio-Rad Labs, Richmond, California). The detector (Model 56V, Glenco, Houston, Texas) monitors differential absorption (525 nm relative to 440 nm) in a 10 mm flow cell. Usually 0.25–0.5 ml sample volumes are injected onto the columns.

URINE SAMPLES FOR DPPH CHROMATOGRAPHY

Urine samples were obtained from melanoma patients being cared for or seen in consultation, at the University of California Melanoma Clinic, San Francisco. The patients were classified either as having metastatic disease, or as having no evidence of disease (NED) by physical examination or conventional laboratory tests and scans. The NED category thus includes patients at high risk for developing metastases, as well as those who have been surgically "cured" and who are normal for all practical purposes.

The urine samples were aliquots from 24-hour collections, which were kept under refrigeration during collection, without added preservatives. Aliquots were acidified to pH 2.5 with HCl, and then stored at–75 C pending analysis.

RESULTS

INFLUENCE OF MELANOMA ON THE THYMUS

The thymus is the key organ in the processing of T cells.[12,50] Such thymus-derived lymphocytes are, of course, the primary cellular elements responsible for cell-mediated immunity, which is probably the most effective immunological surveillance factor in the control of malignant cells. Numerous investigators have demonstrated either the beneficial or the adverse influences of the functional status of the immunological apparatus upon the course of melanoma in patients, and the therapeutic role that cell-mediated immunity can play under some circumstances in the survival of the patient.[11,17,21]

Previously unpublished data (Riley, 1978) have demonstrated that progressively growing B-16 melanomas in mice have a potent suppressing influence upon the thymus. This is expressed most conspicuously by thymus involution as shown in Figure 9-1, where more than a 60% weight loss of this vital immunological organ occurs during 25 days of progressive melanoma growth.

Figure 9-1 demonstrates that the thymus-suppressing effect increases with time following tumor implantation, and that this time-course weight loss is correlated with increasing melanoma mass. The potentially undesirable immunological consequences to the host of such progressive thymus impairment are obvious.

The biochemical and physiological mechanisms responsible for the thymus destruction observed in this murine melanoma model deserve further study so that corrective therapy may be attempted. From a teleological perspective, the malignant melanocytes seemed to have devised an ingenious biochemical means for nullifying a natural host mechanism that is potentially capable of

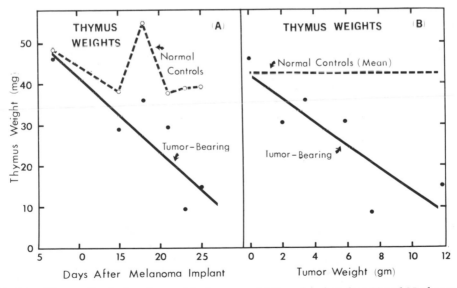

FIGURE 9-1. Thymus involution observed during melanoma growth. A. shows thymus weight decreasing as a function of time following tumor implantation, while B. depicts thymus involution as a function of increasing tumor mass. Thymus weights analyzed on days 23 and 25 after tumor implantation showed a statistically significant difference from the mean of the normal controls. (P < .005; student's t test)

destroying "foreign" cells. This remarkable physiological capability of the transformed melanocyte is further testimony of the diverse means that cancer cells can utilize for their defense and temporary survival.

INFLUENCE OF MELANOMA ON THE SPLEEN

In contrast to the weight loss, or involution, occurring in the thymus during the course of B-16 melanoma growth, the spleen exhibits hyperplasia. Figure 9–2 illustrates this increase as a function of the time following melanoma implant, as well as correlation with increasing tumor mass.

Splenomegaly is not an unusual expression of the neoplastic process in rodents, and it is frequently seen in association with tumors other than melanomas. Its occurrence under experimental circumstances where thymus involution is present, however, is of special interest since the usual cause of thymus weight loss is an elevation of circulating adrenal corticoids.[13,41] Such hormonal effects usually in-

clude a corresponding weight loss of the spleen and peripheral lymph nodes. However, no elevation of plasma corticosterone was observed in mice bearing this melanoma.

A nononcogenic virus infection that also produces opposite effects upon the thymus and spleen has been described.[30,42,43] In this case, the provoking agent was the benign LDH-elevating virus (LDH-virus).[30,34,36] It has been demonstrated that the observed involution of the thymus following this virus infection is caused by a temporary rise in plasma corticosterone, which is the rodent equivalent of cortisol in human subjects.

In a conversation with G. Dalldorf, 1962, he described the splenic hyperplasia in the LDH-virus infected mouse as being suggestive of early leukemia, even though the splenomegaly never proceeds to overt malignancy.[42] This hyperplasia results from a virus-induced physiological mechanism apart from the elevated plasma corticosterone level that causes the thymus involution. In fact, there is a dual effect of LDH-virus infection upon the spleen and lymph nodes: (1) an early and continuous immunoblast proliferation in the

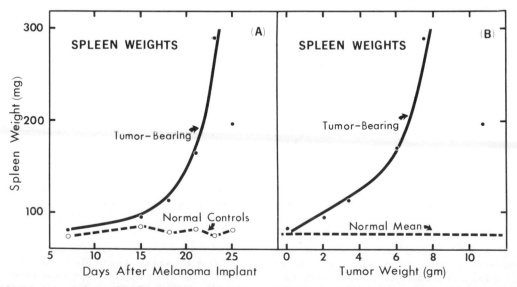

FIGURE 9–2. Spleen weight increase observed during melanoma growth. A. shows spleen weight increasing as a function of time following tumor im- plantation, while B. shows spleen weight increases as a function of increasing tumor mass.

thymus-independent regions, concomitant with (2) a corticosterone-induced destruction of small lymphocytes in the thymus-dependent regions.[23,26,31,42,43] The tumors employed in these studies were not contaminated with the LDH-virus (see Chap. 10).

INFLUENCE OF MELANOMA GROWTH ON THE LYMPH NODES

Figure 9–3 shows that the peripheral lymph nodes of melanoma-bearing mice exhibit a statistically significant hyperplasia, which is analogous to that observed in the spleen. Enlargement of both organs probably result from the same nonmetastatic physiological mechanisms. The lymph node hyperplasia shows a good correlation with increasing tumor size, as indicated by a correlation coefficient of 0.98. Various statistical tests gave P values of 0.01 to 0.001 for the differences

observed between the nodes from tumor-bearing and control mice. It is relevant to note that both gross and microscopic examination indicated that the peripheral node and spleen enlargements are not due to pigmented metastases (G. Dalldorf, Sloan-Kettering Report, 1962).

INFLUENCE OF MELANOMA GROWTH ON THE LIVER

Liver weights were also increased significantly in melanoma-bearing mice, as illustrated in Figure 9–4. Both the spleen and liver showed continuing weight increases up to tumor weights of 8 gm; these organ weight increases then levelled off or decreased as the mouse entered the terminal stage of the disease. The lymph nodes, however, continued to increase in size throughout all stages of tumor growth.

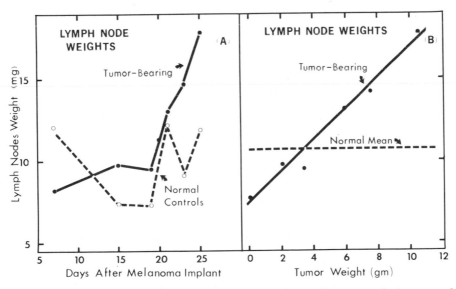

FIGURE 9–3. **Increase in the weight of the peripheral lymph nodes as a function of time, following melanoma implant (A) and tumor mass (B). Lymph node weights obtained on days 21, 23, and 25 after melanoma implant differed signifi-** cantly from the mean of the normal controls (P < .001; student's t test). Note the linearity of node weight increase as a function of tumor mass. (Correlation coefficient = .98)

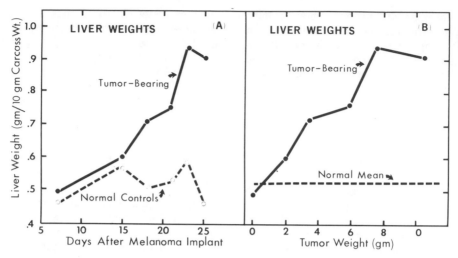

FIGURE 9-4. Increase in liver weight as a function of time following melanoma implant (A) and tumor mass (B). Liver weights obtained on days 23 and 25 after melanoma implant showed a statistically significant difference from the mean of the normal controls (P<.001; student's t test). Liver weight is plotted as grams per 10 grams of carcass weight, because of the influence of animal size upon the liver mass.

TUMOR–INDUCED CACHEXIA

In contrast to the systematic increases in various organ sizes, the net weight of the carcass exhibited a decrease, as shown in Figure 9-5. The net carcass weight was established by subtracting the tumor weight and excess spleen and liver weights from the total body weight. Thus, although the total weight of the tumor-bearing mouse increases rapidly, there is a net decrease in the weight of most carcass tissues. As a consequence, the tumor-bearing mouse, like the cancer patient, exhibits a substantial loss in structural body weight. The observed cachexia appears to be, at least partially, the consequence of a tumor-induced anorexia, as shown in Figures 9-6 and 9-7. The rapid increase of tumor mass, plus the weight increases in the liver, spleen, and nodes, seem particularly remarkable in view of this decrease in food consumption.

TUMOR–ASSOCIATED ANOREXIA

One of the most provocative findings resulting from these studies was that the B-16 melanoma induces a rapid and conspicuous

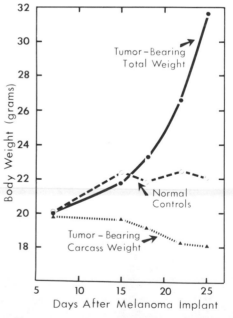

FIGURE 9-5. Cachexia observed during melanoma growth. When the weight of the tumor, plus the tumor-associated increase in the liver and spleen weight of the tumor-bearing mice is subtracted from the total weight, a significant decline in carcass weight becomes apparent.

anorexia in mice that is manifested by a systematic voluntary decrease in food and water consumption in direct correlation with increasing tumor mass.

As can be seen by inspection of Figures 9–6 and 9–7, food consumption in the mice bearing the B-16 pigmented tumor was linearly reduced as a function of increasing tumor size. This observation has been confirmed in several independent experiments. Other observations indicate, however, that various tumor types have different characteristics in this regard.

AMINO ACID PROFILES

Previously published results from our laboratory have shown that changes occur in a variety of both plasma and urinary amino acids during the course of melanoma growth.[39]

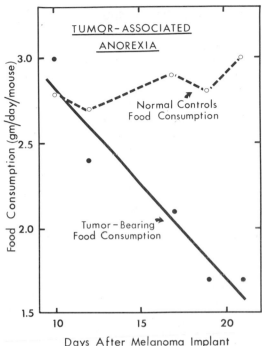

FIGURE 9-7. Comparison of food consumption of melanoma-bearing mice and normal controls held in the same protective facilities. Line showing food consumption of tumor-bearing mice was fitted by least squares method.

Because of the large number of plasmas, urines, and tissues analyzed in these studies, and the 30 to 50 amino acids present in each sample, we have explored various means to present the resulting complex data in a graphical manner that will allow both similarities and differences in the samples to be more readily identified. We have consequently developed a new version of the "amino acid profile." In such profiles, amino acids from a normal or reference sample are collocated and prioritized, or ranked, in order of their descending concentration to form a smooth concave reference curve. Similar plots of the amino acids from other samples are then arranged in the same order and, as a consequence, individual amino acids readily exhibit their concentration departures from the reference curve. The graphic results of this treatment are demonstrated in several of the following figures.

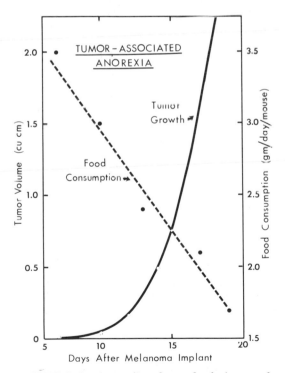

FIGURE 9-6. Anorexia observed during melanoma growth. This figure shows a rapid decline in food consumption occurring simultaneously with the growth of the B-16 melanoma. Food consumption line was fitted by least squares method.

AMINO ACID ALTERATIONS

Mouse Plasma. The amino acids assayed in plasma from B-16 melanoma-bearing mice show many deviations from normal concentrations, as shown in Figure 9-8. Significantly elevated amino acids in this prioritized "profile" are taurine, proline, and phenylalanine. Other significant elevations include alanine, glycine, valine, threonine, and histidine. Conversely, several amino acids exhibit lower plasma concentrations in the melanoma-bearing mice. These are glutamine, serine, arginine, and tryptophan. These amino acid concentration changes increase or decrease systematically as the tumor grows. This is in-

dicated by Figure 9-9, which shows a simultaneous decrease in arginine and an increase in proline concentration in the plasma as a function of time after melanoma implantation. Figure 9-10 depicts a decrease in plasma glutamine and an increase in plasma alanine during melanoma growth. Essentially identical observations have been made in two independent experiments.

Mouse Urine. The most conspicuous amino acid alteration in the urine of melanoma-bearing mice is a dramatic decline in taurine concentration during tumor growth. This is illustrated in Figure 9-11. This chart also shows, inversely, an increase in creat-

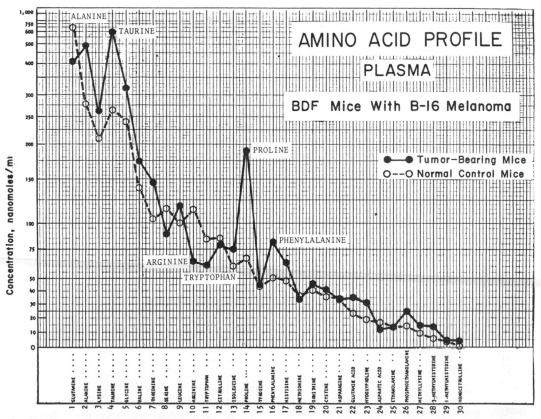

FIGURE 9-8. Amino acid profile, comparing the concentrations of all the amino acids in the plasma of melanoma-bearing mice with those in the plasma of normal BDF mice. Departures from normal are readily apparent due to the novel method of plotting. Data was obtained on day 25 of tumor growth.

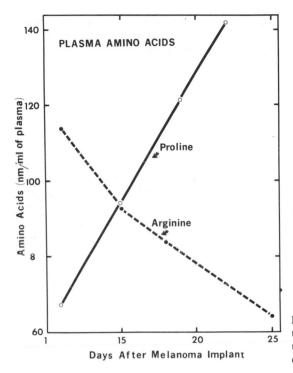

FIGURE 9-9.   Opposite alterations in the concentrations of two amino acids, proline and arginine, in the plasma of melanoma-bearing mice as a function of time following melanoma implantation.

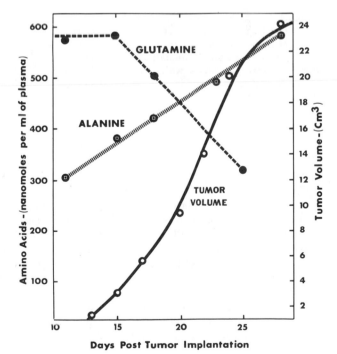

FIGURE 9-10.   Opposite alterations in the concentrations of two amino acids, glutamine and alanine, in the plasma of melanoma-bearing mice, as a function of time following melanoma implantation.

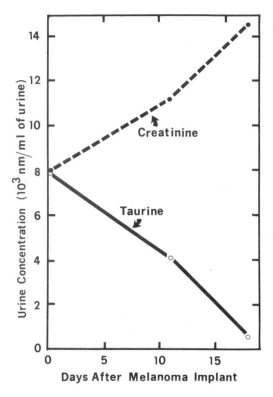

FIGURE 9-11. Simultaneous alterations in the concentrations of taurine and creatinine, in the urine of melanoma-bearing mice, as a function of time following melanoma implantation. The excretion of taurine decreases while creatinine is excreted in higher concentrations in the urine of the melanoma-bearing mice.

inine concentration in the urine during the same time period. These results have also been confirmed in two separate experiments.

Taurine is the most abundant amino acid found in B-16 melanoma tissue, as well as in all normal tissues of the mouse. It is the principal excretion form of sulfur in this mammal, and its decreased excretion in the melanoma-bearing animal may be a direct reflection of the progressively decreased food consumption shown in Figures 9-6 and 9-7.

Creatinine has no known metabolic function and is the end product after the energy from phosphocreatine has been utilized. Creatinine excretion is usually fairly constant in an animal, mainly reflecting muscle metabolism. Its progressively increased excretion rate during the growth of this tumor may thus reflect the increasing energy needs of the growing tumor mass.

Free Amino Acid Concentrations in Mouse Melanoma Tissues. A free amino acid concentration profile of the B-16 pigmented melanoma tissue is shown in Figure 9-12. For comparison of the melanotic and amelanotic tumors, Figure 9-13 shows an analogous profile of the B-16 nonpigmented genetic variant. Although the similarities are more striking than the differences, the pigmented tumor exhibited larger proline and hydroxyproline peaks, while the nonpigmented variant displayed a larger cystine peak, as well as a decrease in phosphoethanolamine concentration, which was not observed in the pigmented tumor.

The relative amino acid concentrations of the Cloudman S91 melanoma are shown in Figure 9-14. This tumor tissue exhibits the typical low glutamine and aspartic acid concentrations that are common to many tumors. However, in contrast to the two B-16 tumors, the Cloudman melanoma exhibits relatively lower concentrations of lysine and cystine; and higher concentrations of arginine.

Glutamine. Figures 9-12, 9-13, and 9-14 compare the concentrations of amino acids in three types of melanoma tissue with those of normal mouse tissues. One of the most conspicuous differences between the melanoma tissues and normal tissues is a much lower concentration of glutamine in the melanoma tissues. This is also the case with other tumors that have been tested, such as the EL-4 lymphoma and the Ehrlich carcinoma. In apparent correlation, the glutamine concentration in the plasma of mice bearing the B-16 melanoma also is less than that of normal mice. This may be seen in the plasma amino acid profile shown in Figure 9-8, while Figure 9-15 shows the decline in plasma glutamine

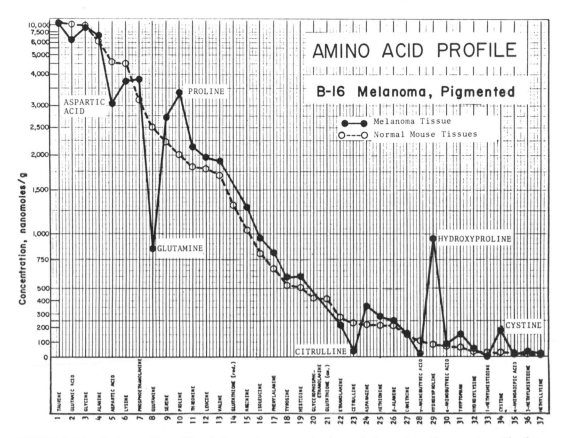

FIGURE 9-12. Amino acid profile of the amino acids in B-16 melanoma tissue, compared with those found in normal mouse tissues. Conspicuous amino acid differences in tumor tissue are low concentrations of glutamic acid, aspartic acid, glutamine, and citrulline, and higher concentrations of proline, hydroxyproline, and cystine. Note the log scale.

during the time course of tumor growth, together with a simultaneous increase in glutamine excretion in the urine.

TUMOR INFLUENCES ON DRUGS

Following the establishment of an in vitro reaction between an accepted tumor metabolite and an exogenous compound such as para phenylenediamine (PPDA),[33] the obvious question was whether there would be any measurable biological or therapeutic consequences if such a reactive compound were injected into tumor-bearing animals. Tumor in-

hibition was observed, as shown in Figure 9-16. In the process of establishing proper dosage and routes of administration, another biological response was observed; specifically, that the presence of a growing melanoma partially protected the host from the toxicity of p-phenylenediamine, as shown in Figure 9-17.

In order to explore this phenomenon, a simplified experimental design was employed. Control and tumor-bearing mice were injected with identical toxic doses of the test compounds on a milligram per kilogram basis, and the survival time was recorded to the nearest minute. If the challenging compound is distributed uniformly throughout the carcass and the tumor, and reacts in the same manner with both control and tumor-bearing mice, the survival time should be the same within experimental limits. These limits have been determined with appropriate controls, and the differences reported between tumor-bearing and control mice have been analyzed and found to be statistically significant.

These experiments have demonstrated that a positive relationship exists between the protection conferred by the tumor against PPDA toxicity, and tumor size.[29] If survival time following injection with PPDA, for example, is plotted against tumor weight, a sigmoid curve is obtained representing an increasing protection with increasing tumor mass. It has also been noted that the presence of pigment is not essential for protection, since a nonpigmented variant of the Cloudman S91 melanoma also gives protection. If two methyl groups are substituted for the hydrogens of a PPDA amino group, as in N,N-dimethyl-PPDA, the behavior of the compound is altered sufficiently so that the tumor-bearing host is no longer able to detoxify it.

It has been useful to compare the differences

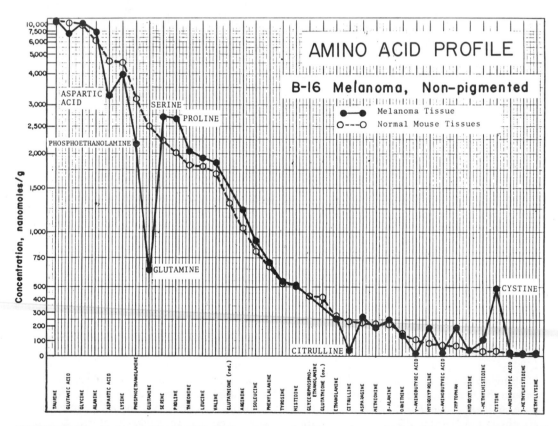

FIGURE 9–13. Concentration profile of 37 amino acids present in the nonpigmented, variant B-16 melanoma tissue, compared with amino acid concentrations found in normal mouse tissues. Similarities to the original pigmented tumor shown in Figure 9–12, include low concentrations of glutamic acid, aspartic acid, glutamine, and citrulline; and elevations of proline, hydroxyproline, and cystine.

in toxicity of the three isomers of phenylene-diamine. Thus far, the para and the ortho isomers have been the most completely studied. It will be noted that the toxicities of the three isomers are widely different. With an acute dose in mice, the para is about ten times as toxic as the ortho, while the meta occupies an intermediate position in this regard.

The experiment illustrated in Figure 9–18 compares the response of normal and mela-noma-bearing mice (Cloudman S91) when challenged with the para compound in con-trast to the ortho isomer. It may be seen that the presence of the tumor has opposite effects

on host survival time if the molecular arrange-ment of the drug is only slightly altered. The tumor protects the host against para phe-nylenediamine (PPDA), while the toxicity of ortho phenylenediamine (OPDA) is increased by the same tumor-host system. It may be noted also that both of these compounds have antitumor effects against this melanoma. See Figure 9–16.

Frequently, from casual observations of the increased vulnerability of tumor-bearing ani-mals to drugs come the explanation that this is due to a "weakened" condition. These ex-periments establish that it is a matter of

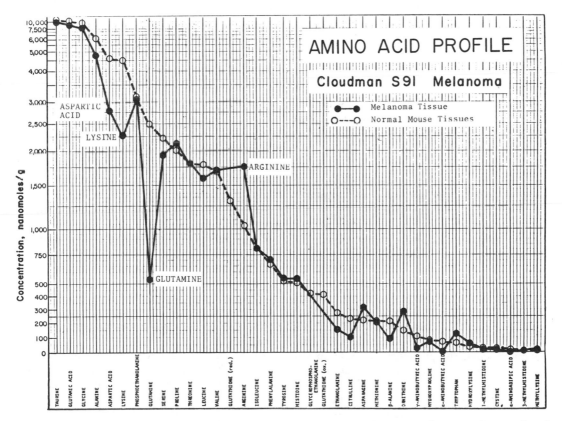

FIGURE 9–14.   Concentration profile of 37 amino acids in the pigmented Cloudman S91 melanoma. While some amino acids show a pattern similar to those seen in the B-16 melanoma, pigmented and nonpigmented, the S91 tumor tissue also exhibits a prominent arginine peak.

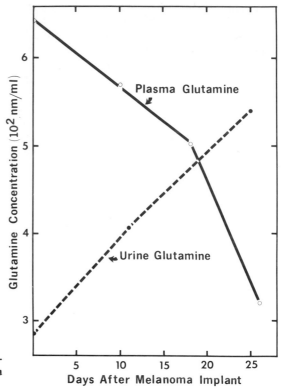

FIGURE 9–15. Decrease in glutamine concentration in the plasma of melanoma-bearing mice, and a simultaneous increase of glutamine in the urine.

specific tumor-host biochemistry, and that in some instances, the tumor-bearing animal is in a "strengthened" condition.

If the same drug system is employed, but substituting a different tumor type, the Ehrlich ascites carcinoma, the metabolic effects of the two phenylenediamine isomers are reversed, so that the presence of the Ehrlich tumor becomes a handicap for the host when PPDA is administered, but protects against the toxicity of OPDA. This tumor thus reverses the effects upon phenylenediamine toxicities observed when the pigmented Cloudman S91 was the host's tumor. This is illustrated in Figure 9–19.

To further show that these phenomena are not restricted to melanomas and the phenylenediamines, Figure 9–20 illustrates the findings with another tumor-host-compound system. This model used Sarcoma-180 and two closely related compounds that have

antitumor activity against this mouse malignancy.[10] As indicated in Figure 9–20, 6-diazo-5-oxo-L-norleucine (DON) and azaserine have a molecular difference of only one atom in the carbon chain; an oxygen is substituted for a carbon, with its two hydrogens in the 4 position. It is seen that DON behaves similarly to PPDA in being detoxified by or through Sarcoma-180, whereas azaserine is analogous to OPDA in that this sarcoma-host system enhances its toxicity.

There are several possible mechanisms to account for the foregoing phenomena. The most straightforward explanation is that the intraperitoneally injected compound goes into the peripheral circulation and, as it passes through the vasculature of the tumor, is acted upon by the unique enzymes or special metabolites localized there. By further analogy, one may think of the tumor as an ex-

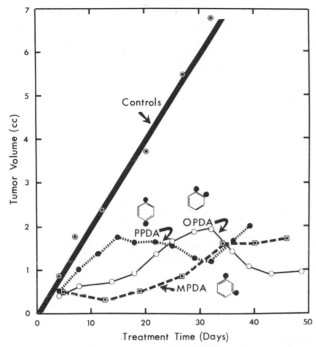

FIGURE 9–16. Inhibition of melanoma growth brought about by the intraperitoneal injection of either ortho, meta, or para phenylenediamine. The tumor was the Cloudman S91 pigmented melanoma. These phenylenediamine compounds are too toxic for clinical use in their present form.

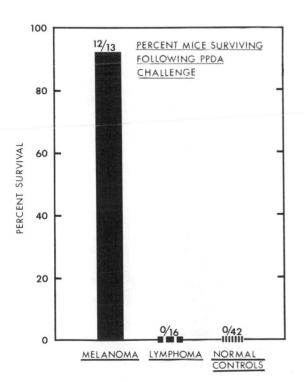

FIGURE 9–17. Protective effect of a transplanted melanoma against a normally lethal dose of p-phenylenediamine (PPDA). Over 90% of the melanoma-bearing mice survived a PPDA dose that was fatal for both nontumor controls and mice bearing a transplanted lymphoma.

tra transplantable organ in reference to its special capacities to engage in the biochemical transformation of appropriate compounds. The altered compound then expresses itself by increased or decreased toxicity and is thus either more or less lethal to the vital functions of the host. It is also theoretically possible, of course, that an alteration of the compound may occur without being detected by this experimental design, if toxicity values are not affected.

Since tumor metabolites, as well as special enzymes, are transported out of the cells into the peripheral blood, it is possible for the biochemical reactions to take place in the host vascular system without the necessity of tumor cell penetration. However, when PPDA is combined with a melanoma extract in vitro and incubated for a short time, the toxicity of PPDA is diminished. This indicates that the tumor cells are capable of converting PPDA to a less toxic compound in the absence of assistance from the host.

Alterations in liver catalase[20] and recent unpublished evidence of other enzyme altera-

tions in the liver (V. Riley, unpublished data, 1979) as consequences of an animal being host to a tumor, are further evidence of the roles that tumors play in phenomena involving altered drug toxicity.

DPPH CHROMATOGRAPHY OF URINES

An automatic ion-exchange chromatographic system has been developed over the past few years for separating and detecting dihydroxyphenylalanine (DOPA) and related metabolites in the urine of patients with melanoma. This system is similar to the automatic amino acid analyzer, but uses the stable free radical diphenylpicrylhydrazyl (DPPH) as the post-column colorimetric reagent, rather than ninhydrin. The new system has its own unique set of operating parameters.

DPPH reacts with a wide range of reducing compounds of physiological origin, including the hydroxy- or methoxy-substituted indoles

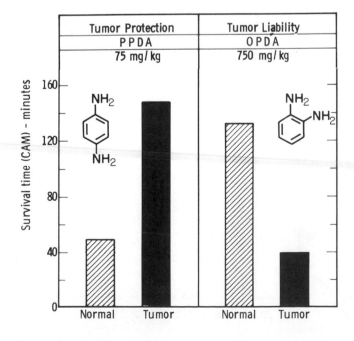

FIGURE 9-18. Influence of the Cloudman S91 pigmented melanoma on the survival time of mice challenged with lethal doses of either ortho or para phenylenediamine. The presence of the transplanted tumor provides either protection, as shown in the case of the para compound (PPDA), or survival liability as in the case of challenge by the ortho compound (OPDA). (CAM) is the cumulative average median in minutes.

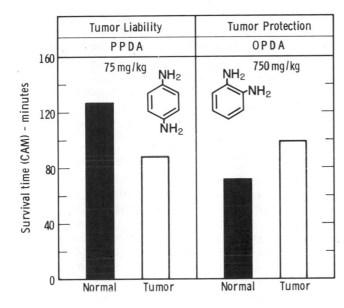

FIGURE 9-19. Influence of the Ehrlich ascités tumor upon phenylenediamine toxicities. This tumor afforded partial protection for the host with respect to the ortho isomer of phenylenediamine (OPDA), or survival liability when challenged with the para compound (PPDA). The influence of this Ehrlich tumor is thus opposite to that of the Cloudman melanoma shown in FIGURE 9-18.

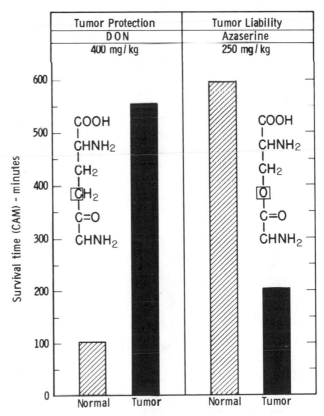

FIGURE 9-20. Influence of the Sarcoma 180 against the toxicity of the chemotherapeutic drug, 6-diazo-5-oxo-L-norleucine (DON), as compared with the opposite effect of the tumor when azaserine was the challenging drug.

and phenols, which are the intermediates in the formation of both phaeomelanin and eumelanin. DPPH is particularly useful as a colorimetric indicator of elevated levels of these melanin metabolites, the melanogens, in the urine of melanoma patients.

The DPPH chromatography system has been used to obtain elution profiles of a series of urine samples from normal subjects and melanoma patients, yielding generally similar patterns for healthy individuals and for patients with no evidence of disease (NED), as well as for most patients with local primary melanoma. In contrast, chromatograms of urine from patients with disseminated metastatic melanoma are quite different, exhibiting a number of major peaks in the catechol-indole elution range that are not found in the urine of healthy individuals. The following figures demonstrate these findings.

Metabolism of L-DOPA. Since L-DOPA (3,4-dihydroxyphenylalanine) is the parent compound for the formation of both melanin pigments and the neurogenic amines, its metabolism has been thoroughly studied.[19] It is well known that the ingestion of L-DOPA, as in the clinical management of Parkinson's disease, leads to the urinary excretion of its major metabolic products: DOPAmine (dopamine), DOPAC (dihydroxyphenylacetic acid), and HVA (homovanillic acid), through the action of intestinal, circulatory, and hepatic enzymes. Ingested DOPA is largely decarboxylated to DOPAmine, which is metabolized further to DOPAC, HVA, and other products. The rapid and extensive loss of DOPA, the active agent that crosses the blood–brain barrier, is one reason for the inclusion of a decarboxylase inhibitor, such as carbidopa, along with DOPA in the current treatment of patients with Parkinson's disease.[54] Goodall[19] estimated that approximately two-thirds of infused DOPA is converted to catecholamines and their related metabolites. The DPPH chromatogram shown in Figure 9-21 of the urine from a normal volunteer who had ingested L-DOPA clearly shows the major metabolic peaks of DOPAC and homovanillic acid (HVA), with DOPA itself a relatively minor constituent. DOPAmine is not displayed in this type of chromatogram. Interestingly, acidic metabolites of the catecholamines subsequent to DOPAmine, such as

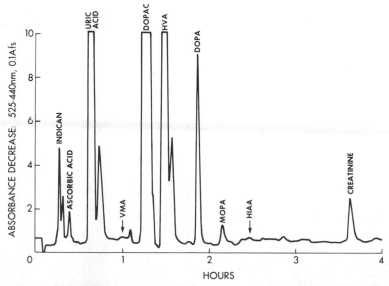

FIGURE 9–21.   DPPH chromatogram of a urine sample from a normal volunteer, eight hours after ingesting 250 mg of L-DOPA.

vanillactic acid (VLA) from norepinephrine, do not appear to be elevated following the ingestion of DOPA. For comparison, Figure 9-22 shows a DPPH profile of a normal human urine.

One of the striking observations about the urine of patients with advanced melanoma is that their DPPH chromatograms, as indicated by Figure 9-23, bear almost no resemblance to those of normal individuals ingesting

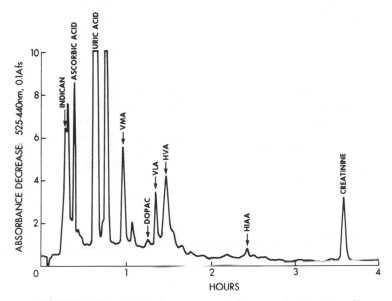

FIGURE 9-22.   DPPH chromatogram of a normal urine (0.5 ml).

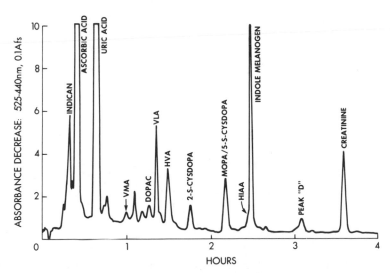

FIGURE 9-23.   DPPH chromatogram of the urine (0.5 ml) from a patient with disseminated melanoma.

L-DOPA, aside from the typical urinary constituents, such as indican, uric acid, 5-hydroxyindole-3 acetic acid (HIAA), and creatinine. Despite earlier reports on the elevation of DOPA[53] and homovanillic acid (HVA) in urine from melanoma patients, later results show that urine concentrations of both DOPA and HVA,[5] as well as DOPAmine,[22] correlate poorly with the extent of disease. These findings suggest that the pigment cell itself, rather than the circulatory system or the liver, is the major source of these metabolites observed in the urine of melanoma patients.

Although it is necessary to rely on more than one pigmentary intermediate found in urine to estimate the clinical status of melanoma patients,[8] 2-S-cysteinyldopa (2-S-CD) alone shows good correlation with the extent of disease. Figure 9–24 compares the histograms of 2-S-CD concentrations in urines from melanoma patients with no evidence of disease (NED) and patients with disseminated melanoma. All of the patients with disseminated disease have 2-S-CD values at the top of the scale; no values from such patients are found at the low end of the scale. Most of the NED patients have 2-S-CD urine concentrations that cluster at the bottom of the histogram. Two of the urines from NED patients have distinctly higher 2-S-CD concentrations, but they still fall below the range of values for patients with metastatic disease.

The vanillactic acid (VLA) histograms shown in Figure 9–25 show that this compound is nearly as reliable an indicator of metastatic disease as 2-S-CD. Most of the urine samples from patients with metastatic disease have high VLA concentrations, with

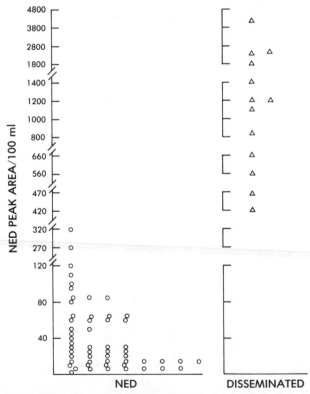

FIGURE 9–24. Histograms of 2-S-cysteinyldopa (2-S-CD) concentration in the urine of melanoma patients with no evidence of disease (NED), and melanoma patients with disseminated disease. Concentration values in close proximity to one another have been grouped together at a common ordinate value.

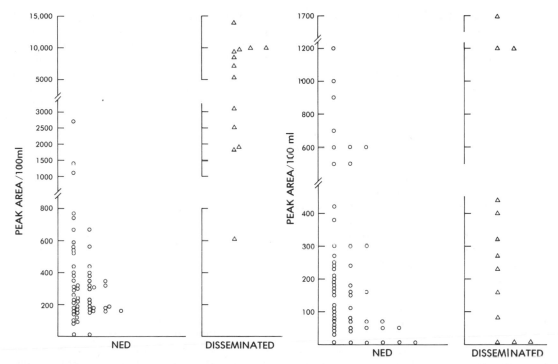

FIGURE 9-25. Histograms of vanillactic acid (VLA) concentration in the urine of melanoma patients with no evidence of disease (NED), and melanoma patients with disseminated disease. Concentration values in close proximity to one another have been grouped together at a common ordinate value.

FIGURE 9-26. Histograms of homovanillic acid (HVA) concentration in the urine of melanoma patients with no evidence of disease (NED), and melanoma patients with disseminated disease. Concentration values in close proximity to one another have been grouped together at a common ordinate value.

only one such urine showing an intermediate value. A few urine samples from patients with no evidence of disease (NED) have high VLA concentrations, which intermingle with those of patients with metastatic disease, but most NED samples have low values and cluster towards the bottom of the histogram.

The homovanillic acid (HVA) histograms shown in Figure 9-26 fail to show any significant separation between the concentrations in urine samples from metastatic patients and patients with no evidence of disease. HVA concentrations in both categories intermingle throughout the entire range of values, although some clustering of the values from NED patients is evident at lower concentrations. Our finding of a low diagnostic value for HVA is contrary to the reported use of this compound in evaluating melanoma patients and monitoring their therapy.[51] Our accumulated evidence thus shows that homovanillic acid is a poor choice as an indicator for melanoma metastases.

Variability in Urinary Excretion of Pigmentary Intermediates by Melanoma Patients. One of the earliest conclusions to come from the DPPH chromatographic screening of urine samples from patients with metastatic melanoma was the variability in excretion patterns of the pigmentary intermediates, even in patients with similar clinical pathologies such as hepatic metastases. This variability has continued to be observed through several changes in analytical instrumentation and technique, and is no longer considered to be the result of uncontrolled variability in the new DPPH detection system, but is rather considered as evidence indicating the individual biochemical differences in the types of melanoma cells proliferating in patients with metastatic melanoma.[8] Thus, it appears that no single pigmentary metabolite in the urine is pathognomonic of melanoma metastases.

The urinary pigmentary intermediates that appear to be tumor-related include: VLA (vanillactic acid), 2-S-CD (2-S-cysteinyldopa), MOPA (3-methoxytyrosine), 5-S-CD, and indoles. Both VLA and an indole melanogen, purportedly 5-methoxy-6-hydroxyindole-2-carboxylic acid, were reported many years ago by Duchon and his co-workers[14,15] as urinary markers for melanoma. DPPH chromatographic analyses confirm the importance of these compounds. A number of years ago, 5-S-cysteinyldopa was first noted as the precursor for the formation of red-brown melanins (phaeomelanins) by Prota and Nicolaus[27] and was observed in urine from melanoma patients by Rorsman, Bjorklund, and co-workers.[7] DPPH chromatography showed that MOPA[3] and 2-S-CD[4,8] were also major constituents in the urine of melanoma patients. The influences of organ systems outside the tumor cells cannot be completely ignored, however, since at least two urinary DOPA metabolites that show good correlation with extent of disease, MOPA and vanillactic acid, require transformations (3-O-methylation, deamination, oxidation) that may occur in many tissues.

Unidentified Cancer-Associated Urinary Constituents Detected by DPPH Chromatography. In addition to the pigmentary intermediates already mentioned, other urinary constituents, presently unidentified and termed peaks "D" and "E",[8] and a postcreatinine peak,[4] have been detected by DPPH chromatography, which also correlate with the extent of neoplastic disease.

These three peaks do not appear to be pigment-related for the following reasons: They are not observed in extracts of melanoma tissue; they cannot be synthesized by the enzymatic oxidation of DOPA or DOPA-cysteine;[4] and they are found in the urine of patients with metastases from other categories of tumors, such as adenocarcinoma metastatic to the liver (P. W. Banda, unpublished observations, 1978). These peaks do not correspond to other urinary markers indicating rapid cell growth, such as polyamines or t-RNA derived nucleosides. The origin of these DPPH-positive compounds in urine samples from melanoma and other cancer patients remains to be determined.

DISCUSSION

TUMOR CHARACTER

The amino acid data indicate that there are certain common biochemical features characteristic of tumor-bearing hosts, such as the striking decrease in plasma glutamine. However, the most impressive aspect of the overall data is the demonstration of the highly individualistic character of the biochemistry and physiology of the various tumor types. This uniqueness of each tumor's biochemical personality is exhibited not only in the amino acid fingerprinting, but is also shown by the differential patterns of the metabolites appearing in the urine.

BIOCHEMICAL IMPLICATIONS

A therapeutic implication of this metabolic individuality suggests that each tumor variety carries special vulnerabilities, which, if they can be identified, may be biochemically exploited. The recognition of these essential physiological differences lies easily within present technical capabilities. Prototype possibilities are indicated by the prioritized, collocated amino acid concentration profiles, and by the metabolic fingerprinting of the urine of patients and tumor-bearing animals. The observed differences clearly inform us of the tumor-induced biochemical peculiarities found in the plasma and urine that are awaiting therapeutic and diagnostic utilization.

MEASURABLE PARAMETERS

With 30 to 50 amino acids as reflective parameters in the plasma, and probably over 1,000 characteristic metabolites in mammalian urine, it is apparent that such generous differential biochemical patterns found in health and disease deserve interfacing with appropriate computer technology for optimum recognition and specific identification of the various physiological and pathological patterns that are uniquely associated with a given disease.

TUMOR–HOST INFLUENCE ON METABOLISM OF DRUGS

The potential therapeutic consequences of tumor influences, direct or indirect, upon the fate of a given anticancer drug are illustrated by Figures 9–16 through 9–20. In these cases, the presence of a tumor in the host has a dramatic effect upon the metabolic processing of drugs by the tumor-host metabolic team.

As demonstrated in the Results section, azaserine and DON are closely related compounds differing only by a CH_2 substitution for oxygen in the molecular structure. Both drugs have been used for cancer therapy. By employing a simple experimental procedure to detect subtle changes in an administered drug or the toxicity of its metabolites, it is possible to demonstrate the capability of a tumor to function essentially as an auxiliary "organ" in metabolically processing the therapeutic drug or test compound. The data derived from these studies demonstrate that the presence of a given tumor can either increase or suppress the toxicity of the administered drug, which is probably an expression of tumor-directed biochemical changes in the drug metabolites. This phenomenon is of special relevance when the therapeutic features of a drug lie in its metabolic products, rather than in the drug itself.

It has been further established that different tumor types will process the same drug quite differently. Thus, again, an intimate knowledge of the physiological and metabolic characteristics of the tumor that is being treated will place the therapist in a stronger position to exploit vulnerable tumor characteristics.

The individualistic amino acid patterns in the plasma and in the urine of tumor-bearing subjects, together with the variety of substances detected in the urine of melanoma patients, found when using DPPH chromatography, is undoubtedly related to the above metabolic phenomena.

DPPH CHROMATOGRAPHY OF URINE SAMPLES FROM MELANOMA PATIENTS: UNSOLVED PROBLEMS

The adoption of a chromatographic approach, coupled with a unique colorimetric detecting reagent, DPPH, has permitted the assembly of data that yields a comprehensive picture of the excretion of pigmentary intermediates, as well as other metabolic products, in urine of melanoma patients. This chromatographic approach to the detection of urinary melanogens has provided valuable clinical information, often unavailable by any other test, which may assist in evaluating the clinical status of melanoma patients. Although the less than perfect correlation between urinary melanogens and the clinical status of melanoma patients may at first appear confusing, the evidence suggests that these results involve fundamental biochemical and biological problems that accompany the growth of metastatic melanoma, rather than a failure of the analytical chromatography.

METABOLIC DIFFERENCE OF LUNG AND LIVER

In assembling the preliminary DPPH chromatographic data, it was noted that a number of patients with small pulmonary nodules, of less than 1 cm, appeared to have normal concentrations of urinary melanogens, while hepatic metastases of a similar size were detected early and reliably by DPPH chromatographic screening.[8] It was believed at the time that this was due partly to the high sensitivity of lung tomography in detecting small lesions, and partly to the less than optimal sensitivity of the earlier prototype chromatographic detectors. Although recent analyses, which employ more sensitive methodology, have narrowed the range of false negatives, patients with known pulmonary metastases, and exhibiting normal patterns of urinary melanogens, have continued to be observed. These puzzling cases do not represent a lack of sensitivity of the analytical chromatography, but rather, elevated concentrations of pigmentary intermediates in fact appear to be absent from urine sample of these patients. Data from three separate areas of research may shed some light on this apparently anomalous situation.

CLONAL NATURE OF MELANOMA METASTASES

The experiments of Aubert et al.[1] are particularly intriguing. They have observed, with melanoma cells in culture, that some strains of pigmented cells release 5-S cysteinyldopa into the surrounding media, while other pigmented strains do not. It was suggested that differences in the structure of the melanosomes might be responsible for the release or nonrelease of this pigmentary intermediate. It has also been recently reported, in a mouse melanoma model,[16] that certain clones of cells preferentially metastasize to certain organs; for example, to the lung only. Observations of a melanoma-bearing dog show that, while the primary tumor on the leg was highly pigmented and pigmented metastases were present in the lung, only amelanotic metastases were found in the liver (P. W. Banda, unpublished data, 1976). As in the case of the mouse melanoma model,[16] the apparent ability of biochemically different clones from a primary canine melanoma to metastasize to different organs was suggested.

Since the polyclonal nature of human primary melanoma has long been recognized,[9] one may speculate that the absence of melanogens in the urine of certain patients with pulmonary metastases is a consequence of the preferential metastasis of clones of cells whose melanosomes are incapable of releasing pigmentary intermediates, or that the physiological environment of each organ may impose different metabolic responses upon its tumor metastases. The variation in the excretion of urinary melanogens in disseminated cases may also be due to clones of differential susceptibility to adjuvant therapy. The rate of tumor growth and various environmental factors may also influence the amount of melanin that is produced, in either primary or metastatic lesions.[24]

STRESS AND METABOLISM

An important factor affecting tumor growth and development that is widely unappreciated is the effect of either subtle or overt environmental factors that induce acute, chronic, or intermittent anxiety stress. This can be biochemically measured, and substantially controlled by appropriate environmental modification of animal housing facilities and animal handling techniques.[35] Application of such stress measurements and stress control in man is, of course, a more complex and difficult undertaking.

The most immediate and dramatic consequence of psychosocial or anxiety stress is the elevation of plasma glucocorticoids in the blood plasma. In mice, a twofold increase in plasma corticosterone occurs within five to ten minutes following a mild stress stimulus, and tenfold increases may be observed within 15 to 20 minutes.[47,48] The relevance of stress in these studies has to do with the significant metabolic alterations that mild anxiety stress can bring about.

Since the comparative metabolism of normal and tumor-bearing subjects is a primary subject of this report, any uncontrolled factor that may generate background biochemical "noise" is of significance to these studies. In the case of the animal experiments described in this report, stress was carefully controlled, both through the use of special low-stress housing facilities, and the utilization of minimal-stress animal handling techniques.[35]

Physiological Consequences of Stress. Following are some of the physiological parameters that glucocorticoids can influence, especially in a stress-induced elevated phase: Carbohydrate metabolism is altered and blood glucose is increased. Gluconeogenesis is increased, with a decrease in the use of glucose by tissues. Fat mobilization is enhanced. Of special relevance to the present studies are the changes induced in protein metabolism, particularly the mobilization of proteins and amino acids from tissues and cells. Another stress-associated factor that could contribute to the metabolic observations made in these studies, is the corticoid effect upon an increased permeability of capillary membranes, which would permit a more rapid transfer of amino acids and various metabolites between cells and extracellular physiological fluids.

Stress and Amino Acids. Figure 9–27 illustrates some of the physiological consequences of a mild rotation-induced anxiety

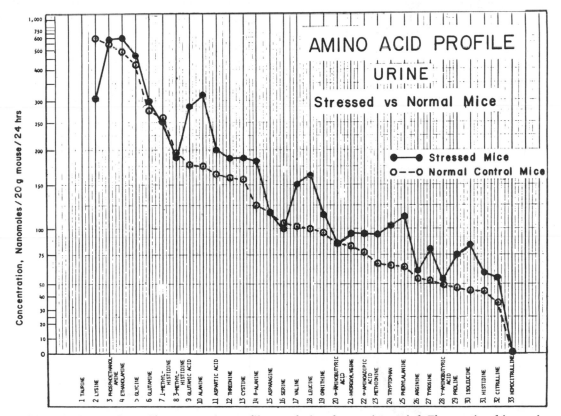

FIGURE 9–27. Amino acid concentration profiles of the urine of mildly stressed mice as compared with normal quiescent control animals. The anxiety stress was quantitatively induced under highly controlled experimental conditions, using a slow-speed rotational device at 45 rpm intermittently for 24 hours. The urine was a 24-hour sample collected during the rotation period. The rotational intermittence was controlled automatically and was programmed for ten minutes rotation and 50 minutes rest each hour. Food and water were available at all times during the 24-hour period. The centrifugal force of the rotation was less than 1 g, which permitted the mice to move about their cage at will.

stress,[35] as indicated by significant alterations in the amino acid profile of the urine of normal mice compared with analogous stressed animals. Some of the more conspicuous changes that may be noted are the decreased concentration of lysine, and in contrast, the elevations of glutamic acid, alanine, valine, leucine, tryptophan, phenylalanine, tyrosine, and isoleucine.

These observations demonstrate the sensitivity of the concentration-prioritized amino acid profiles for detecting subtle physiological changes. Of equal importance, the combined data illustrate the remarkable sensitivity of the organism in responding to both its internal and external environments.

Stress and Tumor Bahavior. The theoretical question arises, when discussing the influence of various environmental factors upon

animal physiology, as to whether such factors have either beneficial or harmful effects upon neoplasia. In order to examine the specific question as to whether controlled anxiety stress can influence the cancer process, a tumor-host model was established that was relatively sensitive to subtle alterations in the immunocompetence of the host. Since it is known that stress may have adverse effects upon cell-mediated immunological capabilities,[31,35,36,46] the tumor-host model was specifically designed to detect such effects, if indeed they existed.

Figure 9-28 illustrates an experimental consequence of the exposure of such an animal model to a mild pulse of anxiety stress during the early stages of tumor establishment and growth. Under these experimental circumstances, the normal quiescent mouse was able to cope with the incipient neoplasia and bring

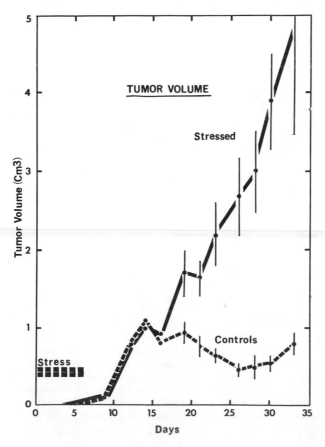

FIGURE 9-28. Influence on subsequent tumor growth of host exposure to an intermittent course of mild anxiety stress. The stress was induced by slow rotation at 45 rpm for ten minutes out of each hour during the first six days following tumor implantation. The tumor was the 6C3HED ascites. lymphosarcoma inoculated subcutaneously into C3H/He female mice about ten weeks old. Food and water were available at all times during the experiment.

about a regression of the developing tumors. In contrast, analogous animals subjected to mild rotational-induced anxiety stress during the early stages following tumor implantation, were not able to reject similar tumors, which went on to progressive growth with fatal consequences for the host.

Reference to Figure 9-27 shows a different biochemical manifestation of the metabolic changes that occurred in similarly stressed mice. Although there is no direct experimental evidence that the observed stress-induced changes in amino acid concentrations are related to the observed tumor growth enhancement, it has been reported that changes in certain amino acid levels have been associated with a reduction in immunological competence.[57]

TUMOR-ASSOCIATED ANOREXIA

The finding of tumor-induced anorexia in an experimental animal model, as shown in Figures 9-6 and 9-7, carries several useful implications. These observations relate to the nutritional problems of cancer patients that result from a loss of appetite followed by weight loss, and in some instances, an eventual lethal cachexia. This murine tumor-host model provides an opportunity to approach these problems experimentally.

The observations suggest that one or more metabolic products released by certain growing tumors may interfere with the host appetite control centers located in the hypothalamus, which are known to control appetite, thirst, and certain other basic physiological processes. An appetite-depressing peptide, which seems to act on receptors localized in the hypothalamic centers controlling appetite, has recently been isolated from the urine of patients with anorexia nervosa.[52] It may also be pertinent that a substantial increase occurs in two unidentified compounds appearing on amino acid chromatograms of urine obtained from mice with growing B-16 melanomas.[39]

It would be appropriate to determine whether these, or related substances, may be responsible for the anorexia that occurs in melanoma patients, as well as in melanoma-bearing mice. Such substances could theoretically be isolated and characterized, which might lead to the use of inhibitory analogs or other means for neutralizing the adverse effects of the anorexia-inducing substances released or induced by the cancer process.

This approach is in contrast to current hypotheses involving taste aversions and other psychologically-oriented explanations for cancer-associated anorexia. The results illustrated in Figure 9-6 and Figure 9-7 provide clues that may lead to the isolation of specific substances produced during the cancer process, which may be quantitatively correlated with increasing tumor mass and decreasing food consumption.

SUMMARY

This chapter emphasizes the biochemical and physiological influences that tumors, both pigmented and nonpigmented, have upon their hosts. Of special significance are the highly specific relationships that exist between individual tumors and their hosts, both in respect to biochemical alterations of normal endogenous components, as well as the physiological handling of administered exogenous substances. These tumor-induced biochemical effects are further manifested by alterations in the integrity and behavior of various organs such as the thymus, spleen, lymph nodes, and liver. Possibly related to some of these tumor-induced alterations in the host organs, is a conspicuous anorexia occuring in melanoma-bearing mice, which leads to cachexia.

The resident tumors also have remarkable abilities to alter the normal balance in the concentrations of various plasma amino acids that make up the usually highly stable circulating pool. The concentration changes in individual amino acids are not necessarily in the same direction; for example, the same tumor can cause a decrease in plasma glutamine and an increase in plasma alanine. Further, each tumor type exhibits characteristic amino acid patterns of the tumor tissue itself, as well as specific patterns in the plasma.

These data indicate that the complex patterns of the metabolic products associated with various tumor categories are unique, and thus provide individual biochemical identifications that may be theoretically useful for new approaches to cancer diagnosis, prognosis, or therapy.

Upon the administration of exogenous compounds, either for therapy or for toxicology studies, the resulting metabolic products processed by the tumor differ depending upon the tumor variety. For example, the data presented demonstrate that certain tumors can protect the host from a given toxic drug, while another tumor type can enhance the drug's toxicity, with subsequent lethal effects. Thus, the growing tumor may be looked upon as an auxiliary organ which enters into the overall metabolism and imposes unpredictable alterations upon normal metabolic processes.

The stable free radical, diphenylpicrylhydrazyl (DPPH) reacts with a wide range of reducing compounds of physiological origin, producing a color reaction that is suitable for the quantitative assay of various urinary metabolites that are associated with melanomas and other malignant processes, employing automatic chromatographic techniques.

Some of these biochemical or anatomical alterations that are produced in the tumor-bearing hosts may be useful as neoplastic markers for diagnostic purposes, or as physiological clues that may provide new exploitable opportunities for experimental cancer therapy.

REFERENCES

1. Aubert C, Lagrange C, Rorsman H, et al.: Catechols in primary and metastatic human malignant melanoma cells in monolayer cultures. Eur J Cancer 12:441–445, 1976
2. Banda PW, Sherry AE, Blois MS: An automatic analyzer for the detection of dihydroxyphenylalanine metabolites and other reducing compounds in urine. Anal Chem 46:1772–1777, 1974
3. Banda PW, Sherry AE, Blois MS: An automatic analyzer for the detection of urinary melanogens, in Riley V (ed): Melanoma: Basic Properties and Chemical Behavior, Basel. S. Karger, 1976, p 254
4. Banda PW, Sherry AE, Blois MS: Column cation-exchange separation of melanin-related metabolites in urine from cases of melanoma. Clin Chem 23:1397, 1977
5. Banda PW, Tuttle MS, Selmer L, et al.: Data processing of urine chromatograms for the clinical management of melanoma. Comput Biomed Res, in press, 1980
6. Benson JV Jr, Gordon MJ, Patterson JA: Accelerated chromatographic analysis of amino acids in physiological fluids containing glutamine and asparagine. Anal Biochem 18:228–240, 1967
7. Bjorklund A, Falek B, Jacobsson S, et al.: Cysteinyldopa in human malignant melanoma. Acta Derm Venereol (Stockh) 52:357, 1972
8. Blois MS Banda PW: Detection of occult metastatic melanoma by urine chromatography. Cancer Res 36:3317, 1976
9. Clark WH, Mastrangelo MJ, Ainsworth AM, et al.: Current concepts of the biology of human cutaneous malignant melanoma. Adv Cancer Res 24:267, 1977
10. Clarke DA, Reilly HC, Stock CC: A comparative study of 6-diazo-5-oxo-L-norleucine and o-diazoacetyl-L-serine on sarcoma 180. Antibiot Chemother 7:653–671, 1957
11. Cochran AJ, John UW, Gothoskar BP: Cell mediated immunity in malignant melanoma. Lancet I:1340–1341, 1972
12. Comsa J, Hook RR Jr: Thymectomy, in: Luckey TD: Thymic Hormones, Baltimore, University Park Press, 1973 pp 1–18
13. Dougherty TF, Berliner MD, Schneebeli GL, Berliner DL: Hormonal control of lymphatic structure and function. Ann NY Acad Sci 113:825–843, 1964
14. Duchon J, Matous B: Identification of two new metabolites in melanoma urine. Clin Chim Acta 16:397, 1967
15. Duchon J, Matous B, Prochazkov B: Vanillactic acid in the urine of melanoma patients. Clin Chim Acta 18:487, 1967
16. Fidler IJ, Kripke ML: Metastasis results from preexisting variant cells within a malignant tumor. Science 197:893. 1977
17. Fossati G, Colnaghi MI, Della Porta G, et al.: Cellular and humoral immunity against human malignant melanoma. Int J Cancer 8:344–351, 1971
18. Glick D, Von Redlick D, Levine S: Fluorometric determination of corticosterone and cortisol in 0.02–0.05 milliliters of plasma or submilligram samples of adrenal tissue. Endocrinology 74:653–655, 1964

19. Goodall McC, Alton H: Metabolism of 3,4-dehydroxyphenylalanine in human subjects. Biochem Pharmacol 21:2401, 1972
20. Greenstein JP: Biochemistry of Cancer, ed 2, Academic Press, New York, 1954
21. Hellstrom I, Sjogren HO, Warner G, Hellstrom KE: Blocking of cell-mediated tumor immunity by sera from patients with growing neoplasms. Int J Cancer 7:226–237, 1971
22. Hillier KA: Catecholamines in melanoma urine, MS thesis, Univ of Cal, San Francisco, 1978
23. Howard RJ, Mergenhagen SE, Notkins AL, Dougherty SF: Inhibition of cellular immunity and enhancement of humoral antibody formation in mice infected with lactic dehydrogenase virus, Transplant Proc 1:586–588, 1969
24. Hu F: Proliferation and melanin production in melanoma cell cultures, in Riley V: Pigmentation: Its Genesis and Biologic Control, New York, Appleton, 1972, pp 479–496
25. Jose DG, Good RA: Quantitative effects of nutritional essential amino acid deficiencies upon immune responses to tumors in mice. J Exp Med 137:1–9, 1973
26. Proffitt MR, Congdon CC: Effect of a large dose of LDH-virus on mouse lymphatic tissue, Fed Proc 29:559, 1970
27. Prota G, Nicolaus RA: Struttura e biogenesi delle feomelanine. Gass Chim Ital 97:665, 1967
28. Riley V: Adaptation of orbital bleeding technique to rapid serial blood studies. Proc Soc Exp Biol 104:751–754, 1960
29. Riley V: Demonstration of differences between normal and tumor-bearing animals. Proc Soc Exp Biol Med 97:169–175, 1958
30. Riley V: Lactate dehydrogenase in the normal and malignant state and the influence of a benign enzyme-elevating virus, in Busch H (ed), Methods in Cancer Research, vol 4, New York, Academic Press 1968, pp 495–612
31. Riley V: Persistence and other characteristics of the lactate dehydrogenase-elevating virus (LDH-Virus). In Hotchin J (ed), Slow Virus Diseases, New York, S. Karger, 1974, pp 198–213, Progress in Medical Virology, vol 18, Melnick JL (series ed)
32. Riley V: Protective ventilated shelves for experimental animal storage. Proc 23rd Annu Sess Am Assoc Lab Anim Sci 1972
33. Riley V: Synergistic reaction between p-phenylenediamine and melanoma components. Proc Soc Exp Biol Med 98:57–61, 1958
34. Riley V, Lilly F, Huerto E, Bardell D: Transmissible agent associated with 26 types of experimental mouse neoplasms, Science 132: 545–547, 1960
35. Riley V, Spackman DH: Housing stress. Lab Anim 6:16–21, 1977
36. Riley V, Spackman DH: Modifying effects of a benign virus on the malignant process and the role of physiological stress on tumor incidence, in Chiragos MA Fogarty International Cancer Proceedings, No 28, US Government Printing Office, 1977, pp 319–336
37. Riley V, Spackman DH, Fitzmaurice MA: Critical influence of an enzyme-elevating virus upon long-term remissions of mouse leukemia following asparaginase therapy, in Grundman E, Oettgen HF: Experimental and Clinical Effects of L-Asparaginase, New York, Springer, 1970, pp 81–101
38. Riley V, Spackman DH, Fitzmaurice MA: Influence of asparaginase and glutaminase upon free amino acids in normal and tumor-bearing mice, in Boiron M: La L-Asparaginase. Paris, Centre National de la Recherche Scientifique, 1971, pp 139–158
39. Riley V, Spackman DH, Fitzmaurice MA: Plasma and urine amino acid changes associated with melanoma. Proc 8th Int Pig Cell Conf, Basel, S. Karger, 1973, vol 1, pp 331–345
40. Riley V, Spackman DH, Santisteban GA, et al.: The LDH-virus: An interfering biological contaminant. Science 200:124–126, 1978
41. Santisteban GA, Dougherty TF: Comparison of the influences of adrenocortical hormones on the growth and involution of lymphatic organs, Endocrinology 54:130–146, 1954
42. Santisteban GA, Riley V, Fitzmaurice MA: Thymolytic and adrenal cortical responses to the LDH-elevating virus. Proc Soc Exp Biol 139:202–206, 1972
43. Snodgrass MJ, Hanna MG Jr: Histoproliferative effects of rauscher leukemia virus on lymphatic tissue. Alterations in the thymic-dependent area induced by the passenger lactic dehydrogenase virus. J Nat Cancer Inst 45:741–759, 1970
44. Spackman DH: Improved resolution in amino acid analysis in cancer therapy studies. Fed Proc 28:898, 1969
45. Spackman DH, Riley V: E-N-monomethyllysine and other plasma amino acids in leukemic mice, and effects of asparaginase. Fed Proc 30:1067, 1971
46. Spackman DH, Riley V: The modification of cancer by stress: effects of plasma corticosterone elevation on immunological system components in mice. Fed Proc 35:1693, 1976

47. Spackman DH, Riley V: True adrenal gluco-corticoid values in experimental animals: Implications for cancer research. 12th Int Cancer Congress, Buenos Aires, 1978 in press

48. Spackman DH, Riley V, Bloom J: True plasma corticosterone levels of mice in cancer/stress studies. Proc Amer Assoc Cancer Res 19:57, 1978

49. Spackman DH, Stein WH, Moore S: Automatic recording apparatus for use in the chromatography of amino acids. Anal Chem 30:1190–1206, 1958

50. Sundberg RD: Lymphocytes and plasma cells. Ann NY Acad Sci 59:671–689, 1955

51. Trapeznikov NN, Raushenbakh MO, Ivanova VD, et al.: Clinical evaluation of a method of quantitative determination of homovanillic acid for the estimation of degree of tumor dissemination process in melanoma of the skin, Cancer 36:2064, 1975

52. Trygstad OE, Reichelt KL, Johansen JH, Foss I: First International Colloquium on Receptor, Neurotransmitters, and Peptide Hormones, in Internal Med News 16:3, 1979

53. Voorhess ML: Urinary excretion of DOPA and metabolites by patients with melanoma. Cancer 26:146 1970

54. Yahr MD (ed): Current Concepts in the Treatment of Parkinsonism, New York, Raven Press, 1974

CHAPTER TEN

PRINCIPLES OF CLINICAL EVALUATION AND TREATMENT OF MALIGNANT MELANOMA

IRVING M. ARIEL

Recent data define various forms of malignant melanoma with different natural histories and different prognosis.

HUTCHINSON'S MELANOTIC FRECKLE

Jonathan Hutchinson in 1892 described a lesion of the face that is almost always associated with severe solar degeneration of the skin. Occasionally, however, it may appear in younger people without solar degeneration. This suggests that individual susceptibility is necessary for solar action to be effective in causing melanotic changes. Hutchinson noted that the lesion has a tendency to advance and recede like an infection, which he believed it was, and on occasion may disappear but recurs after a month or even years. This lesion is usually impalpable before invasive nodules appear, which takes 10 to 15 years, occasionally longer. The nodules can be malignant as in a case described by Hutchinson (his case 1). In 1894, he altered the name to lentigo melanoses and stated that he had seen the lesion on the lips and prepuce.

Dubreuilh, in 1894, described lesions also occurring in the younger groups, termed *mélanose circonscrite précancéreuse*, meaning any melanotic area of the skin or mucous membrane that in time would undergo malignant changes.

Portions of Hutchinson's freckle may consist of malignant melanoma, while other portions are premalignant. The prognosis after excision is usually very good.

This tumor has been termed *lentigo maligna melanoma* by Clark et al[12] and described in detail by Kopf and Bart.[35]

MAJOR TYPES OF MALIGNANT MELANOMA

Two major types of malignant melanoma are: (1) superficial spreading melanoma with and/or without invasion, and (2) nodular invasive melanoma. These designations have been utilized for many years. Recent categories defining levels of invasion or thickness of the melanoma have permitted a better understanding of growth patterns, treatment policies, and prognosis (Fig. 10–1) (Chap. 6).

SUPERFICIAL SPREADING MELANOMA

This most frequent form of melanoma, with varying colors and irregular borders, usually occurs in younger and middle-aged people[15] (Fig. 10–2). It tends to remain superficial and grow horizontally several years after which it develops a vertical growth phase with nodules becoming apparent. Many of these melanomas arise from preexistent nevi. During the early epidermal phase, pathologists may call them nevi with atypical cells, or active junction nevi, or atypical melanocytic hyperplasia.

LEVELS

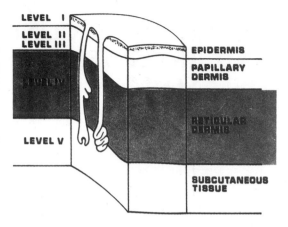

FIGURE 10-1. Levels of invasion of melanoma as described by the Clark classification. Level I tumors are intra-epidermal, i.e. above the epidermal-dermal junction. Level II tumors penetrate the loosely woven papillary dermis. Level III tumors fill the papillary dermis and press on the reticular dermis. Level IV tumors penetrate the reticular dermis. Level V tumors invade the subcutis. (From Kopf AW, Bart RS, Rodriguez-Saens RS: Malignant melanoma: A review, J Dermatol Surg Oncol, vol 3, Jan-Feb, 1977, p 54 with permission of author and publisher. Copyright 1977, The Journal of Dermatologic Surgery and Oncology, Inc.)

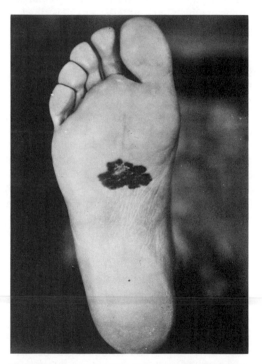

FIGURE 10-2. A spreading superficial melanoma of the sole of the foot.

NODULAR MALIGNANT MELANOMA

These lesions start as nodules that are dark brown to blue-black, occasionally amelanotic,

and they are the most malignant (Fig. 10-3). There is no so-called intraepidermal growth phase without associated dermal invasion, as is seen in the superficial spreading malignant melanoma.

OTHER TYPES OF MALIGNANT MELANOMA

The acral-lentiginous melanomas, described by Arrington et al.,[4] refer to melanomas occurring on the palms and soles, and the subungual lesions. In early phases in certain sections pathologists may call them simply benign melanocytic hyperplasia, whereas other sections may represent pure malignant melanoma. From a clinical standpoint we separate the subungual lesions from the others as we are convinced that all subungual malignant melanomas must be treated by amputation of the digit (see Chapter 22).

Malignant melanoma of the mucous membrane (Fig. 10-4) occurs more frequently in Orientals and Negroes than in whites, and usually has a poorer prognosis.

Ocular melanoma is a special entity treated by ophthalmological surgeons[28] (see Chapter 18).

Metastasizing malignant melanomas occasionally arise in the usually benign blue nevus of Jadassohn.

Juvenile melanoma (Spitz nevus) occurs most frequently in children but occasionally in adults. It usually involves the face and often is of a pale pink color (see Chapter 5).

Amelanotic melanomas are discussed in Chapter 14.

Desmoplastic and spindle-cell nevi and ma-lignant melanoma usually refers to histologic diagnoses.[18]

Pseudomelanoma of Ackerman consists of atypical melanocytic hyperplasia that recurs after incomplete excision of some nevi. It is a benign lesion.

The differential diagnosis in the clinical

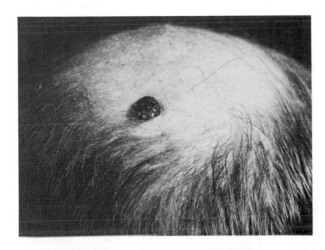

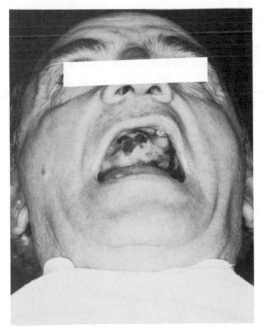

FIGURE 10–3. Nodular melanoma of the scalp.

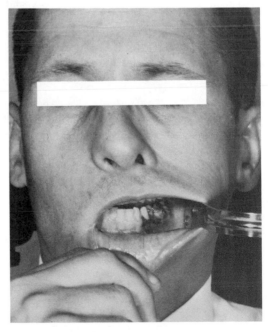

FIGURE 10–4. Left: Diffuse melanoma involving the hard and soft palate. Right: Extensive melanoma invading the left lower gingiva.

evaluation of malignant melanoma includes all pigmented lesions, some of which are: the B.K. moles, solar keratoses, hemangiomas, pigmented Bowen's disease (squamous-cell carcinoma in situ), pigmented basal cell carcinoma, and benign nevi, as well as dermatofibromas, and others.

A generalization regarding differential diagnosis of melanomas from benign nevi is that melanomas are usually variable in size, shape, boundaries, and color, and softer in consistency while nevi are usually uniform in color, with a regular outline and firm consistency. Multiple melanomas in the same patient are not rare.[6]

LOCATION

Melanomas may occur anywhere in the body. The distribution of cutaneous melanomas seen by the Pack Medical Group are presented in Table 10-1. Figures 10-5 and 10-6 are scattergrams denoting the relative frequency of benign nevi and malignant melanomas. They also occur in the mucous membrane, eyes, and other locations, but less frequently. The increased incidence of malignant melanoma of the head and neck and lower extremities, especially the feet, is noteworthy. Figure 10-7

shows the pattern of melanoma distribution, which does not correlate with the incidence of malignant melanoma.

AGE

Age, per se, is no contraindication when considering the possibility of a melanoma in a pigmented lesion. While no age is exempt from developing malignant melanoma, the vast majority of cases occur between the ages of 35 and 60. It occurs at a lower age than do most carcinomas. Although extremely rare in children, it may occur in the infant, transmitted through the placenta from a mother with disseminated melanoma, or de novo in a preadolescent child. Table 10-2 presents the types of pigmented lesions related to age. Figure 10-8 graphically displays the age distribution of patients with malignant melanoma seen at the Pack Medical Group. The ontogenetic relationship of the various pigmented lesions are shown in Figure 10-9.

COMPLEXION

Although no racial group is immune from developing melanomas, the majority occur in

TABLE 10-1. The Location of Malignant Melanomas. Pack Medical Group (1939-1967 inclusive)

	Number	Percent*
Trunk	1122	34.0
Chest wall	640	
Abdominal wall	482	
Head and neck	772	23.0
Lower extremity	673	20.0
Upper extremity	487	15.0
Subungual (toes and fingers)	72	2.2
Female genitalia	48	1.5
Gastrointestinal tract	22	0.7
Miscellaneous or undetermined primary	109	3.3
Total	3305	100.0

* The total is less than 100% as most figures are rounded to whole numbers.

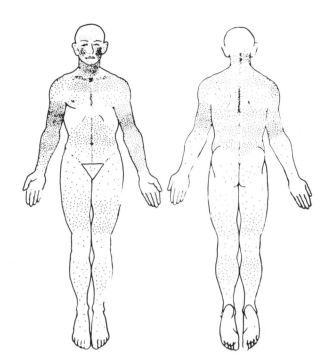

FIGURE 10-5. Regional distribution of nevi found on general examination, based on 1,000 adult patients. Each dot represents five nevi.

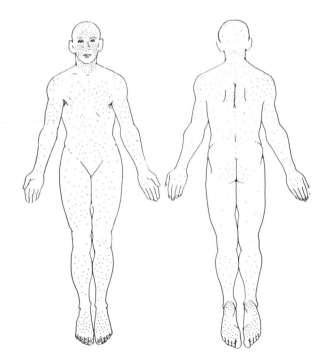

FIGURE 10-6. Regional distribution of malignant melanomas, based on 1,225 patients. Each dot represents one malignant melanoma.

TABLE 10-2. Incidence of Pigmented Lesions Related to Age

Age	Infancy 1–10 Months	Childhood 10 Months to 8 Years	Pre-Sexual 8–14 Years	Pubertal Male-28 Yrs. Female-24 Yrs.	Maturity Varies	Senescence Marked Chronological Variance
Shakespeare	"At first the infant mewling and puking in the nurse's arm"		"And then the whining schoolboy, with his satchel and shining morning face, creeping like a snail unwillingly to to school"	"And then the lover sighing like furnace with a woeful ballad made to his mistress eyebrow"	"Then the soldier full of strange oaths, and bearded like the Bard, and then the justice, in fair round belly with good capon lined"	"Second childishness and mere oblivion, sans teeth, sans eyes, sans taste, sans everything"
Definition	Birth to independent nutrition	To development of senses	Intermediate stage between childhood and adulthood	From puberty to end of growth period	From end of growth to sexual decline (male), menopause (female)	From menopause (female), sexual decline (male), to demise
Pigmented Tumors Benign*	Mongolian spot Bathing trunk nevi Beginning of some nevi (2%)	Spontaneous disappearance Early junction nevus First compound nevi Benign juvenile nevus		Nevi tend to enlarge slowly Incidence decreases Halo nevus (usually in girls), Dermal nevus, enlargement and darkening of compound nevi	Further decrease Enlargement and darkening of nevi, areola, etc., during pregnancy	Nevi may fall off, or undergo necrosis or fibrosis None to rare Absence of nevi Increase lentigo
Tumors Malignant	Juvenile melanomas (rare) Malignant melanoma transmitted thru placenta from mother (3 cases reported)	Juvenile melanomas (most common age bracket) Melanoma very rare (Approximately 100 cases reported)		Incidence decreases (15% of juvenile melanomas) Beginning increased incidences of malignant melanoma	Highest incidence of malignant melanoma	Decrease in incidence of malignant melanoma

* Any rapid change in a nevus (size, pigmentation, itch, bleeding) warrants its immediate removal.

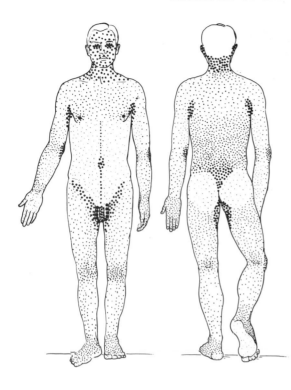

FIGURE 10-7. Pattern of primary melanin distribution, when unaffected by sunlight or other melanin-provoking exposure, based on spectrophotometric data (courtesy of Dr. Edward A. Edwards, Department of Anatomy, Harvard Medical School).

patients with fair complexion, blue eyes, and red or strawberry blond hair. They are also frequent in patients who freckle easily after exposure to the sun and do not tan. Of our 3,305 patients, 85% fell into this complexion category. About 10% of all people in this geographic region exhibit these features. Individuals with mixed background, such as mulattos, are more prone to develop melanomas than those with a purely dark background. A pigmented lesion that is primary in the skin of a Negro is virtually

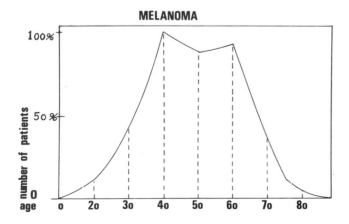

FIGURE 10-8. Age distribution of 3,305 melanomas of the Pack Medical Group.

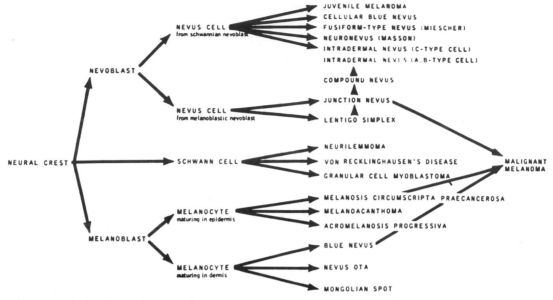

Figure 10-9. Pathogenesis of melanotic tumors from neural crest. (With permission from Mishima Y: Macromolecular changes in pigmentary disorders. Arch Dermatol 91:519, 1965. Copyright 1965, AMA.)

never a malignant melanoma, except on the soles of the feet, palms of the hands, and mucous-cutaneous junctions.

SEX

The number of men in different series exceedes the number of women in every site except the lower extremities, where the reverse is true.

HISTORY

The history of a patient who presents with a pigmented lesion should include a number of questions that will be helpful in determining the diagnosis as well as the prognosis.

1. Did the lesion arise de novo, or did a preexisting mole that had been present for many years change in character (size, color, itching, or bleeding). In either of these cases, the possibility of a melanoma must be considered.

2. Had the patient received any therapy elsewhere? Had another lesion been removed from the skin? This is particularly important if the patient presents with a metastasis to the regional lymph nodes with an occult primary. The appearance of satellites in a lesion previously excised without histology strongly suggests that a malignant melanoma had been previously excised.

3. A family survey should be included, especially if a parent or sibling has been treated for malignant melanoma.

4. The patient should be queried as to other lesions that may have changed or appeared de novo, inasmuch as multiple melanomas may be present in the same patient.

5. Questions should include symptoms that refer to the possible presence of another lesion, inasmuch as the incidence of a second primary cancer is somewhat higher in patients bearing melanoma than in the average individual.

The incidence of multiple primary malignant melanomas in patients is difficult to evaluate because of the paucity of reported data (Fig. 10–10). The incidence increases somewhat in patients with familial melanomas over those who have developed sporadic melanomas without a preceding etiologic factor. Greene and Fraumeni[22] combined data from different reports, and determined an incidence of multiple melanomas to be 197 of 7,233 patients (2.7%). The multiple lesions occurred slightly more frequently in females (84 females; 74 males). Site distribution fluctuated according to those factors determining the sites in patients with sporadic melanomas, and the mean number of primary melanomas per patient, determined by Greene and Fraumeni, was 2.4. Incidence is higher in hereditary familial melanomas than in sporadic ones. Fifty of 406 patients with hereditary melanomas (12.3%) showed an almost equal distribution between the sexes. The mean age at the time of diagnosis was 35.8 years, as compared with 42.9 years for those with single tumors. Females with multiple primaries were younger than the males (33.4 years vs 39 years). The site distribution of the hereditary multiple tumors revealed a greater frequency in the trunk in females, and the arms of both sexes. Inasmuch as the role played by hereditary factors in the melanoma syndrome is uncertain, the physician should perform a complete check of the family of a patient with malignant melanoma. Multiple primary melanomas may coexist with multiple basal cell carcinomas, especially in patients with xeroderma pigmentosa (Figure 10–11). Melanoma may also be associated with coexistent pigmentary disorders (Figure 10–12).

It is of interest that the hereditary multiple primaries were of the superficial spreading type in 86.1%.

The history should also include exposure to sunlight, as well as possible trauma to the site, which may have had an influence either in the development of the melanoma or in causing the clinical changes that drew attention to the pigmented lesion.

Despite the number of factors that focus attention on melanomas and the differential diagnosis that must be evaluated, the only way a melanoma can be diagnosed is by biopsy.

BIOPSY

All pigmented lesions should be biopsied if the physician is concerned regarding the diagnosis. A pigmented lesion that requires therapy should never be treated by ointments, escharotics, electrocoagulation, irradiation, or any other form of treatment. All excised pigmented lesions of the skin should be carefully reviewed by a pathologist knowledgeable in the field of melanoma (Figs. 10-13 through 10-20). (Despite having seen and studied several thousand malignant melanomas, I am still foiled in considering certain lesions as malignant melanoma that prove to be benign; I have also evaluated lesions as benign only to get a report back from the pathologist that they are malignant.)

The biopsy should consist of a complete excision. Incisional biopsies are reserved for bulky or diffuse lesions where one wants to fortify clinical diagnosis by histologic confirmation. It is essential to remove the entire lesion, where possible, in order to give the pathologist significant tissue to determine the nature of the surrounding tissues. This will permit him to make a diagnosis of malignant melanoma, to differentiate between primary or metastatic melanoma, to evaluate the level of invasion, whether invasion of lymphatics or blood vessels has occurred, and the thickness of the tumor.

A local bloc anesthesia is preferable to infiltration of the melanoma site, after which the tumor can be removed conservatively by means of an elliptical incision and the wound closed with interrupted, nonabsorbable suture material. We do not depend upon frozen section analysis since we have never found any danger in delaying several days to permit the pathologist to examine several sections of the specimen. We are encountering more and more evaluation of depth of invasion based on

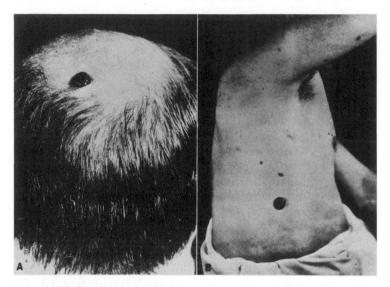

FIGURE 10-10.   Multiple primary melanomas in a white male. A. In the scalp. B. In the trunk.

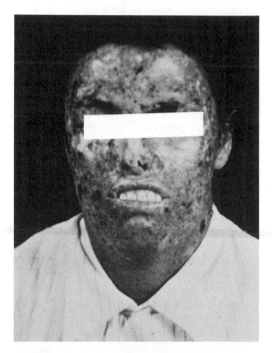

FIGURE 10-11.   A young girl with xeroderma pigmentosa who developed multiple malignant and multiple basal cell carcinomas on the facial skin.

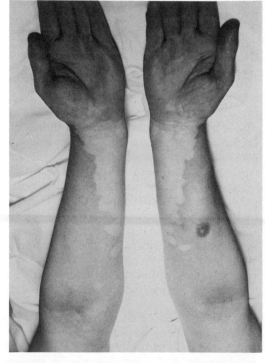

FIGURE 10-12.   Malignant melanoma of the right arm associated with vitiligo.

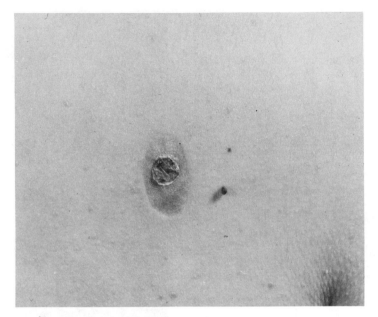

FIGURE 10-13.   Differential diagnosis. Basal cell carcinoma.

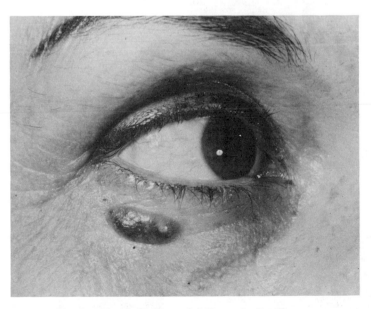

FIGURE 10-14.   Differential diagnosis. Papilloma.

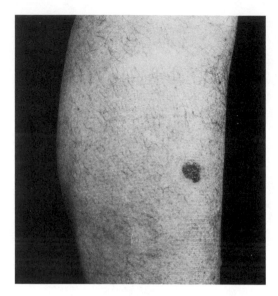

FIGURE 10-15. Differential diagnosis. Kaposi's sarcoma.

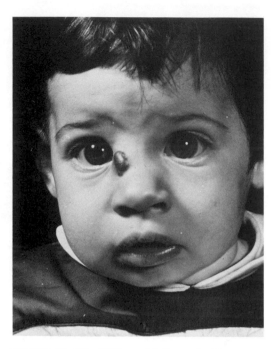

FIGURE 10-17. Differential diagnosis. Cavernous hemangioma.

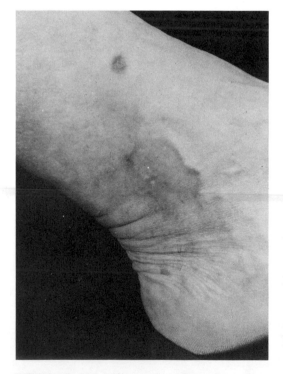

FIGURE 10-16. Differential diagnosis. Dermatofibroma.

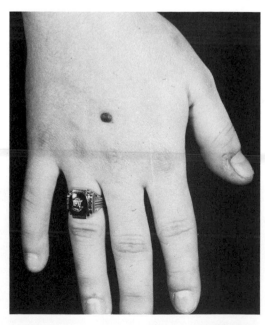

FIGURE 10-18. Differential diagnosis. Pappillary nevus.

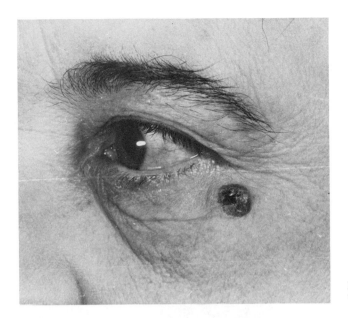

FIGURE 10-19. Differential diagnosis. Verrucous.

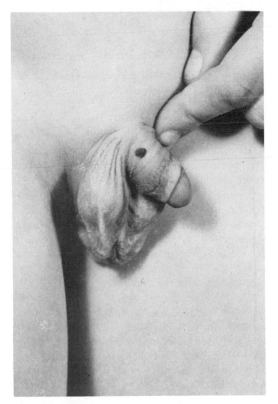

FIGURE 10-20. Differential diagnosis. Resting dermal nevus of penis in a preadolescent boy.

one slide submitted to the consulting pathologist. This leads to incorrect evaluation and the practice is to be condemned.

PRINCIPLES OF THERAPY

PRETHERAPY EVALUATION

Once the diagnosis has been established, studies should be performed to aid in determining whether the tumor is localized or whether it has metastasized. In the latter case, radical surgical intervention would be contraindicated, and the treatment would then be palliative. Figure 10-21 shows the incidence of metastases to different organs of patients dying from malignant metastases (Figs. 10-22 and 10-23).

The routine evaluation consists of a complete physical examination with roentgenograms of the lungs and a roentgen survey of the skeletal system.

Additional diagnostic procedures available for undergoing clinical evaluation are: certain biochemical markers (discussed in Chapter 9), and the use of isotopic techniques for the detection of melanoma or its metastases (discussed in Chapter 11).

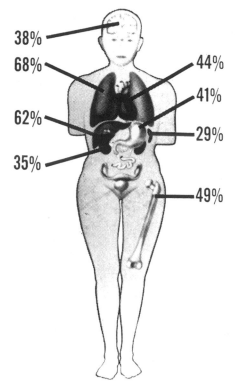

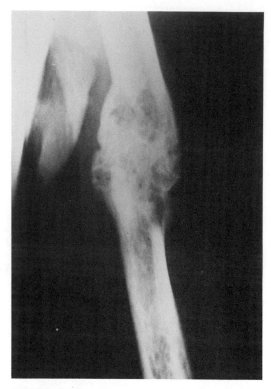

FIGURE 10–21. Topographic chart showing incidence of distribution of metastatic melanoma found on postmortem examination. (Pack Medical Group)

FIGURE 10–22. Metastatic melanoma to humerus.

Urine Examination. Urine examination for melanogenuria as a test for the presence of melanoma or metastases by either the ferric chloride test, Thormählen's test, or the Erhlich test have been found unsatisfactory and positive only in the presence of very extensive metastases, which would in any case have been determined by other tests.[7]

Thermography in Malignant Melanoma. Thermography is used to diagnose many cancers; several authors, including Hessler and Maillard,[26] believe that melanomas and other lesions such as inflammation and angiomas are hyperthermic. They feel the best application of thermography is in detecting metastases or local spread not visible by ordinary clinical evaluation.

On the other hand, Bodenham, in 1968, found that melanomas, if they were hyperthermic, were only slightly so, being exceeded by other malignant tumors in this regard.[9]

Computerized Axial Tomography (CAT Scan). The use of computerized axial tomography will gain more and more use in the detection of metastases from melanoma. Diagnosis of an amelanotic melanoma was reported by Menzer and colleagues in 1975.[44] We have diagnosed metastatic melanoma with CAT scanning of the brain in several patients with melanoma, and have found it to be the best method of diagnosis in a patient who has been treated for melanoma and who develops symptoms of central nervous system involvement. It is being used extensively for diagnosis of melanomas of the thorax and abdomen.

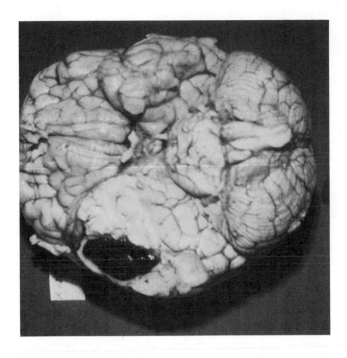

FIGURE 10-23. Metastatic melanoma to brain.

Radionucleid Photoscanning. Radiopharmaceuticals are widely used in the detection of space-occupying lesions of the lungs, liver, kidneys, and other organs. They are particularly useful in detecting lesions of the skeletal system, which appear many months before the lesion is visible roentgenographically.

Roth and colleagues[58] have reported the use of isotope scanning of the liver, bone, brain, and entire body during the initial evaluation of patients with stage I and II malignant melanoma (Fig. 10–24). They concluded that the yield was so slight that the procedure was not indicated because of the great expense to the patient and the fact that it may delay initiation of definitive therapy. In their series of 100 patients, scanning resulted in change of staging or therapy in only one individual.

I routinely perform radioactive technetium liver scans and bone scans on my patients with malignant melanoma. Our findings are similar to those of Roth and colleagues in that the scanning of the patient did not influence the overall treatment policies. However, the use of the scans has been found to be most useful in repeat followup of the patient. For example,

in a number of patients with normal livers at the time the patients were first treated, a space-occupying defect developed later. Although treatment of metastases of melanoma to the liver has had poor results, the knowledge that a space-occupying lesion exists influences the diagnosis and plan of treatment for the patient. The hope of better modalities for treatment in the future makes earlier diagnoses desirable. The use of the hepatic scan has been found to be particularly helpful for patients who later developed such entities as hepatitis, or parenchymal hepatic disorders. The scan combined with a profile of the blood chemistries permitted us to make a diagnosis that the patient was suffering from an extramelanoma malady.

Similarly, the use of bone scans has been found particularly helpful in the case of patients who have been followed for a prolonged period who develop back pain or other pain related to the osseous system. Having the scans available as a bank of background data will be useful in future evaluation and treatment. One such patient had severe pain in both hips, but negative scans eventually

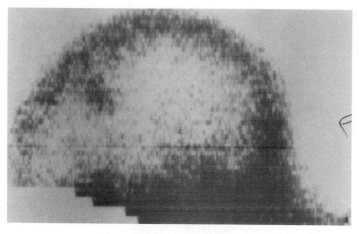

FIGURE 10–24.   Metastases to brain as determined by brain scan. Only complaint of the patient was headache. Note abnormal pick-up of isotope in the anterosuperior aspect.

pointed to a diagnosis of arthritis; she had a hip replacement performed on both sides and remains well.

Refer to Chapter 11 for more information on radionucleid photoscanning.

Gallium Scanning. Gallium-67 is an isotope that is preferentially concentrated by inflammatory sites, abscesses, and some tumors. In 1973, Milder and colleagues[45] reported total body scanning in 44 patients with malignant melanoma proved by biopsy. They concluded that if one could rule out infection, and if the patient had not been operated upon recently, the number of false positives was only 2%. False negatives occurred in 45% of the patients. They suggest that gallium scanning be combined with other techniques, and have found that the degree of pigmentation had no influence on the pickup, but that size did. Masses larger than 2 cm in diameter were positive in 75% of their cases, whereas those 2 cm or less were positive in only 17%. Accordingly, they conclude that a negative scan has no clinical significance, but a positive scan in the absence of inflammation or infection is useful in evaluating the presence of metastases.

We have performed ^{67}Ga scans in 50 patients with melanoma, including those with known metastases, and have found the test positive in 20 individuals with especially large metastases. Individuals with known metastases to the inguinal region did not show an abnormal pickup of the gallium. Those with pulmonary metastases did show unusual pickup of gallium for large lesions but no pickup in the same lung of smaller lesions. Patients with hepatic metastases who have a space-occupying defect that is "cold" by routine liver nucleoid scans may be "hot" on gallium scan. Gottschalls diagnosed numerous subdermal metastases on ^{67}Ga scans in a patient who presented only one metastases clinically (personal communication).

Splenomeglia or Increased Spleen Scans.[8,49] Liver scans performed with 99m Tc-sulphur colloid are often performed on patients with cancer to rule out metastases to the liver (Fig. 10–25). In 1974, Goldman, Braunstein, and Song, while performing liver scans on patients with malignant melanomas, noticed that of 22 patients who did not have any abnormalities of their livers, ten showed an augmented splenic activity.[20] As controls, they used 54 patients with cancers from other sites without hepatic involvement, and only one of these had increased splenic uptake.

Chandra and colleagues[11] demonstrated increased splenic uptake in C–57 black mice bearing B–16 melanomas as compared with

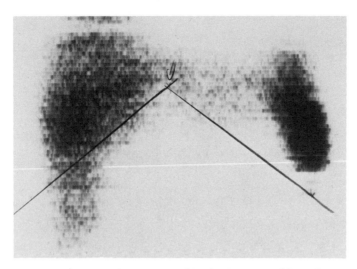

FIGURE 10-25. Liver/spleen scan (anterior view) in a patient treated for melanoma of the back. The spleen (left) is somewhat enlarged and denser than normally observed.

C-57 control mice bearing mammary carcinomas. The cause for this increased uptake is unknown.

Sober and co-workers,[62] in a combined study from New York University and Harvard, reviewed scans of 150 patients with malignant melanoma with no evidence of visceral involvement, and found that the prognosis of certain patients who initially showed augmented splenic activity as the only abnormal finding to be significantly worse than those of patients who did not demonstrate those findings (Figs. 10-26 and 10-27). Chandra et al. injected three groups of mice for splenic study: one group with melanoma implants, another with mammary carcinoma implants, and a third without any implants. Both the mammary and melanoma implanted animals showed increased uptake. The uptake was significantly greater in the animals with melanoma.

Nathanson and Kahn[50] reported on 24 patients, and in an answer to a letter to the Journal of Nuclear Medicine by the New York University Medical Center group, they presented evidence of a number of patients with increased splenic uptake who on autopsy were found to have metastases. They stated:

The clearcut answer to the question of whether increased splenic uptake of 99m Tc-sulfur colloid represents a remote effect of melanoma, presumably mediated by some humoral mechanism, or whether it simply indicates diffuse micrometastases in the spleen, will be resolved only when it is possible to carry out histopathologic examination on a significant number of spleens in these patients.

In our experience with 50 patients with malignant melanoma, some with evidence of metastases and some without, ten revealed an increase in splenic activity (Fig. 10-25).

If micrometastases within the spleen can be ruled out,[48] and if the claim of increased pickup by the spleen as a body response to the presence of a malignant melanoma is substantiated, splenomegalia represents an important diagnostic and prognostic index.[24,32] Further investigations are indicated.

TREATMENT POLICIES

After the biopsy has confirmed the diagnosis of melanoma, complete surgical resection should be performed (Fig. 10-28). A generous portion of normal tissue, approximately 5 cm

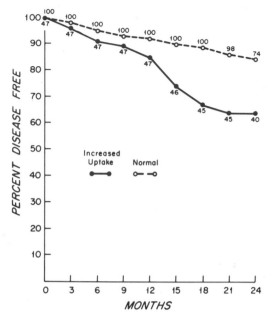

FIGURE 10-26. Life-table analysis of recurrence of disease in patients with malignant melanoma separated on basis of uptake status of spleen. Numbers associated with each item point represent number of patients followed that length of time. Curve of patients with normal scans differ from curve of patients with augmented splenic uptake (p < 0.02). (From Arthur J. Sober, et al.: The significance of augmented radiocolloid uptake by the spleen in patients with malignant melanoma, Journal of Nuclear Medicine, 20(12):1979, with permission of author and journal.)

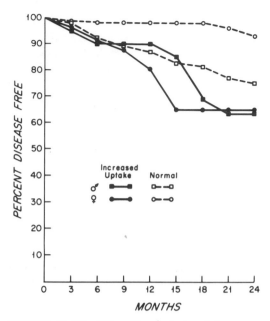

FIGURE 10-27. Life-table analysis of frequency and time of recurrence by sex and scan status. Curve for women with normal scans differs from curve of women with augmented splenic uptake (p < 0.05). (From Arthur J. Sober, et al.: The significance of augmented radiocolloid uptake by the spleen in patients with malignant melanoma, Journal of Nuclear Medicine, 20(12):1979, with permission of author and journal.)

surrounding the initial lesion, should be resected down to naked muscle, including the fascia. On rare occasions the muscle may be found to be involved by the melanoma, in which case it should be extensively resected. When the excision is performed on the torso, the defect may be closed by sliding flaps or the H-type incision. If the lesion is on an extremity, it is necessary to remove a large margin of tissue with the closure being effected by split thickness skin graft (Fig. 10-29).

If the regional lymph nodes are involved, the resection should include, wherever possible, an incontinuity dissection of the regional

lymph nodes[53] (Fig. 10-30). If the lesion involves the lateral aspect of the foot or the heel, the popliteal nodes may be involved and should be resected, in conjunction with a radical groin dissection (Fig. 10-31). There are several cases on record where the lesion remained localized to the lymph nodes, grew to an enormous size, and doomed the extremity. Cures of up to 45% were obtained by radical amputation such as hip-joint disarticulation with lymph node dissection, or hemipelvectomy. Before performing a radical amputation of the lower extremity, the abdominal contents can be inspected through the groin incision to rule out the possibility of metastases. If metastases are present, the procedure should be abandoned, unless it is being performed for purely palliative purposes. With the upper ex-

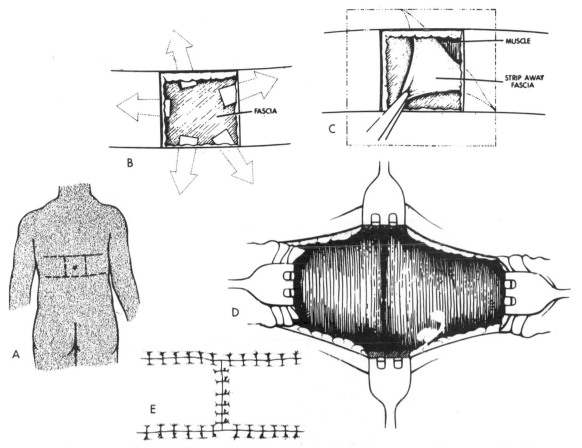

FIGURE 10-28. A. Type of incision to be made about the malignant melanoma of the back. B. The square of skin is excised, at least 4–5 cm equidistant from the melanoma. Skin flaps developed laterally will permit exposure of the underlying fascia. C. The fascia is stripped off the underlying muscle, and the dotted line demonstrates the amount of fascia to be excised. D. Completed excision showing the underlying muscle. E. The closure obtained by the sliding lateral flaps. (From Ariel IM: Surg Gynecol Obstet 139:1974, by permission of Surgery, Gynecology, & Obstetrics.)

tremity, an axillary dissection should be performed in conjunction with a resection of the primary site, preferably in continuity. For all subungual melanomas, an amputation of the digit and the proximal metacarpal or metatarsal bone should be performed. For those melanomas involving the chest wall, if the lower chest wall is involved, the ipsilateral axilla should be resected of its lymph nodes; if the involvement is in the region of the clavicle, then a combined axillary and cervical resection should be performed.

At our present stage of knowledge, chemotherapy and immunotherapy have very little to offer in the way of cure.

The question of lymph node dissection for clinical stage I melanoma (i.e., where no evidence of metastases to lymph nodes exists) is in a state of controversy with no definite rules applicable to date. With a diagnosis of malignant melanoma of Clark's Level I or Breslow's thickness less than 0.75 mm, then one can dispense with any thought of a regional lymph node dissection. If the diagnosis

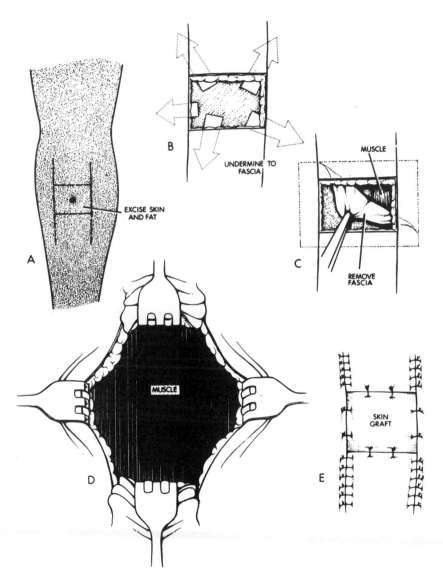

FIGURE 10-29.   Type of excision to be performed for a malignant melanoma of an extremity. A. Type of incision to be made, with extensions of the incision extending superiorly and inferiorly above and below the block of skin which is to be dissected. B. Development of the skin flap exposes the underlying fascia. C. The fascia is then stripped free with the specimen en bloc. D. Completed operation, demonstrating the underlying musculature. E. Partial closure of the defect with sliding flaps is shown, and the remainder of the defect is closed with a split thickness skin graft. (From Ariel IM: Surg Gynecol Obstet 139:1974, by permission of Surgery, Gynecology, & Obstetrics.)

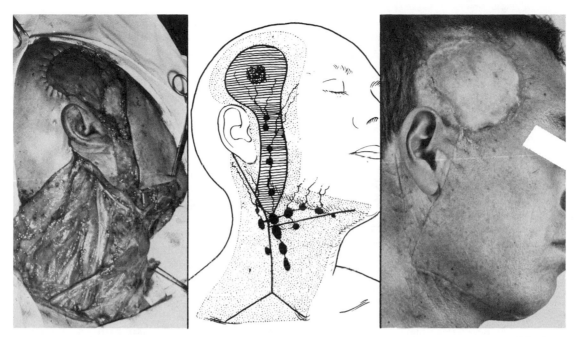

FIGURE 10–30. Illustration showing extent of resection of melanoma of temple metastatic to preauricular and cervical lymph nodes. Left: Operative view of dissection. Middle: Diagram showing extent of dissection. Right: Postoperative appearance.

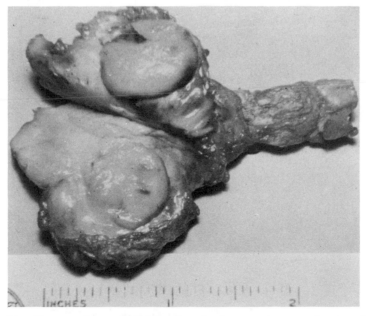

FIGURE 10–31. Metastases to popliteal lymph nodes from a primary melanoma of the lateral aspect of the foot. The popliteal artery and veins were resected and repair effected by vascular grafts.

is Clark's Level II, then the advisability of a dissection is questionable. Level III is an indeterminate value but seems to behave like a level IV thus far in our observations. We have observed level II and III metastasizing to regional lymph nodes, and unless contraindications exist, we prefer to do an elective lymph node dissection, either of the groin or the axillary lymph nodes, especially for those lesions adjacent to the lymphatic draining basin. For levels IV or V, an elective lymph node dissection should be performed in all instances, in our opinion. These surgical principles have been adopted by us after seeing 3,305 patients with malignant melanoma. The validity of current more conservative measures must be critically evaluated, as better education of both the medical profession and the laity now permit earlier diagnoses.

The behavior of untreated or unsuccessfully treated melanoma is unpredictable. It may remain localized for many years and grow to large size before metastases occur (Fig. 10–32 and 10–33). The metastases may remain regionally localized for long periods. One unusual case was recorded where the metastases of the melanoma involved only one side of the body (Fig. 10–34). A small primary melanoma may produce huge metastases to the regional lymph nodes with no further dissemination. Some of these can be cured by radical amputation (Fig. 10–35). A metastasis may produce such severe pigmentation as to "blacken" the patient (Fig. 10–36).

NONSURGICAL MEASURES FOR TREATING MALIGNANT MELANOMA

Cancer chemotherapy (Chapter 15) and immunotherapy (Chapter 8) are discussed in separate chapters. Other modalities include the following.

Lazer Radiation. Kozlov et al.[36] reported on the effects of malignant melanoma in animal tumors and they discovered that the more highly pigmented the tumor, the greater the reaction, and the less firm the consistency, the better the response. They suggested

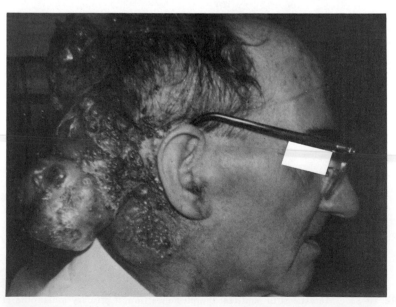

FIGURE 10–32.   A huge localized melanoma of the scalp which remained localized and killed the patient by invasion to the brain.

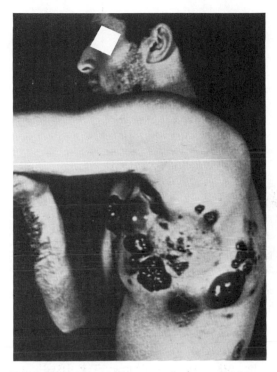

FIGURE 10-33.   Malignant melanoma which remained regionally localized with metastases to the chest wall for many years before dissemination occurred.

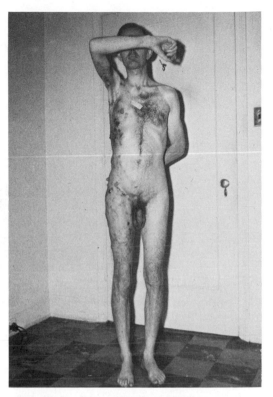

FIGURE 10-34.   Extensive metastases of a melanoma invading only the right side of the body.

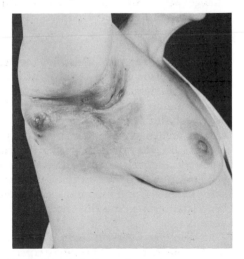

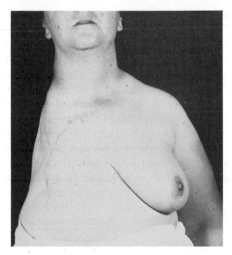

FIGURE 10-35.   Left: Extensive metastases to axilla involving the right breast. Right: Status after interscapulomammary amputation. The patient enjoyed palliation for four years before dissemination became manifest.

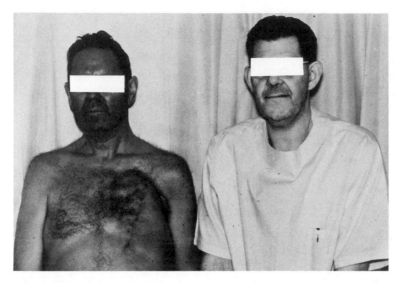

FIGURE 10–36. The patient with disseminated melanomatoses, who was originally a blond with a very light complexion, gradually became more pigmented. The resident at the right was originally darker than the patient.

that a lazer beam might be useful for surface neoplasms. They further found that high-speed electrons plus the lazer beam had a greater effect than either of these values alone.

Goldman[20,21] has reported interesting clinical trials of the utilization of surgery by lazer for malignant melanoma with preliminary promising results. He uses a CO_2 lazer and may repair the resulting defect with a split-thickness skin graft. Almost complete lack of bleeding after lazer excision enhances the graft take. He concludes that lazer is useful especially in the elderly and debilitated, for whom extensive surgical resection is contraindicated. He has found destruction of metastatic melanoma with combined chemotherapy and irradiation, but states: "More clinical investigative studies are required to determine the place of the lazer, particularly in the treatment of visceral metastases." He has found it most useful in treating metastatic animal lesions.

This modality should be used only in the hands of an expert until its exact role is determined.

Chemosurgery has been utilized by Mohs, Bloom, and Sahl[47] to treat three patients with the B.K. mole syndrome. The fixed-tissue chemosurgical technique provided a microscopically controlled, safe, effective, and conservative means of removing the numerous lesions. Atypical moles suspected of malignant change were removed by biopsy-excision, as this technique is contraindicated for malignant melanoma.

Radiation Therapy. Radiation therapy has a limited place in the overall treatment of melanoma. Melanomas are considered radioresistant tumors, and we have not used it in recent years for curative purposes. In the past, certain malignant melanomas, such as those of the vulva, were treated by radiation therapy. However, the resistance of the tumor and the poor radiation bed, a result of the often senile skin, kerarosis, and moistness, precluded any beneficial results, and this method was abandoned.[34]

Low-voltage x-rays utilizing the Miescher's technique, that is, 200 rad every three or four days for five treatments with x-rays generated at 12 KV filtered through 1 mm of cellon (equivalent to a HVL of 52 microns of AL) were delivered at a target to skin distance of 20 cm. The half-dose depth was 1.3 mm. This technique was utilized at the skin and cancer unit of the New York University Medical Center previously for the treatment of Hutchinson's freckle (lentigo maligna melanoma) as reported by Petratos and Kopf.[55] They quote 16 patients who were treated with the (soft) x-rays, of whom seven developed recurrences of lentigo maligna and three developed metastases of lentigo maligna melanoma. They have, accordingly, abandoned this technique.

In earlier years, we treated five patients with lentigo maligna melanoma with a slightly different technique utilizing x-rays of 20–50 KV volts with a total dose of 2,000 rads over a period of three weeks. The results were unsatisfactory and we have abandoned this technique for over 20 years, and have substituted surgical resection.

Several authors, including Arma-Szlachzic et al., continue to advise treatment of the melanotic freckle with radiotherapy.[3]

Pack and Livingston reported 217 patients with melanoma treated by irradiation with beneficial results in only five patients, and they abandoned its use. Ackerman and delRegato[1] found beneficial results in only 2% of the cases they evaluated.

A significant report was made by Dickson[17] in 1958 of a combined study from the Toronto General Hospital, the Johns Hopkins Hospital, and the Baltimore Public Health Hospital, using combined surgery and radiation therapy with a retrospective analysis of 254 patients. The irradiation was administered by various techniques including interstitial irradiation, teleradium to both primary and metastatic nodes (4,800–6,500 rads in four to six weeks), and roentgen therapy at 100 KV (5,000 rads in ten days to the primary site, and 4,500 in five weeks to the lymph node regions at 200–400 KV, and subsequently super-voltage radiation to the primary site and draining lymphatics). The 234 patients were divided into three treatment groups for evaluation. Forty-two were treated with a wide local excision, 71 with limited excision or the application of caustics, and 121 received radiation therapy. Five-year survival rates were 26.2% for those treated with wide local excision, 19.7% for

those who received limited local therapy, and 41.3% for those who received radiation therapy. The disparity of the different groups do not warrant any definite conclusion, but the study does suggest some beneficial effect from radiation therapy if judiciously used.

Pearson[54] reported, from the Christie Hospital in England, 48 patients treated with radiation therapy but without histologic confirmation. Results regarding radiation therapy without histologic confirmation cannot be accepted.

A randomized investigation of adjuvant radiation therapy for regional nodal metastases from malignant melanoma from the Mayo Clinic led to the following conclusion:[14]

> After nodal metastasis from malignant melanoma, approximately 80% of patients die from disseminated disease. To clarify the role of radiation therapy (XRT) following node dissection, 56 patients with biopsy-proven nodal metastasis participated in a randomized, prospective clinical trial which compares radiation therapy to the regional lymph node area following lymphadenectomy (27 patients) with lymphadenectomy alone (29 patients). Interesting differences in the survival curves (p = 0.09) and in the disease-free interval curves (p = 0.08) for the two treatment groups proved to be attributable to imbalances in the age and nodal distributions in the treatment groups. Covariate analysis identified age and sex as the factors having the most significant (p < 0.04) effect on survival and identified the number of positive nodes as the covariate having the most significant (p < 0.02) effect on disease-free interval. Treatment did not have a significant effect upon survival or disease-free interval.

Danger of complications from extensive irradiation must concern the therapist. Milton[46] calls attention to the fact that massive primary melanomas would not penetrate healthy periosteum, but he records a patient with melanoma of the mucous membrane treated by radiation therapy, which resulted in extensive bone necroses.

Radiation therapy is used more frequently in Europe than in the United States. Hellriegel[25] reported on 289 patients with melanoma (68%

proved by biopsy). Stage I lesions had a 62% five-year survival when irradiation was part of the treatment. He advises preoperative radiation therapy. Lissner and Von Lieven[41] evaluated 1,900 stage I melanomas from the literature. They record a 50% five-year cure for surgery alone (1,110 patients), 67% for irradiation alone (289 patients), 69% for preoperative irradiation (175 patients), and 48% for postoperative irradiation (326 patients).

Melanomas of the mucous membrane are usually more radio sensitive than cutaneous ones.

Dickson[17] gave postoperative irradiation to the primary site and lymph nodes of a series of patients and obtained a five-year survival of 41%, compared with 26% by surgical extirpation alone.

Radiation Therapy for Palliation. Radiation therapy can produce rewarding results as a palliative treatment.[59] Milton calls attention to the fact that metastases to the bone will respond very readily to radiotherapy. Habermalz and Fischer treated a series of patients with high-dose radiation therapy. They delivered over 600 rads of supervoltage rays once or twice a week, which at times produced complete or extensive regression in 29 of 33 melanomas so treated. It is interesting that in 11 lesions the individual doses of 200–500 rads did not produce a satisfactory response, although a total dose of 5,000 rads or greater was given.

Vogler et al.[64] noted gratifying response from radiation therapy to metastases to the bone. Poppe[56] and Windeyer[66] also advocate irradiation as a palliative measure and claim beneficial results. Ackerman and del Regato believe that, although melanoma is usually a radioresistant tumor, some cases will show an unexpected radiosensitivity with marked relief, but seldom are curable. They record one patient with metastases to the liver who survived over five years.

Hilaris et al.[27] record their experience at Memorial Hospital from 1956 through 1961, during which period 139 courses of radiation therapy were given to 73 patients with metastatic melanoma. Their conclusions are as follows:

> Improvement at the end of treatment was obtained in 57% of the case, which compares favorably with 53% obtained in the treatment of all other distant metastases during the same period. Bone and brain metastases showed the most striking improvement. Radiation therapy is a simple and effective way to provide worthwhile palliation without significant side reaction for many patients with metastatic malignant melanoma.

This should dispel the pessimism regarding the benefits of radiation therapy for palliation as advocated by Snelling and Greeves.[61]

I have reported control of an extensive malignant melanoma of the vagina by means of interstitial radiation therapy for a period in excess of six years (see Chapter 28).

Radiation therapy plays a major role in the treatment of malignant melanoma of the uveal track.[40] Because melanomas are radioresistant, external radiation therapy has not been utilized. Accordingly, efforts have been made to control the uveal cancer with gold radon seeds or cobalt 60 plaques to deliver about 10,000 rads to the tumor. The result is a fibrous scar at the site of the previous tumor. These techniques have been advocated by Davidorf et al.[16] and by Long et al.[42]

Proppe[57] has recently commented on the use of radiotherapy in malignant melanomas, claiming beneficial palliation, in the treatment of Hutchinson's freckle, but indeterminate results in superficial spreading melanomas.

Kaha and colleagues[30] have reported some encouraging results with the use of surface therapy of malignant melanoma by high-energy electrons. The results are preliminary.

Cooper, Kopf, and Bart[13] report benefits from palliative irradiation in two-thirds of their patients; 26 patients with brain metastases were irradiated; in 12 marked improvement occurred, in nine slight to marked improvement, and in five no improvement. Objective signs of improvement were observed by computerized axial tomograms of the brain in some of their patients.

Chapter 13 describes internal irradiation. The data to date indicate that the use of higher individual doses (500–600 rads) per treatment, and the use of the newer equipment such as betatrons and linear accelerators may favorably alter the role of radiation therapy in the treatment of malignant melanoma.[5,10,23,28,31]

PROGNOSIS

Melanoma was considered previously to be universally fatal. Ewing,[19] whose monumental book, *Neoplastic Diseases*, served to classify all cancers into their distinctive categories and thus paved the way for "divide and conquer" cancer, stated:

It has perhaps the most sinister reputation among malignant tumors, and the prognosis is almost universally regarded as hopeless.

Hutner, a famous pathologist, in 1949, wrote: Melanomas are generally considered the most malignant of all tumors because of very rapid and widespread growth, once metastases appear. The spread is by the lymphatic system and blood stream, the latter being a late event and often absent until late in the course of the disease. When spread does occur, it is usually so extensive that hardly a tissue or organ escapes. For this reason the prognosis is usually grave, the average duration of life being two or three years.

Stout, the famous oncological pathologist, 48 years ago stated:

The writer has never come in contact personally with any case of malignant skin melanoma which has remained more than six years without evidence of metastasis or local reappearance.[63]

When I first became interested in melanoma (1936), I was taught that melanoma was akin to pregnancy. Just as you cannot have a touch of pregnancy, so you cannot have a touch of melanoma. Increased knowledge regarding the natural history of melanoma indicates that different types exist and different stages of variable degrees of malignancy exist. One can have a "touch of melanoma," e.g., Hutchinson's freckle, lentigo maligna, etc. Certain melanomas do possess a very malignant potential and often a poor prognosis. There are factors that help differentiate the various types for which treatment policies may be developed and prognoses evaluated.

The prognosis for patients with malignant melanoma has been steadily improving.[2] At Memorial Hospital, prior to 1931, a 12% survival rate was reported for 267 patients. In 1952, Pack, Gerber, and Scharnagel[52] reported a 40.5% five-year survival with stage I melanoma and 14.5% with stage II. In 1964, McNeer and Das Gupta[43] reported a 71% five-year survival in 359 determinant patients with stage I and 19% in 295 patients with stage II. Goldsmith, Shah, and Kim[21a] studied 1,552 patients treated between 1950 and 1965 with an overall 53% survival rate. A survival rate of 85% was reported for stage I and 38% for stage II.

Different survival rates are reported from different institutions, often based on the nature of the patient load and the pathologic evaluation of the lesion. Uniformity is the present goal, with a correlated system of reporting prospective randomized evaluations.

FACTORS INFLUENCING PROGNOSIS[38]

Some of the known factors influencing prognosis include: (1) *Tumor type*—cellularity, mitotic index, thickness, level of invasion, size, color, lymphocytic response, cell type, ulceration, invasion of dermal lymphatics and/or blood vessels, lateral junction spread; (2) *history*—extensive exposure to sunlight, previous inadequate treatment (ointments, escharotics, electrodessication, etc.), change in size and color, age and sex; (3) *physical exam*—Color and location, macular or papulary, location, size, discharge, bleeding, satellites, regional lymphadenopathy; (4) general condition of the patient; (5) the patient's immune status; and (6) the extent of previous surgery.

Some of these can be measured, and efforts have been made to create a prognostic index. However, melanomas may at times be most unpredictable in their behavior and defy all laws of prognostication.

Level of Invasion.   The studies of Clark and his colleagues have contributed greatly to an understanding of the natural history of melanomas (Fig. 10–1). Level I are those melanomas limited to the epidermal-1 dermal junction, which have an extremely good prognosis. Level II are those that invade the papillary dermis. Level III go through the papillary dermis and press against the reticular dermis. Level IV melanomas invade the reticular dermis. Level V represents invasion into the subcutaneous tissues. Levels III, IV, and V are far more malignant with a higher propensity to metastasize than level II. Level I is not considered by us to be a true metastasizing melanoma. Nodular melanomas are usually within levels IV and V, whereas the superficial spreading melanomas, in their earlier horizontal growth phase, are levels II to III. After the vertical component of growth occurs, they extend into levels IV and V. It thus becomes important to make an early diagnosis during the more favorable portion of the histologic development of these abnormal melanocytes.

Another classification, which has been largely chronicled by Breslow (Chap. 6), represents the thickness of the melanoma as measured from the top of the epidermis to the deepest melanoma cells in the dermis. If the melanoma is less than 0.76 mm the prognosis is excellent. In patients with lesions from 0.76 mm to 1.5 mm in thickness, metastases may develop; thus it is called the *gray area* from a prognostic standpoint. With melanomas thicker than 1.5 mm, metastases are frequently found and the prognosis is worse (Chapter 6).

The incidence of the different types of melanomas varies from institution to institution. Of the 3,305 melanomas studied at the Pack Medical Group, the most frequent types were the invasive melanomas, levels IV to V,

and possibly level III, in contrast to reports from most institutions where the most frequent form is the superficial spreading melanomas, which extend to levels II and possibly III. This may be due to the retrospective nature of our analyses, during which period patients presented themselves with melanomas in an advanced stage.[51] Education tends to lead to earlier diagnoses, less invasive melanomas and hopefully improved results.

Staging of Melanomas.   Melanomas are staged by us into four categories: Stage I represents a primary lesion without evidence of metastases to regional lymph nodes. These would include small satellites within the immediate vicinity of the primary melanoma (a melanotic halo). Stage II represents those that have metastases to the regional lymph nodes. Stage III are those that, in addition to metastases to regional lymph nodes, also have metastases to the afflicted limb—either satellites or metastases intransit. Stage IV represents blood-borne metastases.

Wanebo, Woodruff, and Fortner,[65] of Memorial Hospital in New York, conducted a clinicopathologic study in 151 patients with melanomas of the extremities and correlated the level of invasion with the incidence of metastases to regional lymph nodes and survival. They concluded:

There was a correlation between the depth of invasion by Clark's levels and the incidence of lymph node metastases in patients with stage I melanoma who had elective node dissection. The incidence of nodal metastases was 4% for level II, 7% for level III, 25% for level IV, and 70% for level V. There was a correlation between Clark's level of invasion and survival after surgery. The five-year cure rate was 100% for level II, 88% for level III, 60% for level IV, and 15% for level V melanoma. The presence of nodal metastases augured a much worse prognosis than Clark's level per se. In patients with level IV melanoma, the five-year cure rate was 82% in patients with negative nodes and 27% in those with nodal metastases after elective node dissection. Microstaging primary melanoma according to Clark's levels serves as a useful standard with which to compare surgical results. In this series of extremity melanomas there was no difference between local recurrence and lymphadenectomy for level II melanoma. For level III and level IV melanoma, wide excision and lymphadenectomy gave higher cure rates than wide excision only, both at five and nine years after surgery. The results were significant only for patients with level III, however. Use of the measured depth of invasion added significant clinicopathologic information. The incidence of nodal metastases at elective node dissection was 5% to 9% for melanoma showing 0.6 to 2.0 mm of invasion, 22% for melanoma measuring 2.1 to 3.0 mm, and 39% for melanoma invading beyond 3.0 mm. The 5-year cure rate was 100% for melanoma measuring less than 1.0 mm, 83% for melanoma invading 1.1 to 2.0 mm, 58% for lesions measuring 2.1 to 3.0 mm, and 55% for melanoma invading over 3.0 mm. The microstage technique combining Clark's levels and the measured depth of invasion has an important use as a prognostic index and as a standard upon which to select treatment for primary melanoma of the extremities.

Huvos, Shah, and Mike[29] from the same institution compared the various features of 100 patients with melanoma who died in less than five years with 100 long-term survivors (ten years and longer) and found the significant features of the short-term survivors were: male, primary lesion less than 1 cm, ulceration, deep dermal penetration, dermal lymphatics or blood vessel invasion, and a lack of lymphoid reaction around the primary lesion.

Clark and colleagues[12] found that level II has a mortality of 8.3%; level III, 35.2%; level IV, 46.1%; and level V, 52%. Lentigo maligna had the best prognosis of 89.7%, superficial spreading melanoma 68.5%, and nodular melanoma 43.9%.

Knutson, Hori, and Spratt[33] critically evaluated 230 melanomas seen at the Ellis Fischel State Cancer Hospital in Columbia, Missouri, treated between 1940 and 1969. They statistically evaluated 54 variables by the Chi-Square tests to find out if any of them were statistically significant. They concluded that only two of the 54 variables withstood the analysis and remained significant. The patient's sex was the first significant variable (difference was $p < 0.3$). There was a significantly higher incidence of male patients in the metastatic group. In women 29.6% of the melanomas metastasized, whereas 49.8% of the melanomas in men fell into the metastatic group. The second significant variable that existed between the metastatic and nonmetastatic melanomas was the color of the lesion. Of all brown melanomas, 58.6% appeared in the metastasizing group, compared with only 34.8% of all other colors that appeared within the same group (difference was $p > 0.01$). Melanomas with a variegated color were found predominantly in the nonmetastasizing group (90.9%) (difference was $p > 0.1$), which correlates with the better prognosis for Hutchinson's freckles. The other colors (black and unpigmented) were distributed among the metastatic and nonmetastatic groups with similar probabilities.

They further attempted to compare the long-term survivors (ten years or more) with short-term survivors (up to five years) evaluated against the 54 variables. They concluded that no outstanding variable was associated with either a long- or short-term survival. A few significant differences were noted and were summarized as follows:

1. No patient with a melanoma and an outdoor occupation survived ten years (difference was $p > .01$).
2. A strong correlation existed between the clinical diagnosis of a Hutchinson's freckle and a survival of ten or more years (difference was $p > 0.1$).
3. A strong correlation existed between the regional lymph nodes being histologically involved with metastatic tumor at the patient's first evaluation and the survival of five years or less (difference was $p > 0.1$).

They concluded that the difference in the actuarial survival between patients with superficial and invasive melanoma was *not* statistically significant. The recurrence rates for patients with superficial and invasive melanoma were similar, but the time interval between primary treatment and the observed recurrences was longer for superficial melanoma than for invasive melanoma. They question the association of any significant isolated clinical or histologic variable with a favorable or unfavorable prognosis. They do reveal a continued improvement in survival over 20 years, which they attribute primarily to the refinement of surgical techniques and a more sophisticated understanding of the insidious nature of the lesion.

Larsen and Grude,[39] from the University of Oslo, performed a detailed study regarding various parameters relative to prognosis in 669 cases of primary cutaneous malignant melanoma in clinical stage I. They noted that a good prognosis was related to spindle-shaped tumor cells, marked pigmentation, slight atypia, and few mitoses. A poor prognosis was related to epithelioid tumor cells, little pigment, marked atypia, and many mitoses. There was no significant relationship between lymphocyte response and sex and age of the patient and the tumor cell type. There was a highly significant relationship between a dense lymphocytic infiltration and superficial tumor invasion as far as the papillary-reticular interface, in contrast to a weak response associated with deeper invasion. There was no significant relationship between lymphocytic infiltration and tumor cell types, pigmentation, atypia, mitotic count, and sex and age of the patient. They question the prognostic significance of a dense lymphocytic infiltration.

Lane, Lattes and Malm,[37,38] reporting from Columbia University on the clinicopathologic correlation in melanoma, have noticed that a markedly favorable prognostic significance was associated with a pathologic feature term *lateral junctional spread*. The term describes the presence of malignant melanoma cells in junctional and intraepidermal position peripheral or lateral to the central, more deeply invasive portion of the growth. They believe that this feature appears to reflect a tendency toward a restrained superficial type of growth. They further observe that melanomas 2 cm or less in size had a five-year apparent cure rate of 61% as opposed to a 16% five-year cure rate for melanomas more than 2 cm.

A comprehensive multifactorial analysis of melanoma from the University of Alabama was recorded by Balch[5] and colleagues. They analyzed 339 patients with melanoma over a 33-year period, and noted that five of the 13 parameters examined simultaneously were found independently to influence five-year survival rates. These were: (1) pathologic stage, (2) ulceration, (3) surgical treatment (wide excision vs wide excision plus lymphadenectomy), (4) melanoma thickness, and (5) location (upper extremity vs lower extremity vs trunk vs head and neck). The factors considered that had either indirect or no influence on survival were: clinical stage of disease, age, sex, level of invasion, pigmentation, lymphacytic infiltration, growth pattern, and regression. They state that most of these latter variables derive their prognostic value from correlation with melanoma thickness, except sex, which correlated with location. Three of the categories of risk were delineated by measuring tumor thickness (Breslow's microstaging) in stage I patients: (1) thin melanomas (<0.76) were associated with localized disease and a 100% cure rate; (2) intermediate-thickness melanomas (0.6–4.00 mm) had an increasing risk of 80% of harboring regional and/or distant metastases; and (3) thick melanomas (>4 mm) had an 80% risk of occult distant metastases at the time of initial presentation. They observed that level of invasion (Clark's microstaging) correlated with survival was less predictive than measuring tumor thickness. Both microstaging methods (Breslow and Clark) were less predictive factors in patients with lymph node or distant metastases.

The effects of pregnancy on melanoma were evaluated by Shiu and colleagues[60] in 251 surgically treated patients. They concluded that there was no statistical difference in survival in five years for stage I melanoma between nolleparous, parous, nonpregnant, and pregnant women. For stage II melanoma, however, a significantly lower survival rate was observed for pregnant patients (29%) and parous women who had experienced activation of the lesion in a previous pregnancy (22%) as compared with nolleparous patients

(55%) and other patients in the parous group (51%). They conclude that this discrepancy in survival, together with the observed higher frequency of state II cases, melanomas occurring on the trunk, and symptoms such as bleeding, ulceration, irritation, and elevation of the lesion, strongly suggest an adverse influence of pregnancy on women with stage II melanoma.

REFERENCES

1. Ackerman LV, delRegato JA: Cancer; Diagnosis, Treatment, and Prognosis, ed 3. St Louis Mo, CV Mosby Company, 1962. p 101
2. Adair FE: Treatment of melanoma: Report of 400 cases. Surg Gynecol Obstet 62:406, 1936
3. Arma-Szlachzic M, Ott F, Storck H: Zur Strahlen-therapie der melandischen precancerosen. Hautarzt 21:505–508, 1970
4. Arrington JH, Reed RJ, Ichinose H, et al.: Acral lentiginous melanoma: A distinctive variant of human cutaneous malignant melanoma. Am J Surg Pathol 1(2):131, 1977
5. Balch CM, Murad TM, Soong SJ: A multifactorial analysis of melanoma, Ann Surg 188:732–742, 1978
6. Beardmore GL, Davis NC: Multiple primary malignant melanoma. Arch Dermatol 111:603–609, 1972
7. Beeler MF: Melanogenuria—evaluation of several commonly used laboratory procedures. JAMA 60:52–54, 1961
8. Berman RA, Didolkar MS, Parthasarthy KI, et al.: Significance of splenic size by Tc-99mm sulfur colloid scan in malignant melanoma. Proc Amer Soc Clin Onc 19:355, 1978
9. Bodenham DC: A study of 650 observed malignant melanomas in the southwest region. Ann R Coll Surg 43:218–239, 1968
10. Catterall M: Fast neutrons in oncology. Br J Hosp Med 12:853, 1974
11. Chandra R, Bart RS, Mintziz MM, et al.: Distribution of technetium-99m sulfur colloid in mice bearing melanomas or mammary carcinomas. Cancer Res 37:3293–3296, 1977
12. Clark WH, Ainsworth AM, Mihme MC: The clinical manifestations of primary cutaneous malignant mclanoma. In Clark WH et al. (eds): Human Malignant Melanoma. New York, Grune & Stratton, 1979, pp 33–53
13. Cooper JS, Kopf AM, Bart RS: Present role and future prospects for radiotherapy in the management of malignant melanoma. J Dermatol Surg Oncol 5(2): 134–139, 1979
14. Creagan ET, Cupps RE, Ivins JC, et al.: Adjuvant radiation therapy for regional nodal metastases from malignant melanoma: A randomized, prospective study. Cancer 42(5):2206–2210, 1978
15. Das Gupta J, McNeer GP: Superficial melanoma, a clinical study. Arch Surg 99:531, 1969
16. Davidorf FH, Makley TA, Lang TR: Radiotherapy of malignant melanoma of the choroid. Trans Am Acad Opthal Otolaryngol 81:849–861, 1976
17. Dickson RJ: Malignant melanoma: A combined surgical and radiotherapeutic approach. Am J Roentgenol 79:1063–1070, 1958
18. Echevaria R, Ackerman LV: Spindle and epitheloid nevi·in the adult: Clinopathologic report of 26 cases. Cancer 20:175–189, 1967
19. Ewing J: Neoplastic Diseases; a Textbook on Tumors, ed 2. Philadelphia, WB Saunders, 1922, p 253
20. Goldman AB, Braunstein P, Song C: Augmented splenic uptake of ^{mm}Tc sulphur colloid in patients with malignant melanoma. Radiology 112:631–634, 1974
21. Goldman L: Surgery by lazer for malignant melanoma. J Dermatol Surg Oncol 5(2):141–144, 1979
21a. Goldsmith HS, Shah JP, Kim DD: Prognostic significance of lymph node dissection in the treatment of malignant melanoma. Cancer 26(3):606–609, 1970
22. Greene MH, Fraumeni JF: The hereditary variant of malignant melanoma. In Clark WH et al. (eds): Human Malignant Melanoma. New York, Grune & Stratton, 1979, pp 143–144
23. Habermalz HJ, Fischer JJ: Radiation therapy of malignant melanoma. Experience with high individual treatment doses. Cancer 38:2258–2262, 1976
24. Harvey WC, Kopp DT, Podoloff DA, et al.: Reversed liver-spleen ratio and the normal liver-spleen scintigram. J Reticuloendothel Soc 19:19–27, 1976
25. Hellriegel W: Radiation therapy of primary and metastatic melanoma. Ann NY Acad Sci 100:131–141, 1963
26. Hessler C, Maillard GS: Apport de la thermographie dans le diagnostic et le traitement du mélanome maligne. Schweiz Mcd Wochensch 100:972–975, 1978
27. Hilaris BS, Raben M, Calabrese AS, et al.: Value

of radiation therapy for distant metastases from malignant melanoma. Cancer 16(6):765–773, 1963

28. Hutner LM: Death from metastatic melanoma 36 years after removal of probable primary ocular tumor. Calif Med 71:420–423, 1949

29. Huvos AG, Shah JP, Mike V: Prognostic factors in cutaneous malignant melanoma. Hum Pathol 5(3):347–357, 1974

30. Kaha A, Otto O, Krystof V: Surface therapy of malignant melanoma by high energy electrons. Cest Radiol 32(5):333–336, 1978

31. Kirchner JA: Nasal melanoma: Its treatment by a new technique in radiation therapy. Trans Am Acad Ophthalmol Otolaryngol 80:429–430, 1975

32. Klingensmith WC: Resolution of increased splenic size and uptake of ^{mm}Tc sulphur colloid following removal of a malignant melanoma. J Nucl Med 15:1203–1204, 1974

33. Knutson CO, Hori JM, Spratt JS Jr: Current problems in surgery: Melanoma. Year Book Medical Publisher, 1971, pp 1–55

34. Konecny M, Krenarova V: A contribution to the radiotherapy of malignant melanoma. Neoplasma 16:335–337, 1969

35. Kopf AW, Bart RS: Lentigo maligna melanoma. J Dermatol Surg Oncol 5(2):98–99, 1979

36. Kozlov AP, Akimov AA, Moskalik KG, Pertsov OL: Anti-tumor effect of lazer radiation. Acta Radiol (Ther) (Stockh) 12:241–256, 1973

37. Lane N, Lattes R, Malm J: Clinicopathological correlations in a series of 117 malignant melanomas of the skin of adults. Cancer 11:1025–1043, 1958

38. Lane N, Lattes R, Malm J: A multifactoral analysis of melanoma: Prognostic histopathologic features comparing Clark's and Breslow's staging methods. Ann Surg, 1978, pp 732–742

39. Larsen TE, Grude TH: A retrospective histological study of 669 cases of primary cutaneous malignant melanoma in clinical stage I. Acta Path Microbiol Scand Sect A 86:437–459, 513–530, 1978

40. Lederman M: Radiotherapy of malignant melanomata of the eye. Br J Radiol 34:21, 1961

41. Lissner J, Von Lieven H: Die strahlentherapie des malignen melanomas. Chirurge 45:362–365, 1974

42. Long RS, Galin MA, Rotman N: Conservative treatment of intraocular melanomas. Trans Amer Acad Ophthal Otolaryngol 75:84–93, 1971

43. McNeer GL, Das Gupta T: Prognosis in malignant melanoma. Surgery, 56:512–518, 1964

44. Menzer L, Sabin T, Mark VH: Computerized axial tomography. Use in the diagnosis of dementia, JAMA 234:754–757, 1975

45. Milder MS, Frankel RS, Bulkley GB, et al.: Gallium 67 scintography and malignant melanoma. Cancer 32:1350–1356, 1973

46. Milton GW: Malignant Melanomas of the Skin and Mucous Membrane. Sydney Australia, Churchill & Livingstone, 1977, p 93

47. Mohs FE, Bloom RF, Sahl WJ: Chemosurgery for familial malignant melanoma. J Dermatol Surg Oncol 5(2):127–131, 1979

48. Nathanson L: Letter of Reply. J Nucl Med 19:1093–1094, 1978

49. Nathanson L, Hall TC, Farber S: Biological aspects of human malignant melanoma. Cancer 20:650–655, 1967

50. Nathanson L, Kahn P: Splenic uptake of Tc-99m sulfur colloid in malignant melanoma. J Nucl Med 18:1040, 1977

51. Pack GT: End results of treatment of malignant melanoma. Surgery 46:447, 1959

52. Pack GT, Scharnagel IM, Gerber DM: Treatment of malignant melanoma of the skin. Surg Clin North Am 33:517, 1953

53. Pack GT, Scharnagel IM, Morfit M: The principle of excision in continuity for primary and metastatic melanoma of the skin. Surgery 17:849, 1945

54. Pearson D: Radiotherapy in malignant melanoma. Proc R Soc Med 67:96–97, 1974

55. Petratos MA, Kopf AW, et al.: Treatment of melanotic freckle with X-rays. Arch Dermatol 106:189–194, 1972

56. Poppe H: Klinik und Therapie der fortgeschritten Stadien des Melanomalignom. In Meyer H, Becker J: Strahlenforschung und Strahlenbehandlung; Vortrage aus den Gebieten der Strahlenphysik, Strahlenbiologie und Strahlentherapie, Bd 2. Strahlentherapie Sonderbd. 46:1–252, 1960; 3–24

57. Proppe AH: The worth of radiotherapy in malignant melanomas. J Dermatol Surg Oncol 4(8):613–616, 1978

58. Roth JA, Eilber FR, Bennett LR, Morton DL: Radionucleid photoscanning: Usefulness in preoperative evaluation of melanoma patients. Arch Surg 110:1211–1212, 1975

59. Scherer E, Makoski HB: Die strahlentherapie dis malignen melanoms. Langenbecks Arch Chir 342:546–548, 1976

60. Shiu MH, Schottenfeld D, MacLean B, Fortner JG: Adverse effect of pregnancy. Cancer 37:181–187, 1976

61. Snelling MD, Greeves RA: Diseases of eye. In

Carling ER, Windeyer BW, Smithers DW (eds): Practice in Radiotherapy. St Louis Mo, CV Mosby, 1955, pp 350–363

62. Sober AJ, Mintzis MM, Lew RA, et al.: Augmented radionuclide uptake by the spleen in patients with malignant melanoma. Yale J Biol Med 50:583, 1977

63. Stout AP: Human Cancer: Etiologic Factors; Precancerous Lesions; Growth; Spread; Symptoms; Diagnosis; Prognosis; Principles of Therapy. Philadelphia, Lea & Feberger, 1932, p 135

64. Vogler WR, Perdue GD, Wilkins SA Jr: Clinical evaluation of malignant melanoma. Surg Gynecol Obstet 106:586–594, 1958

65. Wanebo HJ, Woodruff J, Fortner JG: Malignant melanoma of the extremities: A clinicopathologic study using levels of invasion (microstage). Cancer 35(3):666–676, 1975

66. Windeyer BW: Treatment of malignant melanoma of skin. In Meyer H, and Becker J: Strahlenforschung und Strahlenbehandlung; Vortrage aus den Gebieten der Strahlenphysik, Strahlenbiologie und Strahlenthcrapie, Bd 2. Strahlentherapie Sonderbd. 46:1–252, 1960; 36–42

LABELLED CHLOROQUINE ANALOGS IN THE DIAGNOSIS AND TREATMENT OF OCULAR AND DERMAL MELANOMAS

WILLIAM H. BEIERWALTES,

AND SATINDER P. GILL

ORIGINAL FEASIBILITY STUDIES IN ANIMALS

The idea for our development of a radioiodinated analog of chloroquine originated from the observation that chloroquine used to treat malaria occasionally caused a retinopathy. Several reports indicated that chloroquine has a marked affinity for melanin and is slowly released from pigmented tissues.[4,18,21]

The results of our feasibility study are shown in Table 11-1. Sixteen black and 16 albino mice were implanted with melanoma subcutaneously. Radioactivity was administered intravenously and animals were sacrificed at 1, 2, 3 and 4 days after injection. Radioactivity increased through 4 days in the eyes of black mice but decreased rapidly in the eyes of albino mice.[2] This difference was presumably because of presence of melanin in the choroids of black mice. Of the other tissues studied, there was high activity in melanin containing transplanted malignant melanotic melanoma in both pigmented and albino mice. The skin of black mice also contained high radioactivity in contrast to albino mice skin, which had negligible radioactivity.

Figure 11-1 shows the structure of ^{14}C-labeled chloroquine and the structure of the other analogs of chloroquine that we have tested in our laboratory to date.[3,7,8] In Table 11-2, tissue distribution of three chloroquine analogs has been compared with that of ^{14}C-chloroquine. For our experimental model,

15 C57 B-16 black mice were chosen. All had B-16 melanoma tumors implanted subcutaneously 8 to 10 days previously. Ten μCi of each analog was given to the mice by oral gavage. The animals were then killed at 6 hours, 1, 2, 3, and 4 days and the radioactivity assays were performed. The concentration of one of the first of the radioiodinated analogs (NM-113) in the implanted tumor was sufficient to delineate the malignant melanoma by scintillation scanning.

DIAGNOSIS OF DERMAL MELANOMAS

We then studied the diagnostic efficacy of this compound (NM-113) in three patients.[1] Figure 11-2 shows the right side of the face of an 83-year-old woman. Note the primary lesion in the right cheek with satellites posterior to it, a nonvisible but palpable preauricular node; a visible black satellite below and behind the ear; and a neck dissection scar without visible or palpable lesions. Figure 11-3 is a photograph of the scintillation scan of the right side of her face. Note the considerable concentration of radioactivity in the region of the preauricular node (which proved to contain metastatic melanoma showing 565 counts/minute).

We have summarized our experience in the diagnostic efficacy of NM-113 in dermal

TABLE 11-1. ^{14}C Chloroquine Tissue Distribution in Mice with Melanomas*

Time after injection (hours)	Melanoma		Eye	
	B-16	H.P.	B-16	H.P.
25	424 ± 17	583 ± 410	911 ± 83	106 ± 26
48	445 ± 58	279 ± 73	954 ± 132	35 ± 2.4
72	376 ± 38.3	178 ± 36	1086 ± 70	13 ± 6.3
96	379 ± 31.6	359 ± 258	1479 ± 239	44 ± 20

Time after injection (hours)	Skin		Liver	
	B-16	H.P.	B-16	H.P.
25	237 ± 49	103 ± 49	222 ± 24	237 ± 34
48	265 ± 40	46 ± 4.6	100 ± 15	138 ± 7
72	260 ± 4	57 ± 12	41 ± 7.1	29 ± 1.7
96	352 ± 32.6	28 ± 3.9	30 ± 3.5	31 ± 5.6

* Four mice were used in each experiment; values are given in counts per minute per milligram. B-16 melanomas in pigmented mice; HP melanomas in albino mice.

melanomas in 30 humans.[6] The radioactivity concentration ratio for melanoma compared with skin, muscle, and fat ranged from approximately 7:1 to 60:1. Amelanotic tissue and the areas of necrosis in melanotic tissue concentrated the compound poorly, if at all, compared with other tissues. No false positive scans were obtained but there were false negative scans in five patients. In one patient, the false negative scans were due to the small size of the lesions. The remaining four patients had amelanotic lesions.

The limitations and indications for the use of NM-113 might be summarized as follows:

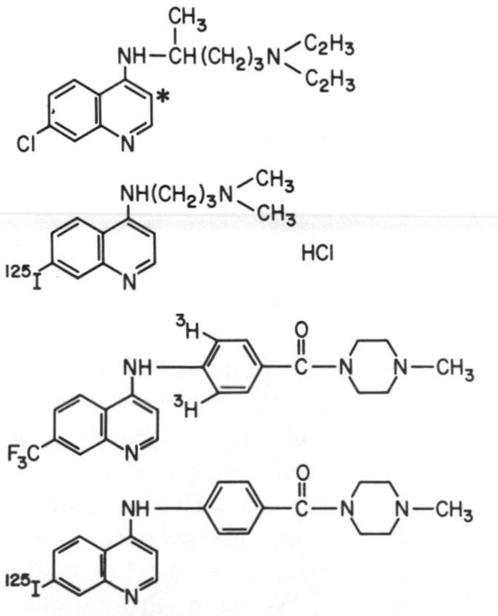

FIGURE 11-1. Compounds used in study.

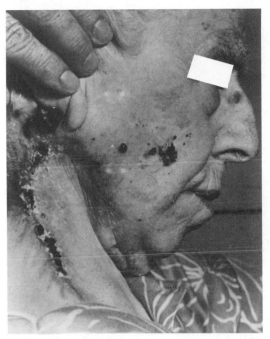

FIGURE 11-2. A woman, 83 years old, with primary lesion in the right cheek with satellites posterior to it; nonvisible but palpable preauricular node; visible black satellite below and behind the ear and neck dissection scar without visible or palpable lesions.

Limitations

1. Uptake in brain metastases is nonspecific.

2. Uptake in normal lungs is too great to allow detection of metastases to lung.

3. Uptake in lung prevents accurate imaging of axillary nodes.

4. Radioactivity excretion in bile and bowel prevents adequate imaging of retroperitoneal metastases.

5. Lesions smaller than 1 cm in inguinal nodal areas cannot be detected.

6. No uptake in amelanotic melanoma.

Indications

1. Can detect presence of melanotic mestases in regional lymph nodes in face and neck, even when the nodes are deep cervical and nonpalpable.

2. Can differentiate melanotic melanoma metastatic to liver from nonmelanotic melanomas.

DIAGNOSIS OF OCULAR MELANOMAS

The compound has found its best use in the diagnosis of ocular melanoma. Ferry has shown that 19% of enucleated eyes with a diagnosis of malignant melanoma do not contain a melanoma.[9] The ^{32}P test is not specific for melanomas and there is a high percentage of false positive and false negative results. There is difficulty experienced in placing the counting probe directly over the lesion and this difficulty may lead to mistaken diagnosis and result in unnecessary enucleation.[12] A small tumor that is not delineated well on funduscopic examination and is asymptomatic can easily be missed.

Figure 11-4, is a photograph of a horizontal section of an eye containing an asymptomatic 7 mm diameter subretinal hemorrhage at the back of the globe, which gave a diagnostically high uptake count with ^{32}P in the operating room under direct probe placement.

Figure 11-5 is a graph showing the results of our first efforts with NM-113 in imaging ocular melanomas in 28 patients.[5] Radioactivity in both eyes of each patient was compared by external counting using a 5-inch diameter sodium iodide detector with a single hole collimator. Radioactivity determinations by external counting were made two to five times in each patient three to 50 days after the tracer dose.

Results were expressed as the average percent difference between the mean counting rates over two eyes using the formula:

$$R = \frac{2 (A-B)}{(A+B)} \times 100$$

(Where A and B are right and left eyes.)

Although relatively large melanomas were detected with this relatively crude geometry,

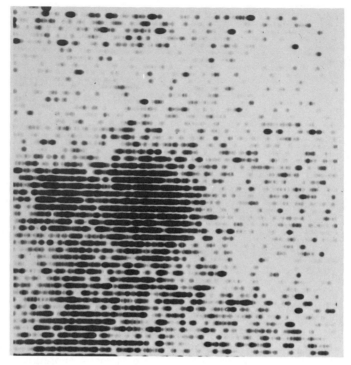

FIGURE 11–3. Photograph of scintillation scan of right side of the face of the 83-year-old woman shown in Figure 11–2.

it occurred to us that if we could decrease the mean percent difference in external counting rate, between eyes, of 7.6% after 14 days following the dose, with an upper limit of 18% (± 2 SD), we could detect much smaller melanomas.

Figure 11–6 is a graph indicating the importance of detecting small ocular melanomas.[10] The mortality rate is threefold greater at a tumor volume of 2.2 cc as compared with 1.2 cc.

There are two populations of ophthalmology patients who deserve close scrutiny because of their high risk of having ocular melanoma: (1) Those having routine refractions where the ophthalmologist sees something that involves a differential diagnosis of choroidal nevus, retinal or choroidal hemangioma, retinal hemorrhage, retinal or choroidal detachment, or retinal or muscular degenerations. (2)

Where opacities present inadequate retinoscopy; corneal, lenticular, or vitreous spacities, secondary membranes, degenerated eye and phthisis bulbi; these blind eyes with opaque media, for some unkown reason, harbor melanomas with disturbing frequency.[13]

The diagnostic dose of 2 mCi usually used in this study would not be expected to produce radiation damage to the retina. Radiation dosimetry shows that the choroidal dose is approximately 46 rads. Harmful permanent effects on the retina from external radiation at much higher dose rates have been seen only with over 3250 to 4500 rads.[19] Furthermore, in our studies of the treatment of dermal melanotic melanomas in dogs,[16] we have shown that it would require a whole-body dose of three times the LD 50/30 to reach a damaging dose of beta radiation to the rod and cone layer of the retina.[15]

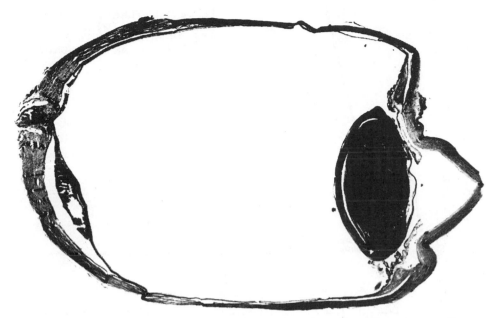

FIGURE 11-4. Photograph of horizontal section of an eye containing a 7 mm diameter subretinal hemorrhage at the back of the eye, which gave a diagnostically high uptake count with ^{32}P in the operating room under direct probe placement.

The 18% upper limit (± 2 SD) of percent difference in external counting rate between the two eyes was attributed to the difficulty in accurately placing the detector and to normal differences in the uptake between the two eyes. Our associate, G. Knoll, then invented an improved, an uncollimated detector, which gives higher detection efficiency and is less sensitive to changes in position than the collimated detector. The standard deviation for controls was reduced to 3% with this improved detector.[14]

In both methods, the radiation from the tumor must be detected above the background coming from the entire choroid. This background can readily mask a small tumor since the *specific* concentration of the chloroquine is higher in the choroid than in the tumor by a factor of about 8:1. The sensitivity of both methods is also reduced by normal differences between the eyes and by variations in probe placement.

For these reasons, a well-collimated scintillation probe was designed by our associate, W. L. Rogers, which can be accurately positioned and aimed by means of ultrasound.[20]

The focused collimator (Fig. 11-7) could be specifically focused on the lesion.[14] Collimation eliminated counts from the surrounding normal choroid. Localization of the eye tumor was achieved by ultrasound examination of the globe. The probe is positioned in such a way that the tumor is directly in front of the probe and at the focal length of the collimator. The axis of the ultrasound transducer and gamma probe intersect at the lesion (Fig. 11-8). This arrangement of combining ultrasound transducer and gamma ray probe in the same assembly enabled localization of the tumor with ultrasound and counting the radioactivity over the lesion at the same time. Positioning of the gamma probe is accurately accomplished within ±1 mm.

Two basic problems were encountered,

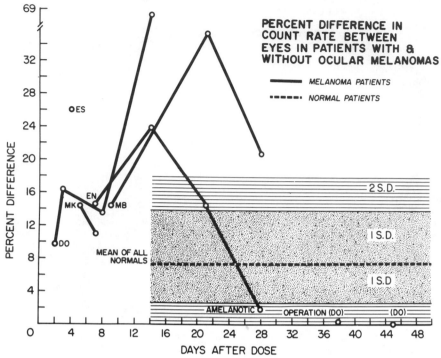

FIGURE 11-5. Graph showing results of our first efforts with NM-133 in imaging ocular melanomas in 28 patients.

RELATION OF TUMOR SIZE TO MORTALITY

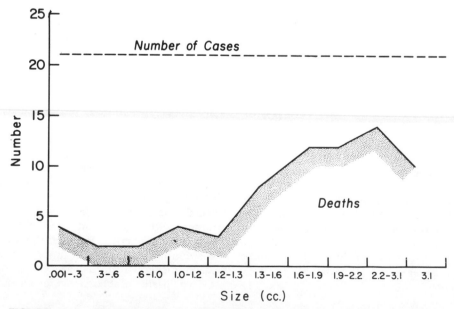

FIGURE 11-6. Graph showing the relationship of mortality to ocular melanoma size.

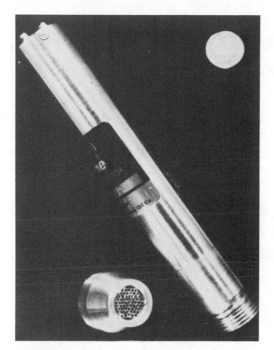

FIGURE 11–7. Gamma ray probe with focused collimator.

however, which reduced the detection sensitivity of the ultrasound-guided probe:[22]

1. Signal was not well localized especially in tumors with necrotic cores.
2. Too much detection efficiency was sacrificed in prototype design for the amount of room-background and retro-orbital background encountered in the clinic test.

However, these problems could be eliminated by a redesign of the detector and collimator.[22]

1. Improved detector shielding will reduce room background to 3 counts/minute.
2. Counting in air using a contact ultrasound scanner to position the gamma-ray probe will improve counting efficiency by a factor of 3 by minimizing the amount of water between the detector and tumor.
3. Redesigning the collimator to give a flat field response will improve counting effi-

ciency by a factor of 3 but with somewhat increased choroidal background.

The observed change of count rate as a function of time agreed with that observed by Knoll et al. with peak count rates after the 14th day. Peak asymmetry was observed in the present group anywhere between the 3rd and 14th day. Counting of the patients was started on the day the dose was given in an attempt to verify an early tumor uptake peak reported by Packer et al.[17] in hamsters. Rogers, Gill, and Wainstock observed rapid appearance in the eye, but no early asymmetry common to the patients diagnosed as having melanoma.[22]

TREATMENT OF DERMAL MELANOMAS WITH RADIOIODINATED QUINOLINE ANALOGS

DOGS[16]

We treated five normal dogs and three dogs with metastatic melanomas with 1.3 to 1.8 mCi per pound of body weight of ^{131}I-NM–113. This dosage was calculated from subsequent studies to give a total body dose of 44 to 223 rads. The concentration of radioactivity in the melanomas ranged from 2.4 to 30.1 μCi/gm of tissue. The calculated absorbed dose in four metastases in three dogs was 177 to 2,880 rads. We showed that to reach a damaging dose of beta radiation to the rod and cone layer of the retina, the whole body dose would have to be three times the LD–50/30.

One dog with a gingival melanoma, recurrent after previous surgical resection and with uptake of ^{131}I from ^{131}I-NM–113 in both the recurrent primary and in palpable regional cervical lymph nodes, was observed to have regression of the size of the primary and metastases beginning at three weeks after his treatment dose. At five weeks, an autopsy with histologic sections of the region of the primary and metastases revealed no evidence of residual melanoma by gross or microscopic examination.

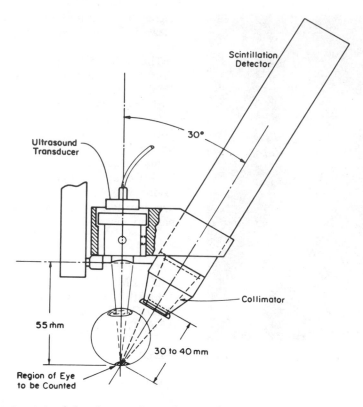

FIGURE 11-8. Axis of the ultrasound transducer and gamma ray probe intersecting at lesion.

HUMANS

In unpublished work, we have treated three patients with metastatic dermal melanomas with a 25 mCi treatment dose of ^{131}I–NM–113, three patients with a 50 mCi dose, and one patient with a 100 mCi dose.

The criteria for selection were that the patients had proved recurrent, unresectable *melanotic* melanoma with a relatively good prognosis for 3 to 6 months (so that they might live to enjoy the benefit of the radiation).

We also found that it was necessary that the patients had no known brain metastases. We asked that the patients have visible and palpable metastases so that these could be directly observed and measured. The patients were also required to have a good uptake of radioactivity in melanoma tissue by scanning and by point counting. These patients had complete blood counts, visual acuity tests, and slit lamp examination before and after treatment, repeated weekly, along with measurements of visible tumors.

Of the three patients treated with 25 mCi, there was no observed beneficial or harmful effect. One patient died 35 days after the treatment dose with a positive brain scan and autopsy. A second was alive 21 months later, and the third was alive three months later.

Of the three patients who had a 50 mCi treatment dose, there was also no observed beneficial or harmful effect. One patient died one month later of brain metastases, proved at autopsy. The second patient died one month later with no autopsy. The third patient died four months later with no autopsy.

The patient treated with 100 mCi was a 57-year-old woman who received her treatment dose on May 5, 1971, was discharged on May 14, 1971, was last seen on follow-up July 23, 1971, and died on December 16, 1971.

Before treatment, the patient had metastases, proved by surgery, to the liver, the left lower pelvis, and lymph nodes in the left thigh recurrent after previous resection (see Fig. 4–9).

During the two weeks in the Clinical Research Unit during her studies preliminary to her treatment dose, the left thigh mass grew from 13 × 5 cm to 15 × 8 cm. Figure 11–9 is a picture of her left thigh mass on April 26, 1971.

Figure 11–10 is a photograph of a rectilinear scintiscan showing the uptake in the pelvic mass and in the left thigh mass on May 4, 1971 (one day after a 2mCi tracer dose), on June 11, 1971 (26 days after the treatment dose), and on June 25, 1971 (40 days after the treatment dose).

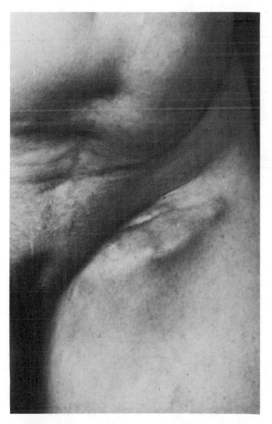

FIGURE 11–9. Melanoma in left thigh recurrent after previous surgery.

After treatment, her hematocrit values fell to the lowest levels at four weeks. These values then returned to the pretreatment level by seven weeks. Special tests of rod and cone function of the retina showed no deleterious effects; dark adaption showed no change and her increment threshold improved during the three-month followup.

At three weeks after therapy, as in the dog, the neoplasm began to decrease in size. The center of this lesion became hot and fluctuant. The border of the inguinal mass shrank and softened. A 10% regression in the size of the mass occurred during the next four weeks. The patient experienced a marked subjective improvement. Nine weeks after the treatment dose, regrowth began.

We have treated no further patients because of lack of funding of this work and because the majority of the patients referred to us have too small a melanin concentration in the lesion for adequate uptake. This finding is probably related to the fact that as the malignant melanoma becomes faster growing and more undifferentiated, the melanin concentration decreases.

OTHER RADIONUCLIDE–LABELLED CHLOROQUINE ANALOGS

The relative tissue distribution of four 4-amino-quinoline analogs (see Figure 11–1 and Table 11–2) in mice with malignant melanotic melanomas was compared with that of ^{14}C-chloroquine.[11] After the oral administration of 10 μCi of each compound (dose in mg, or μg per kilogram body weight), three mice in each group were sacrificed at five different time intervals after each tracer dose, 6, 24, 48, 72 and 96 hours. A new radiolabelled 4-amino-quinoline analog, 4- [p-] (4-methyl-1-piperazinyl)carbonyl[anilino]-7-(trifluoromethyl) quinoline concentrated in the melanoma of mice 4 times greater than ^{14}C-chloroquine and 3 times greater than the iodinated analog of chloroquine 4-(3-dimethyl-aminopropylamino)-7-iodoquinoline ^{125}I–NM–113) even when the ^{125}I–NM–113 had a 3 times greater specific activity than the new compound.

TABLE 11–2. Tissue Distribution of Radiolabelled Quinoline Analogs in Mice with Melanomas at Time of Peak Uptake in Melanoma†

Tissue Samples	% KG Dose/GM ± S.E.M.				Target:Nontarget Ratios			
	¹⁴C Chloro.	¹²⁵I NM–113	NP–45	NP–57	¹⁴C Chloro.	¹²⁵I NM–113	NP–45	NP–57
Tumor	0.04 ±0.01	0.06 ▽	0.18 ±0.02	0.11 ±0.01	—	—	—	—
Eye	0.08 ±0.01	0.13 ±0.01	0.47 ±0.08	0.25 ±0.02	0.5	0.46	0.38	0.44
Liver	0.02 ▽	0.05 ▽	0.03 △	0.02 △	2	1.2	6	0.92
Kidney	0.01 ▽	0.07 ±0.01	0.03 △	0.04 ±0.04	4	0.86	6	2.75
Spleen	0.02 ±0.01	0.07 ▽	0.04 ±0.01	0.04 ±0.03	2	0.86	4.5	2.75
Lung	0.01 ±0.01	0.02 ±0.01	0.01 △	0.01 △	4	3	18	11
Adrenal	0.05 ±0.02	0.04 ±0.02	0.06 △	0.07 ±0.02	0.8	1.5	3	1.57
Intestine	0.01 ▽	0.04 ±0.01	0.01 △	0.04 ±0.02	4	1.5	18	2.75
Skin	0.01 ▽	0.01 ▽	0.04 ±0.01	0.04 △	4	6	4.5	2.75

† 24 hours.
▽ Values obtained were less than 0.01.
△ 1 sample.

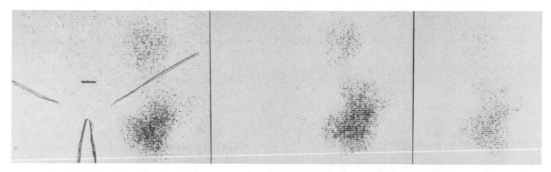

FIGURE 11-10. Photographs of a rectilinear scintiscan showing the uptake of ^{131}I from ^{131}I-NM-113. Left: One day after a 2 mCi tracer dose on 5/4/71. Middle: On 6/11/71, 26 days after a 100 mCi treatment dose. Right: On 6/25/71, 40 days after the treatment dose.

The ^{125}I-labelled analog of our new compound (NP-57), concentrated in malignant melanomas 2 times greater than ^{125}I-NM-113. The ^{3}H activity from the N-demethylated derivative (NP-73) of our new compound concentrated least. Since radioiodinated NM-113 has been used successfully in the diagnosis of dermal and ocular melanomas in the human, the new iodinated analog of the 4 aminoquinoline deserves further evaluation.

ACKNOWLEDGMENT

The authors wish to thank John Wiley and Sons, Inc., and M. N. Croll, MD, editor of *New Techniques in Tumor Localization and Radioimmunoassay* for their reprint permission for our Table 11-1, Figures 11-2, 11-3, 11-4, 11-5, 11-6, and 11-7.

REFERENCES

1. Beierwaltes WH, Lieberman LM, Varma VM, Counsell RE: Visualizing human malignant melanoma and metastases. Use of chloroquine analog tagged with iodine 125. JAMA 206:97, 1968
2. Beierwaltes WH, Varma VM, Lieberman LM, et al: Scintillation scanning of malignant melanomas with radioiodinated quinoline derivitives. J Lab Clin Med 72:485, 1968
3. Beierwaltes WH, Wickrema Sinha AJ: A new radiolabeled quinoline analog in mice with malignant melanomas, Abstracted. Clin Res 22:640A, October 1974
4. Bernstein H, Zvaifler N, Rubin M, Mansour AM: The ocular deposition of chloroquine. Invest Ophthalmol 2:384, 1963
5. Boyd CA, Beierwaltes WH, Lieberman LM, Bergstron TJ: [125]I labeled chloroquine analog in the diagnosis of ocular melanoma. J Nucl Med 12:601, 1971
6. Boyd CM, Lieberman LM, Beierwaltes WH, Varma VM: Diagnostic efficacy of a radioiodinated chloroquine analog in patients with malignant melanoma. J Nucl Med 11:479, 1970
7. Counsell RE, Pocha P, Morales JO, Beierwaltes WH: Tumor localizing agents. 3. Radioiodinated quinoline derivitives. J Pharm Sci 1042, 1967
8. Counsell RE, Pocha P, Ranade VV, et al.: Tumor localizing agents. 7. Radioiodinated quinoline derivitives. J Med Chem 12:232, 1969
9. Ferry AP: Lesions mistaken for malignant melanoma of the posterior uvea, a clinocopathologic analysis of 100 cases with ophthalmoscopically visible lesions. Arch Ophthalmol (Chicago) 72:463, 1964
10. Flocks M, Gerende JH, Zimmerman LE: The size and shape of malignant melanomas of the choroid and ciliary body in relation to prognosis and histologic characeristics (a statistical study of 210 tumors). Trans Am Acad Ophthalmol Otorhinol 59:740-758, 1955
11. Gill SP, Beierwaltes WH, Ice RD, Mosley ST: A new radiolabeled quinoline analog in mice with malignant melanoma. J Nucl Med 16:530, 1975 (abstr)

12. Halger WS, Jarrett WH, Humphrey WT: The radioactive phosphorous uptake test in diagnosis of uveal melanoma. Arch Ophthalmol (Chicago) 83:548, 1970
13. Hogan MJ, Zimmerman LE (eds): Ophthalmic Pathology, ed 2. WB Saunders, Philadelphia, 1962, p 429
14. Knoll GF, Lieberman LM, Nishiyama H, Beierwaltes WH: A gamma ray probe for the detection of ocular melanomas. IEEE Trans Nucl Sci NS-19:76–80, February 1972
15. Lieberman LM: The effects of radiation on the retina of the dog, doctoral dissertation. University of Michigan, Ann Arbor Michigan, 1970
16. Lieberman LM, Boyd CM, Varma VM, et al.: Treatment doses of ^{131}I-labeled chloroquine analogue in normal and malignant melanoma dogs. J Nucl Med 12:153–159, April 1971
17. Packer S, Redvanly C, Lambrecht RM, et al.: Quinoline analog labeled with Iodine 123 in melanoma detection. Arch Opthalmol 93:504–508, 1975
18. Potts AM: The reaction of uveal pigment in vitro with polycyclic compounds. Invest Ophthalmol 3:405, 1964
19. Reese AB, Merriam GR, Martin HE: Treatment of bilateral retinal blastoma by radiation and surgery: Report on 15-year results. Am J Ophthalmol 32:175, 1949
20. Rogers WL, Wainstock MA: An ultrasound-guided gamma-ray probe for detection of ocular melanomas. Ultrasonics Symposium Proceedings, Nov 11–13, 1974, Milwaukee, Wisc #74, CHO 896-150, 1974
21. Sams WM Jr, Epstein UW: The affinity of melanin for chloroquine. J Invest Ophthalmol 45:482, 1965
22. Wainstock MA, Gill S, Rogers WH: Final report to "Flight for light" on an ultrasound-guided gamma-ray probe. Jan 1977

THE LYMPHATIC SPREAD OF MELANOMA AND THE EFFECTS OF METASTASES AND SURGERY UPON LYMPHATIC DYNAMICS

IRVING M. ARIEL

Living lymphography (lymphangio-adenography) is defined as the roentgenography of the lymphatic channels (lymphangiography) and the lymph nodes (lymphadenography) following the injection of a radiopaque material into a lymphatic vessel. Accordingly, we have been provided with a new dimension for visualizing the lymphatic dynamic state when cancerous metastases are transferred via a lymphatic vessel to a lymph node, as well as a means for studying the sequence of events that follow such transmission. The administration of a cancerocidal agent, a radioactive isotope, permits the internal irradiation of cancerous deposits within a lymph node and of in-transit metastases.[1,4-8]

This chapter details some of the lessons learned from living lymphography and describes clinical results in the diagnosis and treatment of certain cancers.

LYMPHOGRAPHY IN DIAGNOSIS OF MALIGNANT NEOPLASMS

Normally, the lymph nodes will concentrate the injected contrast medium, ethiodized oil (Ethiodol), but when metastases of a given size are present, a vacuole remains. Thus, the diagnosis of metastases within the lymph node depends upon the fact that metastases do not concentrate the ethiodized oil.

APPEARANCE OF NORMAL LYMPH NODES

The normal lymph node is usually ovoid with a regular contour, but may also be of V or J shape, and frequently a small notch is present in the margin known as the hilum, the point of entry of the lymphatic trunk. The opacified, normal lymph node has a homogeneous and granular appearance. A false positive diagnosis can be made if a normal lymph node is partially replaced by fat and/or fibrous tissue, lending an appearance similar to that of a cancerous metastasis. Fischer and Thornbury[15] call attention to another defect in normal lymphography that may create a false positive diagnosis of metastasis, that is, when two nodes lie closely adjacent, giving the radiographic appearance of a single node with a small space in the middle. Special studies and oblique views help to delineate these defects.

APPEARANCE OF METASTASES

Metastases will appear as a clear area or vacuole in an otherwise homogeneously filled lymph node (Fig. 12-1). The observed patterns of metastases are numerous and varied. Frequently, lymph nodes containing metastases demonstrate marginal filling defects because of the presence of small metastases in the subcapsular region, presenting a moth-eaten appearance. Usually these nodes are of normal size and do not become enlarged until extensive metastases are present.

Koehler, Wohl, and Schaffer[23] demonstrated that a metastasis must be at least 5 to 10 mm in diameter before it can be visualized roentgenographically. Numerous examples have been observed of completely normal-appearing lymph nodes which, in fact, contained microscopic-sized deposits of cancer.

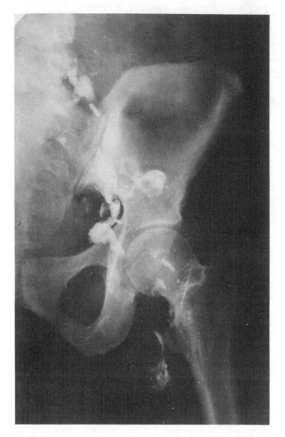

FIGURE 12-1. Metastatic melanoma in lymph nodes. Note vacuolated appearance.

If a lymph node is completely replaced by cancer, the flow of injected ethiodized oil will completely circumvent this node, and it will not be visualized radiographically. Therefore, the absence of opacification may give the surgeon a false sense of security.

Total replacement of a node by cancer will produce an absolute stoppage in the flow of ethiodized oil. Further testament to complete nodal replacement by cancer is the appearance of a pattern of fine reticular collateral lymphatic channels branching off from the area of abrupt obstruction.

Accuracy in diagnosing lymph node metastases by means of lymphography averages 30%. Errors may be made on two points: false negatives in which no metastases are observed in a radiographically normal lymph node; and false positives where defects not resulting from metastases are observed within a node.

Lymphography may provide additional benefits:

1. It permits the oncologist to study both normal and abnormal lymphatic dynamics and to learn more about cancer spread.

2. Since the lymph nodes will retain the radiopaque medium from six to nine months, any change within the lymph node can be observed, such as a response to therapy, or an increase in size caused by cancerous growth.

3. It offers the radiotherapist a landmark for the placement of radiotherapeutic portals.

4. One can study the response to x-ray therapy by observing any change in size of the lymph node, particularly a decrease in size.

5. A repeat lymphogram, especially in patients with lymphoma who must be followed for prolonged periods, will provide an assessment as to the status of the malignant process.

6. When chlorophyll is combined with ethiodized oil, all the opacified lymph nodes are stained light green. Therefore, preoperative lymphography aids the surgeon, especially the surgical resident, in the visualization of the lymph nodes during the performance of a lymphadenectomy for cancer. We have used this technique in the past but have discontinued it since the Federal Drug Administration now prohibits the use of chlorophyll in this instance.

7. It demonstrates to the surgeon the adequacy of his lymph node dissection. A preoperative lymphogram is performed, and on completion of a lymphadenectomy, a repeat roentgenogram taken on the operating table will demonstrate the presence of any retained lymph nodes (Fig. 12-2). It must be borne in mind that a lymph node completely replaced by cancer (unopacified) will not be exhibited on x-ray film. However, such cancerous nodes are usually markedly enlarged and are readily visible to the surgeon at the time of operation.

8. It demonstrates abnormalities of the mediastinum by any alteration in the anatomy of the thoracic duct.

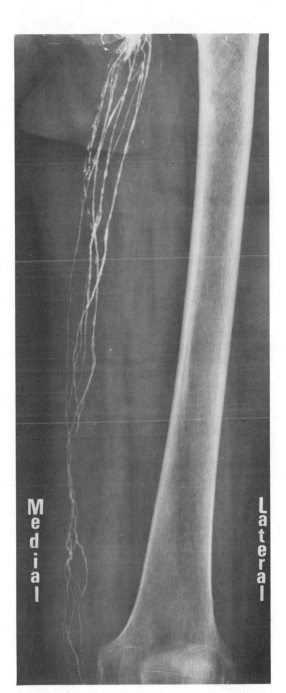

FIGURE 12-2. Normal lymphatic vessels. Note small caliber and regular course.

COMPLICATIONS

In a review of 100 consecutive lymphograms performed, Fischer and Thornbury[15] cite the following complications: (1) fever, 24 patients; (2) radiographically demonstrable contrast embolization in lung, asymptomatic, six patients, and liver, asymptomatic, two patients; (3) extremity edema, worsened, three patients; (4) penile edema, two patients, (5) lymphangitis, two patients; (6) superficial thrombophlebitis, two patients; (7) aseptic incision separation, two patients; (8) allergy to patent blue violet, two patients; and (9) postconization parametritis exacerbation, one patient.

In our series of 300 lymphograms performed by the author and his colleagues, no complications were encountered. Ten patients complained of a transient sense of ill-feeling which they could not pinpoint; five of these patients complained of transient mild nausea. The only reaction we have observed is slow healing of the incision at the injection site. Inasmuch as many of our patients received radioactive isotopes endolymphatically administered with the ethiodized oil, we believe the slow healing to be, in all probability, the result of leakage at the site of incision. The simple procedure of pouring one liter of normal saline solution over the wound before it is closed by suture has obviated this difficulty in the last 50 patients treated.

Spillage of the contrast medium into the lung parenchyma via the thoracic duct is inherent in the technic. As a result, although symptoms are not produced in a patient with normal pulmonary function, a few serious sequelae have been described in patients with extensive pulmonary disease, and two fatal fat embolizations have been reported.[11,16] This complication has been averted in our patients by our limitation of the amount of contrast medium injected. We do not inject more than 4 ml into each lower-extremity lymphatic vessel and a maximum of 3 ml into each upper-extremity lymphatic vessel.

An occasional patient may be sensitive to the blue dye injected intradermally to visualize the lymphatic vessels. At first we used FDC number 1, which we found most satisfactory. However, the Federal Drug Administration has now prohibited its use, so we use a less satisfactory blue dye, direct sky blue. Rarely is a patient sensitive to the iodine; however, one patient of ours did develop a macular dermatitis, which responded readily to treatment.

LYMPHATIC DYNAMICS

Knowledge of the normal lymphatic anatomy and physiology provides us with a better understanding of the changes that may occur as a result of metastasis, or following the performance of certain surgical and radiologic procedures, and will illuminate our understanding as to the best possible course of treatment to follow.

NORMAL LYMPHATIC DYNAMICS

Normally, when ethiodized oil is injected into a lymphatic vessel, the medium will be transported throughout the lymphatic network with only a slight delay before deposition in the lymph nodes that drain the region. The radiopaque material remains within the lymphatic vessels from three to six hours and will drain within 24 hours in almost every instance. In contrast to blood flow, lymphatic flow is either extremely slow or stagnant when the extremity is in the dependent position. With the patient in a horizontal position, it may take from one to two hours to inject 10 ml of ethiodized oil, using a pressure pump. Accordingly, serial roentgenograms will provide an index of the lymphatic distribution pattern following the intralymphatic injection of ethiodized oil.

LOWER–EXTREMITY LYMPHATIC VESSELS

The lymphatic trunks of the lower extremity usually follow the course of the greater saphenous vein (saphena magna system). The lymphatic vessels vary from 0.25 to 1 mm in diameter, usually retaining their caliber as they ascend toward the inguinal region and usually following a straight course to end abruptly (Fig. 12–3A). When a contrast medium is injected into a lymphatic vessel on the dorsum of the foot, the lymphatic vessels are visualized as one or more trunks coursing proximally along the anteromedial aspect of the leg, converging toward the knee, then ascending and dividing into 12 to 16 divisions as they enter the superficial inguinal lymph nodes (injection site 1, Fig. 12–3B).[2] If the opaque material is injected into a lymphatic vessel along the lateral aspect of the foot, the lymphatic vessels are seen to course proximally toward the popliteal fossa (saphena parva system), where one or two popliteal nodes are usually found (injection site 2, Fig. 12–3B); the latter are found routinely in dogs, whereas in the human being they are absent in a significant number of patients (Fig. 12–4). The lymphatic vessels continue to course proximally to the deep lymphatic chain and terminate in the superficial inguinal vessels, which course to the thigh and extend mesially to enter the groin in juxtaposition to the femoral vessels. Valves are found in the lymphatic vessels that tend to prevent backflow. The lymph nodes of the saphena parva system, draining the back of the leg and following the course of the lesser saphenous vein, are said to lie deeper and more craniad than those draining the trunk of the greater saphenous system.

INGUINAL AND ILIAC LYMPH NODES

There are from four to ten inguinal nodes normally, both superficial and deep, presenting a variable pattern. Efforts to divide this group into subgroups based on a relationship to the greater saphenous vein are believed to be of no practical use in clinical radiographic diagnoses.

Rouvier[28] originally described the efferent lymphatic vessels from the inguinal nodes continuing proximally to the external iliac

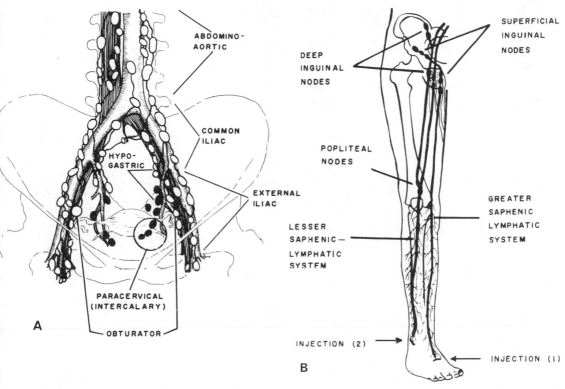

FIGURE 12-3. A. Anatomy of lower abdominal lymph nodes. **B.** Lymphatic vessels of lower extremity. Injection site 1, on dorsum of foot, drains into greater saphenous lymphatic system. Injection site 2, lateral aspect of ankle, drains into lesser saphenous system, into popliteal nodes, and then to inguinal lymph nodes.*

chain of nodes and dividing into three chains: a lateral chain located lateral to the external iliac artery (one to four nodes), a middle group that lies on the posterior surface of the external iliac vein (two to four nodes), and a medial group (three to four nodes) posterior to the external iliac vein usually in juxtaposition to the lateral pelvic wall. The obturator node is considered a part of the medial group of the external iliac chain of nodes; it may lie either in direct continuity with the remainder of the medial chain, or it may be somewhat distant as a solitary node within the obturator fossa, usually between the external iliac vein and the obturator nerve and vessels.

Continuing proximally, the common iliac chain, four to 12 nodes lying in close relationship to the common iliac artery and vein, subdivides into the hypogastric nodes, two to eight in number, and courses along the hypogastric artery; from the common iliac nodes, several trunks course craniad along the aorta and inferior vena cava to form the abdomino-aortic lymph node group (25 to 45 nodes). The abdomino-aortic nodes are divided into four groups: right lateral aortic, left lateral aortic, preaortic, and retroaortic. Efferent lymphatic vessels from the abdomino-aortic chain empty into the cisterna chyli usually at the level of the second lumbar vertebra. Rarely can

* Figures 12-3 through 12-12 are from Ariel IM: Progress in cancer: Lymphography and endolymphatic administration of radioactive isotopes for treating cancer. NYS J Med 68(10): 1248–1268,1968. Reprinted by permission from the New York State Journal of Medicine, copyright by the Medical Society of the State of New York by IM Ariel.

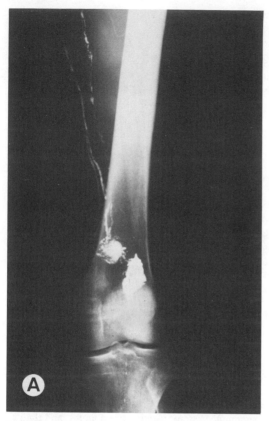

FIGURE 12–4. A. Lymphogram of normal man demonstrating two popliteal lymph nodes. Injection made posterior to internal malleolus (courtesy H. W. Fischer, MD). **B.** Lymphogram of patient with melanoma, performed as in A, demonstrating well-developed chain of lymphatic vessels coursing popliteal space; no lymph nodes present. Dissection revealed one popliteal lymph node completely replaced by fat.

lymph nodes be visualized in the posterior mediastinum, but not infrequently supraclavicular nodes may be seen in the region of the termination of the thoracic duct.

UPPER–EXTREMITY LYMPHATICS

There are usually two groups of lymphatic vessels in the upper extremity, a lateral and a medial, which join above the elbow and usually follow the basilic vein along the inner aspect of the arm to the axillary chain of lymph nodes (Fig. 12–5). The axillary nodes vary in number, are interconnected by many trunks, and their efferents may either drain directly into the subclavian vein or may lead to the supraclavicular nodes and then empty into the subclavian vein. Inconsistently, one to two small lymph nodes may be visualized in the epitrochlear region along the medial aspect.

LYMPHATIC–VASCULAR COMMUNICATIONS

A communication normally exists between the lymphatic and venous systems. Rusznyak,

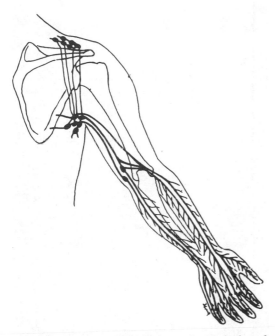

FIGURE 12-5. Lymphatic vessels and lymph nodes of upper extremity. Note communications from axillary to supraclavicular lymph nodes.

Foldi, and Szabo[29,30] have demonstrated an anastomosis between the lymphatic vessels and the veins, especially in the thyroid, kidney, and liver. Blalock et al.[9] demonstrated the presence of numerous connections between the lymphatic vessels and the inferior vena cava, the azygous, and other veins especially after ligation of the thoracic duct. Pressman et al.[27] demonstrated the existence of a communication between the lymph nodes and the blood vessels by injecting air into the lymph nodes of animals; the air was seen in both the lymphatic vessels and the veins. Wallace et al.[39] demonstrated direct lymphatic-venous communications in the normal individual, found most frequently in the cervical region and to a lesser extent in the upper extremity, and the communications were more abundant in those individuals with lymphatic obstruction.

It is not surprising to note these connections between the lymphatic and venous systems, inasmuch as, embryologically, the lymphatic sacs are formed by a process of budding from the blood vascular endothelium. Budding sacs from the anterior cardinal veins give rise to the lymphatic vessels of the head and neck. Sprouts from the mesonephric vein develop paired sacs, which become the precursors of the skeletal lymphatic vessels; two additional sacs are derived from the mesonephric vein, one later becomes the cisterna chyli and the lower thoracic duct, and the other forms the lymphatic vessels of the abdominal viscera.

EFFECTS OF METASTASES: ALTERED LYMPHATIC DYNAMICS

METASTASES IN LYMPHATIC VESSELS

The lodgment of tumor implants either within the lymphatic vessels or the lymph nodes may produce an alteration in the normal lymphatic dynamics often determined by the location and degree of obstruction. The blockage of a lymphatic vessel in either the leg or the arm may produce one or a combination of the following alterations in collateral lymphatic flow: (1) The anterior compartment may be completely blocked, shunting the lymphatic flow into the posterior compartment; (2) the anterior chain may be incompletely blocked, producing a partial shunt into the posterior compartment, resulting in function of both compartments; and (3) both compartments may be functional without evidence of block.

Accordingly, a cancer located on the dorsum of the foot may spread to the popliteal lymph nodes either because of an anatomic shunt to the posterior lymphatic chain or because of an obstruction in the anterior lymphatic chain.

POPLITEAL LYMPH NODES

When present, the popliteal nodes drain the lesser saphenous lymphatic system and may drain the greater saphenous system as well.

Therefore, cancer cells may and do lodge in these nodes. Accordingly, for a malignant neoplasm in the location of drainage into the popliteal nodes, such as directly inferior to the popliteal space, the lateral aspect of the foot, or the heel, the nodes should be included in the therapeutic plan.

It has been stated, "metastasis to the popliteal nodes is so rare that the possibility of its occurrence should not enter into the discussion of the management of melanoma of the lower extremity inferior to the condyles."[24] We are in disagreement with this premise, for we have seen many instances of metastasis of melanoma and other cancers (epidermoid carcinoma and sarcoma) to the popliteal and epitrochlear lymph nodes. Although the popliteal lymph nodes are absent in some human beings, they are, however, present in others. The probability exists that these nodes undergo attrition with advancing age, as do many lymph nodes, and they are present in older individuals in a nonfunctioning, atrophic form.

Our data further suggest that if the lymphogram demonstrates a collateral route from the greater saphenous to the lesser saphenous system, the popliteal nodes should definitely be considered in the therapeutic plan. If lymphograms are not performed, at least a clinical search should be made in the popliteal and epitrochlear regions in all patients seen with either primary or secondary cancers distal to these sites.

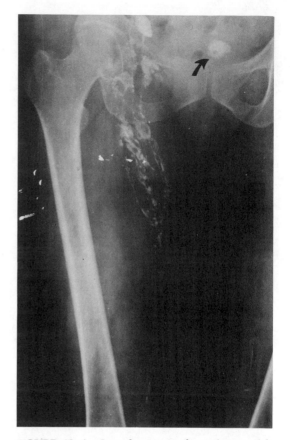

FIGURE 12–6. Lymphogram of patient with metastatic melanoma to left inguinal region, taken five days after injection of ethiodized oil. Note stagnation of lymphatic vessels and development of collateral circulation where presacral node visualized in midline (arrow). Note space-occupying lesions in inguinal lymph nodes characteristic of metastases.

METASTASES IN LYMPH NODES

When metastases in the lymph nodes have reached sufficient size, the resultant blockage will shunt the lymph into alternate channels to maintain the integrity of lymphatic flow. A vast network of potential, not normally functioning lymphatic vessels will be enlisted into service, and those in the immediate vicinity of the obstruction will first become functional. Figure 12–6 is the lymphogram of a patient with metastatic melanoma to the left inguinal region taken five days after the injection of the contrast medium. Stagnation of the lymphatic vessels was present, and collateral circulation developed via the pre-sacral chain of nodes. Eventually metastases were demonstrated in the lymph nodes of the opposite groin. Should this adjacent network prove insufficient, new groups of lymphatic vessels become functional in an effort to reestablish lymphatic flow.

The nature of the collateral lymphatic vessels is often determined by the level or location of an obstruction. Obstruction in the para-aortic lymphatic vessels may produce an atypical collateral network that may extend into the visceral lymphatic vessels. Obstruction at the level of the porta hepatis may produce such stagnation of the lymphatic system distal to the blockage that the lymph nodes may be compressed and destroyed by the back pressure. Wallace et al.[39] demonstrated that obstruction at the thoracic duct produced by posterior mediastinal lesions hindered the normal flow of lymph and induced retrograde filling of the gastrointestinal trunk as well as the intercostal lymphatic vessels.

Those collaterals called into play after an obstruction has become extensive are so eccentric and unpredictable that they defy any effort at interpretation, and the application of therapeutic modalities is nearly impossible. This was demonstrated in an obstruction in the iliac nodes secondary to a carcinoma of the cervix that produced a lymphatic collateral chain in the anterior abdominal wall to the axilla where a metastatic cancer was encountered.[36]

PERIVASCULAR LYMPHATICS

The existence of potential spaces in perivascular locations was recently described by Wallace et al.[39] These spaces were successfully demonstrated by the investigators as an additional collateral route for the transport of lymph and tumor cells. They liken these perivascular spaces to the perineural or endoneural spaces, which have been amply demonstrated to play a major role in the dissemination of tumor emboli. Although they have observed these perivascular spaces, they have been unable to establish their exact anatomy. Are they actual potential spaces between the vessel wall and its surrounding membrane, or do they constitute an integral part of the lymphatic system? However, these authors have shown conclusively the existence of a direct connection between the lymphatic system and these potential spaces to which lymph is transported and which offers a possible route for the unopposed transport of tumor cells. These spaces, located within the perivascular sheath, have been seen in patients with and without edema.

STAGNATION OF LYMPH

When radiopaque material is injected into a lymphatic vessel, normally it will have emptied from the lymphatic vessels in from four to 24 hours. In the presence of obstruction, stagnation ensues and the injected material will remain within the lymphatics for long periods; as long as two and a half months as determined by the authors and perhaps longer, but measurements have not been made.

Clinically, a stagnant lymphatic state may be manifest by the appearance of edema. An impediment to the free flow of lymph causes an increase in lymphatic pressure with the resultant deposition of lymph within the interstitial spaces of the extremities, producing edema; however, stagnation of lymphatic flow has been observed without resultant edema. We interpret stagnant lymphatic flow as presumptive evidence of the existence of an obstruction in either the proximal chain of lymph nodes or within the proximal lymphatic vessels.

Figure 12–7 is the lymphogram of a patient with metastases in the axilla from a primary melanoma of the left lateral side of the chest wall. This patient manifested a direct lymphatic connection between the axillary and supraclavicular lymph nodes, illustrating a route for the passage of tumor emboli from the axilla into the supraclavicular region. The lymphogram showed the presence of metastases within the lymph nodes of the axilla; it demonstrated the retention of the contrast medium within the lymphatic vessels three days after the performance of the lymphogram, indicative of stagnation in the lymphatic flow. In some instances, metastases within the lymph nodes may be of such small size as to go undetected lymphographically. For example, the stagnant state of the distal lymphatic vessels in one patient prompted the excision of a groin lymph node for histologic study, which revealed the presence of metastases.

Lymphatic stagnation with ensuing edema may be only temporary, providing the development of collateral circulation is adequate. Should this occur, then the free flow of lymph within the lymphatic vessels will be re-

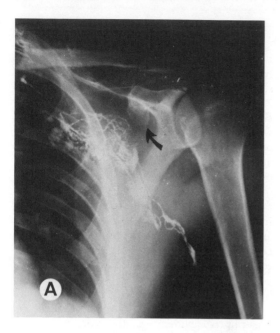

FIGURE 12-7. Lymphograms of patient with metastases in axilla from primary melanoma of left lateral chest wall. A. Note defect in lymph node characteristic of space-occupying lesion or metastasis (arrow). Also note filling of supraclavicular lymph nodes that also contain metastases. B and C. Lymphograms demonstrating retention of dye within lymphatic vessels three days after its injection. Note tortuous course, irregular contour, and variation in caliber of vessels.

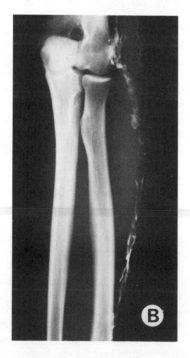

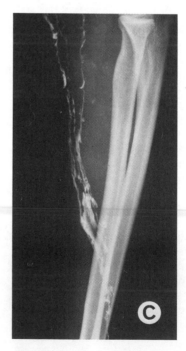

established, and the edema will subside. However, if an adequate collateral circulation has not developed, the edema will become more pronounced as the lymphatic pressure is increased.

Blocker et al.[10] have demonstrated that the normal intralymphatic pressures are subatmospheric in the lower extremity (0 to −16 mm water) with a decreasing gradient upward to the thoracic duct. With blockage, the intralymphatic pressure in the lower extremity is positive, going as high as 60 to 80 mm water. One patient with an inferior vena cava syndrome caused by a mediastinal tumor with generalized edema from the nipple inferiorly had the extremely high intralymphatic pressure of 400 mm water in the lower extremity.

REVERSAL OF FLOW

After a period of failure to establish satisfactory collateral circulation, a reversal in lymphatic flow occurs with the development of a functional superficial chain of dermal lymphatic vessels. In such instances, subsequent regurgitation of lymph occurs distally into a network of dermal lymphatic vessels (Fig. 12–8).

LYMPHATICOVENOUS ANASTOMOSIS

Previous comments have been made regarding the normal existence of lymphaticovenous anastomoses. In the presence of obstruction under the pressure of metabolic necessity, potential, nonfunctioning lymphaticovenous openings become functional, and certain new communications develop in the need to mobilize a collateral circulation for the stagnant lymph, present under an increased head of pressure resulting from obstruction.[15,28,39] Under such circumstances, the transport of tumor cells from the lymphatic into the vascular circulation is probably facilitated.

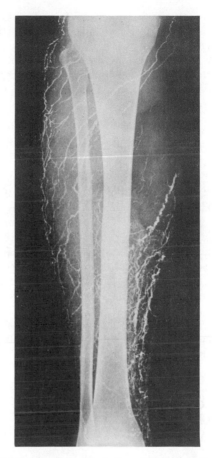

FIGURE 12–8. Marked lymphedema following radical groin dissection for melanoma with development of extensive network of dermal lymphatic vessels.

LYMPHATIC CIRCULATION TIME

We have observed, as have Stehlin et al.,[37] that in the presence of obstruction and following isotopic administration into a lymphatic vessel of the foot, there is a delay in the time it takes for the isotope to reach the inguinal lymph nodes. To ascertain the lymphatic circulation time from foot to groin, a Geiger counter is placed over the groin as the endolymphatic administration of iodine-131 ethiodized oil is begun into a foot lymphatic vessel, and the first recording is taken as the isotope reaches the groin. In six patients without evidence of obstruction, the time averaged five minutes and varied from three to eight minutes. In the presence of clinically detectable metastases in the lymph nodes, the time averaged nine minutes and varied from five to fifteen minutes.

[131]I ETHIODIZED OIL CONCENTRATION IN BLOOD

At the completion of the injection of 10 ml ethiodized oil containing 30 microcuries ^{131}I, the concentration of ^{131}I in the blood could be considered an index of lymphatic-vascular communication. The data are presented in Table 12-1 and demonstrate a significantly increased quantity of ^{131}I in the blood of patients with metastases in the inguinal lymph nodes. Some of this may have been because of spillover via the thoracic duct into the circulation; however, the small volume injected (10 ml) minimizes this possibility.

EFFECTS OF DISCONTINUOUS LYMPH NODE DISSECTION ON LYMPHATIC DYNAMICS

HAZARDS OF THE OPERATION

The performance of a discontinuous operation for melanoma is not without hazard.[2,3] The following sequence of events occurs after the performance of a groin dissection.

There is an extensive escape of lymph through the severed lymphatic vessels resulting in the formation of a lymphocele (Fig. 12-9). A lymphogram was performed three days after the radical groin dissection for a malignant melanoma; a drain was left in situ. Salient in this instance is the observed escape of lymph and ethiodized oil from the lymphatic system into the free tissue spaces of the dissection site because of the innumerable lymphatic vessels severed during the course of the dissection; the drain functions as a suction apparatus for the lymph and ethiodized oil.

When the drainage tube is removed, the ethiodized oil is retained within the free tissue spaces with the formation of a tract along the course of the tube.

Cancer cells in transit within the lymphatic vessels are deposited into the free tissue spaces where they may seed and grow, being revealed as metastases (Fig. 12-10).

Herman, Benninghoff, and Schwartz[18] have demonstrated that a lymphocyst will subsequently become an integral part of the newly formed lymphatic system with the formation of afferent and efferent communicating vessels. However, this is a function of time; the lymph and, presumably, cancer cells will remain in the free tissues for a prolonged period.

A sealing off of the lymphatic vessels next occurs at the incisional site. As a result, one or all of the following mechanisms occur: (1) The lymphatic vessels may seal off and block the incisional region with the resultant retention of lymph in those lymphatic vessels distal to the operative site; (2) reestablishment in continuity may take place by regrowth of the severed lymphatic vessels; (3) the blocked lymphatic vessels may form collateral channels with adjacent lymphatic vessels with the subsequent reestablishment of lymphatic flow (Fig. 12-11); and (4) due to lymphatic blockage, and in the presence of an inadequate development of collateral circulation, a regurgitation of lymph occurs within the subsequently functional superficial or dermal lymphatic channels. As a result, edema of the extremity may occur.

SATELLITOSIS OF MELANOMA

It is not uncommon to find the development of dermal satellite metastases involving the skin of the leg following extensive metastasis to the lymph nodes of the groin or subsequent to the surgical excision of these nodes. Satellite cancers have been noted to occur in those regions of expansive dermal lymphatic development secondary to an obstruction. It is believed that tumor emboli become implanted within the subcutaneous tissue and/or dermis

TABLE 12-1.   [131]I Concentration in Blood Immediately after Endolymphatic
Injection of 30 Microcuries [131]I Ethiodized Oil 10 ml Volume

Groups	Microcuries [131]I
Patients without evidence of lymphatic obstruction or metastases to inguinal lymph nodes (average, 4 patients)	6.5
Patients with evidence of lymphatic obstruction or metastases to inguinal lymph nodes (average, 3 patients)	30

via these dermal lymphatic vessels. Figure 12-12 is the lymphogram of a patient with metastatic melanoma in the left inguinal lymph nodes taken four days after the injection of the contrast medium and demonstrating lymphatic stagnation. A partial groin dissection had been performed two years prior to the development of numerous satellitoses, which involved mainly the medial aspect of the thigh. The lymphogram shows the extensively developed collateral lymphatic circulation with its large number of dermal vessels arising from the deeper lymphatic vessels and extending to the skin at sites of the satellite lesions. This patient was treated by the intralymphatic administration of radioactive isotopes given at the time of the lymphogram, and she remained well eight years after treatment; the satellite metastases disappeared and there were no new skin lesions, but the patient later died from rupture of the spleen due to melanoma metastases.

Malignant melanoma may spread either by direct infiltration or via lymphatic channels into the adjacent tissues, with the resultant deposition of cancer cells in the regional lymph nodes. Stagnation of lymphatic flow, possibly attributable to proximal obstruction, hinders transportation, and the stalled cancer cells implant and multiply to become a fixed metastatic deposit. The latter should be differentiated from the floating cell in transit within the lymphatics. Metastases may be found within the deep lymphatic vessels as well as in the newly developed dermal and subcutaneous lymphatic network. Accord-

ingly, satellitoses may be considered the result of cancer cells presumably traveling in a retrograde manner within the tiny dermal lymphatic vessels, developed in consequence of lymphatic obstruction with failure to promote adequate routes of collateral lymphatic flow; at least this is one mechanism in their development.

Stehlin and colleagues[35,36] have described the lymphatic route as being responsible for satellitoses but have neglected to call attention to the reversal of flow, with the functionally developed network of superficial dermal lymphatic vessels as a probable mechanism attendant with the development of satellite dermal metastases.

Metastases within the lymphatic vessels of the extremity may be present at any depth, and this should be considered in any planned attack on malignant melanoma of an extremity. Consequently, melanoma cells may be found within the lymphatic vessels as (1) floating cells en route to the regional lymph nodes; (2) fixed within the deeper lymphatic vessels where they remain and grow; or (3) within the dermal lymphatic vessels transported in retrograde fashion and coming to a standstill to grow as satellitoses.

CONCLUSION

Lymphography permits the visualization of metastases in the lymph nodes, thereby aiding in planning the policies for treating a cancer;

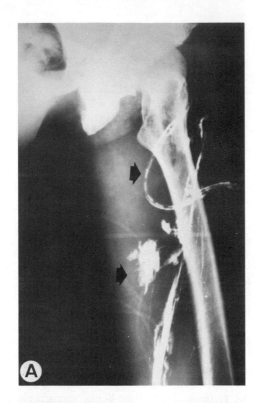

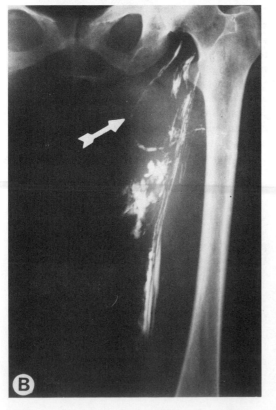

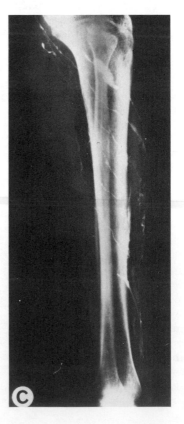

FIGURE 12-9. A. Lymphogram taken three days after performance of radical groin dissection for melanoma. Note injected ethiodized oil removed by means of Hemovac (upper arrow) within wound site. Note lymphocele (lower arrow). B and C. Appearance two and four weeks later (see arrow in Fig. 12-9B.).

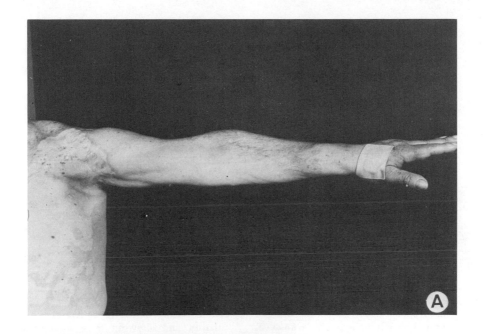

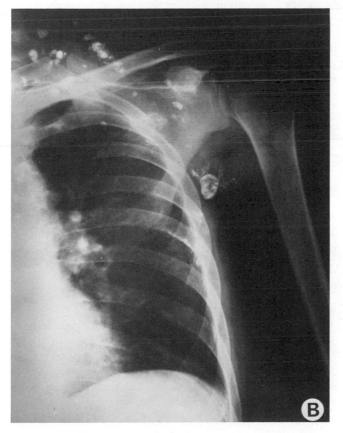

FIGURE 12-10. A. Clinical appearance of melanoma of chest wall and axilla. B. Lymphogram demonstrating reconstituted lymphatic circulation in patient shown in A. Regenerated lymphatic vessels communicate freely with supraclavicular lymph nodes; new collateral circulation developed with internal mammary chain of lymph nodes. Note residual lymph node in axilla harboring metastatic melanoma. Left radical axillary dissection for melanoma performed two years previously elsewhere.

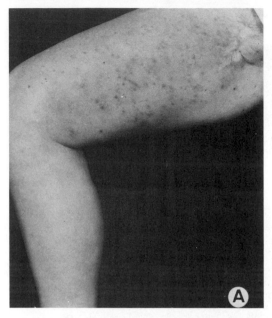

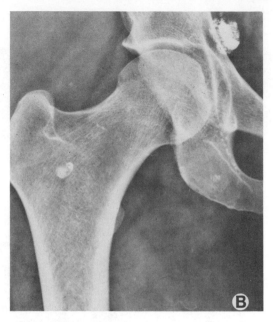

FIGURE 12–11. Patient with metastatic melanoma on whom partial groin dissection was performed two years before lymphography, who developed extensive satellitosis. A. Clinical photograph demonstrating numerous satellite lesions involving chiefly medial aspect of right thigh. B. Lymphogram demonstrating extensive collateral lymphatic circulation and showing large number of dermal vessels arising from deep lymphatic vessels at sites of satellitoses.

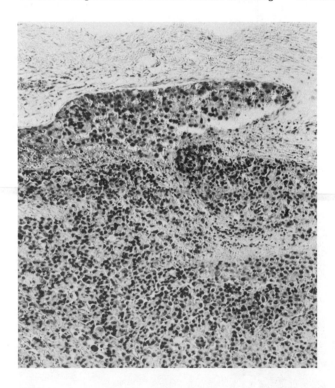

FIGURE 12–12. Photomicrograph demonstrating malignant melanoma within lymphatic vessels of leg amputated for melanoma (hematoxylin and eosin stain).

the overall diagnostic error is 30%, both false positive and false negative.

Since the lymph nodes will retain the radiopaque medium from six to nine months, any change within the lymph node can be observed, such as a response to therapy or an increase in size because of cancerous growth.

It offers the radiotherapist a guide for placing radiotherapeutic ports.

When chlorophyll is combined with ethiodized oil, all the opacified lymph nodes are stained light green. Therefore, preoperative lymphography aids the surgeon, especially the surgical resident, in the visualization of lymph nodes during the performance of a lymphadenectomy for cancer.

It demonstrates to the surgeon the adequacy of his lymph node dissection.

It demonstrates abnormalities of the mediastinum by any alteration in the anatomy of the thoracic duct.

Metastases in the lymph nodes produce the following alterations in lymphatic dynamics: (1) Stagnation of lymphatic flow which may produce edema. The "take" of cancer cells in transit is facilitated, as is the transport of cancer cells into the vascular compartment via lymphatic-vascular communications because of an increased head of lymphatic pressure. (2) Collateral lymphatic channels become so extensive and erratic as to defy interpretation and any anticancer therapeutic program. Cancer cells may be conveyed uninterruptedly for great distances and to almost any region in the body. (3) If the collateral lymphatic circulation is inadequate, a reversal of lymphatic flow occurs via a group of newly developed and functional dermal lymphatic vessels. This is one modus operandi in the formation of dermal metastases (satellitoses of melanoma).

A discontinuous operation for melanoma, that is, the removal of the primary melanoma plus a groin or axillary dissection while completely ignoring the intervening lymphatic vessels, not only aggravates the situation described,[11] but also permits the escape of cancer cells via the severed lymphatic vessels into the free tissue spaces where they may seed and grow.

REFERENCES

1. Ariel IM: Progress in cancer: Lymphography and endolymphatic administration of radioactive isotopes for treating cancer NY State J Med 68:10 (May 15) 1968
2. Ariel IM, Resnick MI: Altered lymphatic dynamics caused by cancer metastases. Arch Surg 94:117 (Jan) 1967
3. Ariel IM, Resnick MI: Altered lymphatic dynamics following groin and axillary dissection: its relationship to treatment policies for malignant melanoma. Surgery 61:210 (Feb) 1967
4. Ariel IM, Bale WF, Downing V, et al.: The distribution of radioactive isotopes of iodine in normal rabbits. Am J Physiol 132:346, 1941
5. Ariel IM, Resnick MI, Caley D: The intralymphatic administration of radioactive isotopes and cancer chemotherapeutic drugs. Surgery 55:355, 1964
6. Ariel IM, Resnick MI, Oropeza R: Effects of irradiation (external and internal) on lymphatic dynamics. Am J Roentgenol 99:404 (Feb) 1967
7. Ariel IM, Resnick MI, Oropeza R: The intralymphatic administration or radioactive isotopes for treating malignant melanoma. Surg Gynecol Obstet 124:25 (Jan) 1967
8. Baum S, Bron KM, Wexler L, Abrams HL: Lymphangiography, cavography and urography. Radiology 81:207, (1963)
9. Blalock A, Robinson CS, Cunningham RS, Gray ME: Experimental studies on lymphatic blockage. Arch Surg 34:1049, 1937
10. Blocker TG Jr, et al.: Lymphodynamics. Plast Reconstruct Surg 25:337, 1960
11. Bron KM, Baum S, Abrams HL: Oil embolism in lymphangiography. Incidence, manifestations, and mechanisms. Radiology 80:194, 1963
12. Burger RH: Lymph node response to high-dose intralymphatic injection of radiochromic phosphate. Bull NY Acad Med 40:142, 1964
13. Chiappa S, Galli G, Palmia C: Observations on intra-lymphatic radiotherapy and general chemotherapy. Clin Radiol 15:202, 1964
14. Fischer HW: Intralymphatic therapy for lymph node metastases of carcinoma of the cervix. An analysis of the proposition and presentation of pertinent experimental data. Cancer 18:1059, 1965
15. Fischer HW, Thornbury JR: Lymphography in the diagnosis of malignant neoplasms. In Ariel IM (ed): Progress in Clinical Cancer, New York, Grune & Stratton, 1965, vol 1, p 213

16. Fuchs WA, Book-Henderstrom G: Inguinal and pelvic lymphography. A preliminary report. Acta Radiol 56:340, 1961

17. Healy RJ, Amory HI, Friedman M: Hodgkin's disease; a review of two hundred and sixteen cases. Radiology 64: 51, 1955

18. Herman PG, Benninghoff DL, Schwartz S: A physiologic approach to lymph flow in lymphography. Am J Roentgenol 91:1207, 1964

19. Hine GJ, Brownell GL: Radiation Dosimetry, New York, Academic Press, 1956

20. Jantet GH, Edwards JM, Gough MH, Kinmonth JB: Endolymphatic therapy with radioactive gold for malignant melanoma. Brit Med J 2:904, 1964

21. Kaplan HS: Presentation at the Symposium on Hodgkin's Disease, French Academy of Hematology and Radiology, Hospital St Louis, February 23, 1965, Paris, France

22. Kinmonth JB: Lymphangiography in man; a method of out-lining lymphatic trunks at operation. Clin Sc 11:13, 1952

23. Koehler PR, Wohl GT, Schaffer B: Lymphangiography —a survey of its current status. Am J Roentgenol 91:1216, 1964

24. McNeer G, Das Gupta T: Routes of lymphatic spread of malignant melanoma, CA 15:168, 1965

25. Molander DW, Ariel IM, Pack GT: Hepatic gamma-scanning as an aid in the management of patients with malignant lymphomas. Am J Roentgenol 99:851 (Apr) 1967

26. Pack, GT, Scharnagel I, Morfitt M: The principle of excision and dissection in continuity for primary and metastatic melanoma of the skin. Surgery 17:849, 1945

27. Pressman JJ, Simon MB, Hand K, Miller J: Passage of fluids, cells, and bacteria via direct communications between lymph nodes and veins. Surg Gynecol Obstet 115:207, 1962

28. Rouvier H: Anatomy of the Human Lymphatic System, Tobias MJ (trans), Ann Arbor, Michigan, Edwards Brothers, 1938

29. Rusznyak I, Foldi M, Szabo G: I: Lymphatics and Lymph Circulation. Physiology and Pathology, New York, Pergamon Press, 1960

30. Rusznyak I, Foldi M, Szabo G: Lymphatic System, Tobias MJ (trans), Ann Arbor, Michigan, Edwards Brothers, 1938, p 318

31. Schwartz SI, Greenlaw RH, Rob C, Rubin P: Intra-lymphatic injection of radioactive gold. A preliminary experimental report. Cancer 15: 623, 1962

32. Seitzman DM, Wright R, Halaby FA, Freeman JH: Intralymphatic radioisotope therapy. Surg Gynecol Obstet 118:52, 1964

33. Seitzman DM, Wright R, Halaby FA, Freeman JH: Radioactive lymphangiography as a therapeutic adjunct. Am J Roentgenol 89:140, 1963 1963

34. Siegel P, Liebner EJ: Intralymphatic radioactive therapy for pelvic cancer. Am J Obstet Gynecol 91:122, 1965

35. Stehlin JS Jr, Clark RL Jr, Smith JL Jr, White EC: Malignant melanoma of the extremities: experiences with conventional therapy: a new surgical and chemotherapeutic approach with regional perfusion. Cancer 13:55, 1960

36. Stehlin JS Jr, Smith JL Jr, Clark RL Jr: Malignant melanoma: diagnosis and current treatment. S Clin North Am 42:455, 1962

37. Stehlin JS Jr, Smith JL Jr, Jing BS, Sherrin D: Melanomas of the extremities complicated by in-transit metastases. Surg Gynecol Obstet 122:3 (Jan) 1966

38. Tubiana, M.: Presentation at the Symposium on Hodgkin's Disease, French Academy of Hematology and Radiology, Hospital St Louis, February 23, 1965, Paris, France

39. Wallace S, Jackson L, Dodd GD, Greening RR: Lymphatic dynamics in certain abnormal states. Am J Roentgenol 91:1187, 1964

CHAPTER THIRTEEN

TREATMENT OF MALIGNANT MELANOMA BY ENDOLYMPHATIC THERAPY

JOHN M. EDWARDS

ENDOLYMPHATIC RADIOISOTOPE THERAPY FOR MELANOMA

Endolymphatic therapy for tumors implies the direct application of therapeutic agents into lymph vessels to treat regional lymph nodes involved with malignant disease. Malignant disease affecting lymph nodes, including primary lymphomas and metastases from solid tumors, have been treated by this method. Particular attention has been directed towards the treatment of melanoma in view of the propensity of this tumor to spread via the lymphatic system.

The ability to demonstrate the lymphatics by the technique described in 1953 by Kinmonth[24] stimulated interest in the diagnostic aspects of lymphography and later to the application of treatment. In 1958 Jantet[22] treated a variety of tumors in lymph nodes by injecting radioactive colloidal gold, [198]Au, into the lymphatics, and later, in 1962, published some encouraging results for the treatment of melanoma.[23] These initial studies with the application of therapeutic substances into lymphatics were made with nonradiopaque substances.

The development of ultrafluid lipiodol (UFL) as a diagnostic agent for lymphography in 1962 enabled lymphatics and lymph nodes to be clearly outlined on radiography. This stimulated the development of therapeutic lymphography, where the combination of radioisotopes with UFL enabled treatment to be combined with a diagnostic view of the lymph node condition. This proved to be a more refined technique than just the therapeutic application of intralymphatic isotopes.

The first agent used in therapeutic lymphography was radioactive iodine, ^{131}I, mixed or bonded to lipiodol, most attention was paid to the treatment of melanoma[15,20] or to the treatment of lymphomas and testicular tumors.[9] Other preparations used for endolymphatic therapy have included radioactive ceramic microspheres, with most of the experimental and clinical work with this material having been developed by Ariel.[34] At the present time the most common agent used for therapeutic lymphography is ^{32}P lipiodol, this having been shown by experimental and clinical studies to be superior to the previous agents used.

RADIOACTIVE ISOTOPE PREPARATIONS USED IN ENDOLYMPHATIC THERAPY

Radioactive Gold ([198]Au). Some of the early studies on intralymphatic therapy were made in 1958 by Jantet[22] with preliminary observations on the use of endolymphatic [198]Au using the method described by Kinmonth[24,26] to achieve the direct application of the isotope to tumor-involved lymph nodes. He demonstrated that the radioisotope could be made to localize in the nodes and that radiobiological decay was slow. In subsequent studies he described clinical methods, particularly with reference to the treatment of patients suffering from melanoma.[23] This group of patients was treated by wide excision of the primary tumor followed by direct intralymphatic injection of radioactive gold to the regional lymph nodes. Following intralymphatic injection the sites of localization of [198]Au were found to be greatest at the regional node area, then the base of the neck and thoracic duct and the liver. Two-thirds of the total radioactivity was found at the first two sites and approximately one-third in the liver, but no correlation was made in the distribution studies with the volume of material injected, and the radioactive dose was also variable.

The physical properties of [198]Au revealed a short half-life of 2.7 days, with emission of β-particles of relatively low energy (mean energy 0.35 MeV) and some low-intensity gamma rays (Table 13–1). The material used was [198]Au in particulate form obtained from the Radiochemical Centre, Amersham, England. This preparation, which has been used in our experimental studies as well as in patients, was a colloidal suspension of metallic gold stabilized with gelatine and glucose (GLS 1 P).[13] The gold particle size in this preparation ranged up to 20 mμ with most of the activity associated with particles of diameter 10 to 13 mμ. This preparation aggregated on contact with tissue protein, developing particles ranging in size from 1 to 5 μ. Following endolymphatic infusion the gold particles were seen clubbed together in the regional nodes, distributed particularly to the regions of the marginal sinuses and hilar vessels. The gold was also distributed to other parts of the reticuloendothelial system and found more especially in Kupffer's cells of the liver. Little was excreted in the urine and feces.[27]

The conclusions of experimental trials on the VX2 tumor of rabbit, between radioactive [198]Au and radioactive ^{131}I lipiodol showed no real difference between the effect of the two products. Both were effective in the treatment of microscopic size metastases. The property of radiopacity of the iodine preparation and the potential danger of hepatic damage from radiogold made radioactive iodine the isotope of choice at that time.[27] This reflected our experience with the clinical application of endolymphatic radiogold. The margin of safety demanded by our present criteria made non-radiopaque products unacceptable for use and led to the discontinuance of radioactive gold treatment.

Radioactive Iodine [131]I Lipiodol. Chiappa was the earliest protagonist of labelled lipiodol, using Lipiodol F tagged with ^{131}I, in treating patients suffering from lymphoma.[8,9] Seitzman was also prominent in early work using ^{131}I labelled lipiodol.[33] The material used in our practice, however, was different to that used initially by Chiappa, as we used ^{131}I triolein, which was mixed with ultrafluid lipiodol.[20] This product was prepared at the Radiochemical Centre, Amersham, at our request. Chiappa in his later work used material similar to our own.

Triolein, in the method used at Amersham, was reacted with iodine monochloride ^{131}I, in a mixture of carbon tetrachloride and acetic acid. The quantity of iodine monochloride was sufficient to saturate about 30% of the double bonds present (as indicated by the iodine value). The iodinated triolein, which was perfectly miscible with ultrafluid lipiodol* was then allowed to dissolve in this material, lipiodol being also an oil, an iodinated poppy seed extract.

The stability of the iodine bond had been confirmed by Balint et al.[5] who found it stable at body temperature in the presence of a range of substances such as gastric juice, pepsin, pancreatin, and saline. A range of pH from 1 to 8 did not cause a breakdown of the iodine bond. Furthermore heating at 100°C for 15 minutes liberated only about 1% of the activity in water-soluble form and the addition of 10% HCl did not liberate iodine.

The quantity of ^{131}I lipiodol supplied for clinical work was:

30 to 35 mCi in 2 ml ultrafluid lipiodol (brachial)
40 to 45 mCi in 4 ml ultrafluid lipiodol (ilio-inguinal)

This dosage was calculated on the basis of experimental and clinical studies evaluating the histological effects of varying dosages.[20,21] The dose was gradually increased to the stated level when destruction of lymph nodes with

---

* Laboratories: A. Guerbet and Cie, 22 rue Landy, St. Ouen, Paris, France; and Mat and Baker, Dogenham, Essex, England.

TABLE 13-1. Physical Characteristics of Some Isotopes

Isotope	Half-life (Days)	Maximum Energy (MeV)	Maximum Range in Tissue (mm)	Kβ β-dose Factor (Rads/ μc.d/g)	Main Energy (MeV)
^{131}I	8.0	0.61	2	110	0.36
^{198}Au	2.7	0.96	4	66	0.41
^{32}P	14.3	1.71	8	730	—
^{90}Y	2.7	2.25	10	183	—

small metastases was noted with regularity.

The actual B-dose in rads was estimated by using β-particle dosimetry formula.[21] By direct measurements of radioactivity on excised nodes and confirming the uniform distribution of the isotope by the histological effect and autoradiographs, the use of this formula had shown the B-dose to reach 100,000 rads, with the dosage quoted for clinical use.[18]

Iodine-131 has a half-life of 8.04 days and is a mixed β and γ-emitter (see Table 13-1). The beta emission of ^{131}I supplies about 90% of the energy useful for therapeutic treatment, the accompanying γ-emission the remainder, and allows the distribution of the labelled product to be evaluated and mapped in the various organs and tissues.

The particle energies of the B-fraction is shown in Table 13-1. It can thus be seen that 0.61 MeV represents 81% of the β-particle and the maximum penetration as calculated in tissue as approximately 2 mm, with mean absorption occurring in the first 0.2 mm.

This range of effectiveness of the β-particle in some respects was advantageous, yet in others rather a disadvantage. The advantageous feature was that if homogeneous distribution was achieved in lymphoid tissue, then a uniform dose was given to the nodes. This had been studied by autoradiographs and the histological effects noted. As the material was confined to this tissue its relatively small range in depth meant that a massive dose was confined to lymphoid tissue. However, it was essential when using this radioisotope that homogeneous distribution be achieved, and this could occur only if the nodes were involved with microscopic-sized metastases. In the primary lymphomas, however, the nodes, though heavily involved, could still be effectively irradiated using this isotope (Fig. 13-1).

Radioactive Phosphorus (^{32}P Lipiodol) (Code PB. 128P). This preparation is sterile oil consisting of a 10% solution tri-n-octyl phosphate (^{32}P) dissolved in ultrafluid lipiodol. Apart from the radioactive component, the physical properties of the preparation are similar to ^{131}I lipiodol. It was initially used in experimental work at London's St. Thomas's Hospital in 1965 and the first patient treated in 1966. The radioactive concentration of the preparation produced by the Radiochemical Centre is 2 mCi/ml and the specific activity 30 to 250 mCi/g octyl phosphate.

The following is the dosage used: For brachial infusion approximately 3 to 4 mCi in 2 ml lipiodol U.F. and for ilio-inguinal infusion 6 to 7 mCi in up to 4 ml lipiodol U.F. ^{32}P is a pure β-emitter. The maximum β energy of ^{32}P is 1.71 MeV with a half-life of 14.3 days. The KB factor used in calculating dosage in rads is 730 rads/uc.d/g (Table 13-1).

Some data on radiation dosage to patients and results of excretion studies may be summarized as follows. They are calculated on the basis of a 6 mCi ^{32}P lipiodol injection to the ilio-inguinal lymph nodes on 50 patients treated with ilio-inguinal infusions.[12]

The average daily urinary excretion of ^{32}P equals 0.3% of administered dose giving a biological half-life of 200 days and effective half-life of 14 days.

A blood content of 0.02 to 0.04%/liter, gives a dose of 2 r to blood and is therefore negligible dose to bone marrow.

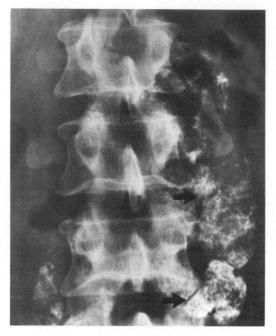 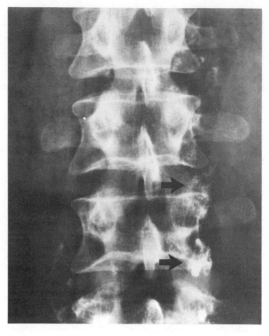

FIGURE 13–1. Lymphoma involving para-aortic lymph nodes treated with ^{131}I lipiodol. Initial ap- **pearance and appearance three months later as denoted by arrows.**

A sample of lymph node dose of 1 mCi in a node of weight 1 with uniform distribution gives β-dose of 730,000 r.

Whole body dose is very small if the area of treated lymphatics or lymph nodes is excluded.

For special organs such as the lungs, the dosage depends to a large extent on the volume of lipiodol injected. This quantity must be monitored carefully and quantities less than 4 ml of ^{32}P lipiodol were given. The lung dosage was usually less than 5% as estimated by scanning studies. With lung dosage of 5% of the administered dose, the B dose would be 200 r to total decay.

No appreciable increase of activity was shown by scanning other organs. Less than 1% of the β energy is converted to *bremsstrahlung*, therefore the γ dose is negligible.

Hb and WBC counts were made on subsequent days while on in-patient and also on out-patient attendances. There was no deviation from the accepted normal range that could be attributed to the effects of ^{32}P lipiodol

in some 50 patients treated and followed up in this way.

The clinical advantages of ^{32}P lipiodol as compared with ^{131}I lipiodol are:

1. Increased maximum penetration of B-particle as compared with ^{131}I (8 mm compared with 2 mm).

2. Pure β-emitter. Safer to handle, with regard to personnel in theater.

3. Increased half-life of 14 days as compared with eight days for radioiodine.

Due to the increased metabolic turnover of lipiodol in the lungs as opposed to the lymph nodes there would be less β-radiation dosage to those organs than with the use of radioiodine.

The major clinical disadvantage is that it is more difficult to scan patients with external scanning devices. Some of the absorbed β-energy of ^{32}P is reradiated as *bremsstrahlung*. This can be detected by external scanning but not as readily as the γ-fraction of radioiodine.

There were obvious theoretical advantages

for the use of ^{32}P lipiodol in clinical practice but before finally adopting this agent a controlled trial on the experimental animal comparing ^{32}P lipiodol and ^{131}I lipiodol was made.[28] The pattern of the experiments was similar to those previously performed for ^{131}I lipiodol.[18,20] The result of the trial showed that both ^{32}P lipiodol and ^{131}I lipiodol were highly successful in treating lymph nodes involved with small metastases. In addition, ^{32}P was marginally more effective with larger metastases lymph nodes and gave a longer survival rate than ^{131}I in the animals treated.

The greater energy potential of ^{32}P lipiodol and the histological effects on nodes excised in clinical studies, together with the factors already mentioned, made this isotope our present choice.

Radioactive Yttrium (^{90}Y). The physical properties of this isotope are given in Table 13–1. In some ways it seemed an ideal agent to use for endolymphatic therapy because it had a greater energy and range than the other isotopes used. Experimental work was performed by Morrison and Young in 1968 using colloidal suspensions of fatty acids and salts of Yttrium in combination with lipiodol for endolymphatic therapy (unpublished data). This material can be combined with lipiodol and could be brought into clinical use. However, for our animal experiments and initial trials with Yttrium, colloidal suspensions have been used. With these materials there were no complications, although the histological study of lymph nodes excised after treatment has shown a marked destructive effect which seemed even more intense than other isotopes. The use of Yttrium in clinical practice, however, has not been actively pursued, partly due to the fact that preparations of ^{32}P were more readily available from the Radiochemical Centre at Amersham and also because of the decision to give this latter preparation a more prolonged trial before considering using another isotope such as Yttrium.

Other radioactive preparations that have been used for endolymphatic therapy include ^{90}Yttrium tagged ceramic microspheres or plastic microspheres. These preparations were recommended in 1964 by Ariel et al.[4] for intra-lymphatic use and have also been used by the intra-arterial route. The microsphere size for intralymphatic use measured one to four micron diameter and to these particles were absorbed radioactive isotopes such as ^{90}Yttrium. The initial results using this agent were promising, but difficulty was encountered in that the microspheres tended to adhere to each other, causing blockage of the cannulating needle during the administration of therapy.

THE TECHNIQUE OF LYMPHOGRAPHY

Lymphography technique for malignant melanoma has to be varied according to the site of the primary lesion, but the basic technique is similar to that for diagnostic lymphography, except that certain modifications were made for safety reasons when using radioactive materials. The aim was to ensure adequate filling of regional nodes likely to be involved with metastatic disease without undue spillover of radioactive material to the lung fields via the thoracic duct or other lymphovenous connections. In the treatment of melanoma lymph node metastases, whenever possible, injection of the radioisotope combination is made just proximal to the excisional area of the primary lesion in order to give therapy to the relevant lymphatic vessels and nodes. Occasionally infusion of the isotope is made from two sites. The infusion of the radioactive material is made slowly, approximately 1 ml every 10 minutes, and the course of the infusion is monitored carefully by radiography.

Early radiography of the limb and regional node areas is essential after injecting a small volume of material in order to ensure satisfactory cannulation of the lymph vessels.

When the radioactive material has filled the proximal group of lymph nodes adequately, with filling also of the efferent lymphatics, then the injection is stopped.[14]

Endolymphatic therapy is particularly relevant to the treatment of stage I and stage II melanoma.

The clinical staging of malignant melanoma used in this discussion is as described below:

Stage I—Primary melanoma (regional lymph nodes not involved)
Stage II—Regional lymph nodes involved
Stage III—Skin satellites that could not be encompassed in primary excision
Stage IV—Distant metastases

Endolymphatic Therapy in Clinical Stage I Melanoma. Therapeutic lymphography is applied two to three weeks after excision of the primary. There are several reasons for this delay: (1) to be sure that the lesion excised proves to be invasive malignant melanoma on histological analysis, (2) to provide time to procure the isotope preparation from the Radiochemical Centre, and (3) to provide an interval for possible tumor metastases in transit to arrive at the regional nodes. This is an idea promulgated by Petersen et al.[32] and by other workers.

The technique of therapeutic lymphography for stage I melanoma is that already described.

Radiographs are taken during and at the end of the infusion. This lymphographic examination is useful mainly in ensuring correct cannulation of lymphatics and also so that the correct volume of radioactive material is administered.

The radiographs taken 24 hours later of the regional area (lymphadenograms) reveal the outline of the lymph nodes filled with radioactive contrast material. These studies are in three planes and enable an assessment to be made regarding metastases. This assessment is more accurate than clinical examination and in certain patients further treatment in the nature of a surgical block dissection has been performed based on the results of these studies (Fig. 13–2).

Should lymphadenograms confirm the clinical impression that there are no large metastases in the nodes, then further treatment is unnecessary.

After scanning the patient on the second postoperative day, the remaining period of five days in hospital is in order to conform to safety precautions with regard to patients receiving radioactive substances. Urine specimens are estimated for radioactive content and blood samples examined with regard to the leucocyte counts.

Subsequently patients attend a special follow-up clinic, when reassessment of the lymph node areas is made on the basis of clinical and radiological examination. The radioactive lipiodol often remains visible and diagnostically significant for periods up to six months, and while it is present further lymphadenogram assessment can be made. Should nodes subsequently become enlarged and show filling defects, then they are excised. Suspicious nodes on the initial lymphadenograms are examined particularly carefully in subsequent radiographs.

Clinical Stage II Melanoma. It is universally recognized that this group of patients presents an infinitely more serious problem than the stage I group, and the prognosis is correspondingly bad by all conventional methods of treatment.

The treatment has been the same as for stage I patients with the addition of block dissection of regional nodes about four to six weeks after the intralymphatic injection, depending on the isotope used, when the isotope has had time to decay to a safe level. The operation is not much more difficult after endolymphatic therapy unless more than six weeks has been allowed to elapse.

Surgical excision of nodes is necessary in this group of patients as the isotope combinations used to date lack the penetration depth of treatment to enable stage II disease to be eradicated. These metastases often measure 10 mm or more in diameter and commonly present as central filling defects in the nodes (Fig. 13–3). The clinical assessment is consequently confirmed by the radiological examination. The addition of endolymphatic therapy to surgery enables more complete treatment and assessment for stage II disease.

RESULTS

There are two large series of patients with results available for analysis. The first series is that treated at St. Thomas's Hospital. The sec-

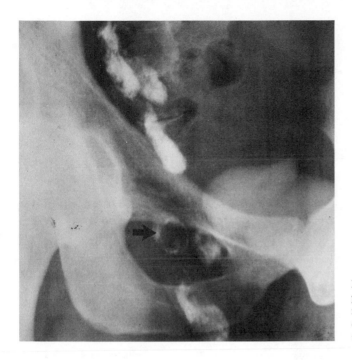

FIGURE 13-2. Occult secondary deposit in deep inguinal lymph node as revealed by lymphadenogram. Block dissection performed as deposit too large to be treated by endolymphatic therapy.

ond is that appertaining to the Medical Research Council trial in Great Britain on endolymphatic therapy for melanoma.

St. Thomas's Hospital Results. The five-year survival rate in a series of 221 patients for stage I disease using a variety of isotopes is 78%. For stage II disease the five-year survival rate is 21% (see Table 13-2). In analyzing the latter group, however, the poor results for stage II patients is really to be expected, as some of these individuals had already been confirmed elsewhere as stage II disease by means of lymph node biopsy. Prognosis for this group of patients is already dismal, but the node biopsy is an additional negative factor.

Lymph node assessment by surgery can be avoided by the diagnostic use of endolymphatic therapy. Should surgical excision be necessary then a full block dissection is performed. Despite adequate eradication of local disease in this group, death often occurred as a result of disseminated disease. It seems obvious in retrospect that disease was already widespread at the time of the initial treatment. However, surgery is still indicated if the

normal methods of investigation, such as body scanning and radiography, fail to reveal disseminated disease. Occasionally long-term survivals occur in the most unpromising clinical situations.[30] However, it must be assumed at present that stage II disease is in many instances a general problem and the main function of endolymphatic therapy and surgery is to remove gross local disease, produce a palliative effect and reduce the total tumor mass.

M.R.C. (Medical Research Council) U.K. Trial for Melanoma. This trial was concerned with the comparison of two methods of management in patients with stage I melanoma of the lower limb: excision of the primary tumor followed by endolymphatic therapy to the regional nodes (ELT group), and excision of the primary tumor followed by other treatment not involving endolymphatic therapy, such as immediate or delayed block dissection (standard group) according to the discretion of the clinician responsible.

Over a ten-year period a group of 146 patients was entered into this trial. Although total results were not significantly affected by

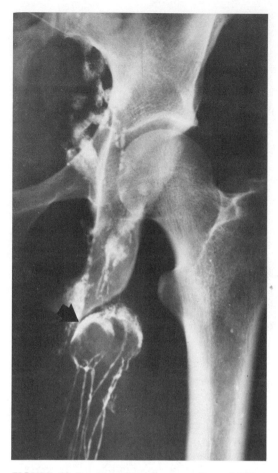

FIGURE 13-3. Stage II melanoma. Central filling deposits in inguinal nodes due to tumor. Surgical block dissection performed as metastases too large for treatment by endolymphatic therapy.

TABLE 13-2. Melanoma all Sites. Treated by Surgery and Endolymphatic Isotope Therapy

Period	Total no. of patients	Survival	Deaths
1–18 yrs	251	174*	77
5–18 yrs	172	Survival rate stage I 78% Survival rate stage II 21%	

* Crude survival rate 1–18 years = 69.32% (Stage I and stage II).

endolymphatic therapy, recurrence in the lymph nodes was largely prevented. More patients in the standard group needed the more major procedure of block dissection, which was done either as a primary procedure or subsequently on lymph node enlargement. The actuarial percentage recurrence rates and survival rates at yearly intervals from 1 to 5 years are shown for standard and endolymphatic therapy in the Table 13-3. Corresponding survival curves are shown in Figure 13-4. Comparison of the recurrence-free and survival occurrence of the two therapies, using the Log rank test, indicated no significant difference between them (P = 0.67 and P = 1.43 respectively).

TABLE 13-3. Medical Research Council Trial. Five-Year Follow-Up

	No.	5-Year Recurrence Free (%)	5-Year Survival (%)
Standard (S)	72	67.7	82.3
Endolymphatic Satisfactory (ES)	42	70.2	78.8
Endolymphatic Unsatisfactory (EU)	32	49.0	57.3

This trial was a multiple center trial; unfortunately at several centers difficulty was encountered in applying the technique of endolymphatic therapy and there was a significant failure rate with regard to this technique. Consequently in the group allocated endolymphatic therapy, there was a large subgroup that did not in fact receive treatment. The group of patients that received endolymphatic therapy on a satisfactory basis, however, did better than the standard method group. Another important factor in the satisfactory endolymphatic therapy group was that the lymph node metastases were markedly reduced as opposed to the standard therapy group (see Table 13-4). It was concluded that the technique, to be ap-

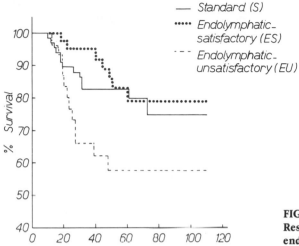

Legend:
— Standard (S)
•••• Endolymphatic_
satisfactory (ES)
--- Endolymphatic_
unsatisfactory (EU)

FIGURE 13-4. Comparison death rates. Medical Research Council Trial. At ten years the results of endolymphatic therapy are better than other methods.

plied successfully, should be done only in the specialized centers, and the results of treatment in these justified the continued use of endolymphatic therapy.

DISCUSSION

The conclusions drawn from the interim results of the M.R.C. trial are described below in terms of survival, recurrence, and pathology.

Stage I melanomas of the lower limb, when the primary lesion has been satisfactorily treated, carry a better prognosis than previous

surveys had indicated. The actuarial percentage survival at five years of 82.3% for the standard group and 78.8% for the endolymphatic group indicates that with early effective primary treatment the outlook is good. It is of note that the crude survival rates over 15 years in the St. Thomas's Hospital series is 87% for stage I and 41% for stage II.[16] In terms of crude survival these figures are significantly better than the standard group in the M.R.C. trial.

The fact that only one patient in the endolymphatic satisfactory group had regional lymph node recurrence illustrates that radioactive isotope endolymphatic therapy destroys microscopic tumor deposits. The pattern of recurrence in the endolymphatic satisfactory group was of skin secondaries occurring in the same limb as the primary. This is of interest in that Veronesi[34] noted in a series of 192 regional lymph node block dissections that 20 cases (10.4%) had these so-called in-transit metastases in the skin of the same limb as the primary. The endolymphatic satisfactory group had a figure of 16% for these in-transit metastases, which is comparable to the group above (see Table 13-4). A probable explanation for this is that neoplastic cells are locked in the limb when the lymphatic pathways are destroyed either by surgery or endolymphatic

TABLE 13-4. Medical Research Council Trial. Failure of Treatment

	Patients		
	No.	Nodal Recurrence	Skin Recurrence
Standard (S)	69	13 (19%)	4 (6%)
Endolymphatic Satisfactory (ES)	48	1 (2.3%)	7 (16%)
Endolymphatic Unsatis-factory (EU)	25	3 (12%)	8 (32%)

therapy. The latter destroys tumor deposits in the lymph nodes, which then undergo fibrosis, and results in partial lymphatic blockage. This fact is borne out by mild lymphoedema of the affected limb that can occur after endolymphatic isotope therapy, although this is usually less severe than after surgical block dissection. Repeat lymphography has been performed on a few cases some years after endolymphatic isotope therapy, and usually shows a mild obstructive lymphoedema pattern.

A major factor that could influence the results of the trial is the pathology of the primary lesion. Unfortunately, the start of the M.R.C. trial predated the newer pathological staging of Clark,[10] with reference to the depth of dermal penetration of the primary tumor. The findings of Breslow[7] indicated that the maximum thickness of the primary lesion when fixed in preservative, together with the histological depth of the dermal penetration, gave an accurate assessment of prognosis. A more detailed pathological survey of the primary lesion is clearly indicated and will be presented in the final analysis of the trial.

The diagnostic accuracy of lymphography in assessing regional lymph node metastases has been questioned. Cox et al.[11] performed a detailed survey of 17 patients with malignant melanoma who had lymphography followed by a block dissection. The x-ray and pathological findings were closely correlated. They concluded that lymphograms were of no help in determining the presence of lymph node metastases, as they described false positive and false negative x-ray findings. However, they studied a relatively small number of cases and only 24-hour lymphadenograms were performed. Lipiodol remains in the lymph nodes for up to six months following either lymphography or endolymphatic therapy. The routine at St. Thomas's is to perform 24-hour, 48-hour, two-week, and four-week lymphadenograms before finally deciding on metastatic involvement of nodes in conjunction with the clinical findings. With nearly 20 years of experience considerable expertise has been achieved in assessing the x-rays, and by close correlation with the clinical findings, the diagnosis of metastases can be made with accuracy.

Other centers that have used endolymphatic radiotherapy[2,29,35] have concluded that the technique of endolymphatic isotopes is of benefit in stage I cases of malignant melanoma. In combination with a block dissection in stage II performed six weeks after the lymphogram it is also of benefit. However, the concensus is that this technique should be employed at specialized centers where it can be performed satisfactorily. The fact that the M.R.C. unsatisfactory group did relatively badly was partly due to incorrect staging and an inadequate dosage of isotope. The last point illustrates a potential hazard of this technique as one could speculate that inadequate dosage of isotope may incompletely destroy tumor and in so doing may cause some tumor enhancement.

The advantage of ^{32}P endolymphatic therapy may be summarized as follows:

1. Diagnostic. A more accurate assessment of regional lymph nodes is possible than by clinical means alone.

2. Therapeutic. In stage I cases it prevents a block dissection by destroying microscopical lymph node metastases. The technique is minimally invasive and the patients suffer very little in the way of side effects. The time spent in hospital is short, four to five days. This compares favorably with the surgical trauma and morbidity sustained by a block dissection.

With stage II melanoma the therapy extends the limit of the block dissection by irradiating lymph nodes that cannot be removed. It reduces the number of viable cells implanted during surgery. The completeness of the block dissection can be checked by an operative x-ray.

The disadvantages are that it is an intricate technique and the injections cannot always be ideally situated. Larger deposits of tumor, which disrupt the flow of lymph through affected nodes, are not destroyed by endolymphatic isotopes. Theoretically by destroying lymph tissue the immune response may be adversely affected.

EXPERIMENTAL AND CLINICAL STUDIES USING ENDOLYMPHATIC BCG

Further work has been done in recent years using and studying the effects of bacterial agents when administered by the intralymphatic route. Some stimulus to this study was prompted by the work of Morton, who showed that intranodal injection of BCG could produce regression of melanoma metastases, and also by reported work where BCG has been used for its immunomodulator effect on the reticuloendothelial system. Consequently it seemed a logical if rather simplistic step to apply BCG directly into lymph nodes involved with malignant disease, both to achieve a direct action on the affected nodes and also possibly to stimulate the endothelial system.

EXPERIMENTAL STUDIES

A series of experiments was embarked on using an experimental tumor, the VX2 tumor in the host animal, the rabbit. The objective was to study the effect of BCG when ad-

ministered directly to the lymphatic system and to study the effect on metastases in the regional lymph nodes from the VX2 tumor.

The plan of the experiment was to inoculate a series of rabbits with VX2 tumor suspension into the right quadriceps femoris muscle (Fig. 13–5). After an interval of 11 days in order to ensure a take of the tumor and also spread to the regional lymph nodes, the primary tumor was widely excised and the wound reconstituted. The rabbits were then randomized into three groups.

One group of 15 rabbits received a dose of 300 μg of lyophilized BCG suspension (Glaxo) directly into the popliteal afferent lymphatics to the regional iliac nodes. In each animal the dose of BCG was followed by the infusion of 0.5 ml UFL (group BCG).

Another group (N = 15), after excision of the primary tumor, received 300 μg of BCG intracutaneously, also 0.5 ml U.F.L. by the lymphatic route, again to opacify the iliac nodes on x-ray in each rabbit (group BCG–X).

The third group (N–15) was given 0.5 ml of lipiodol only via the lymphatics and served as the control group (C).

In all the groups the common denominator

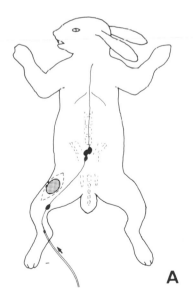 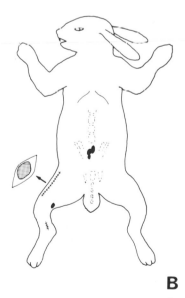

A   **B**

FIGURE 13–5A and B.   Tumor excised right thigh muscle with infusion BCG + Ultrafluid (Group BCG), intracutaneous BCG + Ultrafluid (Group BCG–X), and Ultrafluid only (control group).

was that the iliac nodes were made radiopaque so that the node appearances could be subsequently studied by taking x-rays (so-called lymphadenograms) at appropriate intervals.

The results of the experiments were assessed as follows:

1. Study of serial lymphadenograms
2. Survival rates
3. Histology

(Recurrence of tumor at the primary site excluded the animal from the experiment).

Serial Lymphadenograms. Typical appearances of the lymph nodes in the three groups are depicted as follows:

The control group received ultrafluid lipiodol alone. The typical initial appearance of the lymph nodes showed an enlargement from the normal due to combination of tumor involvement and sinus hyperplasia. Subsequent lymphadenograms revealed a gradual progressive increase in the size of the nodes due to tumor progression (Fig. 13-6).

In the intralymphatic BCG and ultrafluid lipiodol group there was a different pattern of lymphadenogram sequence. The initial appearance was as in the control group with lymph node enlargement. These nodes subsequently showed further enlargement to a peak of 28 days but then began to shrink in size, becoming less than the original size by 71 days (Fig. 13-7).

The intracutaneous BCG group showed essentially similar appearances to the control group but with a slower growth of tumor. Some animals in this group, however, followed the intralymphatic BCG pattern with initial growth followed by gradual decrease in size of the nodes.

The lymphadenograms of the three groups can be summarized in chart form as shown in Figure 13-8. The percent change in lymph node area is depicted, the area on the day of tumor excision being taken as 100%.

Survival Rate. In early work it was found that most animals, following the implantation of VX2 tumor into muscle died between 56 and 70 days.

The survival rate for the three groups in the trial is summarized in Figure 13-9.

In Group C given ultrafluid lipiodol alone the mean survival time was 57 ± 32 days.

For group BCG-X given intracutaneous BCG the survival time was essentially similar, 62 ± 25 days.

Group BCG given intralymphatic BCG fared much better with most of the animals surviving beyond 120 days, in fact cured of tumor. These animals were subject to autopsy after this time and found to be free of tumor.

A few animals $(N = 2)$ that died in the intralymphatic BCG group were found to have died from the effects of lung metastases and also had evidence of viable tumor in the iliac nodes, as was supported from the lymphadenogram appearances in these animals.

Histology. Animals that died during the course of the study and also those sacrificed for histology requirements were subjected to detailed autopsy. In particular the lymph node appearances, both macroscopic and microscopic, were studied in the three groups. The appearance and histology of the lungs was also reviewed as this was one of the common locations for metastases with the VX2 tumor. The following are the results for the different groups:

1. Control Group. Rabbits that died or had to be killed in the control group C all had tumor-involved iliac lymph nodes. The nodes reached massive proportions and often obstructed the bladder. Some tumor nodes spontaneously eroded blood vessels or ruptured, causing hemoperitoneum. In 80% of these animals the lungs were heavily involved with tumor.

2. BCG-X Group. The intracutaneous group showed similar histological appearances to the animals that died of the VX2 tumor in the control group.

3. BCG Group. The intralymphatic BCG group were deliberately sacrificed for histological study in the large majority revealed small iliac lymph nodes. These nodes were macro-

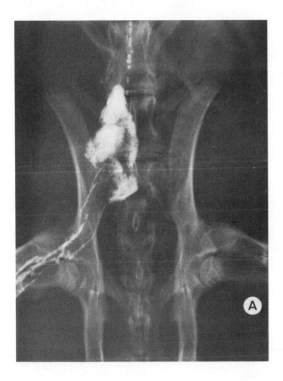

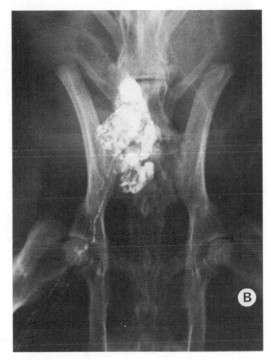

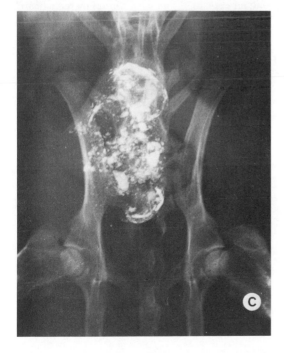

FIGURE 13–6A, B, and C.   Control group. Serial radiographs. Two-week intervals. Progressive increase in size nodes due to growth of tumor.

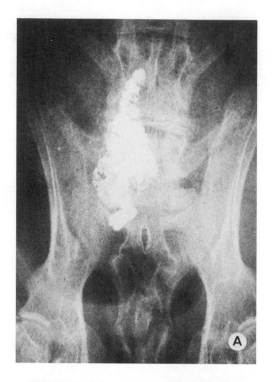

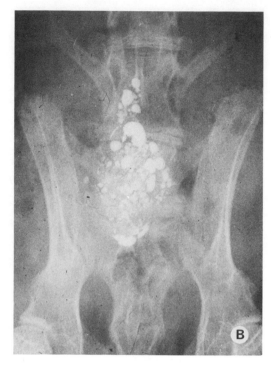

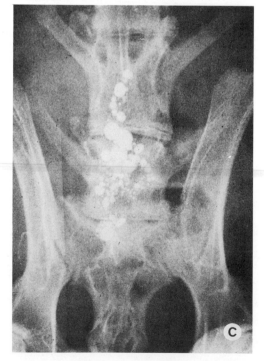

FIGURE 13-7. VX2/BCG group (A and B), and Intralymphatic BCG group (C). Initial increase in size node followed by shrinkage. Sequence of radiographs over period of 145 days.

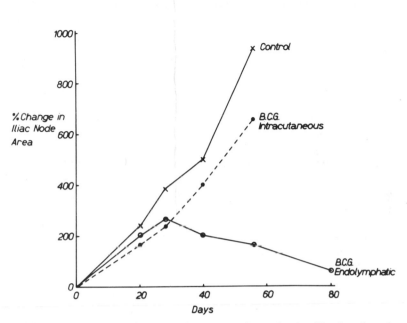

FIGURE 13-8.   Rabbit BCG/VX2. Percentage change in size iliac lymph nodes.

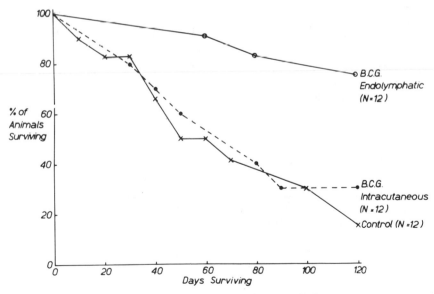

FIGURE 13-9.   Rabbit BCG/VX2. Survival rates.

scopically and microscopically free of tumor. There was also no sign of tumor elsewhere, including the lungs.

Two animals, however, in this group did succumb to VX2 tumor with lung metastases and viable lymph node metastases.

Parallel histological studies have been made of the effects of BCG with sacrifice of animals at different times. In the early stages there is influx of macrophages and giant cells of Langhan's type, as well as polymorphonuclear leucocyte infiltration. Later a very high concentration of eosinophils and granulomata were noted. The tumor necrosis was deduced to be related to the effects of the influx of these cells to the lymph nodes and the chronic inflammatory response provoked by BCG.

The conclusions drawn from the experimental BCG, VX2 study were as follows:

BCG was effective in destroying microscopic sized metastases of the VX2 tumor in lymph nodes.

The route of administration was important, the BCG being much more effective when given directly into the lymphatics.

The effect of BCG appeared mainly mediated by chronic inflammatory response.

Further work on the administration of BCG via the intravenous route had no effect on the survival rate of the rabbits, which corresponded with the survival rate as seen in the control group.

CLINICAL STUDIES WITH BCG— PATIENTS AND METHODS

We have progressed from our animal experiments to applying BCG to patients. We have subsequently given BCG directly by intralymphatic injection.

The clinical experience gained using endolymphatic radioactive isotopes indicated that larger deposits of tumor in lymph nodes were not completely destroyed. The treatment was of limited benefit in cases of advanced stage II or III malignant melanoma. It was decided on the basis of the animal experimen-

tal work referred to in this chapter that the poor prognosis cases might benefit from endolymphatic BCG. Indeed some cases that have received this treatment have had recurrent disease.

Patients with untreated primary lesions had conventional wide excision with a 5 cm margin and skin grafting performed. Prior to receiving the endolymphatic BCG the patients were carefully screened. A full clinical examination, urinalysis, urinary melanin estimation, full blood count and ESR, liver function tests, liver and bone isotope scans, Mantoux time skin test and DNCB* skin tests were performed.

Endolymphatic BCG was given two to four weeks following primary excision or soon after admission if recurrent disease was present. Where extensive skin recurrences were present intralesional BCG was given, as described by Morton[31] as well as endolymphatic infusion. The technique of lymphography was the same as for isotopes. Care was taken to protect the staff from contamination with BCG. To 150 μg of standard intradermal BCG (Glaxo), 2 ml of lipiodol for each brachial infusion and 4 ml of lipiodol for each leg infusion were mixed. Operative x-rays were taken to ensure that enough lipiodol was infused so that the regional nodes were just filled and that no extravasation occurred. At the end of the infusion plain lipiodol 0.5 to 1.0 ml was flushed into the lymphatic to prevent any local reaction. The wound was irrigated with saline and sutured.

Serial lymphadenograms were performed postoperatively. Block dissection of regional nodes was carried out four to six weeks after the infusion where indicated. Further intralesional BCG injections have been given where indicated.

Three brief case reports are described as they illustrate many of the aspects of endolymphatic BCG therapy.

Case 1. Mrs. M.C., date of birth Oct. 3, 1911 This patient was referred to St. Thomas's Hospital with an 18-month history of a brown

* 1-chloro-2, 4-dinitrobenzene

lesion on her right hallux. It had been treated as a fungal infection unsuccessfully until a biopsy had been performed. On admission she had a fungating subungual malignant melanoma of the right hallux with large, clinically metastatic, right inguinal glands (Figs. 13–10A and B). Routine screening revealed no further spread of the disease and a transmetatarsal amputation of the right great hallux was performed. Under the same anesthetic 150 μg of BCG was administered endolymphatically via her right foot. X-rays confirmed extensive involvement of the right inguinal nodes. The patient became febrile and complained of tender groin lymph nodes. One month later a right inguinal and external iliac block dissection was carried out. Histology showed one lymph node with metastatic tumor while all the other lymph nodes had tuberculoid granulomas present. Apart from mild lymphoedema of the right leg the patient has remained well and disease-free.

Case 2. Mr. P.B., date of birth Oct. 8, 1924
A pigmented lesion was removed from his left thigh during a right inguinal hernia repair in 1972. Histologically the lesion was reported as a compound nevus. In 1974 the patient had a severe myocardial infarct and survived a cardiac arrest. He presented in February 1976 with a lump in the left groin, which was biopsied and proved to be a node involved with metastatic melanoma. The histology of the original lesion was reviewed and the diagnosis changed to a malignant melanoma. He was referred to St. Thomas's where no further spread of the disease was detected. He was given endolymphatic BCG, 150 μg to each leg. The plan was to perform a full left inguinal block dissection because the x-rays suggested further disease. However, the anaesthetic risk was considered too great for this to be carried out. Three months following the therapy he developed discharging sinuses in both groins. The discharge was cultured but no growth of tubercle obtained. A groin node was biopsied six months after the endolymphatic BCG. The histology showed the node was full of caseating granulomata. By nine months the sinuses had dried up and healed. Since February 1977

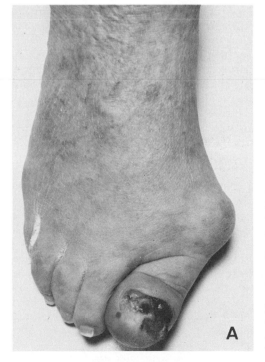

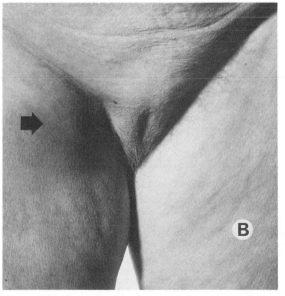

FIGURE 13–10A. Mrs. M.C. Subungual melanoma. Clinical stage II with inguinal node metastases. B. Mrs. M.C. Larger metastatic inguinal lymph nodes denoted with arrow.

the patient has remained reasonably well with no evidence of melanoma recurrence.

Case 3. Mr. G.G., date of birth Sept. 23, 1919
This patient had a malignant melanoma excised and grafted in 1969, he having noticed a mole enlarging on his left ankle for four years. He had a left inguinal block dissection performed in 1970 for metastatic lymph nodes. By 1973 he had developed metastatic skin nodes at his left knee, which were excised and grafted. However, further left leg skin recurrences appeared in 1974. A plain lymphogram was performed at St. Thomas's (Fig. 13–11), which revealed evidence of a previous left groin dissection and collaterals in his scrotum (arrowed). He subsequently developed metastases in this area of his scrotum. He had intralesional BCG and diathermy to the skin metastases, which regressed but only to flare up again in March 1975. This time he had bilateral pedal endolymphatic BCG as well as further intralesional BCG and diathermy. He had a marked reaction in his lymph nodes. The disease regressed satisfactorily until February 1976, including the scrotal lesions, which have not recurred. However, further BCG was administered endolymphatically to his right leg early in 1976. Since then his disease has been controlled by intralesional BCG, diathermy, and DTIC chemotherapy.

RESULTS

The results of giving endolymphatic BCG to cases of advanced malignant melanoma have been ascertained by the following means:

Clinical observations and examination
Routine hematology and biochemical screening tests
Serial lymphadenogram x-rays
Histological analysis of the block dissection specimens
Regular follow-up of patients who have received endolymphatic BCG

The reaction of the patient can be divided into a systemic reaction and a local reaction.

Systemic Reaction. All cases have experienced a postoperative pyrexia of the order of 37.5C to 38C usually for 24 to 72 hours postoperatively. Malaise, sometimes nausea, and vomiting usually coincide with the fever that was experienced. No significant changes were noticed in the differential WBC, hemoglobin, liver function tests, urea, or electrolyte estimation postoperatively.

Local Reaction. The regional lymph nodes became painful and tender to touch some 72 hours later. This effect lasted up to 10 days in some cases. Case 2 was the only patient whose lymph nodes broke down, discharging caseous material. One case developed a severe granulomatous ulcer at the injection site. It has been our practice to cleanse this wound carefully and to flush the BCG/lipiodol mixture as explained earlier in this chapter to prevent this occurrence.

X-Ray Appearances. As mentioned in the experimental work, an initial increase in size of the rabbit iliac lymph node followed by a regression was noticed. Figures 13–12A and B depict a case at the time of lymphogram and two weeks later showing the increase in size of the inguinal nodes (arrowed).

We have also noticed that the BCG/lipiodol mixture has been cleared from the lymph nodes at a faster rate than in patients who have received plain lipiodol and ^{32}P lipiodol.

Histology. The effect of BCG on lymph nodes in the patients who have had block dissections can be summarized as follows:

1. Nodes with large deposits often not seen on lymphograms are largely unaffected.
2. Nodes with lesser deposits show necrotic melanoma cells with caseating granulomas.
3. In nodes apparently without deposits, the histology shows caseating granulomas with an intense chronic inflammatory response. One must speculate that some of these nodes contained smaller tumor deposits that have been destroyed by the chronic inflammatory response.

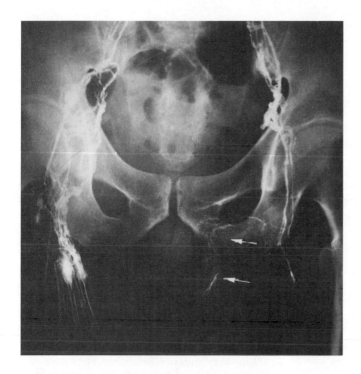

FIGURE 13-11.   Mr. G.G. Melanoma
left leg. Previous surgical block dissection left inguinal. Collateral pathways
in scrotum shown (by arrows).

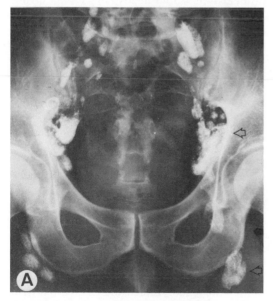

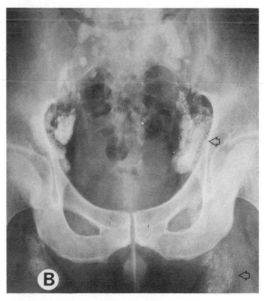

FIGURE 13-12 A.   Mr. C.W. BCG endolymphatic
to ilio-inguinal nodes. Enlarged nodes as denoted
with arrows. B. Mr. C.W. BCG endolymphatic to
ilio-inguinal nodes. Lymph nodes enlarge due to
chronic inflammatory changes.

4. Ziehl-Nielsen stains have been performed but no BCG organisms have been seen in human sections, whereas they were detected in the intralymphatic BCG group of rabbits.

Follow-up. Nineteen patients have received endolymphatic BCG over a three-and-a-half year period. Of the cases that died, three were males with trunk melanomas and the other a female with a very advanced disease. Of the surviving cases all but three are disease-free, see Table 13-5, the mean follow-up time for the 11 disease-free patients is ten months.

TABLE 13-5.   **Endolymphatic BCG**

	Patients	Mean Follow-up
Total number	19*	
Disease-free	11	10 months
Recurrent skin tumor	3	22 months
Died	4	9 months
		(mean survival)

* One patient lost to follow-up.

Complications. Apart from the effects already mentioned under the general and local reactions the complications have been few. One patient developed a granulomatous ulcer at the injection site. This occurrence has been prevented as the BCG lipiodol mixture has been flushed through the lymphatic by a small volume of lipiodol. Also the wound has been carefully cleaned with antiseptic solutions. No patient has ever contracted systemic tuberculosis of granulomatous hepatitis.

DISCUSSION

The results of the Rabbit VX2 tumor experiments using endolymphatic BCG showed that:

1. BCG was effective in destroying microscopic metastases of VX2 tumor in lymph nodes.

2. The route of administration is important as BCG has a much greater effect when given by direct intralymphatic injection.

3. The effect of the BCG was to destroy tumor cells by an intense inflammatory response.

As mentioned above the pathological staging is now a more accurate guide to prognosis so that after the primary melanoma has been excised, the clinician can make a reasoned judgment as to the further treatment required. Indeed Barclay[6] suggests that by using the prognostic index, poor-risk cases with a high prognostic index should be considered for adjuvant therapy.

Our clinical experience with endolymphatic BCG has been with such poor-risk cases. Any interpretation of our results must be anecdotal in that there are no controls to compare with the endolymphatic BCG. However, by using the prognostic index the cases described have been doing extremely well.

From the evidence presented above we can say that endolymphatic BCG causes necrosis of metastatic tumor deposits in lymph nodes. The intense inflammatory response destroys the lymph node tumor metastases where they are small enough to allow the BCG/lipiodol mixture to come into contact with them. The increase in size of the lymph nodes on x-ray and the increased rate of clearance of the lipiodol can be explained by the ensuing inflammation. No systemic nonspecific immunological stimulation has been observed. The local effect on the lymph node is presumably the so-called bystander effect, where an inflammatory response destroys the tumor cells as they are caught in this destructive inflammatory process.

At present endolymphatic BCG can be given in the hope of eradicating advanced local disease in conjunction with surgery and as in Case 3, as a method of palliation when combined with intralesional BCG. Patients seem to tolerate endolymphatic BCG better than systemic chemotherapy in terms of nausea and malaise.

We have detected no undesirable effects in

terms of tumor enhancement or systemic tuberculosis. Our dilemma now is to decide which cases of stage II melanoma should receive endolymphatic BCG or endolymphatic ^{32}P.

We are at present investigating the relative merits of ^{32}P and BCG in the hope of finding the clinical indication for their use. Also under investigation is the use of *Corynebacterium parvum* when administered by intralymphatic injection.

REFERENCES

1. Andrews GA, Root SW, Kerman HD, Bigelow RR: Intra cavitory colloidal radiogold in the treatment of effusions caused by malignant neoplasm. Ann Surg 137:375, 1953
2. Ariel IM: Results of treating malignant melanoma intralymphatically with radioactive isotopes. Surg Gynecol Obstet 139:726, 1974
3. Ariel IM, Flynn W, and Pack GT: Second International Symposium on Regional Therapy of Tumours, Rome, 1967
4. Ariel IM, Resnick MI, Galey D: The intralymphatic administration of radioactive isotopes and cancer chemotherapeutic drugs. Surgery 55:355, 1964
5. Balint J, Pendower J, Ramsey NW: The stability of radio-iodinated olive oil. Clin Sci 19:2, 1960
6. Barclay TL, Crockett DJ, Eastwood DS, et al.: Assessment of prognosis in cutaneous malignant melanoma. Brit J Surg 64:54, 1977
7. Breslow A: Thickness, cross-sectional areas and depth of invasion in the prognosis of cutaneous melanoma. Ann Surg 172:902, 1970
8. Chiappa S, Galli G, Barbaini S, Ravasi G: Endolymphatic radiotherapy: Preliminary result of a new method. Radiol Med (Torino) 48:663, 1962
9. Chiappa S, Galli G: Considerazioni critiche mi MC: The histogenesis and biologic behaviour of primary human malignant melanoma of the skin. Cancer Res 29, 705, 1969
10. Clark WH Jr, Frome L, Bernardino EA, Mihm MC: The histogenesis and biologic behaviour of primary human malignant melanoma of the skin. Cancer Res 29:705, 1969
11. Cox KR, Hare WSC, Bruce PT: Lymphography in melanoma. Correlation of radiology with pathology. Cancer 19, 637, 1966
12. Croft D, Gaunt JI, Edwards JM: Data on P^{32} lipiodol given to M.R.C. Working Party on use of endolymphatic therapy in melanoma. 1969
13. Edwards JM: Melanoma and skin cancer. McCarthy WH (ed): Proceedings of International Cancer Conference, Sydney, 1972, p 441
14. Edwards JM: Malignant melanoma. Treatment of endolymphatic radio-isotope infusion. Ann Roy Coll Surg Engl, 44:237, 1969
15. Edwards JM, Kinmonth JB: Endolymphatic therapy for malignant melanoma. Brit Med J 1:18, 1968
16. Edwards JM, Kinmonth JB: Treatment of melanoma by endolymphatic therapy. Panminerva Med 18:183, 1976
17. Edwards JM, Kinmonth JB: Radio-isotopes in lymph node tumours. Progress in Lymphography. G Thieme Verlag, Stuttgart, 1967, p 243
18. Edwards JM, Gimlette TM, Clapham WF, et al.: Endolymphatic therapy of tumours with particular reference to the VX2 tumour in lepus cuniculus. Brit J Surg 53:969, 1966
19. Edwards JM, O'Donnell TF Jr, Johnson H, et al.: The effect of BCG on regional node metastases from the VX2 tumour in rabbits. Surg Forum 26:147, 1975
20. Edwards JM, Rutt DL, Kinmonth JB: Effectiveness of endolymphatic radioactive lipiodol on metastatic nodal deposits from the VX2 tumor of rabbits. Brit J Surg 52:69, 1965
21. Hine GJ, Brownell GL: Radiation Dosimetry, Academic Press, New York, 1956
22. Jantet GH: Ninth Scientific Meeting, Surgical Research Society, London, 1958. 1959 Trans 9th Internat Congress Radiol
23. Jantet GH: Direct intralymphatic injections of radio-active colloidal gold in the treatment of malignant disease. Brit J Radiol, 35:692, 1962
24. Kinmonth JB: Studies of the Lymphatics in idiopathic lymphoedema. Report 2nd Congress of the International Society of Angiology, Lisbon, 1953
25. Edwards JM. In JB Kinmonth (ed), The Lymphatics: Disease, Lymphography and Surgery. Baltimore, Md., Williams & Wilkins, 1972, pp 364–390
26. Kinmonth JB, Taylor GW, Harper RA: Lymphangiography. A technique for its clinical use in the lower limb. Brit Med J 1:940, 1955
27. Lloyd-Davies RW, Edwards JM, Kinmonth JB: Endolymphatic radiotherapy. Cancer, 24:938, 1969
28. Lord RSA, Kinmonth JB: Histologic effects of endolymphatic radiotherapy. Cancer 23:440, 1969

29. Makosi H, Magnus L, Heissen F, et al.: Klinische Ergebnisse nach Endolymphatischer radionuklidtherapie bei der Behandlung · des Malignen Melanom. Strahlentherapie 148:1, 1974

30. May ARL, Edwards JM: Surgical excision of visceral metastases from malignant melanoma. Clin Oncol 2:233, 1976

31. Morton DL, Eilber FR, Joseph WL, et al.: Immunological factors in human sarcomas and melanomas. A rational basis for immunotherapy. Ann Surg 172:740, 1970

32. Peterson NC, Bodenham DC, et al.: Malignant melanoma of the skin. A study of the origin, development, aetiology, spread, treatment and prognosis. Brit J Plast Surg, 15:49, 1962

33. Seitman DM, Wright R, Halaby FA, Freeman JH: Radioactive lymphangiography as a therapeutic adjunct. Am J Roentgenol 89:140, 1963

34. Veronesi U, Cascenelli N, Balzarina GP, Predo F: Melanoma and skin cancer. Proceedings of International Cancer Conference Sydney, VCN Blight, Government Printer, 1972, p 147

35. Weissleder H: Indikationen, Kontraindikationen und Nebenerscheinungen der Endolymphatischen Radionuklidtherapie (Indications, contraindications, and secondaries in endolymphatic radionuclear therapy). Med Welt, 25: 1028, 1974

CHAPTER FOURTEEN

AMELANOTIC MALIGNANT MELANOMAS

IRVING M. ARIEL

Malignant melanoma has always been associated with the pigmented nature of the lesion, which varies from light brown to deep black with an intermingling of the hues, often in the one lesion. However, certain malignant melanomas are not pigmented. Because physicians seldom suspect nonpigmented lesions of being malignant melanoma, long delays often results before the lesion is excised adequately and studied histologically so that a proper diagnosis can be established and proper definitive therapy instituted.

This chapter analyzes the results of the Pack Medical Group, New York, NY, where 77 amelanotic melanomas were discovered consisting of 2.3% of 3,305 melanomas seen during the period of investigation.

CLINICAL FEATURES

Of the 77 patients, 45 were males and 32 females. Their average combined age was 44 years, varying from 24 years to 73 years with no significant difference in the age of either sex. No site was immune to the development of amelanotic melanomas. Their distribution is presented in Table 14-1. An increased incidence of amelanotic melanoma of the head and neck is noted.

Analysis of the 77 patients according to stage is summarized in Table 14-2. Twenty-seven patients were listed as stage I (no metastasis to lymph nodes), 48 as stage II (metastases to regional lymph nodes), and two patients were catalogued as stage III, presenting with satellitoses and in-transit metastases between the leg and the regional lymph nodes. There were an additional ten patients who presented amelanotic melanomas with metastases with no known primary. These patients are not included in this analysis in that therapy was only palliative, the average duration of life being only 15 months. The possibility exists that a nonpigmented lesion of the skin may have been excised or cauterized, obscuring its presence after metastases had occurred, or that the lesion was so indistinguishable, being further camouflaged by the lack of pigment, that it represented a truly occult lesion. It is possible that the primary lesion was pigmented for we have seen pigmented melanoma produce metastases that are amelanotic.

LEVEL OF INVASION

Each of these melanomas was an infiltrating lesion (Clark's level IV or V). The prolonged delays before treatment may have permitted the horizontal growth phase to progress to the vertical growth phase in many instances.

CLINICAL APPEARANCE

None of our patients presented with a macular lesion with various degrees of vitiligo. All lesions were papular, lighter than the surrounding skin. Three patients presented a ring of an inflammatory reaction surrounding the lesion but most presented a sharp line of demarcation between the lesion and surrounding skin, suggesting a paucity of host reaction (Fig. 14-1). Twelve patients presented ulceration in the center giving the appearance of a basal cell carcinoma. Bleeding was rare, existing in only two patients. Pruritis was common (70 of 77 patients) and was the most frequent reason the patients sought medical attention.

TABLE 14-1. Incidence and Location of Amelanotic Melanoma—Pack Medical Group, New York City

Site	Total Number of Patients	Number of Amelanotic Melanomas	Percent of Amelanotic Melanomas
Thoracic wall	640	12	2
Abdominal wall	482	10	2
Upper extremities	487	6	1
Lower extremities	673	15	2
Head and neck	660	30	4.5
Miscellaneous	251	4	1
Total	3,305	77	2.1

TREATMENT

Each of the patients was treated by a wide resection after the diagnosis had been established, with the defect being closed by skin graft. A radical node dissection was performed for all patients with melanomas of the lower extremities, upper extremities, and thoracic wall. Half of the patients with melanomas of the head and neck were treated by a neck dissection. The ten patients with amelanotic melanoma of the abdominal wall were divided: six were treated by resection of the regional lymph nodes because of the location of the melanoma; in four patients the location was in the midline, and rather than

doing a bilateral groin dissection, none was accomplished—two of these patients survived the ten-year period. Twenty of the patients had been treated previously by their local physicians by ointments, escharotics, or electrodesiccation, not suspecting a melanoma (Fig. 14-2).

RESULTS

The overall ten-year survival for the 77 patients was 30% (23 patients).

Of the 27 patients in stage I classification, 15 (55%) survived the ten-year period without evidence of melanoma. Only eight of the 48

TABLE 14-2. Survival of Amelanotic Melanomas Analyzed According to Stage—Pack Medical Group, New York City

Stage	Total Number of Patients	Number Surviving 10 Years	Percent Surviving 10 Years	Remarks
1	27	15	55	Ten patients presented with dissemination of amelanotic melanoma with no known primary. The average duration of life was 15 months after our evaluation.
2	48	8	17	
3	2	0	0	
4	10	0	0	

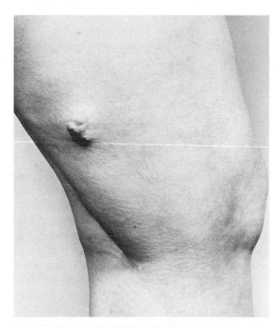

FIGURE 14–1. Amelanotic nodular melanoma of lower thigh, treated by tridimensional resection and incontinuity extended radical groin dissection. Patient developed extensive metastases four years later, from which he succumbed.

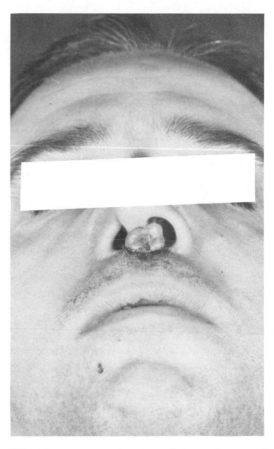

FIGURE 14–2. Amelanotic nodular melanoma of the mid-inferior skin of the nose. Attempted excision unsuccessful. Metastases to cervical lymph nodes, central nervous system, and elsewhere resulted in death of the patient two years after diagnosis.

patients in stage II (17%) survived the ten-year period. The two patients in stage III died 16 and 19 months following therapy. Analysis of the results by location revealed all melanomas of the lower extremities (including the pigmented ones), of which there were 438 determinate patients, yielded a 63% ten-year survival (276 patients) in contrast to the 15 amelanotic lesions of this location, of which only four (27%) survived ten years or longer. The breakdown by stage of these lesions was as follows: pigmented lesions Stage I—157 patients, Stage II—259 patients, and Stage III—22 patients. For the amelanotic lesions there were four stage I, ten stage II and two stage III. Patients with amelanotic melanoma of the upper extremity, of which there were six, showed a 33% (two patients) ten-year survival. Of the ten patients with amelanotic melanoma of the abdominal wall, three (30%) survived and three of the twelve patients

(25%) whose amelanotic melanoma was located on the thoracic wall survived ten years and longer.

There was an average delay of 13 months from the time the patient first noted the lesion until therapy was instituted; the physicians accounted for approximately 50% of the delay. The ten patients (not included in this overall series) who presented with metastases of melanomas, but an occult primary, all died an average of 15 months after being seen at our clinic.

DISCUSSION

The absence of pigment in a lesion almost universally associated with pigmentary changes suggests that the tumor was so anaplastic that it could not differentiate into its functional capacities.[2,3,4] Elder, Ainsworth, and Clark[5] believe that a few flecks of pigment are usually present and can be detected after careful inspection with a hand lens. Complete absence of pigment suggests some other lesion, either a Spitz lesion or a pyogenic granuloma.

It has been suggested by Speece et al. that a deficiency of tyrasinase may be the cause for the lack of the melanotic pigment. Fitzpatrick[6,7] and Comstock et al.[3] state that small amounts of melanin are produced in the amelanotic melanoma but are invisible for detection. In this series special staining with silver, ferric-ferricyanide, and others did not reveal any pigmentation. Huvos et al.[8] called attention to a striking difference in the amelanotic melanoma in humans, observed by electron microscopy, which consists of an absence of ribosomes with their distinctive cytoplasmic pigment granules in the amelanotic tumors as compared with numerous ribonucleoprotein particles and numerous pigment granules of the pigmented tumors. In hamster colonies, when a transplanted pigmented melanoma becomes amelanotic, it manifests increased virulence by augmentation of heterologous transplantability and propensity to metastasize widely in the alien host, according to Huvos and co-workers. A supposition that the amelanotic tumors represent a more anaplastic type of cells, which have sacrificed function for growth, seems to have been borne out. However, certain tumors in human oncology reveal selective functional capacities or lack of them with no relationship to their degree of malignancy, such as carcinoids, neuroblastomas, and others of the APUD series.

The suggestion of the increased aggressiveness of the amelanotic melanoma is further substantiated by the high incidence of patients who presented with evidence of metastases and overall poorer results, especially the precipitous drop in survival of patients who have evidence of metastases to their regional lymph nodes.

A pertinent question is the role of delayed diagnosis or improper treatment by a physician misled by the absence of pigmentation in the observed lesion.

All of the patients in our series had infiltrating lesions. The unavailability of fresh sections for further evaluation precluded our cataloging them according to Breslow's classifications. Practically all of them had a nodular component that varied from a somewhat papillary excrescence over the skin to a pure nodule, often with ulceration. This possibly represented vertical growth, either de novo or after a period of horizontal growth.

In a report of 28 patients (1.9% of 1,483 melanomas) studied at Memorial Hospital, New York City, Huvos, Shah, and Goldsmith[8] recorded a preponderance of females (19 females, 9 males), in contrast to our series, where the incidence of males was slightly higher. The combined average age of their group was 47 years, similar to our average age of 44 years. Their results revealed a singular effect of staging. The five-year survival for those in stage I equalled 71%, comparable to that attained for pigmented melanomas. Their figures are too low for statistical evaluation in that they had only seven patients in stage I, of whom five survived five years and longer. Only two out of 13 patients in their stage II survived (15% survival versus 42% five-year survival of their group with pigmented melanomas). They also revealed a higher incidence for stage II melanomas than stage I for amelanotic melanomas, in contrast to their series of pigmented lesions where the incidence of stage I lesions predominated. In eight of their patients no known primary lesion was discovered, and the patients presented with widespread amelonotic metastases.[9,10]

Balch et al.[1] from the University of Alabama performed a multifactorial analysis of 339 melanoma patients. They found that 18% of their patients had amelanotic melanomas that lowered chances of survival; 36% five-year survival with depigmentation versus 69% with pigmented lesions. They found the survival of patients with amelanotic melanomas was a secondary variable that correlated with thickness.

SUMMARY AND CONCLUSIONS

Amelanotic melanoma comprised 2.3% of the 3,305 melanomas seen at the Pack Medical Group. The 77 patients so observed presented melanomas throughout all parts of skin of their bodies, no site being immune. None were found originating in the mucous membranes. A slightly higher incidence occurred in males (45 patients) than in females (32 patients). The average age of the patients was 44 years, varying from 24 to 73 years of age. There were ten patients (not included in this review) who presented themselves with metastatic amelanotic melanomas with no known primary. The patients with stage II melanomas exceeded those ordinarily seen in that 48 of the 77 patients (62%) had metastases to their regional lymph nodes when first observed.

The overall survival was 30% for the 77 patients observed. Those in stage I had a survival rate of 55%, which dropped to 17% for those with stage II (metastases present in the regional lymph nodes).

The reason for the lack of pigmentation in these relatively few melanomas is unknown, but it has been hypothecated that it represents an anaplastic form of cancer in which function is sacrificed for aggressive growth. Because of the benign clinical appearance and the fact that practically all physicians associate pigmentation with malignant melanoma, the diagnosis is generally not suspected for some time. Increased awareness of this entity, early biopsy, and more expedient therapy may per-mit earlier diagnoses (before metastases have occurred), more definitive treatment, and better results.

REFERENCES

1. Balch CM, Murad TM, Seng-Jaw S, et al.: A multifactorial analysis of melanoma. Ann Surg 188(6):732–742, 1978
2. Clark WH Jr: Four types of cellular fine structure associated with human amelanotic melanoma. Yale J Biol Med 46:428, 1973
3. Comstock G, Wynne E, Russell WO: Dopa oxidase activity in differential diagnosis of amelanotic melanoma tissue. Cancer Res 19:880–883, 1959
4. Costa J, Rosai J, Philpott GW: Pigmentation of "amelanotic" melanoma in tissue culture. Arch Pathol 95:371–373, 1973
5. Elder DE, Ainsworth AM, Clark WH Jr: The surgical pathology of cutaneous malignant melanoma. In Clark WH (ed): Human Melanoma. New York, Grune & Stratton, 1979, p 65
6. Fitzpatrick TB: Human melanogenesis. Arch Dermtol 65:379–391, 1952
7. Fitzpatrick TB, Kukita A: Tyrosine activity in vertebrate melanocytes. In Gordon M (ed), Pigment Cell Biology. New York, Academic Press, 1959
8. Huvos AG, Shah JP, Goldsmith HS: A clinicopathologic study of amelanotic melanoma. Surg Gynecol Obstet 135:917–920, 1972
9. Shah JP: Amelanotic melanoma. In Ariel IM (ed) Progress In Clinical Cancer. New York, Grune & Stratton, 1975, pp 195–197
10. Shah JP, Goldsmith HS: Prognosis of malignant melanoma in relation to clinical presentation. Am J Surg 123:286–288, 1972
11. Speece AJ, Chang JP, Russell WO: A microspectroprotometric autoradiographic study of tyrosine activity in human melanoma. In Gordon M (ed), Pigment Cell Biology. New York, Academic Press, 1959

CHAPTER FIFTEEN

CHEMOTHERAPY OF MALIGNANT MELANOMA

IRVING M. ARIEL

In 1958, the late Dr. George Pack and I edited nine volumes of books entitled *The Treatment of Cancer and Allied Disease.* In the foreword to the entire series, we wrote the following:

> The editors paradoxically hope that these volumes may soon become obsolete with the discovery of more efficient means of curing cancer *such as a chemotherapeutic remedy* or better yet by the creation of an immunity against the disease. In the meantime, these manuals of present day therapy are offered with the wish that the best treatment plan now available can be instituted for any patient bearing any form of cancer.[38]

Now, 23 years later, chemotherapy of malignant melanoma remains provocative, with some encouraging results being reported. The fact that malignant melanomas will respond to chemotherapy with objective shrinkage of the tumor and marked but often transient palliation to the patients evokes hope that these beneficial results may be consolidated and improved by more efficient drugs and immunotherapy.

The accomplishments of cancer chemotherapy must be judged in the light of the natural history of malignant melanoma, which is one of the most unpredictable diseases afflicting the human being. There is a constant ebb and flow of tumor growth and spread, on one hand, and immunologic attempts by the host to counter the growth, on the other. The cancer may lay dormant after local excision of the primary lesion, only to manifest itself in another organ, blood-borne to that organ, after a prolonged period—as long as 27 years in one of our patients, and then to grow wildly throughout the body and to kill the host in a period—as short as six weeks.

Age, sex, location of the primary tumor, genetic factors, and other as yet unknown features play a role in determining the natural history of a given melanoma. In fact, the same host may bear several primary melanomas, one that may be slow growing and remain localized, and another that may grow vertically, infiltrate deeply, and metastasize early.

Judging the effectiveness of cancer chemotherapy at present is further complicated by the fact that it is mainly used for patients with far-advanced disease. Aust[4] calls attention to the fact that if a tumor weighs approximately 10 gm, it will have approximately 10 billion cells. If an agent is 99.9% effective in killing the tumor, it would still leave a million cells for regrowth. This clearly demonstrates the burden placed upon cancer chemotherapy for patients with far-advanced disease, located in different organs.

This chapter presents melanoma chemotherapy in the following categories: (1) systemic prophylactic (adjuvant) chemotherapy following hoped-for surgical cure of the primary neoplasm; (2) systemic chemotherapy for advanced cancer; (3) isolated perfusion for a) prophylaxis (adjuvant) therapy, and b) for treatment for regional metastases in the offending limb; and (4) intra-arterial infusion cancer chemotherapy.

HISTORY

Historically, many agents (toxins, hormones, immunologic, and chemotherapeutic) have been utilized in an attempt to treat malignant melanoma.[25] One of the first was Coly's mixed toxins (1894),[15] which consisted of killed cultures of streptococci from patients with erysipelas, which met with some mild, temporary results. Another was the Shear's polysaccharide, which consisted of bacterial filtrates of Bacillus *Prodigiosus* and showed regression but was abandoned because of its severe toxicity.[41] Pack (1950)[37] noted a patient who had been bitten by a dog and received rabies vaccine for such treatment, and who had spontaneous disappearance of her disseminated melanoma. He, accordingly, advocated rabies vaccine for treatment of melanoma, and it was used rather extensively for awhile, but since has been largely abandoned.[37] Various antibiotics were used in earlier years including an endotoxin from killed trypanosoma cruzi (K–R).

An immune factor was tried by Sumner (as reported by McCune) who treated two patients with malignant melanoma, one of whom had a spontaneous regression; the second was transfused with the blood of the first and had complete disappearance of the tumor. Stimulated by this result, McCune transfused a patient who had malignant melanoma and pulmonary metastases with the blood of another patient who had been free of disease ten years after surgical therapy for malignant melanoma. There was complete disappearance of the leg lesion. When that patient developed metastases to the brain, she had another transfusion out of the immune donor blood extract, with temporary subsistence. When the patient died, autopsy revealed hemorrhage into the cerebral metastases.[34]

Hormones have been used without effect, namely the male sex hormones.[26] Cortisone has been utilized, as well as thyroxin, without any effect. Orchiectomy, adrenalectomy, hypophysectomy, have been useless.[29,30,33,42]

CHEMOTHERAPEUTIC AGENTS

Bellet, Mastrangelo, Berd, and Lustbader[6] utilized statistical methods for evaluating the observed response rates. A search of the literature from 1950 to 1975 by them yielded 232 references. They accepted a minimal acceptable response criterion of 50% decrease in the sum of the products of the perpendicular diameters of all measured lesions for at least one month. On this basis, only 128 articles and abstracts were acceptable for evaluation. They evaluated 28 single agents that met the above criteria, of which six were alkylating agents, four antimetabolites, four antibiotics, three spindle inhibitors, and 11 had unknown or miscellaneous actions.

The pooled response data for each single agent was subjected to analysis to identify those agents that are therapeutically effective: at least a 95% probability of the true response rate equal to or greater than 29%. Results of their analyses yielded only one drug, DTIC, that met this requirement. In 1,188 evaluable patients, 278 objective responses were reported, yielding an observed response rate of 23.4%. Since none of the other drugs met the criterion, they concluded that DTIC is the most effective single agent in the treatment of malignant melanoma, and state that it can serve as a benchmark for other single and multiple-drug therapy regimes. They further found that BCNU, MeCCNU, and Thio-Tepa revealed a probability of a true response rate equal to or greater than 10%. The following drugs they classified as potentially useful: BCNU, MeCCNU, and Thio-Tepa. Drugs they classified as possibly useful were: TMCA, TEPA, L-Pam, DBD, Mito-C, and MTX. They listed eight drugs as probably not useful alone: Streptz, TIC-Must, CTX, ARA-C, Leukeran, VLB, VCR, and CCNU. Drugs considered to have had adequate clinical trials and found to be nonuseful where : 5FU, 6—MP, ICRF-159, HXM, HN₂, HU, BLEO, ADRIA, ACT-D, and Pregnane.

They selected a 5% improvement by a combined regime as the minimum improvement and response rate that would justify subjecting patients to the additional toxicity and other nonacceptable factors. (Table 15–1). Of the 22 combination drug regimes that they tested for objectivity, 15 contained DTIC. They felt that of the 22 combination drugs tested, only the combination consisting of DTIC plus BCNU plus VCR plus HU could be classified as having a superior activity. Three combinations

TABLE 15-1.   Drug Abbreviations and Full Names

DTIC	Imidazole carboxamide
DBD	Dibromodulcitol
MTX	Methotrexate
L–PAM	Melphalan
STREPTZ	Streptozotocin
TMCA	Trimethylcolchicinic acid
VCR	Vincristine
TIC–MUST	Cyclophosphamide
ARA–C	Cytosine arabinoside
MITO–C	Mitomycin-C
VLB	Vinblastine
6–MP	6-Mercaptopurine
HXM	Hexamethylmelamine
HN$_2$	Nitrogen mustard
HU	Hydroxyurea
BLEO	Bleomycin
ADRIA	Adriamycin
ACT–D	Actinomycin-D
PROCARB	Procarbazine
6–TG	6-Thioguanine
DDP	Cis-diaminedichloroplatinum
PREGNANE	Pregnanetrione
CIS PT	Cis-Platinum dismine dichloride

Reprinted with additions from Bellet et al., in Clark, WH (ed): Human Malignant Melanoma, Grune & Stratton, New York, 1979, p 359.

were classified as active: (DTIC + BCNU + VCR + HU), (VLB + PROCARB + ACT–D), and (CCNU + VCR).

Their final recommendation for current treatment is as follows: Presently DTIC is the drug of first choice in the treatment of patients with metastatic malignant melanoma. A nitrosourea (BCNU, or MeCCNU) constitutes a second-line treatment. They currently recommend the addition of VCR to BCNU or MeCCNU because of the data suggesting some improvement in response rate, without additive toxicity. The third-line treatment is problematic. The clinician can choose from among the following: (1) Thio-Tepa or one of the potentially useful single agents; (2) a combination regime that does not contain either DTIC or a nitrosourea; or (3) administration of untried drugs.

We have recently utilized *cis*-Platinum in the treatment of malignant melanoma with suggestive early promising results, but every new drug seems to have early promising good results. Hence we mention this as a drug now being tested, for which no definite statement can be made. We have further used it in combination with DTIC, and VCR.

SYSTEMIC CHEMOTHERAPY

Systemic chemotherapy via the intravenous route is the form most frequently used. Due to the fact that approximately 9,000 individuals develop cutaneous melanoma in the United States each year, in a five-year period there would be approximately 45,000 cases of melanoma. Considering that approximately 50% of these people are not cured, there exists a period, from the time that curative surgical therapy has been found to be unsuccessful until the patient eventually succumbs to the cancer, during which there would be approximately 25,000 people in the United States bearing melanomas, practically all incurable, who would be candidates for systemic chemotherapy. The great demand made on systemic chemotherapy makes this method an extremely important socioeconomic factor, as well as a medical modality of tremendous importance.

ADJUVANT THERAPY

The use of systemic chemotherapy for adjuvant therapy (i.e., the treatment of a patient with high-risk melanoma by the administration of various cancer chemotherapeutic agents systemically administered over a prolonged period) has been tried with various drugs.[48]

Kaufman et al.[31] randomized patients to receive DTIC, BCG, or both. In their report, there have been five recurrences and four deaths in 19 patients treated with DTIC alone; four recurrences and two deaths in 24 patients receiving BCG; and no recurrences or deaths in patients receiving the combination. El Domeiri et al.[21] reported five of 15 patients alive and free of disease after two years of being treated with DTIC, in contrast to eight of 15 who received BCG alone. McPherson[35] compared combination therapy of DTIC + oral BCG with a combination of BCNU, Hydroxyurea, and DTIC + BCG in 30 patients. Those receiving the combination chemotherapy have had survival superior to that experienced by an historical control group, but neither group showed a prolongation of disease-free interval. Hill et al.[28] in a composite evaluation studied the effects of adjuvant DTIC and showed a disease-free survival of 40 weeks for treated patients, versus 73 weeks for the control group—a better survival for the control group. Benjamin[9] believes that their poor results might be due to the fact that the DTIC was given only every three months and only for four courses. He also calls attention to the fact that nine protocols involving immunotherapy and chemotherapy showed an overall response rate of 28%, somewhat higher than the 22% for DTIC alone, or the 24% for nitrosaureas.

Combined chemotherapy and immunotherapy seems to be somewhat promising as an adjuvant combination modality, but the overall results leave very much to be desired.

PALLIATION THERAPY

Every conceivable drug has been utilized for the treatment of disseminated melanoma. Table 15-1 lists many of these drugs with their abbreviations, which are the expressions most commonly used in clinical cancer chemotherapy. The full name of the drug is listed adjacent to the abbreviated form.

All chemotherapeutic agents attempt to destroy the cell during its life cycle, and efforts are made to adapt certain agents to affect the cell during different periods of its cycle. The different cycles are shown in Table 15-2, and the times that have been estimated for the various functions of the different cycles to be completed are also shown in this table (determined by two separate investigators). Thus the alkylating agents affect rapidly multiplying cells causing abnormalities in DNA. These

TABLE 15-2.   Human Melanoma Cell Cycle Time

G.O.—Resting	
G.1. (DNA synthesis; ingredients)	16.3 hours*
S (replication of genome)	
G2 (RNA and protein synthesis)	5.3 hours†
Mitosis	21.0 hours†

* Entire cycle = 36 hours. Sherakawa et al.: Cell proliferation in human melanoma. J Clin Invest 49:1188–1199, 1970
† Hagemann RF, Schiffer LM: Cell kinetic analyses of a human melanoma in vitro and in vivo–vitro. J Nat Cancer Inst 47:519–526, 1971.

have not been successful, for the most part, in melanomas. The antimetabolites act during the S-phase (DNA synthesis), and have also not proved to be very active. The Vinka-alkaloids act on G-2 protein and on RNA synthesis and mitosis, and have shown some activity against melanoma. The drug that has shown the most effectiveness against melanoma is DTIC, which is also probably an alkylating agent; it has shown response rates varying from 17% to 35%. Various unknowns exist pertaining to the use of DTIC. For example, smaller doses produce better results than larger doses in one series; females do better than males; patients with visceral metastases do more poorly than those with nonvisceral metastases. But the results, for the most part, seem to be transient.

SYSTEMIC CHEMOTHERAPY WITH AUTOGENOUS MARROW TRANSFUSION

Ariel and Pack[2,3] treated 31 patients with phenylalanine mustard. In order to obtain the high dosage of the drug without hematologic complications, they withdrew 300–500 cc of bone marrow containing blood, prior to the administration of blood, and retransfused it intravenously six hours after the chemotherapeutic agent had been administered. Most of the phenylalanine mustard had been absorbed in the six-hour period, and studies with tagged cells revealed that most of the intravenously administered marrow found residence in the bone marrow. About two-thirds of the patients

THE MULTIFACETED MANIFESTATIONS OF MALIGNANT MELANOMA

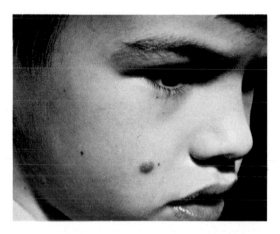

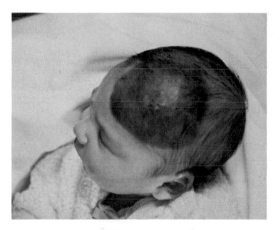

FIG. 1.   Juvenile melanoma of the cheek on a prepubertal boy. This lesion is benign with typical dome
shape.   *(Courtesy of Dr. Alfred W. Kopf)*

FIG. 2.   Large congenital nevus of the scalp of an
infant. Malignant changes are frequent in these lesions.

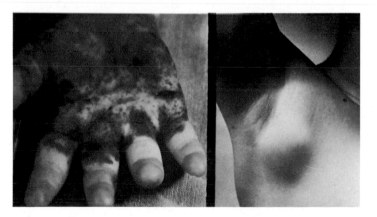

FIG. 3.   Left. Congenital melanoma of the palm of an infant which
metastasized. Right. Axilla of same child showing metastases to axillary
lymph nodes.

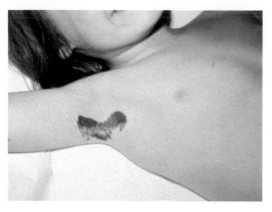

FIG. 4. Benign congenital linear nevus of the axilla of a prepubertal child treated by conservative excision.

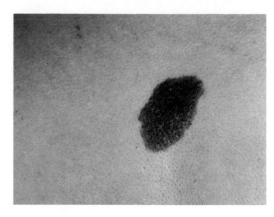

FIG. 5. Benign compound nevus with uniform color and sharp margins, treated by conservative excision.

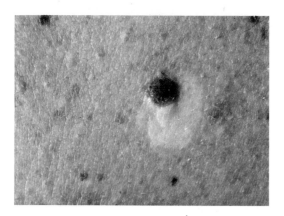

FIG. 6. Halo nevus. Flat surface with well-circumcised edges surrounded by a white ring. The nevus may in time disappear.

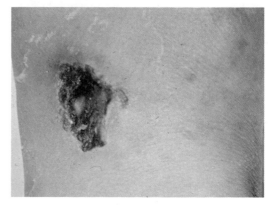

FIG. 7. Nodular malignant melanoma. These are deeply invasive and very malignant.

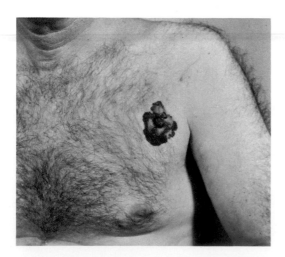

FIG. 8. Advanced phase of a "superficial" spreading melanoma which had metastasized to the axillary lymph nodes. Variation in color, outline, and surface are demonstrated.

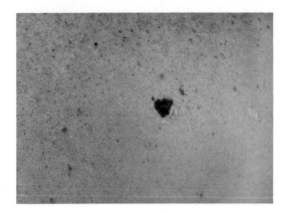

FIG. 9. Early phase of a superficial spreading melanoma.

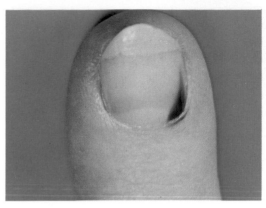

FIG. 10. Early subungual melanoma. The lesion was asymptomatic. Pigmentation was the only sign of the melanoma.

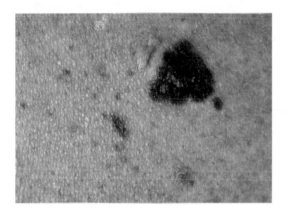

FIG. 11. Superficial melanoma surrounded by benign nevi. Beginning phase of peripheral depigmentation is shown.

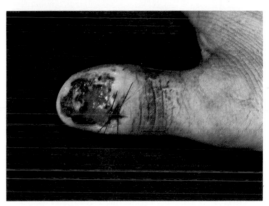

FIG. 12. Advanced stage of a subungual melanoma of the thumb.

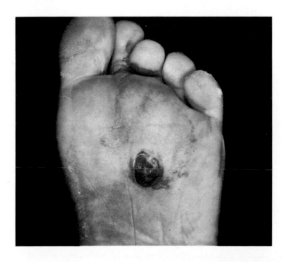

FIG. 13. Nodular melanoma of the plantar aspect of the foot.

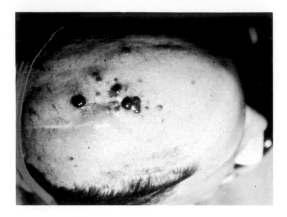

FIG. 14. Malignant Jadassohn nevus of the scalp which had produced numerous satellitoses.

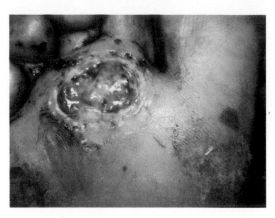

FIG. 15. Amelanotic melanoma of the foot. Absence of pigment often obscures the diagnosis.

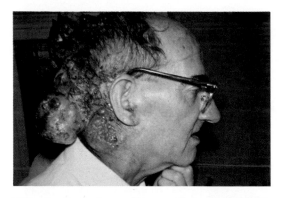

FIG. 16. Extensive melanoma of the scalp which remained localized to the scalp region and finally killed the patient by infiltrating into the brain.

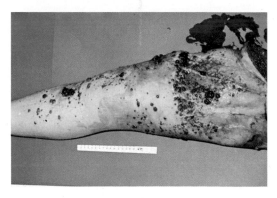

FIG. 17. Amputated leg for massive melanoma to the groin nodes and extensive satellitoses.

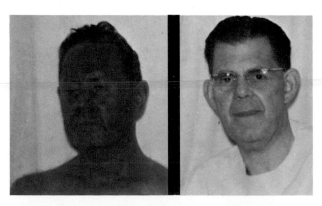

FIG. 18. Extensive pigmentation the result of circulating melanin from extensive metastases. The patient (left) was lighter than the resident (right) before he developed metastatic melanoma.

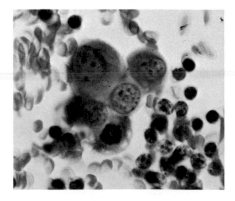

FIG. 19. Melanoma cells in the peripheral blood.

benefited, both subjectively and objectively, from the treatment, but the improvement was all temporary, lasting from one to ten months without significantly affecting longevity. Histologic studies of melanoma after this treatment revealed acute necrosis in metastatic melanoma within lymph nodes. Adding Methotrexate to this regime did not improve the results.[3]

Between 1972 and 1978, a number of studies using DTIC in combination with other drugs have been tried for patients with stage IV melanoma with relatively poor response rates.[5,6] Cohen and co-authors reported a response rate of 20 to 30% lasting from over 30 weeks, with some responders living over a year. They believe their combination of drugs is not significantly better than DTIC alone.[14]

Several studies using combinations of chemotherapy, not including DTIC, have shown similar results to those with DTIC.[8] Didolker et al., using a combination of CCNU and Procarbazine, had a response rate of approximately 25%.[20] A combination of 5FU and Procarbazine by Nordman et al.,[36] and a combination of Cyclophosphamide, Vincristine, and Procarbazine by Byrne,[11] as well as a study of CCNU, Vincristine and Bleomycin by DeWasch[19] have shown response rates of between 35 to 48%. Hersh et al.[27] believe that these results suggest that the emphasis in future studies of combination chemotherapy should be on drugs other than DTIC. Their conclusion regarding systemic chemotherapy is:

> The response to chemotherapy of malignant melanoma is determined by the site of metastatic disease. Soft tissue and lymph node metastases respond best, pulmonary metastases respond next best, while disease in liver, bone marrow, and bone respond least well. Brain metastases, which are a frequent cause of death, are not affected by chemotherapy, even with drugs such as nitrosoureas that cross the blood–brain barrier.

Davis, in discussing a report by Hersh et al., states:

> I agree that chemotherapy used as adjuvant therapy in poor risk patients and as treatment in

advanced or recurrent cases has been disappointing. A response rate of 20% and a response duration of approximately 5 months can be obtained on some occasions with no treatment and without the discomforts of chemotherapy.[18]

Accordingly a number of drugs and drug combinations are available for systemic administration to offer meaningful palliation and possibly some prolongation of life, but these results are not too dramatic.

Gutterman et al.[24] have reported on 89 patients with disseminated melanoma who were treated with DTIC intravenously and BCG administered by scarification, and compared them with 111 patients treated with DTIC alone. The chemoimmunotherapy-treated patients with metastases to the lymph nodes had a remission rate of 55% compared with 18% for those treated with chemotherapy alone (P = 0.025). The duration of the remissions was longer, and chemoimmunotherapy was well tolerated without serious morbidity. They advocate this combination instead of chemotherapy as the sole modality. Thus, the addition of immunotherapy appears to enhance the effects of chemotherapy.

REGIONAL ARTERIAL PERFUSION

The principle of this technique is to administer, for a short period, a large dose of a cancer chemotherapeutic agent introduced into the artery, which is attached to a pump oxygenator, and the limb perfused with the drug for approximately two hours. It was hoped that isolation could be accomplished, but there was always some escape, and therefore the term regional perfusion is preferred. This technique has been utilized for the arm (forequarter), the leg (hindquarter), the head and neck (carotid artery infusion), and for the pelvic area and lower extremities (aortic infusion). The drug most frequently used has been phenylalanine mustard (alkeran). Most of the reports describe the surgical removal of the primary lesion, with the perfusion being utilized as adjuvant therapy to prevent metastases from occurring. In some instances, the patient suffered from stage III melanoma, in that the limb contained numerous deposits of melanoma. Hyperthermia has been used to enhance the effectiveness of the drug perfusion.[44,45]

Rochlin, Wagner, and Rochlin reported before the 1972 International Melanoma Project in Sydney, Australia, a total of 452 patients, of whom 238 were without evidence of metastases, 44 contained local recurrence within a distance of 5 cm, 142 were classified stage III with multiple recurrent lesions scattered throughout the area included in the regional perfusion, and 28 patients whose melanoma had spread beyond. They were quite optimistic about their results, and showed 92% response of stage I group, who were free of melanoma; 71% of the stage II group; and 43% of the stage III group, at the three-year period.[39]

Krementz et al. reported on 714 patients with malignant melanoma who were treated, from 1957 through 1977, by chemotherapy administered by isolated regional perfusion of the limbs, and 56 patients who were treated by intra-arterial infusion.[32] They stated:

Excisional surgery and adjunctive perfusion in 286 patients with Stage I disease resulted in cumulative survival rates of 87% at 5 years and 75% at 10 and 15 years. With recurrent or metastatic regional disease treated by perfusion alone or in combination with surgical excision, the survival rates were 36%, 34%, and 31% at 5, 10, and 15 years, respectively. Even in the least favorable group, those with nodal and soft tissue involvement, the survival rates were 27% at 5 years and 22.5% at 10 and 15 years. Analysis of 121 patients with Stage I melanoma according to level of dermal invasion showed recurrence in 2 of 42 (4%) patients with level III lesions, 11 of 75 (15%) with level IV tumors, and 2 of 4 (50%) with level V lesions. Recurrence rates by pathologic type were 2 of 49 (4%) patients with superficial spreading melanoma, 6 of 30 (20%) with nodular melanoma, and 5 of 14 (36%) with acral lentiginous melanoma, the latter including subungual, plantar, or palmar lesions.

As an adjunct to surgical treatment, chemotherapy by isolation-perfusion offers improved survival rates without prolonged treatment or the risks associated with systemic chemotherapy. As primary therapy for advanced regional disease, chemotherapy by perfusion produces survival rates superior to those obtained by surgery alone or systemic chemotherapy.

Their results are summarized in the following tables.

Results for adjuvant regional chemotherapy by regional arterial perfusion for 12 patients are summarized in Table 15–3. The results of chemotherapy for advanced skin, node, and soft tissue metastases are summarized in Table 15–4. There was only one death secondary to cerebral hemorrhage. An autopsy was not permitted, hence the cause of the hemorrhage remains unknown. Collected results of treatment by regional perfusion in the literature are summarized in Tables 15–5 and 15–6.

Davis, Ivins, and Soule, reporting from the Mayo Clinic in 1975, stated that 269 patients with melanoma of the extremities were treated by regional hyperthermic perfusion.

Wide excision of the primary lesion or a biopsy site and regional node dissection was performed at the time of perfusion in 68 patients, prior to perfusion in 32 patients, and after perfusion in 10 patients. Regional nodes were not excised in 1 patient.[17]

Recurrences developed after perfusion in 35 patients. The mean length of time to recurrences was two years, with a range up to nine years from the date of perfusion. They state the rate of complications was relatively high and consisted of lymph sluffing and edema, which might be related to the surgery. Five amputations were the direct result of complications of perfusion, and five additional patients had significant loss of limb function due to muscle contractures and sympathetic dystrophy. No patient had bone marrow depression severe enough to produce secondary infection or breathing difficulties. In 18 patients, further surgical procedures were necessary to deal with the complications. They concluded that of the 111 patients who were available for analysis, 78 survived 4–13 years after their initial perfusion. Complications developed in 94 patients and were per-

TABLE 15-3. Results of Adjuvant Regional Chemotherapy by Intra-arterial Infusion in 12 Patients

Drugs	Patients Treated	Response/Duration
DTIC	5	3 No evidence of disease, 19–44 months
		2 Local recurrence, 2 months
MTX	1	1 No local recurrence; dead of distant disease at 5 years
1–PAM	1	1 Local recurrence at 5 months
1–PAM, MTX, and/or TSPA	4	1 No local recurrence; dead of distant disease at 6 years
		3 Local recurrence at 2, 3, and 4 months
TSPA, MTX, Act-D	1	1 No local recurrence; dead of distant disease at 8 months

Reproduced from Krementz et al.: The use of regional chemotherapy in the management of malignant melanoma. World J Surg, Vol 3, No 3, 1979, pp 289–304, with permission of author and publisher.

manent in 34. Survival was correlated with both depth of invasion of the primary lesion and stage of disease at the time of perfusion.

At the Ninth International Pigment Cell Conference, where the above data were presented, the authors stated that this pro-cedure is no longer being used at the Mayo Clinic.

It may be noted that, in the Mayo experience, hyperthermia was applied to increase the efficacy of the chemotherapeutic agents. In 1967, Cavaliere et al.[12] suggested

TABLE 15-4. Results of Chemotherapy by Intra-arterial Infusion for Advanced Skin, Node and Soft Tissue Metastases

Drug	Number Treated	Complete Response	Percent Objective Response*
DTIC	11	1	63.6
MTX	10	2	80.0
1–PAM	2	—	50
Combination— 2 or more 1–PAM, TSPA, MTX Act-D	7	1	56
TSPA, MTX, Act-D	4†	—	66
HN₂	1	—	Objective response
TSPA, DTIC	1	—	No objective response

* No patient survived more than 12 months.
† One chemotherapy death.
Reproduced from Krementz et al.: The use of regional chemotherapy in the management of malignant melanoma. World J Surg, Vol 3, No 3, 1979, pp 289–304, with permission of author and publisher.

TABLE 15-5.   Collected Results of Treatment of Primary Melanoma of Limbs by Excision and Chemotherapy by Regional Perfusion

Author	Number of Patients	Regional Lymph Node Dissection	% Survival
Stehlin (1975)	70	No	83.5(5 yrs)
Koops (1975)	30	NS*	77.0(4 yrs)
Sugarbaker and McBride (1976)	199	14/199	88.0(5 yrs)
Golomb (1976)	61	No	72.0(5 yrs)
Wagner (1976)	133	NS	94.0(5 yrs)
Davis (1976)	72	NS	90.0(4 yrs)
Jochimsen (1977)	21	Yes	100.0(2 yrs)

* Not stated.
Reproduced from Krementz et al.: The use of regional chemotherapy in the management of malignant melanoma. World J Surg Vol 3, No 3, 1979, pp 289–304, with permission of author and publisher.

TABLE 15-6.   Collected Results of Chemotherapy of Metastatic Melanoma Confined to the Limb by Regional Perfusion

Author	Stage*	Number of Patients	Surgical Therapy	5-Year % Survival
McBride (1971)	II		Excision	57
Koops (1975)	II & III	35	RLND† in some; number not stated	23
Shingleton (1975)	III	43	RLND if not done previously	28
Stehlin et al. (1975)	II & III	73	Excision if appropriate	48.2
Golomb (1976)	III	85	Excision if appropriate	22
Wagner (1976)	II	41	Most with RLND	68
Davis (1976)	III	39	Excision and RLND	33.3
McBride (1978)	IIIA	40	Excision if appropriate	51
	IIIB	16	Excision if appropriate	33
	IIIAB	14	Excision if appropriate	14

* M.D. Anderson staging.
† RLND = regional lymph node dissection.
Reproduced from Krementz et al.: The use of regional chemotherapy in the management of malignant melanoma. World J Surg, Vol 3, No 3, 1979, pp 289–304, with permission of author and publisher.

hyperthermia without chemotherapy. Stehlin[44] routinely believes that hyperthermic perfusion is superior, and Golomb[22] uses it exclusively, increasing the circulating blood temperature to 43C, and he also increases the duration of perfusion up to two hours. His complication rate is an acceptable one.

Stehlin et al.,[45] who instituted the method of hyperthermia, have reported the benefits as follows:

> Since 1967, we have used a system of hyperthermic perfusion with melphalan to treat patients with melanoma of the extremities. This report presents additional follow-up data on 165 patients, first reported on in 1975, who underwent 185 perfusions. The 70 patients classified as stage I (Stehlin classification system) had a 5-year survival rate of 86.3%. The 5-year survival rate for the 73 patients with stage II and stage III disease was 52.5%. There was a dramatic increase in the 5-year survival rate for patients with stage IIIA disease, from 22.2% prior to the use of heat to 74% for 30 patients undergoing hyperthermic perfusion.

Sugarbaker and McBride[47] performed an analysis of the results at the M.D. Anderson Hospital of Houston, Texas where isolation perfusion with L-phenylalanine mustard was administered to 199 patients with invasive stage I melanoma of the extremities. Determined survival among patients followed for five to 15 years was 83%. They state the Berkson-Gage survivals were 98% in two years, 88% in five years, and 84% in ten years. Failures consisted of local recurrence in 2%; 3% developed in-transit recurrence; 13% developed positive regional lymph nodes; 8% developed systemic metastases; and one developed a local recurrence plus positive regional nodes. Of the 49 patients failing treatment, 15 (31%) are surviving for an unknown period after treatment of their recurrence. The authors believe that, using historical controls in the literature, survival has probably been improved by their therapy. The absolute proof of their method of therapy was evaluated in 14 patients treated by perfusion alone, without local excision. They state that in the regional control the survival was poor, and they conclude that the primary should be locally excised, widely, but that the regional perfusion may be effective in controlling regional subclinical disease (Figs. 15–1 through 15–4). In addition to the figures the following reinformation was also obtained at the M. D. Anderson Hospital:

Stage O — Superficial melanoma
Stage I — Localized primary melanoma
     A. Primary intact
     B. Primary locally excised
     C. Multiple primaries
Stage II — Local recurrence or primary lesion with local peripheral nodules ≤ 3 cm*
Stage III — Regional metastases
     A. In-transit(s)†
     B. Node(s)
     AB. Intransits, plus nodes
Stage IV — Systemic metastases

Shingleton et al.[43] reported the following from the Duke University Medical School:

> Two forms of therapy were employed for treatment of patients with recurrent melanoma limited to the extremity. Perfusion of the involved extremity with phenylalanine mustard has resulted in a 5-year survival rate of 28% in 43 patients. A second group of 25 patients has been treated by a four-stage immunotherapy program consisting of sensitization with intradermal, BCG, followed in 6 weeks by intra-tumor injection of BCG. A third stage involved the activation of the patient's lymphocytes, after removal by a blood cell separator, incubated in vitro with irradiated neuraminidase-treated melanoma cells and reintroduced into the patient either by subcutaneous or intratumor injection. The fourth stage of immunotherapy involves injection of an inoculum of irradiated neuraminidase-treated autochthonous tumor cells plus BCG injected intratumorally or subcutaneously. Sixteen of 24 patients receiving immunotherapy treatment program have experienced arrest of their disease lasting from 5 to 42 months.

* Satellite(s) are locally metastatic nodules ≤ 3 cm periphery of primary lesion or excision site.
† In-transit(s) are defined as tissue metastases that result from implantation and growth of "in-transit" cells between primary and regional nodes.

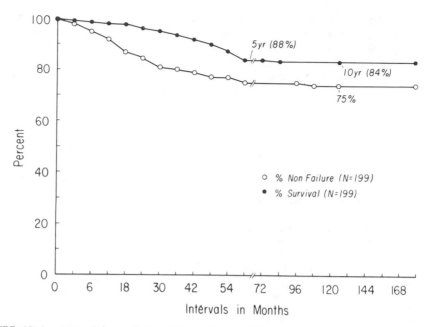

FIGURE 15-1. Actuarial survival and nonfailure in 199 cases of stage I extremity melanoma treated by excision of the primary and perfusion. The date of first recurrence in cases failing initial treatment is used to calculate the "nonfailure" curve. The difference between the two curves reflects the patients salvaged by treatment of their recurrence. (Reproduced from Sugarbaker EV and McBride CM: The results of isolation-perfusion for invasive stage I melanoma of the extremities. Cancer 37(1): 188–198, 1976. Reprinted with the permission of the authors and the American Cancer Society, Inc.)

In Golomb's series, 66 patients with recurrent melanoma limited to one extremity were perfused. Forty-four (60%) had complete disappearance of detectable tumor. The disease eventually recurred in two-thirds of these, but 13 (30%) are still free of tumor 6 to 176 months later. Today 17% are alive 5 to 14 years since recurrent disease was perfused. Eleven of those whose disease recurred were perfused a second or third time (Fig. 15–5).

Golomb's conclusion is:

Based on the disease-free interval data and the parallel survival data, I believe that perfusion should be employed as an adjunct to surgical treatment of melanoma of the distal extremities in patients who have microscopically positive regional lymph nodes, or in whom the probability is high of having occult regional lymph node metastases.[23]

.It does seem that regional perfusion of cancer chemotherapeutic agents plays a role in delaying the onset of metastases and possibly curing small metastases. The method is of limited use, however, because it is cumbersome and has a high rate of complications. It has been used for over 20 years, but in relatively few institutions.

Ariel developed a simple pump by which he perfused phenylalanine mustard without the bubble-oxygenation of the perfusate. He treated 40 patients with this technique, perfusing for ± 30 minutes, 18 who had stage I or

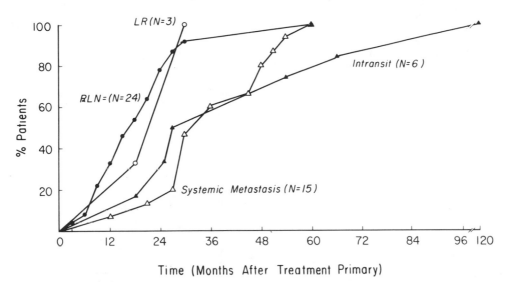

FIGURE 15-2. The site and timing of the first recurrence after excision of the primary and perfusion. Local recurrences and regional node metastases occur earlier. Intransit and systemic failures in large measure account for the biologic variability in melanoma. (Reproduced from Sugarbaker EV and McBride CM: The results of isolation-perfusion for invasive stage I melanoma of the extremities. Cancer 37(1): 188–198, 1976. Reprinted with the permission of the authors and the American Cancer Society, Inc.)

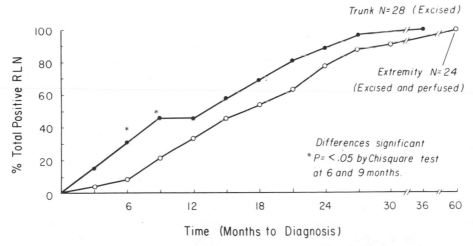

FIGURE 15-3. Comparison of the time of occurrence of regional node metastases from stage I trunk and extremity melanoma. (Reproduced from Sugarbaker EV and McBride CM: The results of isolation-perfusion for invasive stage I melanoma of the extremities. Cancer 37(1): 188–198, 1976. Reprinted with the permission of the authors and the American Cancer Society, Inc.)

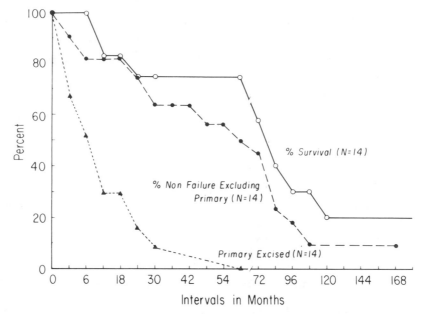

FIGURE 15-4. Survival and failure of extremity melanoma after perfusion without excision of the primary. (Reproduced from Sugarbaker EV and McBride CM: The results of isolation-perfusion for invasive stage I melanoma of the extremities. Cancer 37(1): 188–198, 1976. Reprinted with the permission of the authors and the American Cancer Society, Inc.)

II melanomas and 22 who had regional satellitoses (stage III). The results were more or less similar to those advocated by those who utilized oxygenation.[1]

INTRA–ARTERIAL INFUSION

Intra-arterial infusion differs from intra-arterial perfusion in that a catheter is placed in an artery proximal to the area to be infused. Using a pressure pump, a continuous infusion is given to the extremity over a prolonged period, varying from several days to several months. Techniques have been described by Creech et al.,[16] Bierman et al.,[10] and Golomb et al. The sites most suitable for infusion are both extremities and the pelvic region. The technique originated and advocated by Sullivan[46] is to infuse a dose of 50 mg of Methotrexate over 24 hours while 6 mg of

Citrovorum factor (Leukovorum) is given intramuscularly every 4 to 6 hours. Many drugs have been utilized for infusion, but the one we have used most frequently has been phenylalanine mustard, and more recently, cis-Platinum.

Complications that may occur are dislodgment of the catheter and sepsis. The utilization of a heparinized infusate will prevent clogging of the catheter. Systemic toxicity is greater than for perfusion.[40]

Clark[13] reported on 17 patients with advanced regional malignant melanoma who were treated with intra-arterial infusion therapy with DTIC for isolated inoperable lesions. He quoted six partial objective responses and one complete remission for an overall response rate of 41%. Toxicity was less than that usually seen with systemic chemotherapy of DTIC, and the local response was higher.

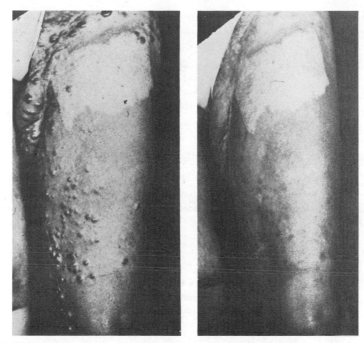

FIGURE 15–5. Left: Leg of a 52-year-old woman with extensive recurrent malignant melanoma. Right: The same patient seven months after perfusion with actinomycin-D. (Courtesy of Dr. Fred Golomb)

We have treated 55 patients with intra-arterial infusion for extensive melanoma of the extremities with an objective response in 35, and an apparent complete response in 5. There was no increased longevity. We have not used infusion as an adjuvant following surgery for the primary lesion with or without lymphadenectomy. The collected results of treatment by intra-arterial infusion are shown in Table 15–7.

Krementz et al.[32] believe that intra-arterial infusion can be used for those patients in whom isolation perfusion therapy is not suitable, such as those with an unacceptable operative risk or those who have failed to respond to perfusion or direct intralesional immunotherapy or chemotherapy. They consider it the treatment of choice for disease confined to a region that cannot be isolated by tourniquet, such as the head and neck area, proximal limb, or liver. They further believe that

infusion is required for utilization of agents requiring prolonged or continuous administration, such as the antimetabolites, and it can be used for palliation of regional diseases, or for making advanced diseases operable. The drugs they have used are summarized in Table 15–8.

Golomb[23] has treated 62 patients with primary melanoma by surgery plus infusion. Seven were of the upper extremity and 54 of the lower. Today 54 patients (72%) are free of disease; eight (13%) are living with disease; and nine (15%) have died of recurrent melanoma with distant metastases. Of the 35 patients treated more than five years ago, 23 (66%) are living. Of these patients 19 were in stage III, that is, with regional lymph node metastases at the time of operation five or more years ago. Furthermore, of these stage III patients, eight (42%) are living. Ten of these patients received Actinomycin-D as a chemotherapeutic agent; of these, two recurred. Five

TABLE 15–7.   Collected Results of Chemotherapy of Melanoma by Intra-Arterial Infusion

Author	Drug	Patients Treated	Complete Response	%Objective Responses
Westburg (1967)	Epodyl, mitopodozide (podophyllin derivative), procarbazine	75	4	69(32/46)
Oberfield and Sullivan (1969)	MTX, 5–FU	33	1	59(17/29)
Savlov, Hall, and Oberfield (1971)	DTIC	6	2	33(2/6)
Einhorn et al. (1973)	DTIC	17	1	41(6/17)
Jortnay (1977)	DTIC	4	—	50(2/4)

TABLE 15–8.   Drugs Used in 56 Patients Who Underwent Regional Chemotherapy by Intra-arterial Infusion

Agent	Number Treated	Daily Dose
DTIC	20	3–4.5 mg/kg × 7–12 day
MTX	13	4–10 mg/day to toxicity
TSPA		3 mg/day to toxicity
MTX	7	3 mg/day to toxicity
Act-D		0.3 mg/day to toxicity
1–PAM		2–5 mg/day to toxicity
MTX	4	3–5 mg/day to toxicity
1–PAM	3	5–10 mg × 10 days
HN_2	1	2 mg dose twice daily × 10 days
Misc.		
Comb	8	

were given Thio-Tepa alone, and four were given TSPA and Melphalan combined. The rest received Melphalan alone. There is accordingly moderate palliation and a suggestion in delaying or even preventing the onset of metastases but no spectacular result in curing metastases and a suggestion that some micrometastases could be destroyed by this technique.

SUMMARY

1. Chemotherapy does produce objective responses in shrinking and partially destroying melanoma, but no cures of existing melanomas can be attributed to chemotherapy.

2. A wide variety of drugs have been used. Imidazole Carboxamide (DTIC) appears to be the best available to date. Other drugs either in

combination with DTIC or without it have been useful.

3. Systemic adjuvant chemotherapy have not been successful in controlling dissemination of melanoma.

4. Regional perfusion may be useful in delaying or preventing regional metastases from developing. It has also proved useful in controlling some cases of regional spread. The complexity of the method has resulted in its use in relatively few institutions.

5. Intra-arterial infusion has resulted in debatable accomplishments both as an adjuvant or therapeutic method of chemotherapy.

6. A combination of chemotherapy and immunotherapy appear promising. The accomplishments to date of chemotherapy in controlling or combating malignant melanoma are meager.

7. The utilization of regional chemotherapy for in-transit metastases or satellitoses has been a welcome substitute for amputation, often used previously for treating these lesions.

REFERENCES

1. Ariel IM: A simplified method of isolation perfusion of anticancer drugs. Am J Surg 104:82, 1962

2. Ariel IM, Pack GT: Treatment of disseminated melanoma with phenylalanine mustard (melphalan) and autogenous bone marrow transplants. Surgery 51:583, May 1962

3. Ariel IM, Pack GT: Treatment of disseminated melanoma with systemic melphalan, methotrexate and autogenous bone marrow transplants. Cancer 20:77, Jan 1967

4. Aust JB: Melanoma and chemotherapy. In Ariel IM (ed): Progress in Clinical Cancer, Vol 6, Grune & Stratton, New York, 1975, pp 199–204

5. Banzet P, Jacquillat D, Civatte J, et al.: Adjuvant chemotherapy in the management of primary malignant melanoma. Cancer 41:1240, 1978

6. Bellet RE, Mastrangelo MJ, Berd D, Lustbader E: Randomized prospective phase III trial of methyl-CCNU (NSC-95441) alone versus methyl-CCNU plus vincristine (NSC-67574) in the treatment of patients with metastatic malignant melanoma. Proc Am Soc Clin Oncol 18:284, 1977

7. Bellet RE, Mastrangelo MJ, Laucius JF, Bodurtha AJ: Randomized prospective trial of DTIC (NSC-45388) alone versus BCNU (NSC-409962) plus vincristine (NSC-67574) in the treatment of metastatic malignant melanoma. Cancer Treat Rep 60:595, 1976

8. Bellet RC, Mastrangelo DB, Lustbader E: Chemotherapy of metastatic melanoma. In Clark WH, et al. (eds): Human Malignant Melanoma, Grune & Stratton, New York, 1979, pp 325–354

9. Benjamin RX: Chemotherapy of malignant melanoma. World J Surg 3:321, 1979

10. Bierman HR, Shimkin MB, Buron RL Jr, et al.: The effects of intra-arterial administration of nitrogen mustard, abstracted. Fifth Int Cancer Cong, Paris, 1950, p 186

11. Byrne MJ: Cyclophosphamide, vincristine and procarbazine in the treatment of malignant melanoma. Cancer 38:1922, 1976

12. Cavaliere R, Ciogatto EC, Giovanella BC, et al.: Selective heat sensitivity of cancer cells: Biochemical and clinical studies. Cancer 20:1351, 1967

13. Clark RH: The evolution of therapy for malignant melanoma at the University of Texas, M.D. Anderson Hospital and Tumor Institute 1950 to 1975. In Riley V (ed): Melanoma: Basic Properties and Clinical Behavior, New York, S Karger, 1977, pp 365–378

14. Cohen SM, Greenspan EM, Weiner MJ, Karakow B: Triple combination chemotherapy of disseminated melanoma. Cancer 29:1489, 1972

15. Coley WB: The treatment of inoperable malignant tumors with the toxins of erysipelas and the bacillus prodigiosus. Tr Am S A 12:183, 1894

16. Creech O Jr, Krementz ET, Ryan RF, Winblad JN: Chemotherapy of cancer: regional perfusion utilizing an extracorporeal circuit. Ann Surg 148:616, 1958

17. Davis CD, Ivins JC, Soule EH: Mayo Clinic experience with isolated limb perfusion for invasive malignant melanoma of the extremities. In Melanomas: Basic Properties and Clinical Behavior, Vol 2, Proc Ninth International Pigment Cell Conf, Houston Texas, 1975. New York, S Karger, 1976, p. 379

18. Davis NC: Invited commentary on: Hersh JT, et al.: Combined modality therapy of malignant melanoma. World J Surg 3:329, 1979

19. DeWasch G, Bernheim J, Michel J, et al.: Com-

bination chemotherapy with three marginally effective agents, CCNU, vincristine, and bleomycin, in the treatment of stage III melanoma. Cancer Treat Rep 60:1273, 1976

20. Didolkar MS, Baffi RR, Catane R, et al.: Use of methyl-CCNU and procarbazine in advanced malignant melanoma resistant to DTIC therapy. Cancer Treat Rep 61:1738, 1977

21. El-Domeiri AA, Das Gupta TK, Trippon M, et al.: Adjuvant therapy of melanoma. Proc Am Assoc Cancer Res 18:178, 1977

22. Golomb FM: Invited commentary on: Krementz ET et al.: Chemotherapy for malignant melanoma. World J Surg 3:302, 1979

23. Golomb FM: Perfusion. In Andrade R et al. (eds): Cancer of the Skin: Biology, Diagnosis, Management, Vol 2, Philadelphia, WB Saunders, 1976, p 1623

24. Gutterman JU, Mavligit G, Gottlieb JA, et al.: Chemoimmunotherapy of disseminated malignant melanoma with dimethyl triazeno imidazole carboxamide and Bacillus Calmette-Guerin. N Engl J Med 291:592, 1974

25. Gutterman JU, Mavligit G, McBride C, et al.: Active immunotherapy with BCG for recurrent malignant melanoma. Lancet 1:1208, 1973

26. Herbst WP: Malignant melanoma of choroid with extensive metastasis treated by removing secreting tissue of testicles. JAMA 122:597, 1943

27. Hersh EM, Jordan W, Gutterman MD, McBride CM: Combined modality therapy of malignant melanoma. World J Surg 3:329, 1979

28. Hill GJ, Moss S, Fletcher W, et al.: DTIC melanoma adjuvant study: final report. Proc Am Assoc Cancer Res 18:309, 1978

29. Howes WE: Castration for advanced malignant growth—short historical review and case report. Radiology 43:272, 1944

30. Howes WE: Removal of testes in treatment of melanoma. JAMA 123:304, 1943

31. Kaufman SD, Carey RW, Cosimin AB, Wood WC: Randomized trial of adjuvant therapy for high-risk primary malignant melanoma. Proc Am Assoc Cancer Res 19:374, 1978

32. Krementz ET, Carter RD, Sutherland CM, Campbell M: The use of regional chemotherapy in the management of malignant melanoma. World J Surg 3:289, 1979

33. Krieger H, Abbott WE, Levey S, Babb L: Bilateral total adrenalectomy in patients with metastatic carcinoma. Surg Gynecol Obstet 97:569, 1953

34. McCune WS: Discussion of Ochsner A, Harpole DH: Malignant melanoma. Ann Surg 155:636, 1962

35. McPherson TA, Paterson AH, Willans D, Watson M: Malignant melanoma (stage 111B): a pilot study of adjuvant chemo-immunotherapy. In Salmon WE, Jones SE, (eds): Adjuvant Therapy of Cancer, Amsterdam, Elsevier/North Holland Biomedical Press, 1977, pp 439–446

36. Nordman EM, Mantyla M: Treatment of metastatic melanoma with combined 5-fluorouracil and procarbazine. Cancer Treat Rep 61:1709, 1977

37. Pack GT: A note on the experimental use of rabies vaccine for melanomatosis. Arch Dermatol Syphilol 62:694, 1950

38. Pack GT, Ariel IM: Principles of treatment. In Treatment of Cancer and Allied Diseases, Vol 1. Paul Hoeber & Co, 1958, p 18

39. Rochlin DB, Wagner DE, Rochlin S: The therapy of malignant melanoma as treated by regional perfusion. In Melanoma and Skin Cancer. Proc Int Cancer Conf, Sydney, Government Printer, 1972, p 443–451

40. Savlov ED, Hall TC, Oberfield RA: Intra-arterial therapy of melanoma with dimethyl triazeno imidazole carboxamide (NSC–45388). Cancer 28:1161, 1971

41. Shear MJ, Turner FC: Chemical treatment of tumors: nature of hemorrhage–producing fraction from Serratia marcescens (Bacillus prodigiosus) Culture filtrate. J Nat Cancer Inst 5:81–97, 1943

42. Shimkin M: Effects of surgical hypophysectomy in many with malignant melanoma. J Clin Endocrinol 12:439, 1952

43. Shingelton, WW, Seigler HF, Stocks LH, Downs RW Jr: Management of recurrent melanoma of the extremity. Cancer 35:574–579, 1975

44. Stehlin JS Jr: Hyperthermic perfusion with chemotherapy for cancer of the extremities. Surg Gynecol Obstet 129:305, 1969

45. Stehlin JS, Jr, Giovanella BC, Ipolyi PD, Anderson RF: Eleven years' experience with hyperthermic perfusion for melanoma of the extremities. World J Surg 3:305, 1979

46. Sullivan RD, Miller E, Sykes MP: Antimetabolite-metabolite combination cancer chemotherapy. Effects of intra-arterial methotrexate-intramuscular citrovorum factor therapy in human cancer. Cancer 12:1248, 1959

47. Sugarbaker EV, McBride CM: The results of isolation-perfusion for invasive stage I melanoma of the extremities. Cancer 37:188, 1976

48. Wood WC, Cosimi AB, Carey RW, Kaufman SD: Randomized trial of adjuvant therapy for "high-risk" primary malignant melanoma. Surgery 83:677, 1978

CHAPTER SIXTEEN

PRIMARY CUTANEOUS MELANOMA: A REPORT FROM THE QUEENSLAND MELANOMA PROJECT*

NEVILLE C. DAVIS, G. RODERICK McLEOD,
GRAEME L. BEARDMORE, JOHN H. LITTLE,
REDMOND L. QUINN, AND JOHN HOLT

In Queensland, the average annual incidence rate of malignant melanoma per 100,000 population in 1976 was 14 for males and 17 for females, an average annual rate of 16 new patients per 100,000 population. It is now (1980) 33 cases per 100,000 of population per annus. This is the world's highest reported incidence.

No aborigines have been treated for melanoma in Queensland since the study began in 1963. No marked predilection was found in persons with a fair complexion, blue eyes, blond or red hair. Unlike squamous cell carcinoma, no particular concentration of melanoma on exposed sites was noted.

An environmental factor is probably responsible for the high incidence of malignant melanoma in Queensland; sunlight is the most likely etiologic agent, and possibly exerts both a direct and an indirect effect on the development of this skin cancer.

SURGICAL TREATMENT

EXTENT OF SURGERY

Not all patients with malignant melanoma should undergo the same treatment. The clinical and pathologic features of the tumor, its anatomical site, as well as the age and sex of the patient influence the prognosis and should be considered before deciding on the extent of excision.

PROGNOSTIC FACTORS

Patients with melanomas on the limbs fare better than those with melanomas on the back (Fig. 16-1). Tumors less than 2 cm in size have a better prognosis than larger ones. Flat lesions have a better prognosis than pedunculated or polypoid tumors. Ulceration is associated with poor prognosis. Women, particularly of premenopausal age, always survive longer than men, if other factors are equal (Figs. 16-2 and 16-3). However, the depth of tumor invasion and the profile of the tumor cells are probably the most important factors in prognosis. If the tumor cells are confined to the epidermis (melanoma in situ) or invade only to the papillary layer of the dermis (superficial malignant melanoma), the outlook is excellent (Fig. 16-4). If the melanoma has arisen from a Hutchinson's melanotic freckle (lentigo maligna) the prognosis is usually good. In contrast, if the melanoma has invaded to the reticular layer of the dermis or beyond, particularly if the dermal lymphatics are involved, the prognosis is poor (Fig. 16-4).

* Reproduced from Davis NC, McLeod GR, Beardmore GL, Little JH, Quinn RL, Holt J, Primary cutaneous melanoma: A report from the Queensland Melanoma Project, Ca—A Cancer Journal for Clinicians, 26(2):80-107, 1976, with permission of authors and the American Cancer Society, Inc.

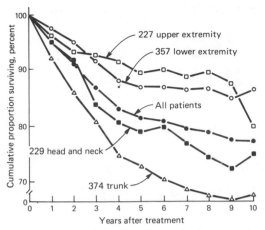

FIGURE 16-1. Age-adjusted survival curves for 1,187 patients with cutaneous melanomas, by site, Queensland, 1963-1967.

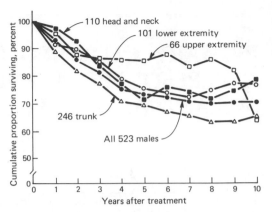

FIGURE 16-3. Age-adjusted survival curves for 523 males with cutaneous melanomas, by site, Queensland 1963-1967.

RECOMMENDATIONS

After considering all factors, the practical problem of how widely and deeply to excise a melanoma in an individual patient should be determined.

The extent of surgery advised in the literature varies widely, with a margin of from 2 to 15 cm. For lesions such as a subungual melanoma, amputation of a digit or extremity has been advocated. Olsen[24] favors preserving the deep fascia, while Cade[4] prefers a three-dimensional excision, which includes the deep fascia. Pack and colleagues[25] go further and recommend the inclusion of routine, elective regional node dissection with excision of the primary skin tumor.

A good standard margin for initial consideration is 5 cm. If the prognosis is thought to be good, the margin may be reduced. For example, a melanoma arising in a Hutchinson's

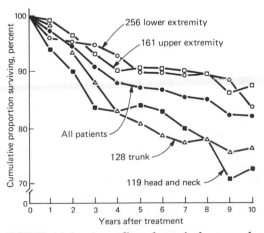

FIGURE 16-2. Age adjusted survival curves for 664 females with cutaneous melanomas, by site, Queenland, 1963-1967.

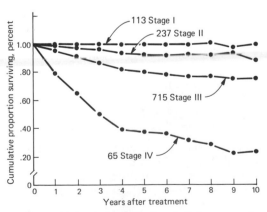

FIGURE 16-4. Age-adjusted survival curves for 1,130 patients with cutaneous melanomas, by stage, Queensland, 1963-1967.

melanotic freckle on the face of an elderly female requires excision with a margin of 1 cm or even less, depending on anatomical considerations. If the prognosis is considered poor, for instance, a melanoma on the back of a male, the width of excision may be increased. However, it has not been proven that this affects the result. All depends on surgical judgment; a 2-cm margin may be adequate for a small, slowly growing superficial spreading melanoma on the leg of a female and yet grossly inadequate for a large ulcerating nodular lesion near the axilla of a male, which may be better treated by excision with a margin of more than 7 to 10 cm toward the axilla and an in-continuity lymph node dissection.

Olsen has shown better results of excision when the deep fascia was preserved than when it was removed. We have not been able to confirm this finding, and the issue may not be of vital importance. We usually include the deep fascia when present, in order to reduce the risk of cutting too close to the deep surface of the tumor. The defect after excision should be covered by a split skin graft rather than a flap, except in special circumstances. Local recurrence is much easier to detect in a split skin graft than under a local flap.

One point must be reemphasized: the initial treatment of a melanoma is the most crucial, as it carries the greatest possibility of cure.

ROLE OF LYMPHADENECTOMY

Therapeutic lymphadenectomy is indicated if the regional lymph nodes draining a primary cutaneous melanoma are clinically involved or suspected. If they are not clinically involved, there is a good deal of controversy on the value of prophylactic (elective) lymph node dissection. We believe there is no place for the routine removal of apparently normal nodes. Obviously, the procedure can be beneficial only when apparently normal lymph nodes contain metastases; unfortunately, there is no way of knowing this information before operation. However, a knowledge of the factors that suggest, on statistical grounds, a good or bad

prognosis, helps forecast whether the lymph nodes contain metastases. For example, we believe that observation, rather than elective dissection, is indicated when the lesion is confined to the epidermis or papillary layer of the dermis. These issues have been discussed elsewhere (see also Chapter 6).

Elective lymph node dissection should rarely be done when:

The lesion is in an area with unpredictable lymph drainage, for example, in the middle of the back

The lesion is at a considerable distance from the regional nodes, e.g. below a knee or an elbow, and an in-continuity dissection is not feasible

The lesion is small, flat, and not ulcerated

The lesion has undergone no change or very little change over a period of a year or more

The lesion arises in a Hutchinson's freckle

The patient is a female or unfit for major surgery

The patient declines

The follow-up facilities are excellent

It is not easy to decide on absolute indications for elective dissection, but it seems reasonable to advocate the procedure when a deeply invasive melanoma or a pedunculated melanoma overlies or is immediately adjacent to the regional lymph nodes.

In patients with a poor prognosis, it may not be significant whether elective dissection is performed or a waiting policy is adopted, provided the follow-up is good. However, many surgeons advocate lymph node dissection for patients with poor prognoses even though some will die of blood-borne metastases. Knowing the statistical frequency of occult metastases in different circumstances may make the decision clearer.

In summary, elective dissection should be considered when:

The primary tumor is in the immediate vicinity of regional nodes or relatively close to a lymph node area

The primary tumor is in an area where it can be expected to have a bad prognosis

There is microscopic evidence of pedunculation or invasion to the reticular dermis or beyond

The lesion is large, ulcerated, nodular or pedunculated and rapidly growing

The lesion was previously inadequately excised or treated by cautery

The patient is a male or fit for major surgery

The patient requests the procedure after discussion of its pros and cons

The follow-up facilities are poor

When possible, the operation should be synchronous with excision of the primary tumor and all tissue between the primary growth and nodes removed in-continuity with radical dissection of the nodes.

SURVIVAL DATA

Data on survival are presented for all 1,187 patients with cutaneous malignant melanoma treated in Queensland between 1963 and 1967, and then subdivided by sex and site, according to the life table method. The closing date of this study was June 30, 1974, giving all patients a minimum follow-up period of five years. The loss to follow-up in the first five years was less than 5%. After the fifth year, those patients with incomplete follow-up were termed as lost for the purposes of this study. Therefore, the statistical significance of the survival rates after five years decreased.

METHODS

Survival data, except for the age-adjusted cumulative survival rate, were computed using the Biochemical Computer Programs software package (program BMDOIS) of the U.C.L.A. Computer Center, and the PDP-10 digital computer of the University of Queensland Computer Center. The input data for the program BMDOIS were constructed from magnetic tape files containing patient records updated to include follow-up information until June 30, 1974. Survival rates were based on time of first treatment. For the pur-

poses of this chapter, all deaths were regarded as the result of the melanoma.

The age-adjusted cumulative survival rate (the fraction of patients alive at a given time, divided by the fraction of controls with the same age distribution expected to be alive at that time) provided a base for comparison of survival from one group of patients to another. In calculating age-adjusted survival, the expected survival rates of the control groups were determined by using the Australia Life Tables for 1966, published by the Commonwealth Bureau of Census and Statistics. Although the great majority of patients were from Queensland, no published life tables were available from this area for any period during 1963–1967. Unpublished 1966 life table data for Queensland revealed no significant difference from the Australia tables, and the latter were adopted.

RESULTS

Anatomical Distribution. Table 16–1 shows the anatomical distribution of cutaneous melanomas by sex. Patients with multiple primary melanomas and with unknown primary tumors have been excluded. The trunk and the lower extremity were the two most common sites.

Sex Distribution. Of the 1,187 patients, 664 (55.9%) were women and 523 (44.1%) were men. The most common sites in women were, in order of frequency, lower leg, upper arm, and back, and in men, the back, face, and lower leg.

Age. The age distribution of all patients is shown in Figure 16–5. The highest incidence for the whole group and for each sex occurred in patients between 35 and 49 years old.

Age-Adjusted Cumulative Survival. The age-adjusted cumulative survival data for the entire series of 1,187 patients is shown in Table 16–2, and the curves in Figure 16–1. As can be seen, 81.6% survived five years.

TABLE 16-1. Anatomical Distribution of Cutaneous Melanomas, by Sex; Queensland, 1963–1967

Site	All Patients		Males		Females	
	No.	Percent	No.	Percent	No.	Percent
Head and neck	229	19.3	110	21.0	119	17.9
Face	132	11.1	58	11.1	74	11.1
Neck	62	5.2	22	4.2	40	6.0
Ear	16	1.3	14	2.7	2	0.3
Scalp	19	1.6	16	3.1	3	0.5
Trunk	374	31.5	246	47.0	128	19.3
Chest	61	5.1	40	7.6	21	3.2
Back	286	24.1	186	35.6	100	15.1
Buttock	6	0.5	3	0.6	3	0.5
Abdomen	21	1.8	17	3.3	4	0.6
Lower extremity	357	30.1	101	19.3	256	38.6
Thigh	87	7.3	41	7.8	46	6.9
Leg	237	20.0	48	9.2	189	28.5
Foot, dorsum	17	1.4	4	0.8	13	2.0
Foot, plantar	11	0.9	6	1.1	5	0.8
Foot, subungual	5	0.4	2	0.4	3	0.5
Upper extremity	227	19.1	66	12.7	161	24.2
Arm	153	12.9	44	8.4	109	16.4
Forearm	61	5.1	17	3.3	44	6.6
Hand, dorsum	6	0.5	3	0.6	3	0.5
Hand, palm	2	0.2	0	0.0	2	0.3
Hand, subungual	5	0.4	2	0.4	3	0.5
Total	1187	100	523	100	644	100

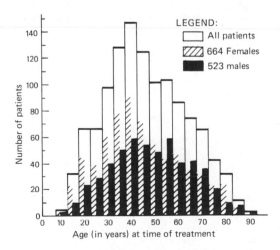

FIGURE 16–5. Age distribution of 1,187 patients with cutaneous melanomas, Queensland, 1963–1967.

Survival of Women. The age-adjusted survival data for the 664 women is shown in Table 16–3, and the curves, subdivided by site, in Figure 16–2. Overall five-year survival for women was 87.7%. Highest survival rates were found in women with melanomas on the limbs, the next highest in those with lesions on the head and neck. Survival was worst for tumors on the trunk.

Survival of Men. The age-adjusted survival data for the 523 men is shown in Table 16–4, and the curves, subdivided by site, in Figure 16–3. Overall five-year survival for men was 73.6%. Five-year survival was highest for lesions on the upper limb, rather than the lower limb, followed by head and neck. It was worst for tumors on the trunk.

TABLE 16-2. Cumulative Survival over 10 Years for 1,187 Patients with Cutaneous Melanomas

Period (in years) after first treatment	0–1	1–2	2–3	3–4	4–5	5–6	6–7	7–8	8–9	9–10
Number alive at beginning of interval	1187	1110	1039	960	885	832	727	513	293	145
Number died during interval	73	67	67	60	32	20	23	11	9	2
Number "lost to follow-up" during interval	4	4	12	15	21	85	191	209	139	108
Effective number exposed to risk of dying	1185.0	1108.0	1033.0	952.5	874.5	789.5	631.5	408.5	223.5	91.0
Proportion surviving	.938	.940	.935	.937	.963	.975	.964	.973	.960	.978
Cumulative proportion surviving (treatment to end of treatment)	.938	.882	.824	.773	.744	.725	.699	.680	.653	.638
Age standardized cumulative proportion surviving	.954	.913	.869	.831	.816	.811	.798	.793	.778	.777
Standard error	.007	.009	.011	.012	.013	.013	.014	.015	.017	.019

Survival Related to Depth of Invasion. The depth of tumor invasion has been subdivided by our pathologists into four histological stages:

1. Tumors limited to the epidermis, i.e., intraepidermal (melanoma in situ)
2. Invasion of the papillary zone of the dermis (superficial malignant melanoma)
3. Invasion of the reticular dermis
4. Invasion of subcutaneous fat

(Staging considered in this section is histological and does not refer to spread of the tumor beyond its primary site.) The description of the depth of invasion in levels, developed in 1969 by Clark and others, was accepted by an international meeting of pathologists in Sydney, Australia. Our histological stages correspond to Clark's levels as follows:

Stage I = Level I
Stage II = Level II or III
Stage III = Level IV
Stage IV = Level V

Of the 1,130 patients whose tumors were staged, 113 (10%) had stage I; 237 (21%), stage

TABLE 16-3. Cumulative Survival over 10 Years for 664 Women with Primary Cutaneous Melanomas

Period (in years) after first treatment	0–1	1–2	2–3	3–4	4–5	5–6	6–7	7–8	8–9	9–10
Number alive at beginning of interval	664	638	610	571	534	509	446	312	182	93
Number died during interval	23	26	31	26	12	10	11	5	7	1
Number "lost to follow-up" during interval	3	2	8	11	13	53	123	125	82	69
Effective number exposed to risk of dying	662.5	637	606	565.5	527.5	482.5	384.5	249.5	141	58.5
Proportion surviving	.965	.959	.949	.954	.977	.979	.971	.980	.950	.983
Cumulative proportion surviving (treatment to end of treatment)	.965	.926	.878	.838	.819	.802	.779	.763	.726	.713
Age standardized cumulative proportion surviving	.978	.950	.914	.885	.877	.873	.861	.858	.829	.829
Standard error	.007	.010	.013	.014	.015	.016	.017	.018	.022	.025

TABLE 16-4. Cumulative Survival over 10 Years for 523 Men with Primary Cutaneous Melanomas

Period (in years) after first treatment	0–1	1–2	2–3	3–4	4–5	5–6	6–7	7–8	8–9	9–10
Number alive at beginning of interval	523	472	429	389	351	323	281	201	111	52
Number died during interval	50	41	36	34	20	10	12	6	2	1
Number "lost to follow-up" during interval	1	2	4	4	8	32	68	84	57	39
Effective number exposed to risk of dying	522.5	471.0	427.0	387.0	347.0	307.0	247.0	159.0	82.5	32.5
Proportion surviving	.904	.931	.916	.912	.942	.967	.951	.962	.976	.969
Cumulative proportion surviving (treatment to end of treatment)	.904	.826	.756	.690	.650	.629	.598	.576	.562	.544
Age standardized cumulative proportion surviving	.926	.866	.813	.761	.736	.731	.715	.707	.710	.708
Standard error	.013	.017	.019	.020	.021	.021	.022	.023	.025	.029

II; 715 (63%), stage III; and 65 (6%), stage IV.

The age-adjusted survival curves for 1,130 patients, subdivided by histological stage, are shown in Figure 16-4. At five years, there were no deaths in patients with stage I melanomas. Five-year survival for patients with stage II lesions was 93.1%; for stage III, 80.6% and for stage IV, 37.8%.

Of 1,187 patients, 79 (6.7%) had confirmed metastases either at the beginning of treatment or within one month. Of these 79 patients, 60(5%) had metastases in the regional lymph nodes; the remainder had distant metastases. This is a remarkably low figure when compared with other series.

A comparison of our survival data with four major well-documented series from the United States, England, and Denmark shows that patients treated for malignant melanoma in Queensland have better survival rates than patients with the same disease in these other countries.

Why? We believe improved survival is due to two factors: public and professional education. The Queensland public is aware of the incidence of skin cancer and the potential danger of any change in a mole, due largely to continual publicity from the Queensland Anti-Cancer Council and the Queensland Health Education Council. Primary physicians are alert to the possibility of melanoma in any pigmented lesion, often make the diagnosis at an early biological stage, and immediately refer the patient for appropriate surgery.

Similar practices in all parts of the world could change the whole spectrum of the disease and significantly improve the outlook of patients with malignant melanoma.

ACKNOWLEDGMENT

The Queensland Melanoma Project is financially supported by the Queensland Cancer Fund and the Clive and Vera Ramaciotti Foundations. We thank Mr. D.Crowley and Mr. R. Fox of the Princess Alexandra Hospital for photographic services and the Queensland Health Education Council for Help in preparing the illustrations.

REFERENCES

1. Cade S: Malignant melanoma. Ann R Coll Surg Engl 28:331–366, 1961
2. Olsen G: The Malignant Melanoma of the Skin. The Finsen Institute and Radium Centre, Copenhagen, 1966
3. Pack GT, Scharnagel I, Morfit M: The principle of excision and dissection in continuity for primary and metastatic melanoma of the skin. Surgery 17:849, 1945

PART TWO

MALIGNANT MELANOMAS OF SPECIFIC ANATOMIC SITES

CHAPTER SEVENTEEN

MELANOMA OF THE HEAD AND NECK

RONALD C. HAMAKER AND JOHN CONLEY

Melanoma is the most interesting malignant neoplasm clinically encountered by the head and neck surgeon. The unpredictability of this enigmatic disease make it a distinct clinical challenge. A fundamental knowledge of the lymphatics with adjunctive pathologic expertise are essential to the surgeon in undertaking effective surgical management of this problem. Once having established the diagnosis, immediate and competent care is essential.

A recent analysis of 772 melanomas in the head and neck from the Pack Medical Foundation was undertaken to add to the biologic understanding of this disease, to review the evolutionary changes in the concepts of its management and to cite the results of treatment.[5] In this 40-year survey completed in 1972 there was sufficient information available in several categories of analysis to produce meaningful results. In addition to a statistical analysis of site variation, the significance of pathology, surgical principles in biopsy, and ablative techniques will be emphasized in this chapter.

Melanomas of the head and neck represented approximately 20% of all melanomas recorded at the Pack Medical Foundation. Ocular melanomas totaled 112 cases but are, henceforth, excluded from this discussion. The statistical information in this chapter has been derived essentially from the detailed analysis of 660 cutaneous and mucosal head and neck melanomas. Mucosal primaries consisted of 59 cases or approximately 9% of the head and neck melanomas, 601 being cutaneous in origin.

GENERAL CONSIDERATIONS

Melanocytes are derivatives of the neural crest and are the cell of origin for melanoma. These cells are distributed widely throughout the body and have a regional distribution of considerable variation. The cheek and forehead have the highest concentration of melanocyte population, having two to three times more than other cutaneous areas. The mucosal surfaces, though devoid of overt pigmentation, have a high concentration of melanocytes. Distributional patterns may explain the wide variation of primary sites as well as the increased frequency of this disease in the head and neck. The facial area accounted for 32.3% of all cases and included the cheek, forehead, eyebrows, eyelids, lips and chin (Table 17–1). Melanomas of the cheek comprised 67% of the entire facial group and represented the most common location, with an incidence of 22% of all head and neck melanomas. Melanoma occurred with equal frequency in the scalp and ear areas, the temporal region accounting for 52% of the scalp lesions or approximately 10% of head and neck melanomas. Postauricular skin accounted for 36% of the ear melanomas with the helix as primary site in 25% of ear melanomas. In the neck, the lateral neck was the most common location, with a 42% occurrence rate for cervical melanomas as compared to the suprasternal, nape, or supraclavicular regions of the neck.

Mucosal melanomas were found in the paranasal sinuses, nose, nasopharynx, middle ear, larynx, and oral cavity. Oral cavity lesions represented 43% of the 59 primary mucosal melanomas, the majority of these being on the hard palate or in maxillary alveolar areas. Middle ear and mastoid sites accounted for ten cases, or 17% of mucosa primaries.

Primary melanoma of unknown origin comprised 3.2% of the head and neck cases. At the time of the review, there were 118 cases of melanoma primaries of this category in the Pack Medical Foundation records. Of these, 21 were in the head and neck and represented approximately 18% of the total unknown

TABLE 17–1. Distribution of Head and Neck Melanoma—Excluding Eye (660 Cases)

	Number of Cases	Percentage
Face	213	32.3
Scalp	130	19.7
Ear	123	18.6
Neck	90	13.6
Mucosal	59	8.9
Unknown	21	3.2
Nose	16	2.3
Miscellaneous	8	1.2

From Conley J, Hamaker RC: Melanoma of the head and neck. **Laryngoscope, 87:760–764, May 1977**

primary tumors or a percentage equal to that of the head and neck melanomas (20% head and neck). Sixteen of the 21 cases presented as involved cervical nodes, five cases were extranodal deposits of metastatic melanoma with three in the cheek, one in the buccal area, and one in the trachea. The incidence of 3.2% of unknown head and neck primaries agrees with Das Gupta et al.[7] who reported an incidence of 3.7% in 992 cases of total body melanomas. The occult primary melanoma again points out the enigmatic qualities of melanoma. This lesion is either masquerading as a benign, innocuous lesion or as a primary melanoma that has undergone spontaneous regression prior to metastasizing. This situation is threatening, but is not an insurmountable problem to the patient if it is possible to remove all detectable melanoma.

Nasal melanomas are relatively rare and constituted only 16 cases or a 2.3% occurrence among the head and neck lesions. Primary site areas were ala (4), dome (5), and nasal dorsum (7).

All age groups were represented in the Pack series. The largest number, 127, was tabulated in the sixth decade. This differed from that cited for the general distribution of melanoma, wherein the fifth decade was the most common age group involved.[13] Tumors occurred with almost equal frequency in the fourth, fifth, and seventh decades and together patients in the fourth to seventh decades comprised over

75% of all the head and neck cases. The disease occurs in the young, and 18 cases appeared in children under the age of 16 with 13 of these ten years or younger. In the case of one male child, nine months of age with melanoma of the face, there was an obvious likelihood of transference of melanoma across the placenta, as the mother died of melanoma shortly after birth. In 32 cases the age was not recorded.

In general, melanoma tends to be slightly more common in females. This, however, has not been the case in the head and neck region. The tumor incidence in females was 256 cases as compared with 380 cases in males, or a 1-to-1.5 ratio. A 2-to-1 male predominance of tumor incidence was noted in the four most common decades of life and there were no age groups with an incidence greater in females than males. Distribution by sex and age is correlated in Table 17–2.

TABLE 17–2. Correlation of Age and Sex

Age (Years)	Female	Male	Total
10 years or less	6	7	13
11–15	2	3	5
16–20	6	14	20
21–30	21	40	61
31–40	46	75	121 (122)
41–50	49	69	118 (121)
51–60	48	78	126 (127)
61–70	47	54	101 (104)
71–80	21	26	47 (48)
> 80	2	5	7
Total	248 (256)	371 (380)	619 (628)

( ) = Number in age or sex group but without correlation. From Conley J, Hamaker RC: Melanoma of the head and neck. **Laryngoscope 87:760–764, May 1977**

Correlation of the anatomical site with sex demonstrated a 3-to-1 male to female ratio in the scalp and ear sites. Nasal and mucosal primaries occurred more often in males (2 to 1), with an equal distribution between the sexes in the cervical melanomas. The face was the only site where the female predominated in tumor incidence, but only by 2%. Largely responsible for this slight shift in frequency of occurrence in the female was the 1.6-to-1 female-to-male ratio in primary melanoma of the cheek. The fourth decade was the peak age for the disease to occur in the ear, fifth decade for the scalp, neck, and nasal areas. The sixth decade was the peak age for facial sites of disease and the seventh decade for mucosal primary melanomas.

Consistent with observations of the occurrence of primary melanomas of other body areas, the blonde, blue-eyed patient with fair complexion predominated in presenting with melanomas in the head and neck. In this large series, there were no blacks reported with melanoma. The usual primary symptom in 65% of the cases consisted of an enlarging mole, a change in pigmentation of a cutaneous lesion, or the presence of an enlarged cervical node.

There were 256 cases of a preexisting mole in 361 cases where this category of analysis was surveyed. This accounted for 70% of the cases analyzed and agrees with many studies that have shown preexisting moles in over half of the melanoma cases.[10] In the majority of cases, once a change occurred in a preexisting mole or birthmark, the diagnosis was made within six months. However, 30% of patients had waited longer than one year before bringing the observation of change to the attention of a physician to establish a diagnosis. Diagnosis was delayed for over two years in 15% of cases.

While change in pigmentation is an important sign, one must be cognizant of the amelanotic melanoma. It is considered relatively rare and often presents extreme difficulty in diagnosis for the pathologist. It is reported to occur in 1.9% of malignant melanoma cases.[12] In 289 cases of the 660 in the Pack series, the pathology was described in detail rather than being signed out as malignant melanoma. There were 30 cases of amelanotic melanoma in the head and neck. This is 10% of 289 cases described in detail or 4.5% of the 660 total cases included in this review. One could surmise that the incidence is close to the 4.5% figure, inasmuch as it is usually the case that amelanotic melanoma will either have a detailed description given or is found to be the true diagnosis from the review of a cervical node. The incidence of 4.5% in the Pack study suggests that amelanotic melanoma may occur more frequently in the head and neck than in other regions of the body.

DIAGNOSIS

Urgency of diagnosis is indicated in all malignant tumors and melanoma is no exception. Clinical diagnostic accuracy in assessing melanoma has been established at 64%.[14] Excisional biopsy is the best mode of diagnosis, and is especially true in melanoma since determination of the level or depth of invasion is essential for prognostication and determination of follow-up appropriate surgical management.

Incisional biopsy in melanoma has been condemned as being harmful to the patient by some who are of the opinion that the procedure causes dissemination of tumor and diminishes the prospect for favorable prognosis. Incisional biopsy has been proven to have minimal negative effect on the prognosis if the lesion is treated appropriately and promptly after biopsy.[9] A disadvantage of incisional biopsy lies in not obtaining a representative sample of the level of deepest invasion of the lesion.

Lentigo maligna melanoma, most common to the head and neck, may contain many foci of invasive melanoma and have different depths of penetration (Figure 17–1). An excisional biopsy of a large lentigo maligna to rule out melanoma could be quite deforming. In this situation, incisional biopsy should be performed in suspicious areas. The sampling may suggest a level II invasion and a definitive treatment would include only wide local excision. The permanent histopathologic section could demonstrate level IV invasion and thus suggest the need for a neck dissection. This deeper level of invasion fortunately is not common. Thus, this lesion points out the problem inherent in the use of incisional biopsy, which is essential here, and the problem of inadequate sampling.

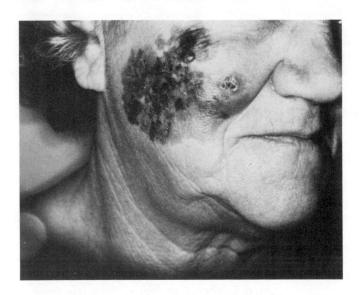

FIGURE 17-1. Lentigo maligna melanoma of right cheek with level II and level IV melanomas in same lesion.

It was possible to determine the method of diagnosis in 457 of the 660 cases. Incisional biopsy was done in only 13% to establish the diagnosis. Excision of a metastatic node established the diagnosis in 11% of the cases and in the latter situations the primary melanoma often had undergone excision without confirmation of a positive diagnosis. If the case was misdiagnosed, the node biopsy then became conclusive. In this group the primary melanoma may have undergone spontaneous regression as well. A thorough search for the primary lesion should be made and in many cases the scalp is likely to be that site. The importance of undertaking a complete examination of the head to include the scalp must be emphasized when a node presents without an obvious primary lesion.

PATHOLOGY

Clark's description of levels of invasion has been a major contribution to the definition of treatment of melanoma over the past eight years.[3] Donnellon et al.[8] correlated the Clark levels with the incidence of neck metastases. No longer does it suffice for the pathologist to state that melanoma is superficially spreading, arising in lentigo maligna or nodular, but rather the specific level of deepest involvement or depth must be recorded. The histopathology report can be utilized to determine if a regional node dissection is necessary.

It was apparent in the review of 772 cases that the diagnosis of malignant melanoma carried with it a wide variation of the degree of malignancy and emphasized the importance of Clark's description of the pathology. Of the 289 cases that could be retrospectively classified by Clark's levels, 19% occurred in level II. The remaining 81% were in levels III through V. This series of head and neck melanomas was weighted toward the highly aggressive, deeply penetrating levels of tumor invasion. Determinate deeply invasive melanomas have a direct correlation with the prognosis as an increase in pathologic regional nodes and distal metastasis occurs. It is unfortunate that in mucosal melanomas no means is available to prognosticate or to indicate predictive regional spread.

The diagnosis was changed in 23 of the 289 cases, an 8% frequency. A review of nodal pathology was utilized for change of diagnosis in ten of the 23 cases and the change of diagnosis most usually involved the amelanotic melanoma, undifferentiated carcinoma, or reticulum cell sarcoma. Similarly, the anaplastic and spindle-cell variance of melanoma added to the pathologist's dilemma. Desmoplastic melanoma is a variant of spindle-cell melanoma that leads to bulky subcutaneous tumefactions, and generally is located in the head and neck. This series contained four cases with only six prior cases reported in the literature.[6] The subcutaneous nodules histologically appeared to be invasive fibrous tumors. The lesion is recurrent locally and often metastasizes. Melanoma may assume many variable and bizarre histological and clinical patterns and the outcome of this variation in form and pathology is usually fatal.

CLINICAL STAGING

The classification of Sylven[15] that stages melanomas into local disease stage I, regional disease stage II, or distal metastases stage III, has been utilized for years but is not adequate. Ballantyne's modification[1] of McNeer and Das Gupta's classification, better adapted to classifying head and neck melanoma, was utilized in our review of the 660 cutaneous and mucosal melanomas. Table 17–3 summarizes this classification and makes note of recurrent stage I disease or recurrent primary disease in stage II. Recurrent primary disease is a more serious entity and is viewed as either an aggressive disease or as an inadequately treated tumor. In the future, a classification similar to the Ballantyne modification, but which incorporates pathologic depths of invasion, will be of more value in prognosis and comparison of treatment.

Of the 660 cases, 478 could be staged. In stage IA were 213 and 50 in stage IB, giving a composite of 56% in stage I. The prognosis for IB is far worse than for IA since there is a greater incidence of nodal metastases in the former. This poor prognosis demonstrated in stage II disease as the primary recurrent (stage IIC) group was indicated in one-third of the cases. The level of invasion of the original lesion bears no relationship to regional metastases when the lesion is recurrent.

It has been reported that local recurrences are more likely to occur in females[1] because of

TABLE 17–3. Clinical Staging of Head and Neck Melanoma

Stage	
I	Local disease
IA	Primary intact or recently incised or excised
IB	Primary recurrent
II	Regional metastases
IIA	With primary intact or recently incised or excised
IIB	Primary controlled
IIC	Primary recurrent
IID	Primary excised node or nodes excised
IIE	Primary unknown
III	Distant metastases

From Ballantyne AJ: Malignant melanoma of the skin of head and neck. Am J Surg, 120:425–431, 1970

the practice of more conservative excisional surgery in women and an increased incidence of superficial spreading melanomas with indiscrete margins in females. In this large series, there was a 2-to-1 predominance of disease in male to female in stages IB and IIC with recurrent primary disease. This could represent an earlier detection of melanoma and consequent allowance for wider excision of smaller lesions in females. It may correlate with the occurrence of more superficial disease in females with less tendency for local recurrence.

Stage II disease represented 33% and stage III disease 11% of all cases staged by Ballantyne classification. It is again apparent that this series of cases is weighted in favor of the more aggressive disease, since 55% of the cases tabulated were stages IB, II, and III, the more aggressive melanoma as seen on initial presentation.

All of the cases under age ten were in stage IA, except for one in IIA. Of the 18 cases of the 17 years or younger age group, three were in stage II. In age group 16 to 20, an increase in regional metastases occurred in six of 20 cases. Two of the six cases were in stage IID wherein a node had been excised and the diagnosis consequently changed. The suspicion of melanoma is low in this age group and represents a warning to be alert to the possibility of dealing with melanoma regardless of the age of the patient.

NODAL DISEASE

There is a high predictability for direction of spread in head and neck tumors. In the majority of head and neck melanomas, the predictability of lymphatic spread to regional nodes is consistent with their clinical behavior. As the surgeon initiates the treatment of melanoma, all potential lymphatic avenues of spread should be reviewed and a fundamental knowledge of all superficial and deep lymphatics in the head and neck is an absolute requirement. Clinical experience enhances the expertise of understanding the behavior of melanoma.

It should be readily understood that a deeply invasive melanoma of the scalp anterior to the auricle (level III to V) will pass through the parotid in its lymphatic dissemination. The occurrence of primary tumor posterior to the auricle requires a posterior neck dissection of the lymphatic structures in conjunction with a routine radical neck dissection. Spread of tumor from the forehead, temporal region, eyebrow, eyelids, nose, cheek, ear, and lips has the potential of passing through the paraglandular parotid nodes. As the site of occurrence of the melanoma approaches the anterior aspect of the face, the tendency for metastasis to be directed to the parotid decreases, the (pre- and postvascular) submandibular node involvement increases. In a review of 100 cases of malignancy in the parotid caused by some secondary extension to it or of metastatic disease, 45% were secondary to malignant melanoma.[4] This points out the importance of inspection of the temporal region, scalp, ear, and face for a primary lesion before removal of a so-called *parotid tumor.*

The locations of the regional metastasis and the primary tumor site of the melanoma were cross-tabulated in 196 cases. Thirty-six of these cases were temporal lesions, and 25 of these (69%) had metastases either solely to the parotid or in conjunction with cervical metastasis. The parotid was involved in metastatic melanoma in 37.7% of the facial areas and in 36.8% of the primary lesions of the auricle. Only 8% of the cervical and 13% of the mucosal primaries could be evaluated in regards to metastatic site, and eventually also involving the parotid.

The incidence of bilateral nodal disease was 5.4% and solely contralateral metastasis occurred in 1.1%. As expected, the bilateral disease was noted in primaries of the scalp, mucosa, and cervical areas.

In Table 17–4, 33.5% of cases had regional metastasis on initial examination, a value, however, which increased to 50% as the interval in time from the date of primary treatment increased. It was possible to correlate the occurrence of nodal disease after the primary lesion had been treated in 179 cases. In patients with regional metastasis, 63% were noted on the initial examination or presented within the first year, 16% occurred in the second year, and 15.6% were noted as occurring in the three- to five-year interval following initial treatment. Only 5% of the cases had regional metastases develop five years after the primary had been treated.

DISTAL METASTASES

In our melanoma series, 11% of the cases presented with distal disease. Evaluation was possible in 188 cases for the occurrence of distal disease after treatment of the primary. Thirty-seven of these cases developed distal disease within the first year or presented initially as stage III, another 20% developed distal disease during the second year, 31% occurred from the third to the fifth year, and 8.5% occurred after five years. In one case, recurrence as distal metastasis was noted 28 years after treatment of the primary. Ocular melanoma quite typically presents with distal disease many years after treatment of the primary and obviously differs from the other head and neck melanomas.

In 219 cases, autopsies were performed and

TABLE 17-4. Classification of Stages

Stage	No. Cases	Percent
IA	213	55.9
IB	50	
IIA	35	
IIB	36	
IIC	52	33.5
IID	22	
IIE	12	
III	50	10.6

From Conley J, Hamaker RC: Melanoma of the head and neck. Laryngoscope 87:760-764, May 1977

distal metastatic sites were recorded. The lung was involved as the only distal site in 9% of the cases, but in combination with other sites in 45% of the cases. The liver in combination with other organs was implicated in 29% of distal metastatic deposits. Cutaneous and subcutaneous deposits were present in 27% of the cases. The brain alone as a metastatic focal area occurred in 4% of the cases, whereas isolated bone deposits were noted in only 1.8% of cases. This data supports the conclusion that the work-up for diagnosis of distal metastatic melanoma of the head and neck requires tomograms of the lung, a thorough examination of the skin, and a liver scan for liver function studies. Brain and bone scans have yielded isolated evidence for metastases in approximately 6% of the cases. Clinical suspicion would warrant inclusion of the latter two studies in the battery of tests to be considered.

TREATMENT

The plan for treatment is determined by the circumstances of the presenting melanoma as well as by the physical status of the patient. Obviously if the patient cannot tolerate therapeutic goals because of a mental or physical disability, then these goals must be varied to best accommodate the problem. Similarly, one plan for treatment is not ideal for all malignant melanomas. Localized or regionalized melanoma of the head and neck is a surgical disease whereas the circumstance of widespread melanotic deposits requires a totally different management rationale. As discussed in the pathology section in this chapter, the consideration of the level of invasion is essential to the decision regarding nodal dissection.

Surgical approaches can be divided into wide local excision, radical neck dissection, composite resection, and isolated distal metastatic excision. Wide local excision varies from excision to a 1 cm margin about a lentigo maligna, level I melanoma, to a 2 to 3 cm margin about a superficial spreading level II melanoma of the face, and to a 5 to 7 cm margin about a scalp melanoma. Lymphatic and hematogenous spread of tumor correlated with the rich vascularization of the scalp, as well as local permeation as observed, require a much wider excision than that required in other areas of the head and neck. It must be emphasized that wide local surgical excision is concerned not only with radial excision of skin but with the vertical depth of excision, which must include the fascia of the underlying muscle in the resection. This could jeopardize deeper structures such as the frontal branch of the facial nerve in the temporal or lateral forehead melanomas. In the scalp, the excision is extended to, but does not include, the periosteum, unless obvious disease is present in the periosteum. In this latter situation the outer table of the skull would necessarily be included in the specimen.

Surgical reconstruction is by primary closure when possible and often can be accomplished in cervical or facial excisions. Split-thickness skin grafting is usually required in frontal, temporal, and nasal areas and always in the melanomas of the scalp. The scalp cannot be closed primarily if adequate resection has been accomplished. Regional or local flaps are utilized to close defects over bone that is devoid of periosteum, i.e. recurrent melanoma of the scalp with excision of the periosteum, or in areas where vital structures require more coverage than that provided by a skin graft.

The need for a neck dissection is obvious in the presence of clinically positive invasive, regional, or nodal disease. It has been shown in head and neck melanomas that if the depth of invasion is at level III or deeper, then a prophylactic neck dissection is beneficial, since the incidence of neck disease varies from 35% for level III to 65% for level V.[8] This potential for extension of the disease justifies the elective neck dissection in primary disease of levels III to V. Technically significant to the neck dissection is the incorporation of the platysma muscle into the resection. This is important in order to resect the superficial lymphatics, which can be permeated by melanoma.

Unfortunately, midline lesions do not lend themselves to a predictable side of secondary involvement. Bilateral posterior neck dissection and/or bilateral radical neck dissections may be warranted in aggressive midline lesions of the occiput or anterior neck. A lesion on the vertex of the scalp in the midline would potentially metastasize to both parotids and bilaterally to the anterior and posterior neck. In this situation, it is best to wait for ultimate manifestation of metastases to determine the appropriate regional nodal therapy. The same rationale applies for management of midline lesions of mucosal areas.

Parotidectomy becomes a major part of the surgical treatment in nodal dissection. In the presence of gross disease, a radical parotidectomy is performed and includes ablation of the facial nerve. Reconstruction of the facial nerve is accomplished by nerve graft or by hypoglossal crossover. If, however, the parotid is removed as a part of an elective or prophylactic dissection, it is recommended that the facial nerve be preserved. The parotid should be resected electively in all lesions of the temporal and frontal areas, auricle, eyelids, eyebrow, and lateral posterior cheek, any of which demonstrates deep invasion.

For ablation of those lesions that require nodal resection, the method of choice includes composite resection of the primary tumor, the cervical lymphatics, and the intervening parotid, if indicated. If discontinuous resection is employed, the intervening superficial and deep lymphatic channels may be lost, resulting in potential permeation of the

melanoma. A composite resection quite obviously cannot be accomplished in certain mucosal lesions, i.e. nasopharynx, nose, and paranasal sinuses. In cases of lesions of the hard palate and maxillary alveolus, resection in continuity would result in major mutilation of the face.

Isolated metastases may be treated with local definitive surgery, recognizing, however, that a solitary lesion could in fact represent a different disease process and must be carefully evaluated in the patient with melanoma. Craniotomy, pneumonectomy, or skin excision for solitary lesions was performed in 33 cases of this series. While the ultimate result was only palliative, in some cases the life of the patient was extended for a considerable period of time.

In certain instances, radiation therapy has been helpful in the treatment of primary disease and in nodal melanoma when surgery was not recommended or could not be utilized. In isolated cases, its use has resulted in cure and is noted in this review of head and neck cases. However, there have been patients in whom the entire area included in the radiation port, after receiving low-voltage radiation, has become melanomatous. Technical advances have been made in radiation therapy and it is anticipated that even newer methods will become available in the future. While radiation therapy has been noted to be a useful adjunct for the management of distal metastatic disease,[11] it is palliative for the most part. The primary and regional melanotic disease remains a process managed ideally by the surgeon.

Electrodessication has played a role in the therapeutic treatment of melanoma, especially in mucosal lesions. The scope of the original surgical resection can be extended by electrodessication of the margins of the resection. This can decrease the extent of oral mutilation yet allow for good local control of the primary disease. Recurrent mucosal lesions can be handled satisfactorily by cautery. Cryotherapy, another thermal tool available, has been found to be of benefit in a limited number of cases of mucosal melanomas.[2]

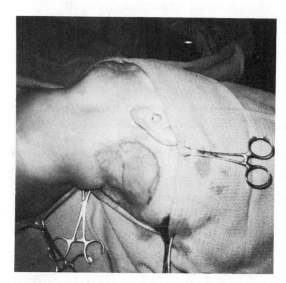

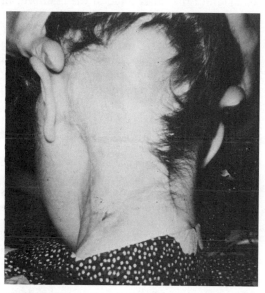

FIGURE 17–2. Patient being prepared for reexcision and radical neck dissection. Her original lesion was level IV melanoma, excised widely but not to periosteum, and the specimen had nodal disease.

FIGURE 17–3. Same patient as in Figure 17–2 after wide reexcision to periosteum and including radical and posterior neck dissection.

Recurrent primary melanoma deserves special attention. A major error can be made in allowing excisional biopsy to supplant the use of more definitive therapy. It must be remembered that biopsy procedures are strictly diagnostic in nature. If by biopsy all margins are shown to be clear of melanoma, a definitive wide local excision is in order as outlined above, with an appropriate margin achieved radially about the incisional scar and deep to include the underlying fascia. Procrastination in the face of a positive biopsy is detrimental to the prognosis of the patient and must be avoided.

Another error results from the acceptance of the diagnosis of malignant melanoma without the indication given of the level of invasion. This point is necessarily reemphasized throughout this chapter to be certain that the nature of the lesion is not underestimated and to ensure that adequate treatment is instituted. When wide local excision demonstrates nodal disease in the specimen, another error has been introduced (Figs. 17–2 and 17–3). Reexcision obviously is required since lymphatics with potential tumor have been crossed, and the entire excisional site is contaminated at its margins both peripherally and deep.

The treatment of recurrent disease, if the primary occurred in level II, is the same as that for level V disease. The disease process (Fig. 17–4) has been changed by the surgical intervention with resulting potential of lymphatic involvement. The original excisional site, whether wide or limited in scope, requires reexcision to include a deeper and wider margin (3 to 4 cm) in composite with a regional node dissection. The depth of excision proceeds to muscle or deeper if the original excision included fascia. Recurrent scalp melanomas represent specific reexcisional problems if the original specimen was taken at the level of the periosteum as recommended for all scalp melanomas. This requires excision of the periosteum and in many cases excision of the outer table of the cranium. In this situation, reconstruction requires a split-thickness skin graft on the exposed diploic surface of the skull, or the rotation into the wound of a large scalp flap. The latter method is usually more conducive to primary healing and presents less of a problem postoperatively.

RESULTS

The overall prognosis of patients with melanoma in the head and neck varies according to the presence of microscopic metastases to the regional nodes. Many published results have not been correlated with the pathology and staging of the disease process. In 119 head and neck melanomas reported by Donnellon et al.,[8] a ten-year actuarial survival rate for disease in level II was given as 86% and in level V as 44%. Ballantyne reported a 76.9% five-year survival rate when an elective neck dissection demonstrated no evidence of disease, as compared with 26% in the presence of clinically positive neck dissections.[1]

In our series, the absolute five-year or greater cure rate was analyzed in 556 of the 660 cutaneous and mucosal melanomas of the head and neck. We report 25.6% of our patients free of disease after five years and an additional 9.3% alive at five years who succumbed to the disease later. Cutaneous head and neck melanomas, excluding the mucosal and unknown primary lesions, showed a five-year absolute cure rate of 27.8%. Mucosal lesions showed an 8% five-year or greater absolute cure rate, with an additional 12% alive at five years who subsequently died of the disease.

The absolute or greater five-year cure rate was 35.4% for all patients who were treated solely at the Pack Medical Foundation. A much more serious prognosis was shown for the patients who were initially treated by the referring physician, but a delay occurred prior to definitive therapy or no further therapy was done until metastatic disease presented itself. In this group was the biopsy excision with clear margins and a wait-and-see approach. The five-year or greater absolute cure rate was

18.8%. This again points out the importance of prompt and appropriate treatment.

Melanotic disease of the scalp had the worst prognosis. While 31.8% were alive at five years, only 16.5% were ultimately determined to be free of disease beyond five years. Nasal lesions, although comprising a small group, had an excellent overall outlook since 60% were observed to be without disease five years or longer. This probably represents early diagnosis with appropriate and prompt therapy. Face and ear sites had identical five-year or greater absolute cure rates of 32.6%. Cervical lesions had a five-year survival rate of 28% while in the cases with unknown primary sites, there were no patients alive over five years. The procedure of elective radical neck dissection was compared with no neck dissection in 175 cases involving melanotic disease stage IA. The absolute five-year or greater survival of all cases with an elective radical neck dissection was 55% as compared with 38.5% with no elective neck dissection. Distal metastases developed in 30% of the cases submitted to elective neck dissection. In contrast, distal disease developed in 70% of the cases treated by therapeutic neck dissections. The absolute five-year or greater cure rate was 12.6% for cases with positive nodes.

SUMMARY

Consistent with our own experiments and those reported by others in the biology and proper management of malignant melanoma, we conclude that head and neck melanoma is a pathologic lesion that can be cured, given an early diagnosis. Success in management is fundamentally dependent upon the surgeon having a thorough knowledge of the lymphatic system of the head and neck and on dependable and reliable pathology consultation.

ACKNOWLEDGMENT

This chapter is dedicated to the late Dr. George T. Pack. He introduced me to the disease of melanoma 32 years ago in what proved

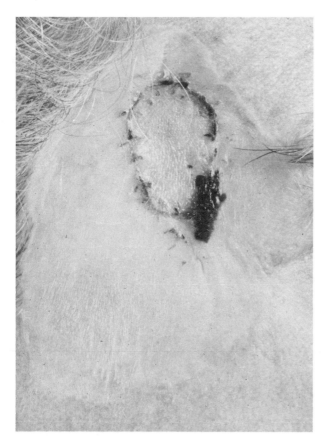

FIGURE 17-4. Recurrent disease in graft site after two operations. Wide local excision of level III melanoma was accomplished originally. Forehead was not paralyzed and obviously a deep margin was not obtained. Recurrent disease locally removed without removal of original graft was similarly inappropriate.

to be an unusual clinical experience with this disease. His energy, searching, and intelligence generated an interest in melanoma that produced a volume of over 3,000 cases over a 37-year period. His associates fully recognized the value of this experience and their indebtedness to his leadership. Seven hundred and seventy-two of these cases of melanoma at the Pack Medical Foundation occurred in the area of the head and neck. Dr. Ronald C. Hamaker studied these melanomas as a Special Fellow in head and neck surgery at the Pack Medical Foundation, abstracted their data, and subsequently carried out this analysis at the University of Indiana. Although it is a retrospective study, it reveals the biological behavior of melanoma, its treatment, and the results produced by one group of workers over three decades of practice.   J.C.

REFERENCES

1. Ballantyne AJ: Malignant melanoma of the skin of head and neck. Am J Surg 120:425–431, 1970
2. Barton RT: Mucosal melanomas of the head and neck. Laryngoscope 85:93–99, 1975
3. Clark WH Jr, Bernardion EA, Mihm MC: The histogenesis and biologic behavior of primary human malignant melanomas of the skin. Cancer Res 29:705–726, 1969
4. Conley JJ: Salivary Glands and the Facial Nerve. New York, Grune & Stratton, 1975
5. Conley J, Hamaker RC: Melanoma of the head and neck. Laryngoscope 87:760–764, May 1977
6. Conley J, Lattes R, Orr W: Desmoplastic malignant melanoma (a rare variant of spindle cell melanoma). Cancer 28:914–936, 1971
7. Das Gupta T, Bowden L, Gerg JW: Malignant melanoma of unknown primary origin. Surg Gynecol Obstet 117:341–345, 1963

8. Donnellon MJ, Mayer T, Huvos AG, et al.: Clinicopathologic study of cutaneous melanoma of the head and neck. Am J Surg 124: 450–455, 1972

9. Epstein E, Bragg K, Linden G: Biopsy and prognosis of malignant melanoma. Arch Dermatol 111: 1291–1292, 1975

10. Franklin JD, Reynolds VH, Bowers DG Jr, Lynch JB: Cutaneous melanoma of the head and neck. Clin Plast Surg 3(3):413–427, 1976

11. Hilaris BS, Raben M, Calabrese AS, et al.: Value of radiation therapy for distant metastases from malignant melanoma. Cancer 16:765–773, 1963

12. Huvos AG, Shah JP, Goldsmith HS: A clinicopathologic study of amelanotic melanoma. Surg Gynecol Obstet 135:917–920, 1972

13. Kopf AW, Bart RS, Rodriguez-Sains RS: Malignant melanoma: A review. Dermatol Surg Oncol 3(1):43–125, 1977

14. Kopf AW, Mintzis M, Bart RS: Diagnostic accuracy in malignant melanoma. Arch Dermatol 111:1291–1292, 1975

15. Sylven B: Malignant melanoma of skin. Acta Radiol 32:33–59, 1949

CHAPTER EIGHTEEN

MALIGNANT MELANOMA OF THE EYE AND ORBIT

IRA S. JONES
AND LAURENCE DESJARDINS

Since pigment is a necessary anatomic and functional part of the visual apparatus, it is to be expected that abnormalities of pigment formation and growth will be encountered (Fig. 18–1). The ocular and adnexal structures are common sites for benign and malignant melanomas, and the frequency of their appearance in this area is greater than that for most other areas of the body (Fig. 18–2). The capability of observation and inspection of these abnormalities by the observer, and the appreciation of the existence of an abnormality by the patient enable early detection and facilitate successful management.

TERMINOLOGY

Melanoma terminology is undergoing transition. The usual nomenclature is probably not the final word, but in general ophthalmologists term melanomas benign or malignant, and divide the latter into low grade and high grade, depending on their clinical behavior and cell type. The greatest confusion is in the naming of melanomas involving the skin and mucous membrane. The nature of the nevus, the necessity for nevus cells to be present, and even whether nevus cells are characteristic are questions that remain unanswered.

MELANOMAS OF THE VARIOUS EYE AND ADNEXAL STRUCTURES

Rather than take the ocular and adnexal structures in the usual front-to-back anatomical survey, it seems preferable to discuss the most

significant melanomas in order of their importance, which will necessitate jumping from one area to another. In the approximate order of importance, these are melanomas of the choroid, melanomas of the iris, melanomas of the iris and ciliary body, melanomas of the skin and of the subcutaneous structures, melanomas of the mucous membrane, and melanomas of the orbit.

NEVUS OF THE CHOROID

It is now common practice to refer to a benign melanoma as a nevus. Some authors prefer to use the name *benign nevus* and avoid the term *benign melanoma*, melanoma being an ominous word often used synonymously with malignant melanoma by Scandinavian workers. The more explicit term benign melanoma might be preferable according to Reese,[12] "nevus" referring to a congenital pigmented lesion of the skin, mucous membrane, and other sites.

Benign choroidal melanomas are easily discovered on routine examination of the eye and are best seen with the indirect ophthalmoscope because of the low contrast between these melanotic spots and the surrounding fundus (Fig. 18–3). With the direct ophthalmoscope, magnification reduces contrast, and often the lesions are found only with the indirect ophthalmoscope with its lower magnification. They are generally ovoid and flat, have feathered edges, and a fairly regular border. The long axis is usually radial to the posterior pole of the eye. There may be overlying white spots or drusen, especially in those

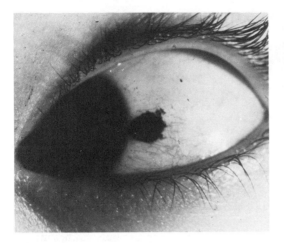

FIGURE 18-1. Pigmented nevus of conjunctiva.

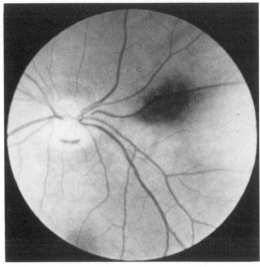

FIGURE 18-3. Benign melanoma or nevus of the choroid.

that have existed for a long time. They are probably not acquired, although the fact that they are seen more often in older individuals leads to the assumption that pigmentation increases with the passage of time. Over long periods of observation, they do not grow in area, although the overlying surface may become thicker and show more drusen. Transillumination is not significantly interfered with.

The B-scan ultrasonogram can be normal or show a slightly elevated lesion if the height of the tumor is more than 1 mm, but the tissue cannot be differentiated, as the mass is too small to have a characteristic echo pattern. However, the ultrasonogram is useful in following the lesion to establish whether the lesion is growing.

Benign choroidal melanomas usually do not produce a visual field defect. Scotomas have

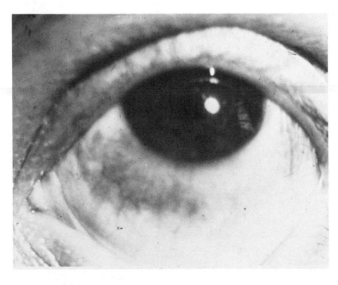

FIGURE 18-2. Partial melanosis oculi.

been reported when the melanoma involves the overlying choriocapillaris, when drusen changes of the lamina vitrea are particularly marked, or when the overlying retina is slightly elevated.

The fluorescein angiogram usually shows no abnormal characteristics with fluorescein dye. However, the tumor can produce a hypofluorescent filling defect in the normal pattern of the background. Some nevi associated with drusen can appear hyperfluorescent angiographically because of thinning of the pigment epithelium and because of dye staining of the subpigment epithelium material.

Congenital hyperplasia of the retinal pigment epithelium, which produces a flat, sharply demarcated, ovoid, dark gray to black lesion, can be mistaken for a melanoma, particularly when it is five disc diameters in size or larger. Small nonpigmented foci are occasionally seen. These lesions have no growth potential. No field defect can be elicited. The pigmented portion of the lesion remains nonfluorescent or hypofluorescent throughout the course of angiography.

MALIGNANT MELANOMAS OF THE CHOROID

Malignant melanomas of the choroid may come to the attention of the patient because of the defect in the visual field, or because of entopic phenomena such as light flashes because of the tenting of the retina around the melanoma as it becomes thicker (Fig. 18–4). There may also be interference with visual acuity as the central retina is involved (Fig. 18–5). The patient may notice dilated vessels on the white of the eye, which correspond to the position of the tumor inside the eye and are caused by the tumor's need for blood circulation. The observer sees a dark subretinal mass that tends to be globular but may be mushroom-shaped or button-shaped. A large base, a thin neck, and then a larger part more central or toward the interior of the eye results from the melanoma's breaking through the elastic lamina of Bruch, which constricts the growth around the neck but allows more

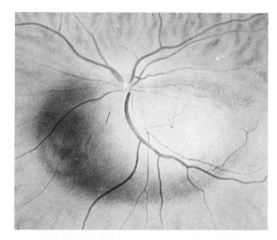

FIGURE 18–4.   Melanoma of the choroid.

growth of the part near the center of the eye. This constriction around the neck also leads to dilatation of the blood vessels in the dome of the melanoma and sometimes to hemorrhage from these dilated vessels. Hemorrhage is not a prominent feature of the usual malignant melanoma. An orange pigment, lipofuschin, is often seen on the dome of these lesions (Fig. 18–6).

Choroidal malignant melanoma gives a visual field defect; transillumination of light

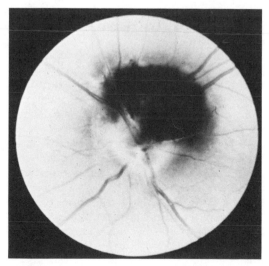

FIGURE 18–5.   Melanocytoma of the optic nerve spilling into adjacent retina and choroid.

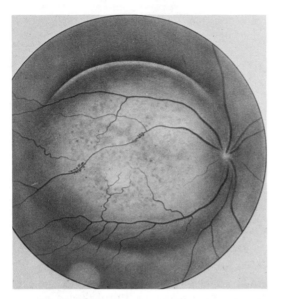

FIGURE 18–6. Melanoma of the choroid. The faint irregular markings on the dome represent orange lipofuschin pigment.

from the outside of the eye on the sclera at the tumor is definitely interfered with, both for the observer looking through the pupil to see the light coming back through, and also for the patient, as the light is passed from uninvolved to involved sectors in moving it along the sclera. The patient's perception is that the light dims or goes out when it gets behind the melanoma.

The differential diagnosis of choroidal melanomas poses some problems. Pigment spots in the fundus that may be confusing are usually retinal pigment spots: These include congenital grouped retinal pigmentation, sometimes called bear tracks; hypertrophy of the retinal pigment of a solitary nature, sometimes called benign melanomas of the pigment epithelium; and proliferated retinal pigment epithelium from irritation such as chorioretinitis. On the optic nerve head and adjacent to it, there may be dark pigmentations, usually benign, due to melanocytes and melanocytomas. Deep hemorrhage under the retinal pigment epithelium can mimic a choroidal melanoma, especially in the early stages when the outlines are sharp and the color is almost

black. Periodic observation over the course of a few weeks will usually eliminate this confusion because the blood does not remain contained but begins to seep, which it would not do in the case of a melanoma. Metastatic neoplasms from distant sites to the choroid may occasionally be misleading, although these are usually light in color and are often multiple. This, in connection with a history of a primary malignant neoplasm elsewhere, such as carcinoma of the breast, is usually sufficient to make the diagnosis clear. Hemangiomas of the choroid, which are benign lesions, are perhaps the most troublesome because they often have irritative pigment proliferation, and it is difficult to distinguish them on clinical grounds from malignant melanoma (Fig. 18–7). It is in this area that the proponents of ^{32}P tests claim the greatest ability to distinguish between benign and malignant lesions.

Ultrasonography is particularly useful in detecting tumors in eyes with opaque media but can also provide helpful information in cases where the tumor can be visualized ophthalmoscopically. In these cases, ultrasonography can differentiate melanomas from other posterior masses, measure the height of the tumor, and follow up the lesion after conservative management. B-scan ultrasonography is the most easily interpreted by the clinician, since its two-dimensional display corresponds to the histologic cross-section of the eye. With the sonometric unit, the A-scan echoes can be displayed simultaneously with the B-scan, thus facilitating the interpretation of more difficult cases. The B-scan ultrasonogram in malignant melanoma shows a dome or mushroom-shaped mass with retinal detachment and strong border echo. An acoustic quiet zone within the tumor is often seen, due to the very homogenous solid tissue. There is a very characteristic choroidal excavation in about 40% of the cases. Shadowing of the orbital fat occurs with large tumors, which occasionally attenuate sounds by their great mass. These B-scan features of the melanomas can differentiate them from metastatic carcinomas, hemangiomas, and subretinal hemorrhage. When a nonrhegmatogenous retinal

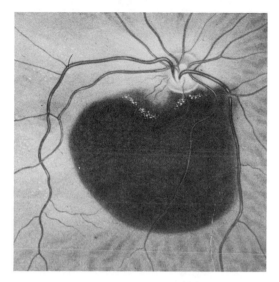

FIGURE 18-7.   Hematoma under the retinal pigment epithelium. This mimics melanoma, but the hemorrhage visible along the central border gives a clue to the diagnosis.

detachment is suspected because of the absence of breaks, smooth bullae, and shifting fluid, elevated intraocular pressure or large iris nevi, ultrasonography should be performed and can visualize the tumor.

The angiographic pattern of choroidal malignant melanomas may vary, depending upon how vascular the tumor is, how much overlying pigment there is between the observer and the vessels containing the dye, and how much pooling there is. The lesion typically shows mottled fluorescence in the arteriovenous phase and prolonged retention of the dye by the tumor. It seems that one of the reasons for the fluorescence observed in choroidal malignant melanomas is the destruction of the retinal pigment epithelium. Fluorescein angiography provides useful information in the evaluation of suspected tumors in most cases.

The ³²P test is somewhat controversial. Some authors think that a ³²P uptake estimation properly performed with precise localization over the tumor itself permits great accuracy in diagnosing malignant tumors of the choroid. Others feel this is not valid. The ³²P

test cannot be considered reliable in distinguishing small benign melanomas from small choroidal melanomas and cannot distinguish between different types of malignancies.

The usual classification from the least to the most malignant pathologically is spindle A, spindle B, mixed, and epithelioid type. The spindle cells have a narrow oval nucleus and an indistinguishable or ill-defined nucleus. Epithelioid cells are round or polygonal and vary considerably in size and shape but are usually rather large; the nucleus is round, large and nucleolated; and multinucleolated forms may be present. The abundant cytoplasm is usually acidophilic. The arrangement of cells is fascicular, tubular, funicular, alveolar, or the growth pattern may be nondescript. Diffuse flat growth occasionally occurs and may involve a wide portion of the uvea or even the entire uvea. Necrosis and its sequelae may be a prominent feature.

In the case of large malignant melanomas, where vision has already been lost or will soon be lost with progression of the tumor, the usual preferred management is removal of the eye. Choroidal malignant melanomas metastasize, and there is a strong correlation between the age of the tumor, the size of the tumor, and the presence of metastases. Consequently, a young individual with a malignant melanoma of the choroid has a greater period of time in which metastases can occur, and the tumor should be either removed or sterilized in order to prevent this from happening. The most easily identified site of metastasis is the liver, and a liver scan should be carried out to determine whether this has in fact already occurred. Smaller malignant melanomas may justifiably be observed for a period of time to determine how rapidly they are growing, since the chance of metastasis from a small lesion is less, and since the growth characteristics are not yet known. It is possible to discourage and, in some instances, probably to sterilize small malignant melanomas of the choroid by radioactive cobalt buttons sewed to the sclera under the base of the tumor. Radon needles have been used, but radioactive cobalt appears to be preferable. Photocoagulation has also been used, and this has proved effective in some instances. The spread of malignant melanomas may be hematogenous to distant sites or by direct extension through the sclera into the orbit. If at the time of enucleation it is apparent that the melanoma has extended through the sclera, it can be presumed that not only is there orbital contiguous spread, but the likelihood of distant hematogenous spread is greater. Nevertheless, local excision of the contaminated orbital tissues may be carried out, and in some instances this will prove to be effective, since the more serious distant spread may not be confirmed. Immunotherapy is discussed in Chap. 8.

The tumor diameter is the single most important clinical and pathological factor in prognosis. The cell type is also an important prognostic factor, with a 15-year mortality as follows: spindle A 20%; spindle B 25%; mixed and necrotic 60%; and epithelioid 70%. Mixed cells are found in 50% of large tumors, and in 20% of small tumors. Other factors have a prognostic importance: mitotic activity of the tumor, tumor height, extrabulbar extension, condition of Bruch's membrane, pigmentation, and location of the anterior border of the tumor. Small melanomas composed of spindle cells with no mitotic activity and no spontaneous necrosis have a good prognosis.

IRIS AND CILIARY BODY MELANOMAS

The iris is highly visible, contains pigment, and often shows pigment spots. These spots may be discrete, flat, and of no significance, such as iris freckles; they may be discrete, slightly thickened, and may represent nevi; they may represent migration or implantation of pigment from the back pigment epithelial layer of the iris onto the iris stroma in front and may appear as very dark, flat spots (Fig. 18-8); they may be sector pigmentation of a congenital nature that is benign. There may even be heterochromia iridis in which the congenital pigmentation of one iris is significantly darker than another, so that the patient may have one brown and one blue eye. Malignant melanomas of the iris, or benign nevi that have undergone malignant transformation, show growth, splinting of the iris or deformation of the iris's normal mobility, pushing aside of the adjacent iris stroma into wrinkles and folds, hypervascularity, and extension onto the back surface of the iris (Fig. 18-9). When identified before reaching the iris root, these can be removed by a sector iridectomy. Malignant iris lesions may extend into the iris root and thence into the ciliary body, and ciliary

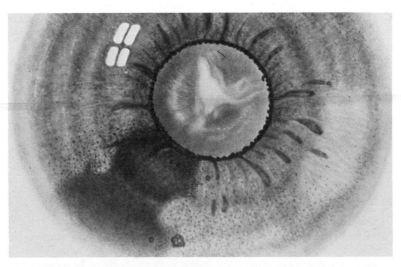

FIGURE 18-8. Sector pigmentation of iris or partial melanosis oculi.

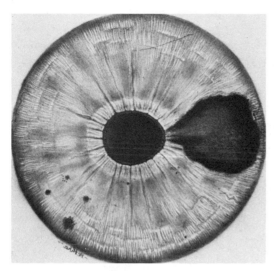

FIGURE 18-9. Nevus of iris. If growth and increased vascularity occur, the diagnosis becomes melanoma.

and nonpigmented nevi, warts, the darker blue nevi, and chemical or foreign body pigmentation such as that engendered by the use of epinephrine or from mascara. If a pigment spot on the skin of the lids shows growth, increased thickness, ulceration or hypervascularity, biopsy or excision is in order. Pigmentation of the skin, particularly near the lid margin, is often part of a process also involving the mucous membrane of the conjunctival sac. Sometimes these pigmentations of the skin and conjunctiva are matched in the upper and lower lids, so that when the lids are closed the nevi coincide; these are called *kissing nevi*. The conjunctiva may have discrete, slightly thickened nevi that early in life may be non-pigmented but during adolescence under hormonal influences will gain pigment; these

body malignant melanomas may extend into the iris root and into the iris itself (Fig. 18-10). Sometimes, melanomas from either source in the root of the iris will prefer to follow the vascular circle of the iris around the iris root, leading to the ring melanoma; this is sometimes difficult to identify because of its position and may become apparent only as glaucoma supervenes. Ring melanomas can be managed only by removal of the eye (Figs. 18-11 and 18-12). Malignant iris and ciliary body tumors that occupy no more than 60° of the circumference of the eye at the limbus may be removed by iridocyclectomy, either with or without an overlying button of cornea and sclera. For properly selected cases, the survival and function have been good.

SKIN AND CONJUNCTIVAL MELANOMAS

The majority of pigment spots on the skin of the lids and on the lid margin are of no significance; these include freckles, pigmented

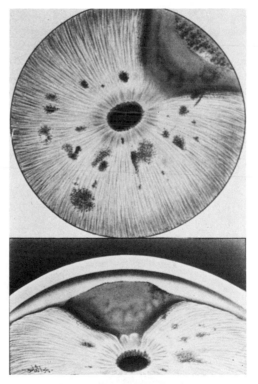

FIGURE 18-10. Melanoma of iris and ciliary body. The latter is assumed because of the obvious angle involvement.

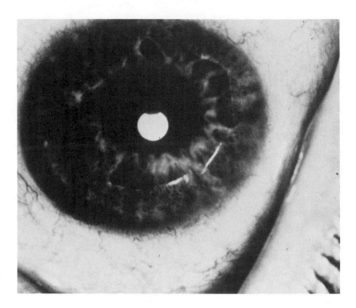

FIGURE 18-11. Ring melanoma of iris.

benign spots may be left alone but often are removed for cosmetic or psychological reasons. There is a remote possibility that they may undergo malignant transformation (Fig. 18-13). In adolescence, very aggressive and dangerous-looking melanosis of the conjunc-

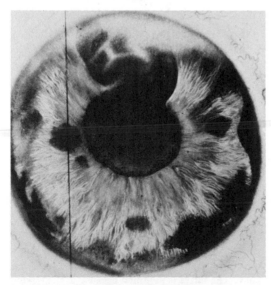

FIGURE 18-12. Ring melanoma of iris with satellite implantations on the iris surface.

tiva may occur, which has hypervascularity, and under the microscope the cells look extremely active. These, however, are benign lesions of short natural history and are called juvenile melanomas. Flat pigmentation of the conjunctiva is usually called melanosis and generally does not pose a threat to the patient. These melanosis areas of the conjunctiva are benign, although they may change their areas, going from one geographic shape to another, with some areas that had previously been pigmented becoming clear and others becoming pigmented. There are apparently pluripotential areas in the conjunctiva where conjunctival melanosis becomes darker and more active, with extensive staining, especially in the fornices. It may represent a transformation into precancerous melanosis, and the precancerous melanosis in time usually goes on to frank cancerous melanosis or malignant melanoma of the conjunctiva. The usual length of time between the first appreciation of precancerous melanosis and the development of frank melanoma averages ten years (Fig. 18-14).

The management of malignant melanoma of the conjunctiva has undergone change in recent years. For a long time, it was felt that exenteration of the orbit with removal of the lids and all of the orbital contents down to bone of-

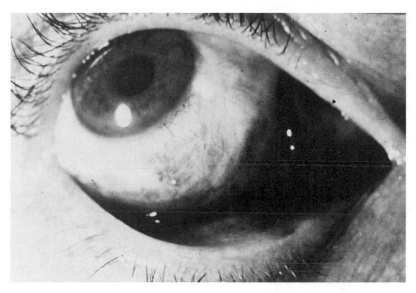

FIGURE 18-13. Precancerous melanosis of lids and conjunctiva.

fered the best chance of recovery. It has gradually become apparent that regional spread through the lymphatics is more likely than distant metastasis of a hematogenous nature, since the malignant melanoma of the conjunctiva usually does not extend deeply but in a pagetoid manner near the surface, and the re

cent development has been to remove the tissues near the front of the eye including skin, lids, conjunctiva and the subjacent tissues, followed by lymphatic dissection in continuity of the face and regional nodes. It is even possible in some cases to preserve the globe, although not as a functioning organ.

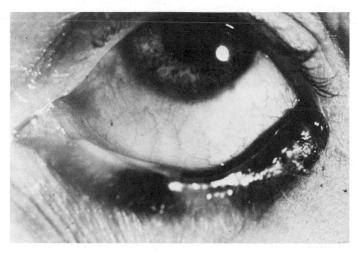

FIGURE 18-14. Precancerous melanosis of lids and conjunctiva that has transformed into malignant melanoma.

Zimmerman's classification of conjunctival pigmented lesions is as follows:

I. Congenital Melanoses
  A. Epithelial
    1. Ephelis
  B. Subepithelial
    1. Ocular melanocytosis (melanosis oculi)
    2. Oculodermal melanocytosis (nevus of Ota)
II. Nevi
  A. Intraepithelial (junctional)
  B. Subepithelial (dermal)
  C. Compound
  D. Spindle/epithelioid (juvenile melanoma)
  E. Blue nevus
  F. Cellular blue nevus
III. Acquired melanoses
  A. Bilateral
    1. Racial
    2. Metabolic
    3. Toxic
  B. Unilateral
    1. Secondary (usually racial)
    2. Primary idiopathic
IV. Malignant Melanomas
  A. In congenital melanosis
  B. In nevi
  C. In acquired melanosis
  D. From uveal melanomas
  E. Metastatic
  F. De novo

Designations recommended by McGovern et al. (1973) are as follows:

Lesions with Radial Growth Phase and Spreading Pigmentation That Give Rise to Invasive Melanomas

I. Hutchinson's melanotic freckle
  A. Lentigo maligna
  B. Senile freckle
  C. Precancerous melanosis
  D. Acquired melanosis
  E. Dubreuilh's melanosis

II. Superficial spreading melanoma, noninvasive
  A. In-situ melanoma
  B. Pagetoid melanoma
  C. Premalignant melanosis
  D. Precancerous melanosis
  E. Acquired melanosis
  F. Dubreuilh's melanosis

The following outline is Zimmerman's Histologic Staging of Acquired Melanosis.

I. Stage I—Benign Acquired Melanosis
  A. With minimal or no melanocytic activity or atypia
  B. With moderate to marked melanocytic activity and/or atypia
II. Stage II—Malignant Acquired Melanosis
  A. With minimal superficial invasion of substantia propria by malignant melanocytes*
  B. With moderate to marked invasion of substantia propria†

CONGENITAL MELANOMAS

Congenital melanomas form a group with similar characteristics. They are benign and usually occur in hyperpigmented individuals (Fig. 18–15). This group includes melanocytoma, blue nevus, cellular blue nevus, congenital ocular melanosis, and congenital dermal melanosis. Congenital melanomas and malignant melanomas that may arise from them have a greater tendency to be familial than other melanomas. Since the blue nevi can be viewed as congenital aberrations, evidence of other associated anomalies of the eye is not

* Idiopathic unilateral acquired melanosis (Synonyms: precancerous and cancerous melanosis; epithelial melanosis; premalignant and malignant melanosis), modified from Zimmerman's Classification of 1966.
† If Breslow's data (Breslow, 1970 and 1975) can be shown to be applicable to conjunctival melanomas, a tumor thickness of < 0.75 mm would serve as the dividing line between IIA and IIB.

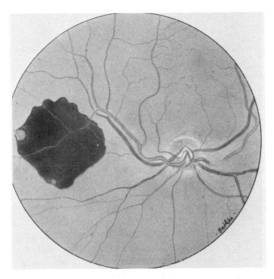

FIGURE 18-15.   Congenital retinal pigment hyperplasia. The flatness and the very dark color differentiate it from choroidal melanoma.

surprising. Remains of the hyaloid system, remains of pupillary membrane, anterior chamber cleavage syndrome, microphthalmos, and ectopic lacrimal glands have been noted in eyes with congenital melanomas.

Clinically, blue nevi are so called because they are often bluish-black. The color is an interference phenomenon due to their greater depth. Their cytologic spectrum ranges from densely pigmented polyhedral cells to densely pigmented fusiform dendritic cells, to sparsely pigmented syncitium of spindle-shaped Schwann cells.

The terms *blue nevus* and *melanocytoma* are used interchangeably, with blue nevus a clinical diagnosis and melanocytoma a histologic diagnosis. The so-called cellular blue nevus, or neuronevus, has growth potential and is viewed as an aggressive variant of the blue nevus.

Melanocytomas of the optic nerve head show some local invasiveness but no orbital extension or metastasis. The differential diagnosis between a juxtapapillary malignant melanoma of the choroid and a primary melanocytoma of the disc rest on four factors: a melanocytoma is usually discovered at routine examination, is characteristically smaller, characteristically stationary, and associated with racial hyperpigmentation.

Blue nevi can be associated with congenital ocular melanosis, also called melanosis oculi. This includes sector pigmentation of the iris, heterochromia iridis, uveal, scleral, and dermal melanosis. The interior of such an eye may be darker than its fellow. The dermal melanosis of the lower, and sometimes the upper, eyelid has been described as a nevus of Ota and sometimes covers a large portion of the face. All these conditions are related and are due to melanocytes in the tissue affected.

Ito in 1952 described dermal melanosis elsewhere in the body associated with ocular melanosis. The full-blown form of the condition, which is a congenital or birthmark condition, is called oculodermal melanocytosis. The condition is benign. It is more prominent in Orientals than in Caucasians. It has been the cause of a great deal of concern and speculation about the prognosis. There is a long-standing concept that melanosis oculi individuals have a greater chance of having a malignant melanoma develop in the choroid than the general population. Consequently, patients having oculodermal melanocytosis, which is easier to diagnose than simple melanosis oculi, have been subjected to intense scrutiny and a good deal of psychic trauma. Recently, various investigators have questioned whether the likelihood of malignant melanoma developing in these individuals is in fact greater. Conservative opinion holds that until the matter is settled more frequent scrutiny of these individuals is in order.

ORBITAL MELANOMAS

A benign or malignant melanoma of the orbit can arise along the sheath of a ciliary nerve as it courses through the orbit (Fig. 18-16). A melanoma arising from a site on the nerve where it passes through the sclera may be

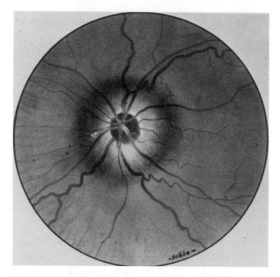

FIGURE 18-16. Melanoma surrounding disc. This may be confused with melanocytoma of the nerve.

located partly in the choroid and partly in the orbit, resulting in an hourglass arrangement.

It is possible that, instead of being primary in the orbit, a melanoma can extend from a tumor in a neighboring structure, such as the adjacent conjunctiva, caruncle, semilunar fold or skin. It can also be a small or flat lesion in the uvea, with early extension to the orbit. However, orbital extension usually occurs in large choroidal melanomas and more often in epithelioid and mixed-cell type and in necrotic tumors. Histopathologic evidence of orbital extension has been found in 10% of enucleated eyes in a recent study. They have a poor prognosis with significant orbital recurrence and metastases. The management of these cases is not clearly established; some think that exenteration should be performed, while others believe it does not significantly increase the survival rate.

An orbital melanoma can also extend from a tumor in the nasal sinus. It can be a metastasis from a malignant melanoma at a distant site.

A progressive infiltrating blue nevus may be primary in the orbit, as well as extending to it from beneath the skin and conjunctiva.

REFERENCES

1. Arnesen K, Nowes R: Malignant melanomas and benign nevus. Acta Ophth vol 53, 1975
2. Blodi FA: Ocular melanocytosis and melanoma. Am J Ophth 80(3), part 1, September 1975
3. Coleman DJ: Ocular tumor patterns: Ultrasonography in ophthalmology. Bibl Ophth 83: 136–140, 1975
4. Callender GR: Trans Am Acad Ophth Laryngol 36:131–142, 1931
5. Davidorf FH, Lang JR: Small malignant melanomas of the choroid. Am J Ophth vol 78(5), 1974
6. Ellsworth RM: The treatment of malignant melanoma of the uvea. Aust Coll Ophth, 1972
7. Hogeweg N, Bod PJ, Greve EL, Hoon AB: Malignant melanomas of the choroid that on fluorescein angiography and perimetry gave the impression of nevi. Doc Ophthalmologica 40:2, 301–318, 1976
8. Jack RL, Coleman DJ: Detection of retinal detachment secondary to choroidal melanoma with B-scan ultrasound. Am J Ophth vol 74(6), 1972
9. McLean IW, Foster WD, Zimmerman LE: Prognostic factors in small malignant melanomas of choroid and ciliary body. Arch Ophth vol 35, 1977
10. Pitts A, Yannoff M: Choiroidal melanoma with massive retinal fibrosis and spontaneous regression of retinal detachment. Survey Ophthalmology 20(4), Jan-Feb, 1976
11. Reese AB: Congenital melanomas. Am J Ophth 77(6), June 1974
12. Reese AB: Tumors of the Eye, ed 3, New York, Harper & Row, 1976
13. Reese AB, Howard GM: Flat uveal melanomas. Am J Ophth vol 64(6), Dec 1967
14. Reese AB, Jones IS: Benign melanomas of the retinal pigment epithelium. Am J Ophth 42:207–212, 1948
15. Reese AB, Jones IS: Hematomas under the retinal pigment epithelium. Am J Ophth 53:897, 1962
16. Reese AB, Jones IS, Cooper WC: Surgery for tumors of the iris and ciliary body. Am J Ophth 66:173–183, 1966
17. Shammos HF, Blodi FC: Orbital extension of choroidal and ciliary body melanomas. Arch Ophth vol 35, Nov 1977
18. Shammos HF, Blodi F: Prognostic factors in choroidal and ciliary body melanomas. Arch Ophth vol 35, Jan 1977

19. Shields JA: Current approaches to the diagnosis and management of choroidal melanomas. Surv Ophth vol 21(6), May–June 1977

20. Shields JA, Zimmerman LE: Lesions simulating malignant melanoma of the posterior uvea. Arch Ophth vol 83, June 1973

21. Shields JA, Annesley WH, Tolino A: Nonfluorescent malignant melanoma of the choroid diagnosed with the radioactive phosphorus uptake test. Am J Ophth vol 79(4), April 1975

22. Smith LT, Irvine AR: Diagnostic significance of orange pigment accumulations over choroidal tumors. A.S.O. vol 76(2), Aug 1973

23. Yannoff M: Glaucoma mechanism in ocular malignant melanoma. Am J Ophth vol 70, Dec 1970

24. Zimmerman LE: Histogenesis of conjunctival melanomas. In Tumors of the Eye and Adnexa. Birmingham Ala, Aesculapius Publishing Co, 1978

25. Zimmerman LE: Problems in the diagnosis of malignant melanomas of the choroid and ciliary body. Am J Ophth vol 75(6), June 1973

DIAGNOSIS AND TREATMENT OF MALIGNANT MELANOMA ARISING FROM THE SKIN OF THE FEMALE BREAST

IRVING M. ARIEL
AND ARTHUR S. CARON

The treatment of malignant melanoma arising from the skin of the female breast poses many problems.[15] We have routinely treated such infiltrating melanomas with orthodox radical mastectomy, removing the entire breast in continuity with the intervening lymphatics and performing a radical axillary dissection.

It may be possible to alter this form of surgery. Can a more conservative procedure, such as removal of the skin in continuity with the intervening lymphatics and radical axillary dissection, be performed? This procedure would theoretically be consistent with the primary tenet of cancer surgery, that is, removal of the primary lesion and the surrounding tissue, the intervening lymphatics, and the first echelon of lymph nodes where metastases can occur. This less-deforming procedure would be much more acceptable to the patient. At the other extreme is a more radical procedure such as extended radical mastectomy in which the internal mammary lymph node chain is also removed. A retrospective analysis of eight patients with melanomas of the breast from a total of 3,305 patients with malignant melanoma seen at the Pack Medical Group is presented.[2]

CLINICAL FEATURES

All of the women were between 25 and 44 years of age, the median being 35 years. Three were blonds, four brunette; in one patient the hair color was not stated (Table 19–1).

PREGNANCY STATUS

Five women had borne children and three were nulliparous. In patient GB the lesion had increased in size during the first pregnancy, 13 years previously, and had then subsided. During the second pregnancy the lesion had increased in size for a period of three months, when it was locally excised and found to be a malignant melanoma. In patient SW the malignant melanoma was discovered during a second pregnancy and was locally excised. This patient remains well three years later.

DELAY IN SEEKING TREATMENT

The neoplasms for which the patients sought medical attention varied from 1.5 to 3.0 cm in diameter. They had been present for prolonged periods prior to initial treatment. Patient SW stated that it had been present all of her life and had enlarged during pregnancy, which caused her to seek therapy. Patient AM stated that the lesion had been present all of her life, but an increase in pigmentation and pruritus caused her to seek medical attention. These changes were unrelated to pregnancy. Two patients (MS and AG) delayed a relatively short period averaging three months before consulting their physician.

Changes in the appearance of the primary lesion that caused the patients to seek medical therapy included an increase in size, an increase in pigmentation, ulceration (during

TABLE 19–1. Clinical Features of Eight Patients with Malignant Melanoma of the Skin of the Breast[2]

Patient, Age (yr.) and Complexion	Pregnancy Status	Duration of Primary Lesion before Treatment	Change in Primary Lesion before Treatment	Size of Primary Lesion (cm)	Location of Primary Lesion	Primary Treatment by Local Medical Doctor	Delay after Primary Treatment before Referral to Pack Medical Group
JM, 41, blond	1 child, age unknown	8 mo	Increased pigmentation	2	Medial aspect of right breast	Local excision	6 wk
GF, 41, brunette	1 child, aged 9.5 yr	Unknown	Increased pigmentation bleeding	2.5	Lateral aspect of left breast	Local excision	2.5 yrs
SW, 25, blond	1 child, aged 6 mo	Present all of life—enlarged during pregnancy	Increase in size, pigmentation	1.5	Medial aspect of right breast	Local excision	10 days
AM, 25, brunette	Nulliparous	Present all of life	Increased pigmentation and pruritus	3	Lateral aspect of left breast	Local excision	1 wk
MF, 27, complexion not stated	1 child, age unknown; 2nd pregnancy 6 mo before treatment of melanoma	3 mo.	Ulcerated: bled during pregnancy	2	Medial upper portion of left breast	Local excision	2 mo
GB, 44, brunette, brown eyes	2 children, aged 13 and 11 yr	All of life	Increase in size	3.5	Medial portion of left breast	Salves	1 yr
RSP, 40, brunette brown eyes	3 children, aged 11, 9, ard 7 yr	1 yr	Increase in size with lateral spread	3	Medial aspect of left breast	Electrodesiccation	1 yr
AG, 36, blond	Nulliparous	3 mo	Increase in size	2	Medial aspect of left breast	Local excision	3 mo

pregnancy in patient MF), lateral spread of the tumor (patient RSP), and pruritus (patient AM). These are the classic signs of change that occur when a benign nevus undergoes malignant transformation.

The left breast was involved in six of the eight patients, but the series is too small to place any significance on this finding. The lateral aspect was involved in two patients and the medial aspect in six.

INITIAL TREATMENT BY THE LOCAL PHYSICIAN

Initial treatment by the local physician consisted of conservative excision in six of eight patients. One physician continued to apply salves of an unknown nature to the tumor for one year (patient GB) and another electrodesiccated the lesion over a one-year period (patient RSP). Both of these patients died of malignant melanoma.

Five patients were referred to us for therapy within three months after the initial local excision. All are alive and free of evidence of melanoma. Two patients were referred for treatment one year after the primary diagnosis and both have died. An additional patient (BM) was referred for therapy two-and-a-half years after therapy because of a huge fixed metastasis to the axilla, which was attached to the latissimus dorsi muscle. A deeply infiltrating malignant melanoma of the breast has been locally excised by the local physician and malignant cells were identified in the lymphatic vessel. This patient was treated by left radical mastectomy plus resection of part of the latissimus dorsi muscle, which was involved by the infiltrating melanoma; she remains well and free of evidence of melanoma 11 years after radical mastectomy despite the presence of cancer cells in the lymphatics and a huge bulky metastasis in the axilla infiltrating the latissimus dorsi muscle. This patient exemplifies what may be accomplished by adequate surgery despite rather extensive spread of malignant melanoma with fixed metastasis in the axilla.

When the patients first presented for therapy, only a scar from the previous local excision with no evidence of residual melanoma or metastases was observed in six of the eight patients. One patient just described had an extensive bulky metastasis involving the axilla. A second patient had a large encrusted ulcerated mass measuring 2 by 3 cm at the site of local excision. She was treated by left radical mastectomy, but died of extensive metastases one year later.

EXTENT OF SURGERY

Treatment in seven of the eight patients consisted of radical mastectomy. In four patients routine radical mastectomy was performed. In three patients radical mastectomy was combined with resection of the internal mammary chain of lymph nodes. In one of these patients a simple excision of several internal mammary nodes was performed for histologic study; on frozen section the nodes were found to be negative for metastases. No additional nodes of the chain were resected. The other two patients had dissection in continuity with removal of the internal mammary nodes combined with radical mastectomy.

In one patient with a superficial melanoma, a tridimensional excision in continuity with axillary dissection was performed. The skin and fascia were dissected from the underlying breast parenchyma. The breast was left intact. This patient remains alive with no evidence of melanoma 11 years after excision without having had to resort to radical mastectomy.

There was no evidence of regional metastases in either the axillary nodes or mediastinal nodes in seven patients. The eighth patient had metastases to the axillary nodes.

PROGNOSIS

The prognosis of female patients with malignant melanoma of the skin of the breast is good. Six of the eight patients are alive without any evidence of melanoma.

One patient (AG) remains well with no evidence of malignant melanoma 5.5 years after radical mastectomy. Of the remaining five patients who are alive with no evidence of melanoma, the length of survival is over 10 years (Table 19–1). Two patients have died of disseminated malignant melanoma. One patient, a 44-year-old woman (GB) who had been treated by the application of salves by her family physician, had extensive local recurrence and was treated by left radical mastectomy. Disseminated metastases developed and she died one year later. The second patient was a 40-year old woman (RSP) whose primary malignant melanoma had been treated by electrodesiccation by her local physician. She was treated by left radical mastectomy with internal mammary node dissection. No residual melanoma was encountered in the breast, axillary nodes, or internal mammary nodes. However, extensive metastases developed throughout the entire abdomen and she died two and a half years after extended radical mastectomy. She was treated with bilateral oophorectomy, intra-abdominal isotopes, and phenylalanine mustard with mild palliation. Incidentally, this patient's mother had died of malignant melanoma. The location of the metastases extensively involving the ovaries and all intra-abdominal organs with no metastases in the lungs or elsewhere suggests that dissemination had occurred via the lymphatic vessels that traverse the rectus abdominus sheath and enter the abdominal cavity.

COMMENTS

LYMPHATICS OF THE SKIN OF THE BREAST

The lymphatic vessels of the mammary skin form an elaborate and intricate network originating under the areola (Fig. 19–1). These lymphatic vessels, as described by Oelsner,[16] communicate freely with the lymphatic vessels of the skin of the chest, neck, and abdomen. There is also a free intercommunication with the lymphatics of the skin of the opposite breast. In fact, metastases may occur from the skin of the breast directly to the axillary lymph nodes of either the ipsilateral or contralateral breast. There is, moreover, an elaborate intercommunication between the lymphatic vessels of the skin of the breast and the breast per se.[24] Most lymphatic vessels of the breast originate from delicate networks around mammary lobules, which collect and follow the mammary ducts to the nipple region where they communicate uninterruptedly with the skin lymphatics in this region.[14] This is evidenced by the fact that many carcinoma cells escape into the lymphatics from a primary carcinoma of the breast and travel towards the subareolar region where they enter the subdermal lymphatics, producing edema of the skin, usually in the infra-areolar region. This connection between the lymphatic vessels of the breast and those of the subcutaneous tissues is an expression of the intercommunication between these two chains. Cancer cells from the dermal region similarly connect freely with the lymphatic vessels of the breast.

The lymphatic vessels of the breast drain directly into the axilla and internal mammary especially those that arise from the medial aspect of the breast or in the vicinity of the areola will drain directly into the internal mammary chain.[6] The lymphatics may extend inferiority through the rectus sheath to enter the intra-abdominal lymphatic vessels.

Several small nodes, the paramammary nodes, are interspersed between the collecting lymphatics of the breast that lie superficially.[23] Metastases from melanoma involving the skin may readily spread to these paramammary nodes.

INCIDENCE OF MALIGNANT MELANOMA

Malignant melanomas of the skin of the breast are rare. There were only eight such cases in a series of 3,305 patients with malignant melanoma seen at the Pack Medical Group in a 40-year period (1930–1970), as incidence of 0.24%.[17,18,22] The area of the skin of

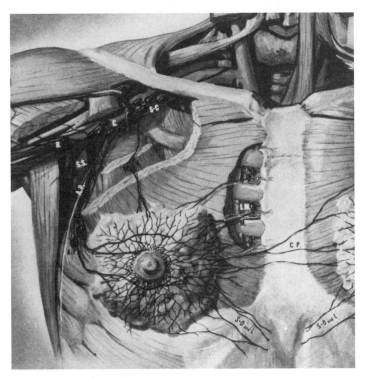

FIGURE 19-1. Lymphatics of the breast revealing the extensive network of dermal and breast lymphatics in the region of the areola. Note the routes of metastases to lymph nodes to the axilla, internal mammary chain, opposite breast, and through the rectus sheath into the abdominal cavity. (Courtesy of Dr. Frank Netter and Ciba Pharmaceuticals, Inc.)

the breast varies considerably in relation to the total body skin.

In most series, melanomas of the skin of the breast are grouped with melanomas of the chest wall.

McLeod of the Queensland Melanoma Project in Australia has estimated that there were six cases of malignant melanoma of the skin of the breast in a series of approximately 2,000 patients with malignant melanoma (personal communication).

CLINICAL FEATURES

The study by Pack, Davis, and Oppenheim[21] in 1963 relative to the race and complexion of patients with malignant melanoma revealed that approximately 90% of such patients had a

light complexion with blond hair and frequently had blue eyes. In this series of eight patients, there was an equal distribution between blond and brown hair color. This series, however, is too small to be significant.

The average age of patients with melanoma reported in a large series from the Pack Medical Group was 36 years.[18] In the present series of eight patients, the ages ranged between 25 and 40 years, with an average of 35. Again, this series is too small for significant evaluation.

INFLUENCE OF PREGNANCY

The effects of pregnancy on pigmentation metabolism are well known as evidenced by the increased pigmentation of the areola of the breast. It is difficult to state from this series whether pregnancy had any effect on the growth of the tumor. Five of the eight patients had borne children. One patient who was pregnant had an increase in the size of a benign nevus that had been present for 13 years. After delivery the lesion became smaller. During a second pregnancy, which occurred two years later, an increase in the size of the lesion resulted in its removal, and it was found to be a malignant melanoma. Patient SW was pregnant with a second child when the lesion was locally excised.

The effects of pregnancy on prognosis cannot be stated. Shocket and Fortner[25] have revealed no effects of pregnancy with other factors being considered. In this series the two patients who were pregnant at the time of discovery of the malignant melanoma are both alive and evidently free of cancer. In one the period is relatively short, it being only three years since operation; in the other patient a prolonged period (11 years) has elapsed with no evidence of cancer.

DIAGNOSIS

Many women have nevi of the skin of the breast, and in this series a change in the state of the nevus caused the patient to seek medical attention. These changes consisted of an increase in size and pigmentation, ulceration and lateral spread of the nevus, and pruritus. These are the classic signs. Despite the rarity of malignant melanomas of the breast, in so-called civilized society the breast is constantly being irritated by the wearing of tight-fitting brassieres (by straps, wires, etc.) and it is suggested that any dark nevus, especially one about the areola or at the site of irritation, be excised.

TREATMENT

The free intermingling of the lymphatics of the skin of the breast with the lymphatics of the parenchyma of the breast suggest to us that radical mastectomy is the treatment of choice for infiltrating melanomas of the breast. Malignant melanomas on the medial aspect of the breast or about the areola were treated by extended radical mastectomy, which includes excision of the internal mammary lymph node chain. It has been determined that lymphatics spread from this area of the breast directly into the internal mammary chain of lymph nodes.[1,27] No metastases were encountered in the lymph nodes of the internal mammary chain in the three patients in whom this was investigated (Figs. 19-2 and 19-3.)

In patients with superficial melanomas, it is justifiable to perform a more conservative operation consisting of excision in continuity with a wide margin of skin and the underlying fascia and axillary dissection. In such instances we prefer to transect the pectoralis major and minor muscles to facilitate axillary dissection, after which we reunite the pectoralis major muscle (Chap. 24).[3] This procedure was performed in one of our eight patients and she remains well three years later (Fig. 19-4).

In a personal communication from R. McLeod, MD in 1971, on the treatment of malignant melanoma of the breast, he stated:

> My present view is that I would treat the patient by radical mastectomy provided frozen section confirmed that the lesion was deeply invasive or if there was definite clinical evidence of spread to the axillary lymph nodes. We have in recent times been becoming less inclined to prophylactic lymph node dissection so that in many of these patients my approach to treatment would either be local excision with a wide margin of normal skin about the lesion or simple mastectomy if the lesion involved the nipple.

This practice presents an opposite view to our own since we believe that the lymph nodes should be resected for infiltrating melanoma (level IV and V and possibly level III) (see Chap. 10). We have demonstrated that the lymph nodes are extremely poor filters and therefore do not act as an adequate barrier to the spread of malignant melanoma. Moreover, the question of their local immunity remains problematic.[3,4,5]

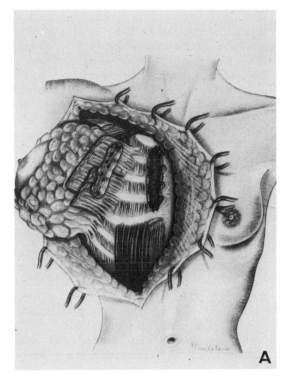

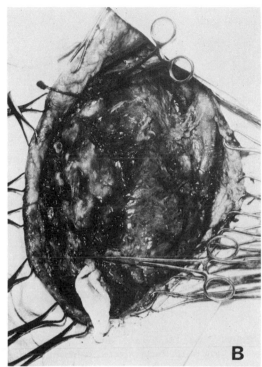

FIGURE 19-2A. A conservative technique for re-secting the internal mammary chain of lymph nodes in continuity with radical mastectomy. B. Clinical photograph demonstrating resection of the internal mammary chain of lymph nodes.

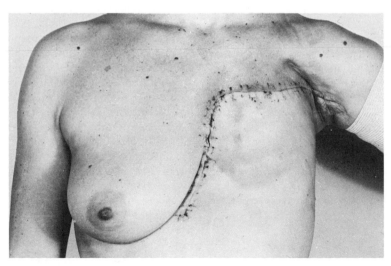

FIGURE 19-3. Surgical scar of patient RSP subsequent to extended radical mastectomy for melanoma (radical mastectomy in continuity with resection of the internal mammary chain of lymph nodes).

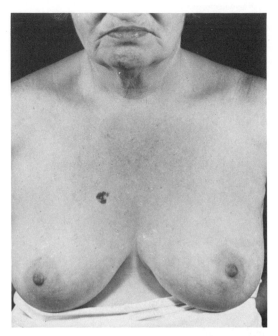

FIGURE 19–4. Malignant superficial melanoma of the skin of the breast treated by tridimensional excision of melanoma in continuity with axillary dissection. Patient is free of evidence of melanoma 11 years later.

PROGNOSIS

The prognosis appears favorable in this small series. Of the eight patients treated, all except two are alive and free of disease over five years (80%). One of these patients who had a bulky axillary metastasis with fixation to the latissimus dorsi underwent resection with apparent cure. Two patients (37%) have died of the malignant melanomas. Death in all probability was the result of a traumatic form of treatment before surgical extirpation. Accordingly, the overall prognosis can be considered good on the basis of these eight patients.[3]

DISCUSSION

The breast is an ectodermal derivative and constitutes an appendage of the skin.

Although it is often considered a parenchymal organ, the entire breast must be considered of ectodermal origin and therapeutic efforts made with this point in view including attention to the extensive lymphatics network.

There have been occasional reports of melanomas apparently arising within the breast parenchyma. One such report by Gatch[9] was believed to arise primarily within the parenchyma of the breast. In a report in 1959 by Stephenson and Byrd[26] a 26-year-old female had widespread malignant melanoma believed to be secondary to a mass that had been noted in the breast for a period of two years, leading to the conclusion that this was a primary melanoma arising from the breast parenchyma. Although melanomas can arise from parenchymous organs such as the ovaries, central nervous system, etc., in view of the fact that in our series approximately 5% of all patients seen have metastases with no known primary, and often there is a history of a primary lesion of the skin that had fallen off or had atrophied to disappearance, one is led to speculate whether these tumors are truly melanomas arising within the parenchyma of the breast, but more likely they represent metastases to the breast from an occult primary.[7]

In a report by Hajdu and Urban,[11] they demonstrate that melanomas represent the most frequent tumor that metastasizes to the breast, after excluding lymphomatous and leukemic infiltration of the breast tissue.

Other reports in the literature are rare regarding the behavior of melanoma of the skin of the breast. Haagensen et al.[10] records four cases: one patient, 63 years old, died 46 months after the first symptoms of melanoma, and a radical mastectomy revealed metastases to the axilla; in two other cases, small melanomas were widely excised and an axillary dissection was performed with no metastases noted in the axilla. Both patients were alive at the time of that report, three and four years, respectively, after the surgery. They record one male cured by local excision and axillary dissection.

In our series, we did not record any of the male patients, inasmuch as it would be difficult to determine exactly where the skin of

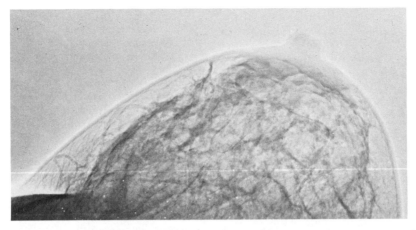

FIGURE 19-5. Two circumscribed lesions on enlarged view of a lateral xerogram that had the radiographic appearance of a fibroadenoma but proved to be metastatic melanoma. (Jochimsen PR, Brown RD: "Metastatic melanoma in the breast masquerading as fibroadenoma," JAMA, 236(24): 2779, 1976. Published through the courtesy of the authors and the AMA. Copyright 1976 American Medical Association.)

the breast tissue begins or ends. Those cases are included as melanomas of the chest wall, of which there were 640 in our series (Chap. 20).

Jochimsen, Pearlman, Lawton, and Platz[12] from the University of Iowa City, reported six cases of malignant melanoma of the breast; five of them were in females; one was in a male who died 19 months after radical mastectomy. One of the women died 28 years after operation for other reasons, with no evidence of melanoma; and two others were alive without evidence of disease five years and nine months after mastectomy (one radical and one modified radical mastectomy). A fifth patient, a 32-year-old female, who was treated by a wide excision, died 32 months after excision; and the sixth was treated by a local excision, developing recurrences 34 months later, which were believed to be in-transit metastases to the breast and which were treated by radical mastectomy. These authors believe that the following important points are brought out by analysis of their data: "(1) All of these melanomas apparently arose in previously existent lesions of the breast skin that had been present for very long periods of time, which suggests that the pigmented lesions occurring on the breast might have a higher rate

of conversion to malignancy than do such lesions in other areas of the body. A nevus of the breast perhaps is not dissimilar from nevi of the genitalia, anal-rectal, or oral regions, and should be removed. (2) Axillary metastases do not preclude surgical extirpation and cure of the disease. (3) Melanomas of the skin of the breast can and do metastasize to the breast parenchyma. Such cases can be cured by total mastectomy and axillary dissection. (4) An even more radical dissection including internal mammary nodes is not warranted in spite of the location of the primary lesion." These authors demonstrated melanoma metastases in the breast parenchyma by xerograms[11b] (Fig. 19-5).

Lee, Sparks, and Morton[13] reported 12 patients with melanoma of the breast region of 186 patients with melanoma referred to the Division of Surgical Oncology of the University of California, Los Angeles Division. Seven of their patients had developed local recurrences, ony one of whom was a female. One cannot consider their report as being truly representative of melanoma of the female breast but rather representative of melanoma of the anterior thoracic skin. Accordingly, we cannot compare their results but rather judge them as representative of melanoma of the skin of the thoracic region as discussed in Chapter 20.

SUMMARY AND CONCLUSIONS

Eight of 3,305 patients with malignant melanoma treated at the Pack Medical Group (0.24%) presented with malignant melanoma of the skin of the breast. Seven of the eight patients underwent radical mastectomy, in addition, internal mammary node dissection was performed in three of the seven patients.

The fact that six patients treated with this procedure over five years ago have remained well and free of evidence of malignant melanoma (75%) suggests that this is the procedure of choice. There is a free communication between the lymphatic vessels of the skin of the breast and the breast parenchyma.

Patients with superficial malignant melanomas of the skin of the breast may be treated by tridimensional excision of the site of the malignant melanoma[8] at times combines with axillary lymph node dissection.

REFERENCES

1. Ariel IM: A conservative method of resecting the internal mammary lymph nodes en bloc with radical mastectomy. Surg Gynecol Obstet 100:623, 1955
2. Ariel IM, Caron AS: Diagnosis and treatment of malignant melanoma arising from the skin of the female breast. Am J Surg 124:384, 1972
3. Ariel IM, Pack GT: Treatment of malignant melanoma of adequate (radical) surgical resection and radical amputation when indicated in: Mulholland JH, Ellison, EM, Friesen SR (eds): Current Surgical Management, Philadelphia, WB Saunders Co, 1957, p 438
4. Ariel IM, Pack GT: Treatment of disseminated melanoma by systemic melphalan, methotrexate and autogenous bone marrow transplants. Cancer 20:77, 1967
5. Ariel IM, Resnick MI: Altered lymphatic dynamics following an axillary dissection: its relationship to treatment policies for malignant melanoma. Surgery 61:210, 1967
6. Ariel IM, Resnick MI: Altered lymphatic dynamics caused by cancer metastases. Arch Surg 94:117, 1967
7. Baab GH, McBride CM: Malignant melanoma, the patient with unknown site of primary origin. Arch Surg 110:896, 1975
8. DeCosse JJ, McNeer J: Superficial melanoma. Arch Surg 99:531, 1969
9. Gatch WD: A melanoma apparently primary in the breast. Arch Surg 73:266, 1956
10. Haagensen CD: Tumors of the skin and accessory glands, in Diseases of the breast, ed 2. Philadelphia, WB Saunders Co, 1972
11. Hajdu SI, Urban JA: Cancers metastatic to breast. Cancer 29:1691, 1972
11b. Jochimsen PR, Brown RD: Metastatic melanoma in the breast masquerading as fibroadenoma, JAMA vol 236, 24:2779, 1976
12. Jochimsen PR, Pearlman NW, Lawton RL, Platz CE: Melanoma of skin of the breast: therapeutic considerations based on six cases. Surgery vol 81, 5:583, May 1977
13. Lee Yeu-Tsu N, Sparks, FC, Morton DL: Primary melanoma of skin of the breast region. Ann Surg,1977
14. Mornard P: Etude anatomique des lymphatiques de la mamelle au pointe de vue de l'extension lymphatique des cancers. Rev Chir 51:462, 1916
15. Nyst MEE: Melanoma malignium mammae. Ned Tijdschr Geneeskd 108:495, 1964
16. Oelsner J: Anatomischer Unter sushungen ueber die Lymphwege der Brust mit Bezug auf die Ausbreitung des Mammacarcinome, Arch klin chir 64:158, 1901
17. Pack GT: End results in the treatment of malignant melanoma Surgery 46:447, 1959
18. Pack GT: The Problem of Malignant Melanoma. Proceedings of the Second National Cancer Conference, 1953. New York, American Cancer Society, 1954, p 54
19. Pack GT, Oropeza R: A comparative study of melanoma and epidermoid carcinomas of the vulva: a review of 44 melanomas and 29 epidermoid carcinomas (1930–1965). Dis Colon Rectum 10:161, 1967
20. Pack GT, Oropeza R: A comparative study of melanoma and epidermoid carcinomas of the vulva: a review of 44 melanomas and 58 epidermoid carcinomas (1930–1965). Rev Surg 24:305, 1967
21. Pack GT, Davis J, Oppenheim A: The relation-

ship of race and complexion to the incidence of moles and melanoma Ann NY Acad Sci 100:719, 1962

22. Pack GT, Lenson N, Gerber DM: Regional distribution of moles and melanomas. Arch Surg 65:862, 1952

23. Rottor J: Zur Topographie des Mammacarcinoms Arch klin chir 58:346, 1899

24. Rouvière H: Anatomie des lymphatiques de l'homme. Paris, Masson & Cie, 1932, p 202

25. Shocket EC, Fortner JG: Melanomas and pregnancy: an experimental evaluation of a clinical impression. Surg Forum 9:671, 1958

26. Stephenson SE, Byrd BF: Malignant melanoma of the breast. Am J Surg 97:232, 1959

27. Urban J: Radical mastectomy in continuity with internal mammary lymph node dissection, in Pack GT, Ariel IM (eds): Treatment of Cancer and Allied Diseases, vol 4, New York, Hoeber, 1964, p 109

CHAPTER TWENTY

PRIMARY MALIGNANT MELANOMA OF THE SKIN OF THE CHEST WALL

IRVING M. ARIEL

Melanomas of the skin of the chest wall, especially those located posteriorly, are away from the field of vision, and hence, often go unnoticed until they have reached an advanced state.

Most authors present their data utilizing the trunk as an anatomic unit. The trunk is divided by us for analytic purposes into the thoracic wall and the abdominal wall. This presentation shall analyze patients with melanoma of the skin of the thorax.

DEFINITION OF ANATOMIC BOUNDARIES

The thorax is presented as all skin inferior to the clavicle and its posterior counterpart and around an imaginary line circumventing the circumference of the trunk at the level of the twelfth rib. This boundary tends to conform with Sappey's lymphatic drainage of the trunk.[17] This delineation attempts to determine which lymph nodes are at potential risk of harboring metastases (Fig. 20–1).

INCIDENCE

At the Pack Medical Group 3,305 patients suffering from malignant melanoma were seen; and of those, 1,122 (34%) had malignant melanoma of the trunk. This category is subdivided into the thoracic skin (640 patients) and the skin of the abdominal wall (482 patients). Melanomas of the thorax comprise 57% of trunkal melanomas and 19% of all melanomas seen.

Melanomas of the skin of the female breast, of which there were eight[2] are not included (Chapter 9.)

In order to evaluate therapeutic accomplishments, the survival analysis is limited to the years 1934–1965, permitting a ten-year evaluation period. Three hundred and eighty-six patients are candidates for this evaluation.

CLINICAL MATERIAL

Practically all patients were Caucasians (81%); 19% did not have race listed on the charts (Table 20–1). There were no patients of the black, yellow, or red races. Of the Caucasians, 44% were of fair complexion, 10% were of dark complexion, and in 5% numerous freckles dominated the complexion. In 41% the complexion was not listed.

Males predominated (71%), while only 29% were females.

None were between the ages of zero and ten, only 3% were between 10 and 20; and the highest incidence (36%) occurred among patients in the 40 to 49 age span. In the 30 to 39 age span there were somewhat fewer patients (27%). There were many fewer numbers of people under age 30 and over age 50.

Thus, all the patients were Caucasians, three-quarters were males, and almost two thirds were in the 30 to 50 year age group.

HISTOLOGIC STAGING

Histologic staging was available in approximately 500 patients. Ten percent were diagnosed as superficial melanomas (Fig. 20–2) and 79% were infiltrating melanomas. In 11% the histologic classification was not recorded.

We had not adhered to the classification of

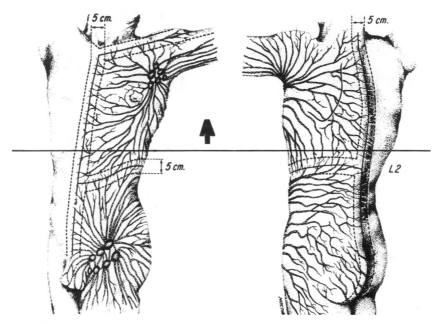

FIGURE 20-1. Illustration of trunk into the thoracic and abdominal segments. The dotted line represents Sugarbaker and McBride's division. The horizontal solid line indicates our division. (Sugarbaker EV, McBride CM: Melanoma of the trunk: The results of surgical excision and anatomic guidelines for predicting nodal metastasis. Surgery 80:22–30, 1976. Reproduced with permission of author and publisher.)

TABLE 20-1. Clinical Characteristics of 640 Patients with Malignant Melanoma of the Skin of the Chest Wall

Clinical Features	Percent of Patients	Sex and Age	Percent of Patients
Race		Sex	
Caucasian	81	Male	71
Unknown	19	Female	29
Other (black, yellow, etc.)	0	Age	
		0–10	0
Complexion		10–20	3
Fair	44	20–29	9
Dark	10	30–39	27
Freckled	5	40–49	36
Unknown	41	50–59	12
		60–69	11
Eye Color		70 +	0
Blue	23	Unknown	1
Brown	10		
Hazel	6		
Unknown	61		

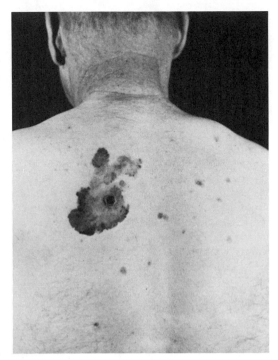

FIGURE 20-2. Superficial spreading melanoma presenting an irregular border and vagaries in color.

Clark–McGovern in the past. We would not consider Clark's level I to be a metastasizing melanoma and is not included in this analysis. Their level's II and possibly III would be our superficial melanoma so designated by the pathologists involved in this evaluation. Their levels IV–V cannot be ascertained separately inasmuch as the designation of *invasive melanoma* as listed by our pathologists include their levels IV and V. The slides are not available for reexamination and more exact interpretation.

LOCATION OF MELANOMA

Of the 640 patients with melanoma of the chest wall, 380 (59%) suffered from melanoma of the anterior chest wall (Fig. 20–3), and 245 (38%) suffered from melanoma of the posterior chest wall. The charts of 15 patients (2%) did not reveal the site of the malignant melanoma.

Approximately 10% of the patients manifested their melanomas in a lateral location (an imaginary line extending inferiorly

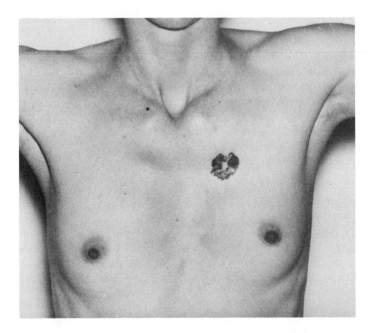

FIGURE 20-3. Superficial melanoma of anterior chest wall that had metastasized to the axilla. No lymph nodes were clinically palpable. An elective axillary dissection revealed occult metastases in the axillary lymph nodes.

between the anterior axillary and posterior axillary lines) (Fig. 20–4) and 12% had melanoma at or in the immediate vicinity of the midline (Fig. 20–5).

TREATMENT POLICIES

A radical tridimensional excision is performed about the primary site of the melanoma including a generous portion (5 cm) of surrounding skin with the development of skin flaps and the removal of about twice the amount of the underlying integument and fascia; the dissection going down to naked muscle. The defect is repaired by sliding flaps (Fig. 20–6)[1] or by split-thickness skin graft (Fig. 20–7). When the melanoma is adjacent to a primary echelon of lymph node drainage, a wide dissection is combined with a radical or modified radical axillary dissection (Fig. 20–8). When the melanoma is situated in the midline, either anteriorly or posteriorly, a tridimensional excision is combined with a bilateral axillary dissection. This procedure was not performed often enough to warrant any conclusions regarding its efficacy. For those melanomas at the level of the clavicle, or the posterior counterpart of this level, where two chains of lymph nodes were at risk, namely the cervical lymph nodes and the axillary lymph nodes, a combined axillary and cervical dissection may be performed. In some instances of melanoma in the parasternal region the axillary dissection was combined with an internal mammary lymph node dissection. These latter procedures were not done frequently enough to warrant any conclusions. The results of resecting the lymph nodes are presented in Figure 20–8.

RESULTS

Of 386 patients treated more than ten years ago, 98 are considered indeterminate inasmuch a they simply came for consultation (Table 20–2). Forty patients died during the interval of evaluation from an intercurrent disease. Determinate patients are the 248 available for ten-year evaluation. Eighty-eight

are known to be alive and free of any evidence of cancer, whereas 160 patients have died from their cancers. The determinate ten-year survival rate is accordingly 35%, which represents those who are alive and free of cancer ten years after treatment, divided by those available for determinate evaluation at the ten-year period (Fig. 20–9). The absolute ten-year survival rate (including all patients treated, regardless of their causes of death) equals 30%.

Additional data are presented in an attempt to evaluate the effects of various parameters upon cure. The absolute figures are evaluated, which include all dead patients regardless of cause and are considered dead due to melanoma, but excludes those 98 patients seen only in consultation and not treated by us.

THE EFFECT OF AGE UPON SURVIVAL

The highest survival rate occurred in the 10 to 20-year-old group in that two of the four patients survived. These data are not significant because of the small numbers. In the other age brackets, there did not seem to be any significant effect of age upon the overall survival (Table 20–3). Many benign nevi occur in the younger age group (Fig. 20–10).

THE EFFECT OF SEX UPON SURVIVAL

The survival rate for females equalled 31%, higher than the 22% for males (Table 20–4).

THE EFFECT OF DELAY UPON SURVIVAL

There is a steady decrease in survival as the delay increases (from the first appearance of the lesion to treatment). The figures vary from 43% for those who delayed from one to three months to a survival rate of 9% for those who delayed from one to two years. An interesting observation is the 20% survival for those pa-

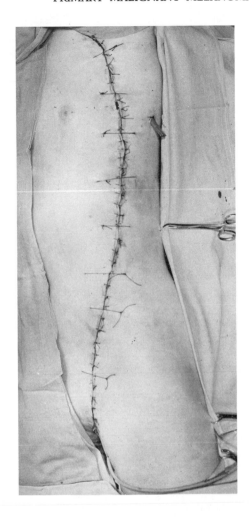

FIGURE 20-4. Surgical scar showing extent of surgical excision of a melanoma of the lateral midline. The melanoma, axillary contents, and groin lymph nodes were excised in continuity. The nodes were found free of metastases.

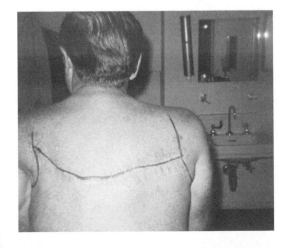

FIGURE 20-5. Surgical scar of an infiltrating melanoma of the midline treated by wide resection and bilateral axillary dissection. Metastases were observed in the left axilla. The patient remains well 12 years later.

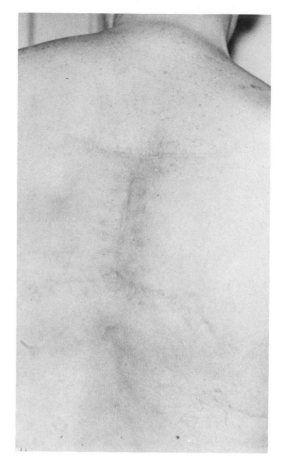

FIGURE 20–6. Scar after wide excision of a melanoma of the midline repaired by sliding flaps. Five years later patient had metastases to right axilla, treated by axillary dissection. Eight years after the primary resection he developed metastases to the left axilla, surgically treated. He died five years later from heart disease.

tients who delayed from three to five years. This, in all probability, represents a biologic determinism that caused the melanoma to remain localized for this period, or it represents a benign nevus that had undergone malignant transformation (Table 20–5).

SIZE OF THE LESION AND ITS EFFECT UPON SURVIVAL

The data here are inconclusive inasmuch as in 175 patients the size was not mentioned in the protocol. For the remainder, there did not seem to be a significant effect of the size of the melanoma on the overall prognosis (Table 20–6).

SITE OF MELANOMA ANALYZED ACCORDING TO SURVIVAL

The patients with melanomas of the anterior chest wall manifested a 30% ten-year survival rate, while patients with melanomas of the posterior chest wall (82 patients) had only a 20% ten-year survival. This may be due to the fact that those lesions located anteriorly can be observed by the patient, whereas those in the posterior location, noticed by someone else, heralds their presence by clinical manifestations such as itching, bleeding, or pain (Fig. 20–11).

Patients with melanoma located at or near the anterior midline (22 patients) averaged a 20% ten-year survival, as did those with

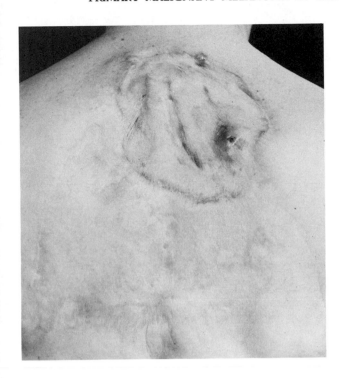

FIGURE 20-7. Superficial melanoma treated by wide excision and split thickness skin graft.

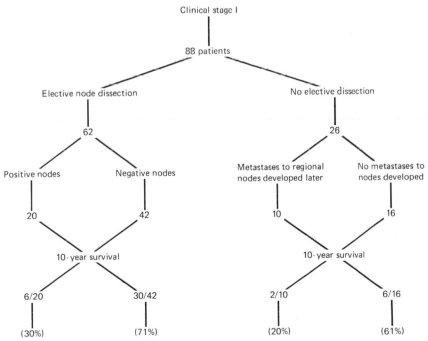

FIGURE 20-8. Melanoma of the skin of the chest wall. Shown here the influence of regional lymph node dissection upon survival.

TABLE 20-2.   Melanoma of the Skin of the Chest Wall. Overall Survival Ten Years after Surgical Resection

	Number
Total number of patients seen	386
Indeterminate patients:	
Patients who came for consultation only	98
Patients known to have died of another intercurrent disease	40
Determinate patients	248
Patients alive and free of cancer	88
Patients known to have died of melanoma	160
Determinate 10-year survival 88/248 =	35%

* **Absolute 10-year survival 88/296 = 30% (Includes the patients presumably dead of another disease but does not include the 98 patients who were seen only in consultation and were treated elsewhere or received no treatment.)**

melanoma of the posterior midline (18 patients) (Fig. 20-6).

Those lesions located on the lateral chest wall (15 patients) showed a poorer survival rate (15%).

THE INFLUENCE OF A PREEXISTING MOLE ON SURVIVAL

One hundred thirty patients (61%) complained of a melanoma developing in a preexisting mole (Figs. 20-12 and 13); their ten-year survival was 36%. Sixty-two patients (21%) stated that their melanomas developed de novo (Fig. 20-14). Their survival rate was somewhat lower, equalling 24%. The data were indefinite for 54 patients whose survival rate was 24% (Table 20-7).

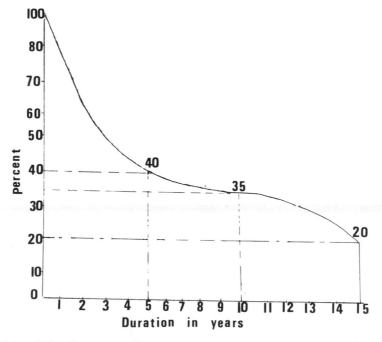

FIGURE 20-9.   Chart showing the survival trend in the determinate patients treated for malignant melanoma of the chest wall.

TABLE 20-3. Melanoma of the Skin of the Chest Wall. The Influence of Age upon Survival

Age	Number of Patients	10-Year Survivors	
		Number	Percent
Under 10	0	0	0
10-20	4	2	50
21-29	30	10	33
30-39	90	22	24
40-49	90	20	22
50-59	40	10	25
60-69	32	8	25
70 +	0	0	0

TABLE 20-5. Melanoma of the Skin of the Chest Wall. The Influence of Delay before Treatment at Pack Medical Group upon Survival

Delay (Months)	Number of Patients	10-Year Survivors	
		Number	Percent
Under 1	10	4	40
1-3	88	38	43
4-6	36	8	22
7-12	56	10	18
13-36	44	4	9
37-60	10	2	20
60 +	0	0	0
Unknown	52	—	—

TABLE 20-4. Melanoma of the Skin of the Chest Wall. The Influence of Sex Upon Survival

Sex	Number of Patients	10-Year Survivors	
		Number	Percent
Male	204	46	22
Female	84	26	31
Unknown	8	—	—

TABLE 20-6. Melanoma of the Skin of the Chest Wall. The Influence of Size upon Survival

Size	Number of Patients	10-Year Survivors	
		Number	Percent
Under 1 cm	26	8	31
1 cm/2 cm	38	14	37
2 cm/3 cm	26	6	23
3+ cm	30	8	27
Unknown	175	—	—

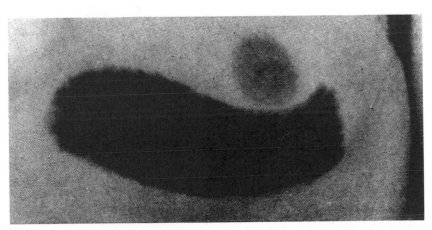

FIGURE 20-10. Benign linear nevus of chest wall in a preadolescent boy. Treated successfully by repeated segmental excision and primary closure.

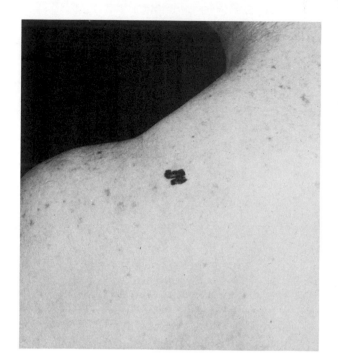

FIGURE 20–11. Recurrent melanoma of the posterior superior shoulder treated two years previously by cauterization. Despite radical surgical resection, the patient died six months after surgical resection from disseminated melanoma. The unacceptable hazards of cautery are demonstrated by this patient.

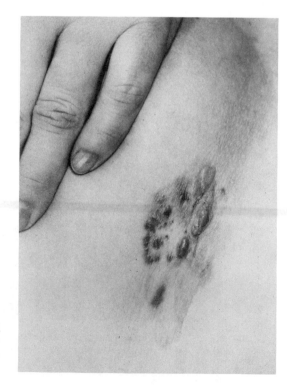

FIGURE 20–12. A close-up view of a superficial melanoma of the chest wall demonstrating body efforts to destroy the melanoma (center of lesion). This melanoma developed on a preexistent mole.

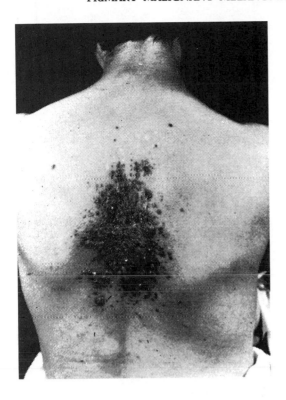

FIGURE 20-13. A large verrucar nevus in which melanoma developed. Despite surgical resection patient developed metastases and died.

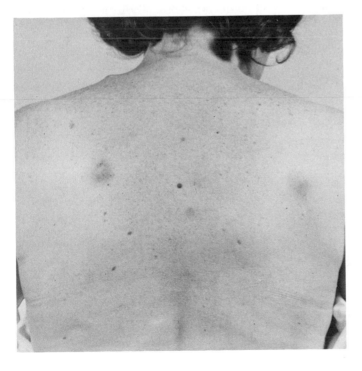

FIGURE 20-14. A small melanoma of the midline of the back whose first symptom was due to metastases to the lung, which killed the patient.

TABLE 20-7.   The Influence of a Preexisting Mole on Survival

	Number	Percent	Number Surviving 10 Years	% 10-Year Survival
Patients with a preexisting mole	130	61	47	36
Patients whose melanomas developed de novo	62	21	15	24
Unknown	54	18	13	24

PRECEDING INJURY OR BIOLOGICAL STRESS ANALYZED ACCORDING TO POSSIBLE EFFECT UPON SURVIVAL

Out of 296 patients with chest wall melanoma, 172 had no history of injury or any other trauma and ten-year survival rate was 24%. Factors which the patients noted are presented in Table 20-8. No conclusions are warranted.

STAGING ANALYZED ACCORDING TO SURVIVAL

Stage I indicates melanomas that are localized to the skin with no clinical evidence of metastases. Stage II are those patients where clinical evidence of metastases to regional lymph nodes exist. Stage III are those where there are satellitoses, intransit metastases, or other signs of regional spread in addition to regional nodal metastases. Stage IV are those patients with evidence of distant blood-borne metastases. Those patients with stage I melanoma, of which there were 90, manifested a 55% ten-year survival, which dropped precipitously for the 150 patients with stage II melanoma to a level of 13%. Those with stage III demonstrated only an 8% survival (Table 20-9).

HISTOLOGIC CLASSIFICATION OF MALIGNANT MELANOMA AS IT AFFECTS 10-YEAR SURVIVAL

Thirty patients were diagnosed as having superficial melanoma (Clark's level II–III) (Table 20-10). The survival rate in this group was 73% (Fig. 20-7). The 210 patients with infiltrating melanomas (Clark's level IV and V) had a 21% survival rate (Fig. 20-15). Among 56 patients whose classification was unrecorded, the survival rate was 18%. Thirty-eight patients (3%) presented amelanotic melanoma; of these, 20 were treated over 10 years ago. Five of these patients (25%) are alive and free of evidence of malignant melanoma (Chap. 14).

THE EFFECT OF TIME OF LOCAL RECURRENCE UPON SURVIVAL

These data are analyzed at the five-year interval. Of 164 patients who did not develop local recurrence, the five-year survival was 41%. Four patients developed local recurrence after one to three months, eight after four to six months, and 12 from 7 to 12 months. All of these patients succumbed from the melanoma. Twelve patients developed a local recurrence between 13 to 36 months, and two such patients survived the five-year span (Table 20-11 and Fig. 20-16A,B).

TABLE 20-8. Melanoma of the Skin of the Chest Wall.
The Influence of Previous Injury or Biological Stress on Survival

Injury or Stress	Number of Patients	10-Year Survivors	
		Number	Percent
None	172	42	24
Brassiere or other irritation	12	3	25
Sun	6	6	100
During pregnancy	10	4	40
Postpregnancy (within 6 mos.)	2	2	100
Other	18	4	22
Familial history of melanoma	12	2	17
Unknown	64	—	—

THE INFLUENCE UPON SURVIVAL OF METASTASES TO THE REGIONAL LYMPH NODES AFTER EXCISION OF THE PRIMARY MELANOMA

Of the 58 patients in whom no metastases developed in the lymph nodes, 79% survived ten years. Metastases developed in lymph nodes after treatment of the primary melanoma in ten patients; the time of appearance varied from one month to 60+ months; and only two of those patients survived the ten-year period (Fig. 20-17). The one patient who developed metastases five years after treatment of the primary lesion survived the five-year span after an axillary dissection (Table 20-12).

THE INFLUENCE OF SATELLITOSES ON SURVIVAL

Ten patients presented satellitoses at the time of the initial consultation, and all of these patients died. One patient developed satellitosis two months after initial treatment, one between four to six months, (Fig. 20-18), and two patients developed satellitosis after one year following the initial treatment. The ten-year survival rate was 4%.

BLOOD-BORNE METASTASES

Blood-borne metastases may occur to any part of the body at any time (Table 20-13). Twenty patients developed metastases be-

TABLE 20-9. Melanoma of the Skin of the Chest Wall.
The Influence of Stage upon Survival

Stage	Number of Patients	10-Year Survivors	
		Number	Percent
Stage I	90	50	55
Stage II	150	20	13
Stage III	48	4	8
Unknown	8	—	—

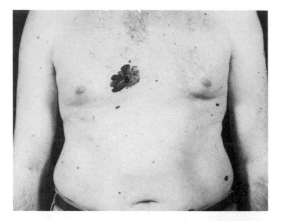

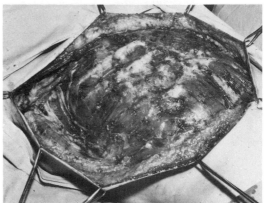

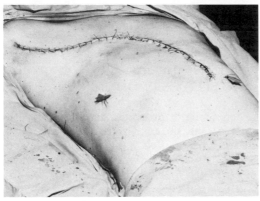

FIGURE 20-15.   Upper left. Infiltrating melanoma of anterior chest wall. Upper right. Operative appearance of resection of the melanoma in continuity with a radical groin dissection. Bottom left. Postoperative appearance of surgical wound.

TREATMENT OF METASTASES

Many methods were utilized to treat blood-borne metastases, varying from surgical resection,[5] various chemotherapeutic measures,[4] radioactive isotopes,[3] immunotherapy in the form of rabies vaccine, BCG and *Bacillus parvum*, and a combination of these procedures. None of these treatments were tremendously effective.

The data are presented as salvage at the five-year interval. Four of eight patients with metastases to the skin survived five years, and one patient with metastases to the liver survived five years after treatment of the primary melanoma. One of 36 patients with metastases to several loci survived five years. (Table 20-14).

tween one and three months; 22 between four and six months; and 50 between the first and second year after initial treatment. Blood-borne metastases may present five years or longer subsequent to initial therapy as manifested by ten patients in this series, one of whom survived five years or longer after resection of the metastases. The site of blood-borne metastases is summarized in Table 20-14.

TABLE 20-10.   Melanoma of the Skin of the Chest Wall. The Influence of Histologic Type upon Survival

Histologic Type	Number of Patients	10-Year Survivors	
		Number	Percent
Superficial melanoma	30	22	73
Infiltrating melanoma	210	44	21
Unknown	56	10	18

TABLE 20-11. Melanoma of the Skin of the Chest Wall.
The Influence of Local Recurrence after Treatment upon Survival

Time of Local Recurrence	Number of Patients	5-Year Survivors	
		Number	Percent
None occurred	164	68	41
Under 1 month	0	—	—
1–3 months	4	0	0
4–6 months	8	0	0
7–12 months	12	0	0
13–36 months	12	2	17
37–60 months	2	1	50
60 + months	1	0	0
Unknown	93	—	—

THE ROLE OF LYMPHADENECTOMY IN THE OVERALL TREATMENT OF MALIGNANT MELANOMA

An analysis of 88 patients with clinical stage I melanoma was made to determine the role of lymphadenectomy on survival (Fig. 20-8). In the group who were subject to an elective node dissection were 40 males and 22 females; the average age was 43 years. Lesions of the an-terior chest wall occurred in 43 patients; posterior in 19 patients. Of those not subjected to a node dissection were 11 males and 15 females; the average age was 45 years. Twelve had anterior lesions and in fourteen, the melanoma was located posteriorly. In 62 patients, an elective node dissection was performed (i.e. the nodes were considered negative on physical examination). In 20 patients the lymph nodes were positive for metastases; and in 42 the lymph nodes were negative on

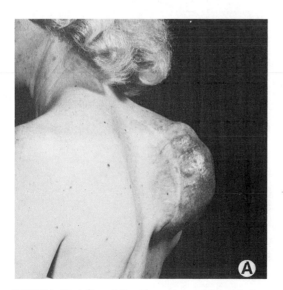

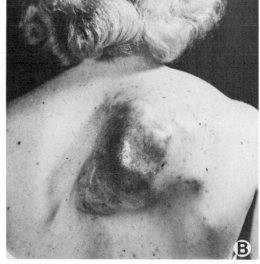

FIGURE 20-16A and B. Posterior and lateral view of a recurrent melanoma, which developed after an incomplete excision. It shows the extent to which untreated or residual melanoma may grow. Patient eventually died from widespread metastases, including metastasis to the brain.

**TABLE 20-12.   Melanoma of the Skin of the Chest Wall.
The Influence of Metastasis (to Lymph Nodes) after Treatment upon
Survival***

Time of Lymph Node Metastasis	Number of Patients	10-Year Survivors	
		Number	Percent
None occurred	58	46	79
Occult metastases discovered at time of elective node dissection	20	6	30
Under 1 month	0	—	—
1–3 months	2	0	0
4–6 months	3	0	0
7–12 months	2	0	0
13–36 months	2	1	50
37–60 months	0	—	—
60 + months	1	1	100

* 198 patients not applicable—stage II or III at consult

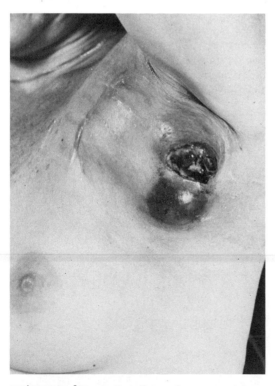

FIGURE 20-17.   Bulky ulcerated metastases to axilla requiring a palliative axillary dissection. Early or elective resection could prevent this severe sequela.

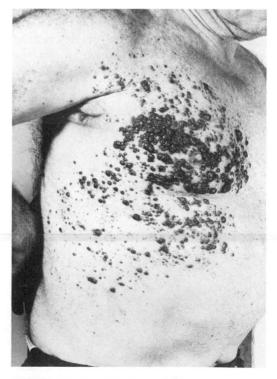

FIGURE 20-18.   Extensive satellitoses of the chest wall after an unsuccessful excision and axillary dissection.

TABLE 20–13.   Melanoma of the Skin of the Chest Wall.
The Influence of Time of Blood-Borne Metastasis after Treatment upon Survival*

Time of Blood-Borne Metastasis	Number of Patients	5-Year Survivors	
		Number	Percent
None occurred	158	145	92
Under 1 month	10	1	10
1–3 months	20	1	5
4–6 months	22	0	0
7–12 months	18	0	0
13–36 months	50	1	2
37–60 months	8	0	0
60+ months	10	1	10
Unknown	24	—	—

* 24 patients not applicable—stage III at consult

histologic examination. The ten-year survival for those with positive lymph nodes was 30% and 71% ten-year survival for patients with no metastases in the lymph nodes. Of twenty-six patients with clinical stage I melanoma in whom no lymph node dissection was performed, ten later developed metastases to the lymph nodes and eight subsequently died of their malignant melanomas after a therapeutic axillary dissection. Sixteen patients did not develop metastases to regional lymph nodes but six patients (39%) of this group developed blood-borne metastases and died of dissemination of the melanoma. The ten-year survival of these 16 patients was 61%.

DISCUSSION

The behavior of melanomas arising from the trunk are divided into melanomas of the chest (thoracic) wall and those arising in the skin of the abdominal wall (Chapter 21). This division is an arbitrary one inasmuch as the vagaries of melanoma spread are so great that one cannot always predict the exact routes of spread. It does, however, offer guidelines which, if interpreted within the realm of its lack of exactness, may be helpful in developing therapeutic policies for a given patient. The division that we have utilized is a circumferential line extending around the cir-

TABLE 20–14.   Melanoma of the Skin of the Chest Wall.
The Influence of Site of Blood-Borne Metastasis after Treatment upon Survival

Site of Blood-Borne Metastasis	Number of Patients	5-Year Survivors	
		Number	Percent
Skin	8	4	50
Lung	16	0	0
Liver	8	1	12
Brain	16	0	0
Bones	14	0	0
Disseminated	16	0	0
Other	4	0	0
More than one of above	36	1	2

cumference of the trunk at the level of the twelfth rib, modified after Sappey.

Sugarbaker and McBride have performed studies delineating the routes of metastases based upon the site of the melanoma. They have utilized the original technique of Sappey, who in 1843, as a medical student, developed the lymphatic distribution within the trunk. Interestingly, Sugarbaker and McBride's studies coincided nicely with the original description of Sappey which is defined as a line running from 2 cm above the umbilicus curving proximally and laterally to the level of the second or third lumbar vertebra. Our guideline extends 3 to 5 cm superior to the umbilicus in the midanterior surface slightly inferior to Sugarbaker's and McBride's boundary. It is slightly inferior in certain regions to that described by Fortner, Das Gupta and McNeer which line runs from the midepigastrium along the twelfth rib to approximately the eight or ninth thoracic vertebra in the midback. Das Gupta and McNeer differentiated the trunk at a somewhat higher level than did Sugarbaker and McBride.

In our series, the site of the metastases to the lymph nodes was predictable in approximately 85% of the cases, utilizing the twelfth rib boundary line. Exceptions which were encountered were as follows:

Four patients with the primary inferior to the clavicle demonstrated metastases to the ipsilateral axilla and the neck, and in two patients metastases to the cervical region occurred and not to the axilla. Of patients with metastases in the midline anteriorly: 8 patients developed metastases to one axilla only, 2 patients with the primary to the right of the midline developed metastases bilaterally, and one patient whose primary melanoma was to the left of the midline developed metastases to the right axilla. One patient who had a primary on the anterior chest wall just above the level of the twelfth rib developed metastases to the groin, and one other patient developed metastases to both the axilla and the groin lymph nodes.

Fortner, Das Gupta and McNeer found relatively little correlation regarding the location of the primary melanoma and the nodes invaded by melanoma. For 46 melanomas of the pectoral region, 18 metastasized unilaterally to the axilla, four bilaterally, four to the neck and axilla, one to the neck. Of five with the primary in the region of the sternum, two metastasized to a unilateral axilla, and one bilaterally to the axillae. Of 12 patients with primaries of the abdomen above the umbilicus, three metastasized to the ipsilateral axilla, one to the ipsilateral groin, and one to both the groin and axilla. Of primaries on the posterior thoracic wall, of 45 in the region of the scapula, 20 metastasized to the ipsilateral axilla, four to the bilateral axillae, two to the neck and axilla and two to the neck. In the interscapular region, of 19 patients, five manifested unilateral metastases, six bilateral metastases to the axillae, and one to the neck and the axilla. On the lateral trunk above the twelfth rib, of 14 patients, 9 had metastases to the ipsilateral axilla and 2 to the neck and the axilla.

Of the melanomas of the trunk reported by Sugarbaker and McBride, they state:

> In this series of 128 patients, a total of 40 patients developed positive nodes at some time during the disease. In two patients nodal metastases developed in association with or after local recurrence and in four patients they occurred after systemic dissemination or as part of "disease explosion." In these six patients regional node dissection would not have been of predictable benefit since other sites of failure preceded nodal involvement and were more significant.

They believe that the unpredictability of the Fortner et al. series may have been due to the fact that many of their patients had positive nodes initially, or that an elective regional node dissection as part of the initial therapy may have affected the location of the metastases to the lymph nodes.[7]

Fortner et al. do not believe that the site of the primary lesion influences its propensity for metastatic spread, or is a determinant of the most likely region for lymph node involvement. Their treatment consisted of a wide excision of the primary site in 76 of the 194 patients (39%). Subsequently, 50 of the 76 patients required a lymph node dissection in one or more regions because of clinically apparent metastases. Their results for all trunkal melanoma reveal that of 85 patients with stage I, the survival rate was 55.2% and for 109 patients with stage II, a 19.2% survival rate was obtained. In their series, elective lymphadenectomy proved most efficacious: 55.5% of the 18 patients with histologically positive but clinically negative nodes survived 5 years, equal to the survival for stage I melanoma. Six (54.5%) of 11 patients who had recurrent local disease without metastases to the regional lymph nodes survived five or more years without cancer. Two of the six died after the five-year period. Only one of 17 patients with recurrent local disease and regional lymph node disease lived five years.

Sylven, from Norway, in 1948 reported a 29% five-year survival of 34 patients with stage I melanoma of the trunk, and a 12% survival of 24 patients with stage II melanoma of the trunk.[19]

The observations that from one-third to one-half of the patients seen with malignant melanoma of the thoracic wall have metastases, or will develop metastases to the regional lymph nodes strongly support the premise that these nodes should be considered in the therapeutic attack. The observation of Sugarbaker and McBride who performed a primary wide excision only, and observed that approximately one-third of those patients later developed metastases, would suggest that excision of the primary lesion only would result in the development of metastases to the regional lymph nodes in a significant number of patients. To deprive one-third of all patients with cancers of the trunk the protection offered by a lymph node dissection in order to spare a slight degree of morbidity would seem to us to be a questionable doctrine. We, accordingly, believe that malignant melanoma of the chest wall, especially infiltrating melanomas, should be treated where possible by resection of the primary tumor in continuity with the regional lymph nodes.

The fact that 58% (21 of 36) of the patients who developed recurrences did so within one year after treatment suggests some inadequacy of the administered treatment. A tentative program for the nodes to be excised during the treatment of a primary malignant melanoma of the skin of the chest wall is shown in Table 20–15.

These suggestions are for infiltrating melanomas (Clark's Level IV and V and possible III, or Breslow's thicker lesions). Further study is necessary to determine treatment policies for stage I, superficial melanomas (Clark's Level II).

SUMMARY AND CONCLUSIONS

1. Melanomas of the trunk constitute 34% of the 3,305 melanomas treated at the Pack Medical Group. Melanomas of the thorax comprise 57% of trunkal melanomas.

2. All patients with melanomas of the thorax seen by us were Caucasians, most with fair skin and blue eyes, three-quarters were males and almost two-thirds were in the 30 to 50-year age group.

3. Of the 296 patients treated, 30% were histologically staged as stage I; 51% were stage II; and 16% were stage III. Ten percent were superficial melanomas (Clark's Level II) and 79% were infiltrating melanomas (Clark's Level IV and V).

4. The treatment is surgical resection. The indications for lymph node dissection and the lymph nodes to be removed are discussed.

5. The determinate ten-year control rate for 248 evaluable patients is 35%. The absolute ten-year survival rate is 30%.

6. Age did not seem to affect cure rate except the four patients in the 10 to 20 year decade fared better. The survival rate for females (31%) is better than that of males (22%).

7. Staging played an important role in the prognosis. For ninety patients with stage I, 55% survived 10 years. The rate dropped to 13% for 150 patients with stage II and precipitously dropped to 4% for 58 patients with stage III melanomas.

8. In elective node dissection when the nodes were found positive, 30% survived, when the nodes were negative, the survival

TABLE 20-15. Regional Lymphadenectomy Predicated on the Site and Clinical Stage of Patients with Infiltrating Melanoma of the Thoracic Cage

Site of Primary Melanoma	Clinical Stage	Treatment
Anterior chest—lateral	I & II	Ipsilateral axillary dissection
Anterior chest wall, 2 in. inferior to clavical & its counterpart posterior	I	Ipsilateral axillary dissection—either simultaneous low-cervical dissection or careful observation of supraclavicular region
	II	Positive axillary nodes—combined axillary and neck dissection
Midline (anterior and posterior)	I & II	Bilateral axillary dissection
Anterior midline or 2 in. lateral	I & II	Ipsilateral axillary and internal mammary lymph node dissection
Lateral chest wall	I & II	Ipsilateral axillary dissection—although groin lymph nodes are at risk, metastases have been so rare that the site may be carefully observed
In the immediate vicinity of the 12th rib: the junction of the thorax and abdomen	I	Careful observation—no lymphadenectomy
	II	Lymphadenectomy of involved region

rate was 71%. When no elective dissection was performed and regional nodes developed metastases that were later resected, 20% survived ten years or longer but when no metastases developed in the lymph nodes 61% survived; the remainder succumbed from blood-borne metastases.

9. A suggested treatment program is offered.

REFERENCES

1. Ariel IM: Tridimensional resection of malignant melanoma. Surg Gynecol Obstet 139:601, 1974
2. Ariel IM, Caron AS: Diagnosis and treatment of malignant melanoma arising from the skin of the female breast. Am J Surg 124:384, 1972
3. Ariel IM, Oropeza R: Intralymphatic administration of radioactive isotopes for treatment of malignant melanoma. Surg Gynecol Obstet 124:25, 1967
4. Ariel IM, Pack GT: Treatment of disseminated melanoma by systemic Melphelan, Methotrexate and autogenous bone marrow transplants. Cancer 20:77, 1967
5. Ariel IM, Pack GT: Treatment of disseminated melanoma with phenylalanine mustard (Melphelan) and autogenous bone marrow transplants. Surgery 51:583, 1962
6. Ariel IM, Resnick MI: Altered lymphatic dynamics caused by cancer metastases. Arch Surg 94:117, 1967
7. Ariel IM, Resnick MI: Altered lymphatic dynamics following groin and axillary dissection: Its relationship to treatment policies for malignant melanoma. Surgery 61:210, 1967
8. Das Gupta T, McNeer G: The incidence of metastasis to accessible lymph nodes from melanoma of the trunk and extremities—its therapeutic significance. Cancer 17:897, 1964
9. Fortner JG, Das Gupta T, et al.: Malignant melanoma of the trunk. Ann Surg 161:161, 1965
10. Goldsmith HS, Shah TP, Kim D-H: Prognostic significance of lymph node dissection in the treatment of malignant melanoma. Cancer 26:606, 1970
11. Haagansen, CD, Feind CR, Herter FP, et al.: Lymphatics of the trunk. In: The Lymphatics in Cancer. Philadelphia, WB Saunders Co, 1972, pp 441–451
12. Holmes EC, Clark W, Morton DL, et al.: Regional lymph node metastases and the level of invasion of the primary. Cancer 37:199, 1976

13. MacDonald EJ: The Epidemiology of Melanoma. The Pigment Cell, Molecular, Biological and Clinical Aspects. New York, New York Acad Sci, 1963, p 4

14. McCune WS, Letterman GS: Malignant melanoma: 10-year results following excision and regional gland dissection. Ann Surg 141:901, 1955

15. McGovern VT, Mihm MC, Baelly C, et al.: The classification of malignant melanoma and its histologic reporting. Cancer 32:1446, 1973

16. McNeer G, Das Gupta T: Routes of lymphatic spread of malignant melanoma. CA 15:168, 1965

17. Sappey MPC: Anatomie, physiologie, pathologie des vaisseaux lymphatiques considérés chez l'homme et les vertébrés. Paris, A DeLahaye & E Lecrosnier, 1874

18. Sugarbaker EV, McBride CM: Melanoma of the trunk: The results of surgical excision and anatomic guidelines for predicting nodal metastasis. Surgery 80:22, 1976

19. Sylven B: Malignant melanoma of the skin. Report of 341 cases treated during years 1929–1943. Acta Radiol (Stockh) 32:33, 1949

CHAPTER TWENTY–ONE

PRIMARY MALIGNANT MELANOMA OF THE SKIN OF THE ABDOMINAL WALL

IRVING M. ARIEL

Malignant melanomas of the trunk comprise approximately one-third of all malignant melanomas. In view of the interrelated connections of the lymphatics from melanomas of the trunk, it is often difficult to determine which lymph node basin is the primary site of drainage, and thus to determine treatment policies; especially the lymph nodes that should be dissected in order to perform a mono block dissection of removing the primary malignant melanoma, the intervening lymphatics, the primary echelon of lymph nodes to which metastases may occur. For example, a malignant melanoma in the region of the umbilicus presents the untenable situation of potential metastases to the lymph nodes of either axilla, either groin, or via the ligamentum teres to the liver.

The overall results for treating malignant melanoma of the trunk have been relatively poor, possibly because of the difficulty in determining the lymph node basins that should be surgically resected. Other possible explanations may be the fact that they may reach a larger size before being noticed because they are not located near the usual line of vision, and they occur more frequently in men, who have an overall poorer prognosis than women.

We have divided the trunk for analytic purposes, into the skin of the thoracic wall, which is being presented in Chapter 20, and those of the abdominal wall.

DEFINITION OF ANATOMIC BOUNDARIES

The skin of the abdomen constitutes that region inferior to the theoretic line surrounding the trunk at the level of the 12th rib. Anteriorly, the abdominal wall extends inferiorly to the groin and to the pubic region. Posteriorly, it extends down to the buttocks but does not include them. This division tends to conform to Sappey's lymphatic drainage of the trunk.[17] It is somewhat more inferior than Sugarbaker and McBride's anatomic division,[18] which is defined as a line running two centimeters above the umbilicus, curving proximally and laterally to the level of the second or third lumbar vertebrae.

The Pack Medical Group saw 3,305 patients suffering from malignant melanoma, and of those, 1,122 (33.9%) had malignant melanoma of the trunk. There were 640 patients who had melanoma of the skin of the thoracic portion of the trunk (57%) and 482 patients (43%) had melanoma involving the skin of the abdominal wall. Those with melanoma of the abdominal wall comprised 14.6% of all melanomas seen in our clinic.

CLINICAL MATERIAL

Caucasians comprised 85% while in 15% race was not listed on the chart (see Table 21–1). None of our patients were either Negro or Oriental. The complexion was listed in 72% of these patients with 52% being of fair complexion, 12% dark, and 8% freckled. Sixty-eight percent were male, and 32% were female. The age distribution revealed that most of the patients (63%) were in the third and fourth decade. The slope decreases on both sides of this plateau. Only 5% of the patients were in the 10 to 20 age bracket while 10% were between 20 to 29 years of age. These patients represent those who presented melanomas as a

351

separate individual entity, and do not include those patients whose melanomas developed upon some other congenital error in metabolism, such as von Recklinghausen's disease, or xeroderma pigmentosa, which were noted in some patients. Thus, all the patients were Caucasian, most were fair-skinned, two-thirds were male, and about two-thirds were in the 30 to 50 age group.

HISTOLOGIC LEVEL OF INVASION

The histologic type was available in 483 patients. We do not consider such lesions as Lentigo nevus or nevi with atypical cells or other such pathologic designations as malignant melanoma, hence none of these entities are included in this study.

In this series 39 patients (9%) were designated as suffering from superficial spreading melanomas, and 344 patients (80%) had infiltrating melanomas. In 47 patients (11%) it was impossible to determine the exact anatomic designation. Twenty-eight patients (6.5%) of the patients were described as having amelanotic melanomas.

We do not consider Clark's level I to be a metastasizing malignant melanoma and hence this subclassification is not included in this investigation. His level III has been found somewhat confusing; hence, our superficial melanomas represent his level II and/or III, and the infiltrating melanomas level IV and V. The slides were not available in sufficient numbers to differentiate between the latter two levels. Our data do not permit an evaluation of Breslow's tumor thickness as a guide for treatment.

LOCATION OF THE MELANOMA

Of the 482 patients, 327 (68%) presented melanomas involving the anterior abdominal wall, of which 12 were in the vicinity of the umbilicus. In 3% the melanomas were located in or adjacent to the midline of the anterior abdominal wall. Thirty percent (145 patients)

TABLE 21-1. Clinical Characteristics of 482 Patients with Malignant Melanoma of the Skin of the Abdomen

	Percent of Patients
Race	
Caucasian	85
Unknown	15
Other (Black, Yellow etc.)	0
Complexion	
Fair	52
Dark	12
Freckled	8
Unknown	28
Eye Color	
Blue	20
Brown	15
Hazel	10
Unknown	55
Sex	
Male	68
Female	32
Age	
0–10	0
10–20	5
20–29	10
30–39	25
40–49	38
50–59	10
60–69	8
70+	1
Unknown	2

presented with their melanomas involving the posterior abdominal wall. The exact location was not listed in ten of the charts reviewed (2%). In 5% of all patients with melanomas of the abdominal wall, the melanomas were situated in a lateral location.

TREATMENT POLICIES

A radical tridimensional excision is performed about the primary site including a generous portion of the surrounding skin with the development of skin flaps and the removal of about twice as much of the underlying integument and fascia with the dissecting going to naked muscle. In most instances closure is effected by sliding flaps.[3] If primary closure is not possible, a combination of sliding flaps, which minimizes the amount of a split-thickness skin graft, is utilized, supplemented by the application of a split-thickness skin graft (Figs. 21-1 and 21-2). In some instances where the melanoma exists in the midline, especially in the lower anterior abdominal wall, a bilateral groin dissection is effected. For those melanomas involving the lateral

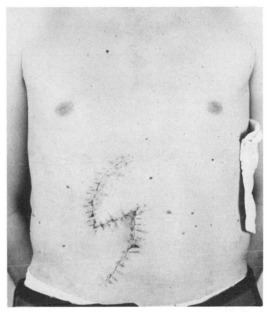

FIGURE 21-2. Surgical repair by Z plasty following tridimensional excision of an infiltrating melanoma of the anterior upper abdominal wall. No lymph node dissection was performed electively. The patient remained free of melanoma for over ten years.

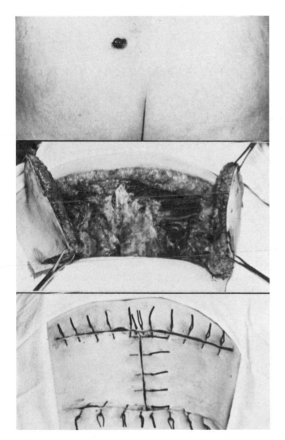

FIGURE 21-1. Top: Malignant melanoma of the posterior inferior abdominal wall. Middle: Extent of tridimensional resection. Bottom: Repair of surgical defect by sliding full thickness skin flaps.

aspect of the abdominal wall, a combined ipsilateral groin and axillary dissection are performed (Fig. 20-4). These have not been performed often enough to warrant any conclusions regarding their efficacy.

RESULTS OF TREATMENT

The survival rates (Table 21-2) evaluate the results obtained in those patients treated more than 10 years ago, of whom there were 260. There were 40 patients who presented themselves for consultation only, of which 10 were in the stage IV category, thus leaving 220 patients available for absolute ten-year survival evaluation. Of these 60 survived the ten-year period, giving a survival rate of 27.3%. In order to evaluate the actual accomplishments of treatment, a relative survival rate is also

TABLE 21-2. Melanoma of the Skin of the Abdomen Overall Survival Ten Years after Surgical Resection

	Number
Total number of patients seen	260
Indeterminate patients:	
Patients who came for consultation only	40
Patients known to have died of another disease	32
Determinate patients	188
Patients alive and free of cancer	60
Patients known to have died of melanoma	128
Determinate 10-year survival 60/188	32%

Absolute 10-year survival rate (includes all patients who have died regardless of cause of death, but excludes those who were seen only in consultation) = 60/220 (27.3%).

presented, which excludes 32 patients who are known to have died of another concurrent disease exclusive of their melanoma. Thus 128 patients were known to have died of their melanomas. Excluding those who came in for consultation only and those who died from another concurrent disease gives a relative survival rate of 32%. Follow-up values were obtained for all patients. The data are analyzed to examine parameters that may have influenced survival. All results are presented in absolute survival terms.

THE EFFECT OF AGE UPON SURVIVAL

The highest survival occurred in the 10 to 30-year age groups. The numbers are so few that they have little or no significance. Of the 50 patients between 30 to 39 years of age, 14 (28%) survived ten years; and of 76 patients between 40 to 49 years of age, 18% survived the ten-year period. There were only two patients over 70 years of age, both of whom died from their melanomas. From these data one cannot make any determination regarding the effect of age upon prognosis in patients with malignant melanoma of the abdominal wall (Table 21-3).

THE EFFECTS OF SEX UPON SURVIVAL

Of the 136 male patients treated over ten years ago, 30 (22%) have survived the ten-year period free of disease, whereas 22 (34%) of the 64 females treated over ten years ago have survived. Females generally have an improved survival rate in melanomas of most locations (Table 21-4).

Fortner and colleagues[7] published a 33% five-year survival of 112 males with melanoma throughout the trunk, and a 42.7% five-year survival for 82 females, a difference they did not consider significant. Our ten-year survival rate is a bit lower than theirs and may be the result of those patients dying between the five- and ten-year period.

SIZE OF LESION AND ITS EFFECT UPON SURVIVAL

In 116 patients where the lesion size was recorded, the best survival rates were melanomas less than 2 cm in diameter. The survival rate then dropped quite precipitously for the larger lesions. This is somewhat in contrast to the melanomas of the chest wall, where the size of the lesion did not seem to exert a dramatic effect upon survival. The nodularity of the lesions was not mentioned frequently enough in this retrospective study to warrant any comment regarding the influence of the macular or papillar characteristics of the lesions upon prognosis (Table 21-5).

SITE OF LESION AND ITS EFFECT UPON SURVIVAL

There were 140 patients whose melanoma occurred on the anterior abdominal wall, of whom 62 patients (44%) survived. Of these were 16 patients whose melanoma occurred at or within 2 cm of the midline, and only four of these (25%) survived the ten-year period. The prognosis is somewhat worse for those mela-

**TABLE 21-3. Melanoma of the Skin of the Abdomen.
The Influence of Age upon Survival**

Age	Number of Patients	10-Year Survivors	
		Number	Percent
Under 10	0	0	0
10–20	4	2	50
21–29	20	10	50
30–39	50	14	28
40–49	76	14	18
50–59	20	4	20
60–69	16	4	25
70+	2	0	0
Unknown	32	—	—

**TABLE 21-4. Melanoma of the Skin of the Abdomen.
The Influence of Sex upon Survival**

Sex	Number of Patients	10-Year Survivors	
		Number	Percent
Male	136	30	22
Female	64	22	34

**TABLE 21-5. Melanoma of the Skin of the Abdomen.
The Influence of Size upon Survival**

Size	Number of Patients	10-Year Survivors	
		Number	Percent
Under 1 cm	20	8	40
1 cm/2 cm	42	18	43
2 cm/3 cm	30	6	20
3+ cm	24	4	17
Unknown	104	18	17

nomas of the posterior abdominal wall, of whom there were 44, with 16 patients (36%) surviving. Of this group were 14 patients whose melanoma involved the midline, and only two (14%) survived the ten-year span. The lateral abdominal wall was involved in 24 patients, of whom six (25%) survived the ten-year span. Twelve patients presented melanomas in the region of the umbilicus, and one of these survived the ten-year period (8%). Two died between the five- and ten-year periods (Table 21-6 and Fig. 21-3).

THE EFFECT OF A PREEXISTING MOLE UPON SURVIVAL

In 124 patients (56%) a preexisting mole was claimd to have existed, whereas in 54 patients (24%) the patient believed that the melanoma arose de novo. For 42 patients (19%) no history was elicited from the chart. Of the 124 with a preexisting mole, 66 patients (53%) survived the ten-year period, whereas only 16 of the 54 patients (30%) who had a de novo malignant melanoma survived

TABLE 21-6. Melanoma of the Skin of the Abdomen. Effect of Location upon Survival

Location	Number of Patients	10-Year Survivors	
		Number	Percent
Anterior abdominal wall	140	62	44
Midline	(16)	(4)	(25)
Umbilical region	(12)	(1)	(8)
Posterior abdominal wall	44	16	36
Midline	(14)	(2)	(14)
Lateral abdominal wall	24	6	25

the ten-year period. This differential suggests a poorer prognosis for patients whose melanomas arose without any history of pre-existing mole (Table 21-7).

THE INFLUENCE OF STAGING UPON SURVIVAL

Of the 96 patients classified as stage I, 58 (60%) survived the ten-year period, which drop to 14% for the 112 patients who pre-

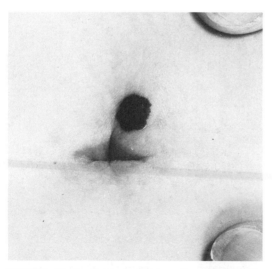

FIGURE 21-3. Benign pigmented nevus in the region of the umbilicus, cured by simple local excision. This is a most dangerous site for a malignant melanoma because of the propensity to metastasize from this site to either axilla, either groin, or via the ligamentum teres to the liver.

sented themselves with stage II melanomas. None of the patients in stage III survived the ten-year period. These figures include all patients who died during the ten-year period regardless of cause of death, and represent 220 patients evaluated (Table 21-8).

THE INFLUENCE OF HISTOLOGIC CLASSIFICATION UPON TEN-YEAR SURVIVAL

Of the 20 patients diagnosed as having superficial melanoma, (Clark's level II or possibly III) 12 (60%) survived ten years, in contrast to the 176 patients who presented with infiltrating melanomas, (Clark's level IV or V) of whom 42 patients (24%) survived 10 years. Of 24 patients whose classification was not listed, ten (42%) survived a ten-year span (Table 21-9).

The data demonstrate that although superficial melanomas carry with them a better prognosis than infiltrating melanomas, they nevertheless constitute a potentially lethal disease, and indicate that one cannot relent in the treatment policy because of a diagnosis of superficial melanoma.

Twenty patients presented with evidence of satellitosis, that is, daughter melanomas surrounding the primary melanoma for varying distances, in addition to metastases to the lymph nodes. Two of these patients survived the ten-year period. Fourteen patients (6%) presented amelanotic melanomas, and four of these (28%) are free of evidence of melanoma ten years later (Fig. 21-4).

TABLE 21-7. Melanoma of the Skin of the Abdomen.
The Influence of a History of a Previous Mole upon Survival

History of Mole	Number of Patients	Percent of Patients	10-Year Survivors	
			Number	Percent
Preexisting mole	124	56	66	53
No preexisting mole	54	24	16	30
Unknown	42	19	8	19

THE EFFECT OF LOCAL RECURRENCE UPON SURVIVAL

Fifteen patients developed a local recurrence at the site of the previous excised melanoma before any evidence of lymph node metastasis or blood-borne metastasis had occurred. Five (33.3%) survived the ten-year period. Local recurrence, per se, is not so ominous as one might think, although it is, of course, not a harmless manifestation.

EFFECT OF METASTASES TO REGIONAL LYMPH NODES UPON SURVIVAL

In 96 patients no metastases were discerned in the lymph nodes, and 67% survived the ten-year period. When metastases occurred within three months after the initial treatment, which occurred in 14 of our patients, none survived ten years. Table 21-10 suggests that the later metastases to the lymph nodes occur, the better the prognosis. Eight patients developed metastases after a five-year period, of whom six survived five years after the lymphadenectomy.

THE ROLE OF LYMPHADENECTOMY IN THE OVERALL TREATMENT OF MALIGNANT MELANOMA

Whether primary lymphadenectomy should be performed on all patients with malignant melanoma is a disputed question. An analysis of 96 patients in clinical stage I of malignant

melanoma of the abdominal wall is summarized in Figure 21-5. In 60 patients with no nodes palpable in the groin, an elective adenectomy was performed, and in 22 patients metastases were found in the lymph nodes of the groin, with a resultant ten-year survival of these 22 patients of 45%. In 38 patients the nodes were negative for evidence of metastases, and the ten-year survival was 79%. In 36 patients no elective dissection was performed; in 16 of these patients (44%) metastases later developed to lymph nodes, for which a lymphadenectomy was performed, with a ten-year survival rate of 25%. In 20 patients metastases did not develop to the regional lymph nodes, and the ten-year survival rate of this group was 70%.

The data demonstrate a 29% error in clinically determining whether lymph nodes are positive in patients with melanoma of the abdominal wall. This is similar to a 32% error in clinically considering lymph nodes to be negative in patients with melanoma of the thorax, whose nodes on histologic examination revealed metastases. The survival rate of patients on whom a delayed lymphadenectomy was performed when clinical manifestations of metastases presented themselves was

TABLE 21-8. Melanoma of the Skin of the Abdomen. The Influence of Stage upon Survival

Stage	Number of Patients	10-Year Survivors	
		Number	Percent
Stage I	96	58	60
Stage II	112	16	14
Stage III	12	0	0

TABLE 21-9. Melanoma of the Skin of the Abdomen. The Influence of Histologic Type upon Survival*

Histologic Type	Number of Patients	10-Year Survivors	
		Number	Percent
Superficial melanoma	20	12	60
Infiltrating melanoma	176	42	24
Unknown	24	10	42

* We do not consider Clark's level I to be a metastasizing malignant melanoma and hence this subclassification is not included in this investigation. His level III has been found somewhat confusing; hence, our superficial melanomas represent his level II and/or III and the infiltrating melanomas levels IV and V. The slides were not available in sufficient numbers to differentiate between the latter two levels. Our data do not permit an evaluation of Breslow's tumor thickness as a guide for treatment.

lower (25%) than those with metastases to lymph nodes whose lymphadenectomy was performed as an elective procedure (45%).

DISCUSSION

This study analyzes the clinical features of 482 patients seen at the Pack Medical Group between 1934 and 1975. Of the 3,305 patients analyzed at the Pack Medical Group, melanomas of the abdominal wall constituted 14.5% of all the melanomas seen, and 43% of the melanomas of the trunk. We have divided the trunk into an arbitrary division of the thoracic portion and the abdominal segment around the trunkal circumference about the level of the 12th rib. Sugarbaker and McBride,[18] following the dissections of Sappey, divided the trunk into an arbitrary division as shown in Figure 20-1. Their divisions are slightly higher for the abdominal wall than ours. Extensive studies regarding the route where metastases to the lymph nodes may occur were performed by Sugarbaker and McBride, and independently by Fortner, Das Gupta, and McNeer.[7] Das Gupta and McNeer use the eighth rib as a landmark for separating the thoracic and abdominal portions of the trunk. We consider this level too high and the large incidence of metastases to the axilla in their series tends to support our opinion.

Fortner and his colleagues found little correlation between the location of the primary melanoma and the lymph nodes that were involved by metastases. Of 12 patients whose primaries were on the abdominal wall above the umbilicus, three metastasized to the ipsilateral axilla, one to the ipsilateral groin, and

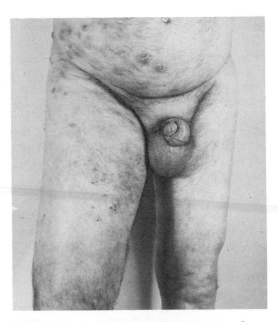

FIGURE 21-4. Extensive subcutaneous and cutaneous metastases to the lower abdomen and thigh.

TABLE 21–10. Melanoma of the Skin of the Abdomen.
The Influence of Metastasis (to Lymph Nodes) after Treatment upon Survival

Time of Lymph Node Metastasis	Number of Patients	10-Year Survivors	
		Number	Percent
None occurred	96	64	67
Under 1 month	6	0	0
1–3 months	8	0	0
4–6 months	10	2	20
7–12 months	8	2	25
13–36 months	20	8	40
60+ months	8	6	75
Unknown	54	—	—

one to both the groin and axilla. Sugarbaker and McBride believe that the location does play a role in determining the routes of the lymph nodes involved, and that the fact that the series of Fortner et al. did not was the result of their patients having had metastases to their nodes initially, or because an elective regional node dissection had been done as part of initial therapy, and that these factors influence the location to which metastases to the lymph nodes may occur. Our studies[2] have demonstrated altered lymphatic circulation after metastases have occurred to regional lymph nodes or after the lymphatic circulation

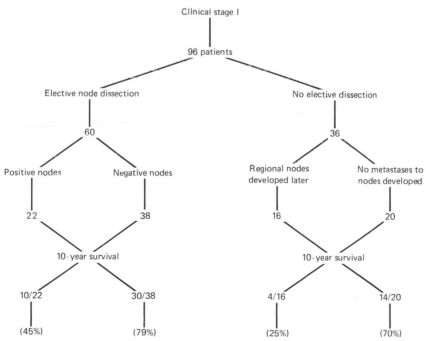

FIGURE 21–5. Melanoma of the skin of the abdominal wall. Shown here is the influence of regional lymph node dissection upon survival.

has been altered by lymphadenectomy. Sugarbaker and McBride believe that regional lymph nodes should be excised with dispatch, and have called attention to the fact that for all melanomas of the trunk, within a median time of ten months after the initial examination, 15 (36.6%) of 41 patients who had not had lymphadenectomy developed metastases to the regional lymph nodes. Thus, 64.9% of their patients with melanoma arising anywhere on the trunk developed metastases to the lymph nodes during their clinical course.

Sylven,[19] from Norway, reported a 29% five-year survival rate of 34 patients with stage I melanoma of the trunk, and a 12% five-year survival rate for 24 patients with stage II malignant melanomas of the trunk.

In our series of patients with melanoma of the abdominal wall, 40% developed metastases to lymph nodes sometime during their clinical course. The sites of metastases to lymph nodes were predictable in approximately 145 patients (75%) of the determinate cases. For those melanomas of the anterior abdominal wall (with the exception of those around the umbilicus), metastases occurred almost exclusively to the lymph nodes in the ipsilateral groin. For those of the midline, metastases usually occurred to one groin, and in 35% of the cases to the opposite groin at a later date, which varied from one to seven years post-treatment for the metastases involving the ipsilateral groin. Synchronous metastases to both inguinal regions were present in 15 patients (3%) of the patients whose primary melanomas involved the midline of the abdomen. When the primary cancer was in the vicinity of the umbilicus, metastases occurred to either axilla, either groin, or via the ligament terres directly into the liver. Spread to the ipsilateral groin and the opposite axilla with involvement of the liver was found in one of our patients, and in one other patient metastases occurred to the right groin and the right axilla, whereas in one other patient metastases were present in both inguinal regions at the time the patient was first seen. The location of the melanoma in relationship to the umbilicus gave no clue where metastases would occur. When the primary melanoma involved the lateral abdominal wall, metastases occurred to either the ipsilateral groin or the ipsilateral axilla. A somewhat surprising and unexplained lymphatic spread of melanoma for those involving the lateral aspect of the abdominal wall and posterior aspect of the abdominal wall was the incidence of metastases to the axilla noted in approximately 8.5% of the patients who developed metastases to lymph nodes. This spread does not fit in exactly with the definition of lymphatic drainage as described by Sappey and adopted by Sugarbaker and McBride. The clinical implication is either a synchronous operation of the groin and axilla, or if the operation is done in the groin, careful attention must be paid to the ipsilateral axilla. We have followed this course in a few patients, but the numbers are to few to warrant any conclusions.

Haagensen[10] depends exclusively upon Sappey's description of lymphatic drainage of the trunk and refers to it as "the watershed at the level of the umbilicus between the lymphatics that drain to the axilla and those that drain into the groin." In his experience with 109 melanomas of the trunk at the Presbyterian Hospital, New York, 64 were situated on the dorsal surface and 39 on the ventral surface. When metastases developed from melanomas inferior to the watershed, they always went to the inguinal nodes. None metastasized to the axillary nodes, which is in conflict with other authors who have described spread to the axillary lymph nodes. He further states that none metastasized to both the axilla and the inguinal nodes, in contrast to our findings. There were only 13 melanomas situated in the midline or within 1 cm of the midline, and his data do not suggest that bilateral metastases to the axilla or inguinal nodes occur frequently enough to justify bilateral prophylactic dissection inasmuch as only one of his patients with a midline lesion was shown to have bilateral axillary metastases. With melanomas situated close to the midline, he had only two patients whose lesions were in the suprapubic area and who developed contra-inguinal metastases at a later date, and one had bilateral inguinal metastases when they first appeared. In

Haagensen's series of patients without clinically involved regional nodes, histologic examination of the resected specimen showed that 23.6% had metastases. Of 55 patients with melanoma of the trunk without clinically involved lymph nodes on admission, on whom lymph node dissection was not done, five developed clinically involved nodes after several years. Thus 31% of patients with melanomas of the trunk developed regional lymph node metastases. The fact that six of his 103 patients with melanoma of the trunk died more than five years after treatment warrants reports of ten-year survival. Haagensen's conclusion is: "Our series of melanomas of the trunk provides significant evidence of the value of lymph node dissection, not only when it is done prophylacticly when there are no clinically involved nodes, but also when it is done for clinically involved nodes." Prophylactic regional node dissection was performed in 43 of his 72 patients without clinically involved nodes on admission more than five years ago. Metastases were found in nine of the 43, and four are still living without recurrences after six to 23 years. Of 29 patients who did not have clinically involved nodes on admission to the hospital and did not have prophylactic regional node dissection, five (19%) subsequently developed clinically involved nodes. He further points out that in three of the patients who were cured, the involved nodes were very large, varying from 3 cm to 9 cm in number, and states that with metastatic melanoma in the lymph nodes, the number of nodes involved is more important than their size.

Mundth and his associates[16] report a five-year survival of 24% for 66 cases, and McLeod and his associates reported a five-year survival of 31% in their series of 90 patients with melanomas of the trunk. For 194 patients reported by Fortner and his associates the five-year survival was 37%. The actual value of regional lymph node dissection in their series of 60 patients in whom an operation was done for melanoma of the trunk is evidenced by the fact that metastases were found in 26 of the 60 patients. Long-term cures without recurrences lasting from six to 23 years resulted in eight

(30%) of the 26 patients. He states that "these results, in our opinion, justify regional lymph node dissection in this disease."

Knutson, Hori, and Spratt[12] report that of 45 of their patients with melanoma of the trunk (including two perianal and one genital melanoma) 17.3% survived the five-year period. In Das Guptas and McNeer's[6] 56% of 194 patients developed metastases to the lymph nodes, and in those instances where no elective lymph node dissection was performed the median interval between the primary excision and the appearance of metastases to the lymph nodes was ten months. In their series of 15 patients with melanoma of the lumbosacral region, four presented in the midline and each of these four had metastases bilaterally to the groin lymph nodes. Five of the remaining had metastases to the ipsilateral lymph nodes and one whose exact location could not be verified had metastases to the ipsilateral axilla and groin.

The reports in the literature, including our data, indicate that melanomas tend to metastasize to regional lymph nodes and that the incidence is high enough to warrant elective lymph node dissection, preferably incontinuity (although studies by Goldsmith, Shah, and Kim[9] have claimed no difference in survival between an incontinuity and discontinuous lymph node dissection—67% five-year survival in both instances of stage I melanoma, 39% five-year survival for incontinuity, and 31% five-year survival for discontinuous operation of patients with stage II melanomas). The vagaries and inconsistencies of the behavior of malignant melanoma must be realized and clinical judgment should evaluate all factors, including staging, depth of invasion, and height, in determining treatment policies.

SUMMARY AND CONCLUSIONS

1. Melanomas of the trunk constituted 33.9% of the 3,305 melanomas treated at the Pack Medical Group. Melanomas of the skin of the abdominal wall comprise 43% of

trunkal melanomas and 14.6% of all melanomas seen.

2. All of the patients with malignant melanoma of the abdominal wall seen by us were Caucasian, most with fair skin and blue eyes, two-thirds were males, and almost two-thirds were in the 30 to 50 age group.

3. Of the 220 determinate patients, 96 were stage I, 112 were stage II, and 12 were stage III. Ten percent were superficial melanomas and 79% were infiltrating melanomas. Ten were amelanotic melanomas.

4. The treatment is surgical resection. The indications for lymph node dissection and for the lymph nodes to be removed are discussed.

5. The absolute ten-year survival rate is 27.3%, and the relative (determinate) ten-year survival rate is 32%.

6. The younger patients in this series seemed to fare better than the older ones. Thus, for the patients between 10 and 30 years, the survival rate was 50%, which decreased to 28% for the 30- to 39-year group, and further decreased to 18% in the 40- to 49-age bracket. The very few patients seen in the 10- to 30-year age bracket do not permit significant evaluation of these figures. The survival rate for females (34%) was better than that for males (22%).

7. The size of the lesion does not seem to affect prognosis, except for those melanomas that are greater than 2 cm in diameter. Our data does not evaluate the role of nodular vs macular melanomas and their effect upon prognosis.

8. The location of the melanomas seems to play an important role in that a 44% ten-year survival rate was observed for the anterior abdominal wall, which decreased to 36% for those of the posterior abdominal wall, and to 25% for those located in a lateral position. Of 12 patients who had melanomas in the region of the umbilicus, none survived the ten-year period.

9. The presence of a preexisting mole that underwent malignant transformation seemed to offer a better prognosis (53% ten-year survival) than did those malignant melanomas that occurred de novo (30%).

10. Staging played a most significant role in prognosis, with a 60% ten-year survival of 96 patients in stage I, in contrast to a 14% ten-year survival of 112 patients in stage II. Of 12 patients in stage III, none survived a ten-year span.

11. The histologic type of melanoma played a role in prognosis in that a 60% ten-year survival was obtained for patients with superficial melanomas (Clark's level II–III), in contrast to a 24% for infiltrating melanomas (Clark's level IV–V). The fact that of the patients whose melanomas were designated superficial melanomas, 40% succumbed, focuses upon the seriousness of this form of melanoma.

12. The time of appearance of metastases to regional lymph nodes after treatment of the primary lesion seems to play a role in that the later the metastases occurred the better was the prognosis.

13. When elective node dissections were performed, as was done in 60 patients with clinical stage I, 22 were shown to have metastases to their lymph nodes. Surgery yielded a ten-year survival rate of 45% for that group in contrast to a 25% ten-year survival for the 16 patients who developed clinical evidence of metastases to regional lymph nodes and on whom a therapeutic groin dissection was performed. An average of 74.5% patients who did not develop metastases to lymph nodes survived.

REFERENCES

1. Ariel IM: Tridimensional resection of malignant melanoma. Surg Gynecol Obstet 139:601, 1974

2. Ariel IM, Resnick MI: Altered lymphatic dynamics caused by cancer metastases. Arch Surg 94:117, 1967

3. Ariel IM, Resnick MI: Altered lymphatic dynamics following groin and axillary dissection: Its relationship to treatment policies for malignant melanoma. Surgery 61:210, 1967

4. Breslow A: Thickness, cross-sectional areas and depth of invasion in the prognosis of cutaneous melanoma. Ann Surg 172:902, 1970

5. Clark WH Jr, Bernardino EA, Mihm MC: The histogenesis and biologic behavior of primary human malignant melanomas of the skin. Cancer Research 29:705, 1969

6. Das Gupta T, McNeer G: The incidence of metastasis to accessible lymph nodes from melanoma of the trunk and extremities—its therapeutic significance. Cancer 17:897, 1964

7. Fortner JG, Das Gupta T, McNeer G: Malignant melanoma of the trunk. Ann Surg 161:161, 1965

8. Goldsmith HS, Shah JP, Kim DH: Malignant melanoma: Current concepts of lymph node dissection. Ca 22:4, July/Aug 1972

9. Goldsmith HS, Shah JP, Kim DH: Prognostic significance of lymph node dissection in the treatment of malignant melanoma. Cancer 26:606, 1970

10. Haagansen CD, Feind CR, Herter FP, et al.: Lymphatics of the trunk. In: The Lymphatics in Cancer. Philadelphia, WB Saunders Co, 1972, pp 441-451

11. Holmes EC, Clark W, Morton DL, et al.: Regional lymph node metastases and the level of invasion of the primary. Cancer 37:199, 1976

12. Knutson CC, Hori JM, Spratt JS Jr: Melanoma in Current Problems in Surgery. Year Book Medical Publishers, Dec 1971, pp 14-15

13. McCune WS, Letterman GS: Malignant melanoma: 10-year results following excision and regional gland dissection. Ann Surg 141:901, 1955

14. McLeod R, Davis NC, Herron JJ, et al.: A retrospective survey of 498 patients with malignant melanoma. Surg Gynecol Obstet 126:99, 1968

15. NcNeer G, Das Gupta T: Routes of lymphatic spread of malignant melanoma. CA 15:168, 1965

16. Mundth ED, Guralnick EA, Paker JW: Malignant melanoma: a study of 427 cases. Ann Surg 162:15, 1965

17. Sappey MPC: Anatomie, physiologie, pathologie des vaisseaux lymphatiques considérés chez l'homme et les vertébrés. A DeLahaye & E Lecrosnier, Paris, 1874

18. Sugarbaker EV, McBride CM: Melanoma of the trunk: The results of surgical excision and anatomic guidelines for predicting nodal metastasis. Surgery 80:22, 1976

19. Sylven B: Malignant melanoma of the skin. Report of 341 cases treated during years 1929-1943. Acta Radiol (Stockh) 32:33, 1949

CHAPTER TWENTY–TWO

SUBUNGUAL MALIGNANT MELANOMAS

IRVING M. ARIEL

A simple discoloration under the nails of the fingers or toes that varies from brown to black color may be a subungual melanoma, which is fatal in almost two-thirds of all cases. This vicious type of neoplasm presents with minimal or often no symptoms except for the presence of the pigmentation. Because of its innocuous appearance it is often misdiagnosed.[22,23]

Although the entity has been known since 1886, when Jonathan Hutchinson[19,20] first described this anatomic type of malignant melanoma as a *melanotic witlow*, the diagnosis is still seldom considered in a differential evaluation and great delays occur before proper treatment is instituted. His description is as timely now as it was then: "The growth was as large as a walnut. It was ulcerated over the whole surface but showed no tendency to sluff or become infected. Just under the overhanging border of the unswollen skin around the nail was a narrow, coal-black margin." This description is one of an advanced melanoma after it has spread beyond the nail to involve the adjacent structures. His description of the pigmentation of the eponychium is pathognomonic criteria that almost universally establish the diagnosis.

Boyer in 1834 thought that a fungus infection might be responsible for subungual melanoma.[6] In 1855, DeMargnay and Monod in France presented an accurate description of the subungual melanoma.[11]

The presentation in this book is a continuation and follow-up report of a series of 72 or 2% of the 3,305 patients seen at the Pack Medical Group, New York, published in 1967.[26] Pack and Oropeza at that time reported 5-year end results. However, some of their patients were not followed for the entire 5-year period.

ANATOMIC DISTRIBUTION

Forty of the subungual melanomas (55.5%) arose in the fingers, and 32 (44.5%) in the toes. A noteworthy feature is the fact that 47 (65%) were located either on the thumb or the great toe (Fig. 22–1). The remainder were more or less evenly distributed throughout the fingers and toes.

Hertzler, in 1922, also stressed the proclivity of melanomas to develop on the great toe and the thumb nail bed.[16]

CLINICAL FEATURES: SEX AND AGE

The sexual distribution was rather even, in that there were 32 males and 40 females. The mean age was 57 years; the youngest patient was a 27-year-old male, and the oldest a 79-year-old male. The age distribution for subungual melanomas is much the same as for melanomas elsewhere (Fig. 22–2).

CLINICAL FEATURES

Most of the patients were of the complexion characteristics noted for other melanomas, namely, fair skin that does not sunburn and freckles easily, blond or sandy hair. Of the patients in this series, 18% were Negro. We have noted in previous chapters that deeply pigmented skin seldom harbors malignant melanoma, and when melanomas do occur they are usually in a less pigmented or non-pigmented region (nail bed, palm, sole, mucoid-cutaneous junction). Forty-seven patients (65%) claimed that the lesion arose in the nail bed de novo. An indeterminate number of patients claimed that trauma pro-

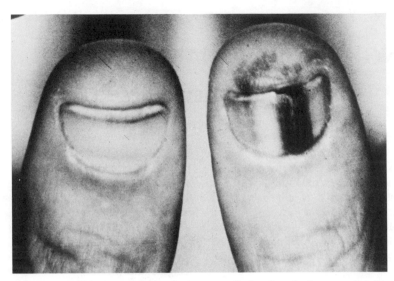

FIGURE 22–1. A subungual malignant melanoma of the thumb that presented as a linear pigmentation.

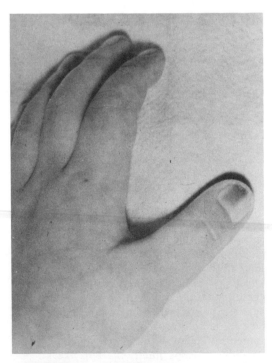

FIGURE 22-2. Subungual benign nevus in a three-year-old child. It was locally excised with complete functional recovery.

duced the pigmentation, but it is highly possible that an asymptomatic and unrecognized pigmented lesion that had increased in size heralded its presence by some traumatic experience. Twenty-one patients (29%) claimed that the subungual pigmentation had been present for many years before the size and color became intensified. The most frequent cause for seeking medical attention was nail deformity, or spontaneous eruption through the nail bed or adjacent to the nail bed. Pain was very rarely a symptom. Five patients presented themselves because of a mass in either the axilla or groin, not aware that the discolored nail bed was the responsible factor.

Because of the innocuous appearance of the early subungual melanomas, the patient and even the physician delay for a prolonged period before instituting proper therapy (Fig. 22–3). They are often diagnosed as a granuloma, infection, hematoma, and treated by ointments, salves, cautery, and other unsatisfactory and often harmful methods. The average delay before the patients consulted us was approximately three years. In only 28 patients was the lesion untreated or simply biopsied before referral for surgical management.[4,5]

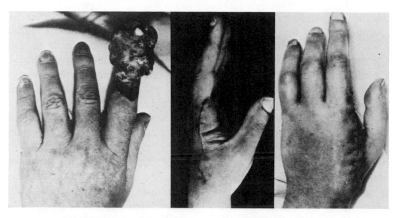

FIGURE 22-3.   Advanced subungual melanoma of the left index finger treated by amputation including the metacarpal bone.

DIAGNOSIS AND BIOPSY

All subungual pigmented lesions should be considered malignant until proved otherwise and the diagnosis established by biopsy. If the tumor has broken through the nail bed, or extended to the perinail structures, a simple incisional biopsy will suffice. If the tumor is under the nail bed, removal of part or all of the nail is the indicated procedure, and incision or excision of the lesion (depending upon its size) should be performed and careful paraffin sections studied by a pathologist skilled in the histologic characteristics of melanomas.

Pigmentation of the eponychium, which was stressed by Hutchinson in 1885,[18] or a history of rapid change in the color, size, or ulceration of the preexisting discoloration, mandates biopsy. We used to depend upon frozen section, but the treatment is of such radical nature that we prefer to obtain paraffin studies, and if a melanoma is established, to institute therapy within a five-day period. The diagnosis may be difficult and confusing because approximately 10% are amelanotic (without pigmentation) and they often have an inflammatory reaction about them, leading to the belief that this is an inflammatory (infectious or fungal) entity instead of a malignant neoplasm.

The differential diagnosis includes:

1. Benign nevus, which is usually more brownish in color and spreads in a longitudinal manner (Fig. 22-2).

2. Subungual hematoma. This causes a difficult differential, but all subungual hematoma pigmentation migrates outward along the nail rather than spreading directly. If the patient has a history of a pigmented lesion at the base of the nail that migrated to the periphery, it is in all probability a hematoma (Fig. 22-12).

3. Paronychia. This is a difficult diagnosis; if one suspects infectious or fungus disease, a slide should be taken for culture and sensitivity, and if it has not completely disappeared within the week of therapy, biopsy is indicated.

4. Pyogenic granuloma. These are usually soft, friable and vascular with a sharp line of demarcation between the lesion and normal skin.

5. Onychomycosis migricans. This fungus infection often mimics malignant melanoma, and in one patient reported by Pack and Adair,[25] was associated with the subungual malignant melanoma.

6. Subungual glomus tumor. This very painful pigmented lesion was first described by Masson in 1935 (Bull Soc Dermat Syph 42:1174, 1935), and occurs most frequently on the fingers and toes. Geschicter, in 1936,

reported 22 subungual finger glomal tumors.[12] The pain and tenderness is almost pathognomonic.

Kopf, et al.[21] have reported several patients with macular pigmented lesions of the digits, which were at first considered benign. The diagnoses were "benign melanocytic hyperplasia," or "atypical melanocytic hyperplasia," or "lentigo maligna-like." They quote Clark, Bernardino, Reed, and Kopf as promulgating a concept of "acral lentiginous melanomas." Included in that group are the subungual malignant melanomas, which are characterized by radial growth phase that simulates but is different from the usual lentiga maligna. They quote the histologic characteristic as containing abnormal (large and spindle) melanocytes situated in the nail bed. Pagetoid cells are not prominent. When the vertical growth phase ensues, such lesions act biologically in the manner of superficial spreading malignant melanomas. (From Clark, et al. (ed), Human Malignant Melanoma, New York, Grune & Stratton, 1979, pp 109–124.)

INCIDENCE OF METASTASES TO THE REGIONAL LYMPH NODES

Of our 72 patients, 25 (35%) presented themselves during their first admission here with metastases to the regional lymph nodes. In 29 patients where the primary tumor was treated by therapy aimed only at the primary lesion with no elective nodal dissection performed, eight (27%) later developed metastases to the regional lymph nodes. Accordingly, 33 (46%) of the 72 patients observed by us developed metastases to regional lymph nodes (Fig. 22–4). The distribution of the incidence of metastases to lymph nodes from the fingers and toes are shown in Table 22–1, with no statistically significant difference between these two primary sites.

TREATMENT

The treatment of subungual melanomas consists of surgical resection, inasmuch as no other method has proved curative. The great distance between the primary tumor and the lymph-node-bearing areas introduces anatomic problems pertaining to the surgery that must be performed. A great deal depends upon the stage of the cancer when the patient is first seen by the surgeon. The situations he may encounter are: (1) the melanoma is limited to the nail bed without clinical evidence of metastases (stage I); (2) the primary tumor is present with clinical evidence of metastases (stage II); (3) a local recurrent melanoma after incomplete resection with or without regional metastases; (4) either of the above situations complicated further by the presence of satellitosis, i.e. metastases to the extremity between the primary tumor and the lymph-node-bearing area (stage III); and (5) any of the above associated with distant metastases (stage IV).

STAGE I MELANOMAS

The best treatment for patients in stage I is the amputation of the involved digit associated with a metacarpal or metatarsal amputation (Fig. 22–5). Conservative amputation of a portion of the digit has resulted in local recurrence in 78% of patients so treated (Fig. 22–6). In addition a resection of the proximal metacarpal or metatarsal bone will give a patient a better structural and functional hand or foot.

The problem is how to treat the regional lymph-node-bearing area. Some surgeons believe that a synchronous groin or axillary dissection should be performed at the time of primary resection. Others prefer a delay of four to six weeks before performing the lymph node dissection, in order to prevent lymph spaces, and to theoretically give the melanoma cells in-transit within the lymphatic vessels a chance to reach the lymph node barrier (which, incidentally, is not a great barrier, as we have demonstrated spread of cancer cells through the lymph nodes). Others prefer no treatment whatsoever to the regional lymph nodes.

There have been no reports to our knowledge regarding the criteria set forth by either Clark's level of invasion or Breslow's

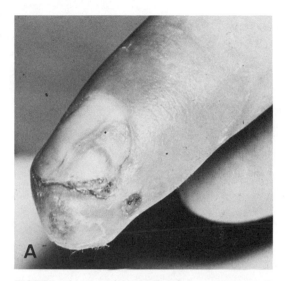

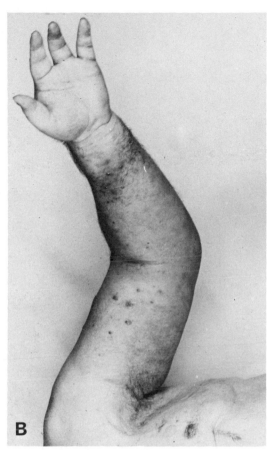

FIGURE 22–4A. Photograph of a nonpigmented subungual melanoma of the left middle finger of a 68-year-old man. He had noticed a "cracked nail" three months before. The finger was amputated through the metacarpal and an axillary dissection done for a rather large node, clinically considered metastatic melanoma, but no metastases were proved. B. Photograph of satellitosis in arm taken four years after operation. The patient also had pulmonary metastases and died shortly thereafter. (Reproduced from Booher RJ, and Pack GT: Malignant melanoma of the feet and hands. Surgery 42:1084–1121, 1957, with permission of authors and publisher.)

TABLE 22–1.   Incidence of Metastases to Regional Lymph Nodes in 72 Patients with Subungual Melanomas

No. of Patients & Location	Metastases to Lymph Nodes on Admission		Metastases Developed in Lymph Nodes after Treatment of Primary Melanoma			Total Incidence of Metastases to Regional Lymph Nodes	
	No.	%	No. of Patients	No. who Developed Mets.	% with Mets.	Total No.	%
Fingers 40	15*	38	17	5	29	20	50
Toes 32	10	31	12	3	25	13	41
Total† 72	25	35	29	8	27	33	46

* This includes one patient whose metastases were discovered during an elective node dissection (one of four elective node dissections performed).
† This number includes all patients observed by Pack Medical Group, but not necessarily treated by Pack Medical Group.

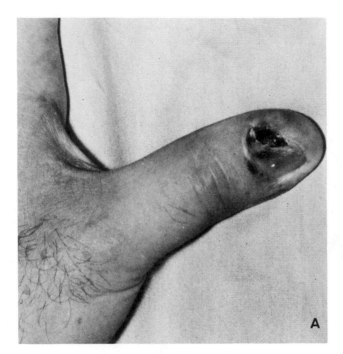

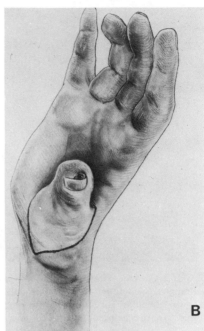

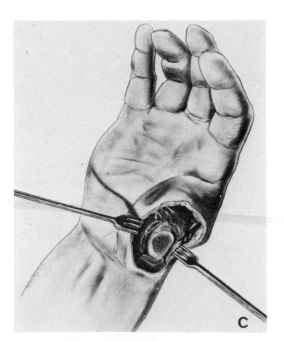

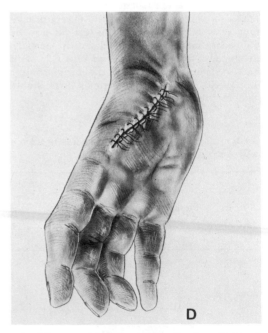

FIGURE 22–5. Subungual melanoma of thumb with illustrations demonstrating technique of amputation. The metacarpal bone is not excised for thumb amputations. Good results are being obtained by autotransplantation of other digits. A. Melanoma. B. Lines of incision. C. Amputation complete. D. Operation completed.

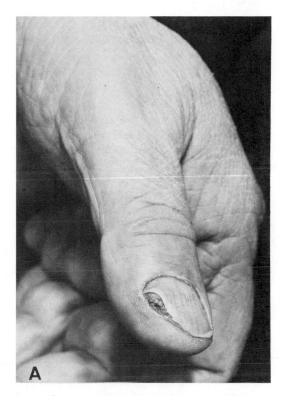

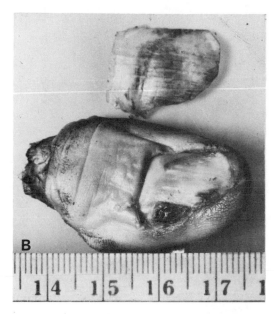

FIGURE 22–6A. Photograph of a small subungual melanoma of a 61-year-old man with a three-year history of his nail "cracking" on the radial side with a subsequent growth of "proud flesh." Despite the long history the lesion is comparatively superficial in the nail bed. B. Photograph of the distal interphalangeal joint disarticulation with the nail removed and showing a small, rather superficial melanoma. The patient remained cured more than ten years. (Reproduced from Booher RJ and Pack GT: Malignant melanoma of the feet and hands. Surgery 42:1084–1121, 1957, with permission of authors and publisher.)

thickness to help determine which course of action to follow pertaining to treatment of lymph nodes (Chapter 6). The fact that approximately 50% of the patients in our series did develop metastases to the lymph nodes indicates that some form of therapy of the nodes should be performed (Fig. 22–7).

One recent patient (not included in this series) with a subungual melanoma of the toe that had spread to the contiguous structures was treated by a metatarsotarsal amputation followed by the endolymphatic injection of radioactive isotopes in the form of ^{32}P lipiodol. Nine months later, because of clinical palpable adenopathy, he was treated by a groin dissec-tion and no nodes were found involved by metastases.

Of the 29 patients treated by amputation alone, metastases later occurred in seven, necessitating repeated operation. Eleven patients (38%) remain alive and well after a ten-year period. Of four patients with stage I melanoma treated by amputation and elective node dissection, one patient with metastases and one without metastases to the regional lymph nodes were dead at five years. One was reported dead of osteogenic sarcoma, but in our analysis he is considered dead of melanoma. One other patient died between the five- and ten-year period.

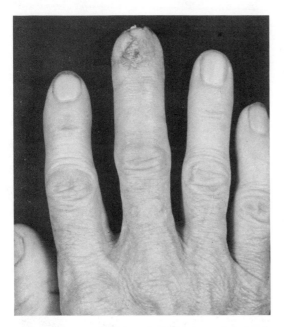

FIGURE 22–7. Amelanotic melanoma of the middle finger which developed metastases to opillary lymph nodes.

STAGE II AND III MELANOMA

Of 23 patients observed with stage II melanomas, four (17%) are alive without evidence of metastases ten years later, but 19 (83%) have died despite the performance of regional lymph node dissection after metastases had occurred.

Of five patients with stage III melanomas, one remained alive ten years after combined nodal dissection, excision of some of the subcutaneous metastases, intra-arterial infusion of phenylalanine mustard and the endolymphatic administration of ^{32}P lepiodol (Chap. 13).

The overall survival rates of the patients treated by us are summarized in Tables 22–2 and 22–3). Of 53 patients, 20 are alive and well after ten years (38%), and 33 (62%) are dead. Of those who are considered dead in this series are four patients who are lost to follow-up and six patients who were classified on their death certificates as having died of other forms of cancer. Three patients (9%) died between the

fifth and tenth year, demonstrating the need to report survival at the ten-year period (Figs. 22–8, 22–9, 22–10).

DISCUSSION

Subungual melanomas are rare lesions comprising about 2.5% of all melanomas in Caucasians, but occur more frequently in Negroes and comprise 15 to 20% of all malignant melanomas in Negroes. The indolent development and the lack of symptoms cause the unwary to treat these potentially lethal cancers for long periods by means of ointments or salves or cautery and thus endanger the patient's life by lack of adequate therapy at the outset.[13]

The differential diagnosis includes many benign lesions; a partial list of lesions as expressed by Kopf et al. includes: nevocystic nevus, keratoechanthoma, Bowen's disease, squamous cell carcinoma, hematoma, glomus tumor, granuloma pyogenicum, foreign body granuloma, Kaposes sarcoma, subungual exostoses, epidermoid inclusions,[23] onychia and paronychia secondary to infections, in growing nails, onychodystrophies, and pigmentations

TABLE 22–2. Subungual Melanoma.
Pack Medical Group: Results of Treatment

	Number	Percent
Total number of patients seen	72	
Total treated by Pack Medical Group	53	100
Patients seen in consultation only and not treated by Pack Medical Group	13	
Patients referred with distant metastases (all died)	6	
Total alive and well ten years or more	20	38
Dead*	33	62

* This number includes four patients lost to follow-up and presumed dead, and six patients who were classified as dying from other causes. Three patients (9%) died between the fifth and tenth year.

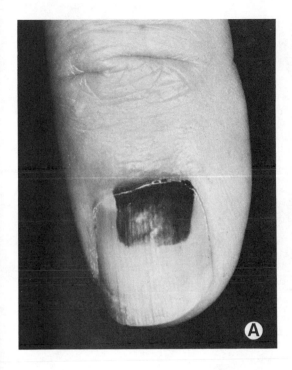

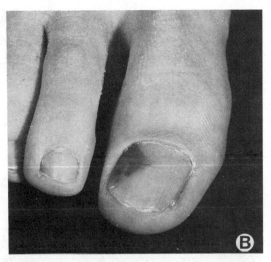

FIGURE 22-8A and B. Earlier stages in the presentation of subungual melanomas of the large toe. (Reproduced from Pack GT and Oropeza R: Subungual melanoma. Surg Gynec Obstet 124: 571-582, 1967, with permission of authors and Surgery, Gynecology, & Obstetrics.)

secondary to Cushing's.[3] Benign clinically insignificant melanotic bands covering the subungual region are not unusual in the blacks and Orientals, as stressed by Higashi and Leyden et al.[17,24] and are very rare in Caucasians (Figs. 22-11 and 22-12).[1]

This presentation is an update of one of the largest series of subungual malignant melanomas which consisted of a report from the Pack Medical Foundation recorded by Pack and Oropeza.[26] The fact that 55.5% of all 72 subungual melanomas seen involved the big toe or the thumb emphasizes the need for extra caution in diagnosing pigmented lesions in these regions. The delay, sometimes two to four years, before adequate therapy was instituted, could be a contributing factor in the high incidence of metastasis to the lymph nodes, which occurred in 46% of all our patients. Fifty percent of the patients with subungual melanomas of the fingers metastasized and 59% of the 32 melanomas of the toe metastasized to the regional lymph nodes. Of the 25 patients, 35% presented metastases to the lymph nodes on admission, and 27% of

29 patients whose digit was amputated later developed metastases to the regional lymph nodes (Table 22-3).

Das Gupta and McNeer[10] also observed metastases in half of their patients with subungual melanomas. Haagenson et al., reporting from the College of Physicians and Surgeons, Columbia University, New York City, recorded 58 melanomas of the upper extremity, of which 12 (20.4%) were subungual.[15] None presented themselves with clinical metastases to the axilla, axillary dissection was performed in seven, and one harbored occult metastasis in the lymph nodes. Of 127 melanomas of the lower extremity in their series, nine (7%) had subungual melanomas, eight arising from the big toe. An elective node dissection was performed in six and in three occult metastases were found in the regional lymph nodes. The high incidence of metastasis in the lymph nodes, especially the frequent delay before optimal therapy is instituted, emphasizes that the lymph nodes should be considered during the initial treatment.

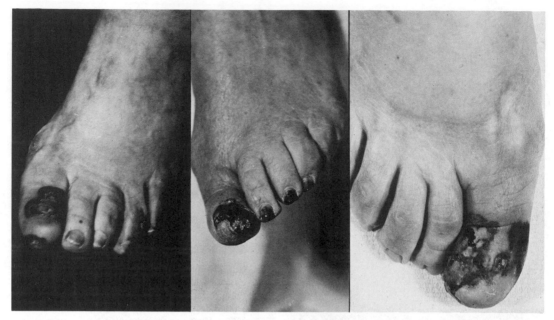

FIGURE 22–9.   Three examples of advanced melanoma of the large toe.

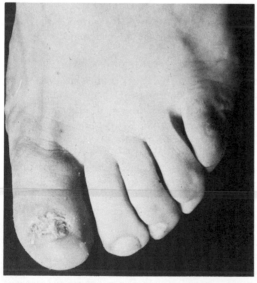

FIGURE 22–10. Amelanotic melanoma of the large toe; disguised as a fungus infection and treated for about one year with salves and ointments. (Reproduced from Pack GT and Oropeza R: Subungual melanoma. Surg Gynec Obstet 124: 571–582, 1967, with permission of authors and Surgery, Gynecology & Obstetrics.)

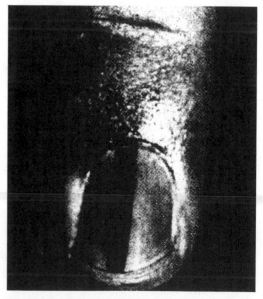

FIGURE 22–11. Photograph showing a linear pigmentation of the right fifth fingernail. This 19-year-old Oriental woman noticed the beginning of this line one year before. No biopsy was obtained. These bands have been observed in certain instances of malnutrition.

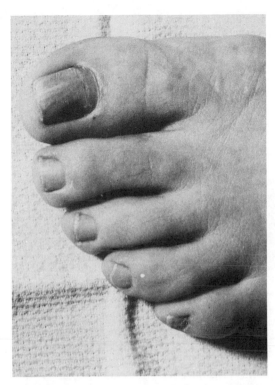

FIGURE 22-12. Subungual hematoma of large toe. Note similarity to melanoma. The pigmented region moves with growth and tends to subside. If in doubt, a biopsy should be obtained.

The best treatment is the amputation of the offending digit and the proximal metatarsal or metacarpal bone. This leads to a good anatomic and good functional status. In light of modern advances of tissue transplant, if the thumb is involved, it is preferable that only the thumb amputation be done so that a transplanted "thumb" from one of the other fingers may later be performed. Anything less than an amputation of the entire digit is unsatisfactory and local recurrences for a lesser procedure have been encountered in approximately 60% of the patients where this has been performed.

The question of synchronous node dissection for stage I melanoma or node dissection electively performed at a later date after treatment of the primary lesion, or whether one should wait for metastases to occur, demands further study.[8]

The fact that metastases occur in approximately 50% of the patients, and that the nodes are distant from the primary site so that an in-continuity dissection cannot be performed, raises the question of the possible harm of a discontinuous form of operation. It has been shown by Ariel[2] that a discontinuous operation may permit cells in-transit either to spill out into the site where the lymphatic vessels have been transsected, or else collateral routes of dissemination may occur to unpredictable areas. If these do not occur, then there is the possibility of regurgitation back with retrograde flow of lymphatics in functional dermal lymphatics, which is one of the methods of producing satellitoses (Chap. 22). In our series, only four patients developed satellitoses, and all of these were of the lower extremity. This may be due to the independent anatomic position of the lower extremities and the resultant venous and lymphatic back pressure but further proof is required.

Studies by Shah et al.[27] demonstrate no

TABLE 22-3. Survival of Subungual Melanoma Patients Seen at the Pack Medical Group: Analyzed According to Stage when Patient Was First Seen

	Number of Patients	No Evidence of Disease		Dead* of Melanoma	
		Number	Percent	Number	Percent
Stage I	40	14	35	26	65
Stage II	23	4	17	19	83
Stage III	5	1	25	4	75

* This includes four patients lost to follow-up and six patients listed as dying from other causes.

significant difference in survival rates of patients who were treated by discontinuous operation from those who were treated by continuous node dissections.

Results are not good, as would be expected, when patients with delayed diagnoses and with a high preponderance for metastases to the lymph nodes are treated. Of the 53 patients treated by the surgeons of the Pack Medical Group, 20 (38%) are alive and free of disease at the ten-year period, whereas 33 patients (62%) have died. This number includes four patients lost to follow-up and presumed dead and six patients who were classified on their death certificates as having died from other causes. Even though the patient may be listed as dying from heart disease, etc., there is the possibility that overlooked metastases may have contributed to death. We thus decided to list all of them as having died from the melanoma. Three of the 32 patients (9%) died between the fifth and tenth year, indicating the need to report survival rate at the ten-year period.

Haagensen et al. report in their series a five-year survival rate of 63.3%. One of their patients developed metastases 12 years later. There were 12 melanomas of the upper extremity (63.6%). Of their nine subungual melanomas of the lower extremity, three of seven patients who had prophylactic inguinal dissection, one who had 14 inguinal nodes involved died of unknown causes after three years, and the other two were apparently cured of their melanomas. One of the two who had 11 inguinal nodes involved died 13 years after operation with ovarian carcinoma and no evidence of recurrence of melanoma. The other patient who had one of ten inguinal nodes involved had no recurrence eight years postoperatively. The remaining two of their nine patients with subungual melanomas had clinically involved inguinal nodes on admission. One died in eight months, the other in two months. They state, in summary, that only two of their eight patients with operable subungual melanomas of the toe were cured by amputation and inguinal lymph node dissection. They further state: "Certainly, all subungual melanomas should be treated by amputation and prophylactic lymph node dissection."

Das Gupta and Brasfield,[9] from Memorial Hospital in 1965, reported a 38% five-year survival for their stage I and stage II subungual melanomas, and Graham,[14] from Pennsylvania, reported a 50% five-year survival in 1973.

CONCLUSIONS

A series of 72 subungual melanomas seen by the surgeons of the Pack Medical Group were reported in 1967. That series, which reported five-year results and contained a number of patients who had not been followed for five years, is reevaluated at the ten-year span. Fifty-three patients were treated by the surgeons of the Pack Medical Group, and of these, 20 (38%) are alive and well after ten years. Thirteen patients were seen only in consultation and were not treated. Six patients were referred with disseminated melanomas with visceral metastases and received only palliative therapy.

Forty of the patients were in stage I, and in this group 14 (35%) were alive and well ten years later, but 26 (65%) had died. Twenty-three patients were stage II, with metastases to the regional lymph nodes and four (17%) survived the ten-year span. Five patients presented in stage III, with dermal or subcutaneous metastases between the primary lesion and the regional lymph nodes, and one of these patients survived after extensive therapy.

In view of the high incidence of metastases to the regional lymph nodes, it seems desirable that an amputation of the involved digit and the proximal metatarsal or metacarpal bone be performed as treatment for the primary lesion and that a discontinuous axillary or groin dissection be performed. Although the discontinuous operation carries with it certain hazards, studies by Shah and Goldsmith have demonstrated no great difference in survival between the continuous and discontinuous operation.

Adjuvant therapy, such as perfusion with or without heat of cancer-chemotherapeutic agents and the endolymphatic administration of radioactive isotopes may afford supplemental means of treating these neoplasms in addition to the necessary surgery.[28,29]

Amputation of the extremity is seldom indicated, but may become necessary depending upon the virulence and the recurrence rate of the melanomas. One such patient of ours who had a forequarter amputation survived the ten-year period.

Palliative major amputations may, on occasion, be necessary.

REFERENCES

1. Allyn B, Kopf AW, Kahn M, Witten VH: Incidence of pigmented nevi JAMA 186:890–893, 1963
2. Ariel IM, Resnick MI: The intralymphatic administration of radioactive isotopes and cancer chemotherapeutic drugs. Surgery 55:355, 1964
3. Bondy PK, Harwick HJ: Longitudinal banded pigmentation of nails following adrenalectomy for Cushing's syndrome. N Engl J Med 281: 1056–1057, 1969
4. Booher RJ: Recognition and treatment of melanoma. Surg Clin North Am 49:389–405, 1969
5. Booher RJ, Pack GT Malignant melanoma of the feet and hands. Surgery 42:1084–1121, 1957
6. Boyer FJ: Fungus hématode du petit doights. Gaz med, Paris, 1834, p 212
7. Clark WH Jr, Ainsworth AM, Bernardino EA, et al.: The developmental biology of primary human malignant melanomas. Semin Oncol 2:83–103, 1975
8. Das Gupta T, Brasfield R: Metastatic melanoma; a clinicopathological study. Cancer 17:1323–1339, 1964
9. Das Gupta T, Brasfield R: Subungual melanoma: 25-year review of cases. Ann Surg 161:545–552, 1965
10. Das Gupta T, McNeer G: The incidence of metastases to accessible lymph nodes from melanoma of the trunk and extremities: its therapeutic significance. Cancer 17:897–911, 1964
11. Demargnay JF, Monod PS: Cancer mélanique du pouce et de l'aisselle. Gaz hop, 1855, p 418
12. Geschickter CF: Glomal tumors. Int Clinics, series 46, 2:1, 1936
13. Gibson SH, Montgomery H, Woolner LB, Brunsting LA: Melanotic whitlow (subungual melanoma). J Invest Dermatol 29:119–129, 1957
14. Graham WP: Subungual melanoma. Pennsylvania Med 76:56, 1973
15. Haagensen CD, Feind CR, Herter FP, et al.: The Lymphatics in Cancer. Philadelphia, WR Saunders, 1972
16. Hertzler AE: Melanoblastoma of the nail bed. Arch Dermatol Syphilol 6:701, 1922
17. Higashi N: Melanocytes of nail matrix and nail pigmentation. Arch Dermatol 97:570–574, 1968
18. Hutchinson J: Trans Pathol Soc, London, 36:468, 1885
19. Hutchinson J: Melanosis often not black: melanotic whitlow. Br Med J 1:491, 1886
20. Hutchinson J: Notes toward the information of clinical groups of tumor. Am J Med Sci 91:470, 1886
21. Kopf AW, Bart RS, Rodriguez-Sains RS: Malignant melanoma: A review. J Dermatol Surg Oncol 3:1 Jan/Feb, 1977
22. Leppard B, Sanderson KV, Behan F: Subungual malignant melanoma: difficulty in diagnosis. Br Med J 1:310–312, 1974
23. Lewin K: Subungual epidermoid inclusions. Br J Dermatol 81:671–675, 1969
24. Leyden JJ, Spott DA, Goldschmidt H: Diffuse and banded melinin pigmentation in nails. Arch Dermatol 105:548–550, 1972
25. Pack GT, Adair FR: Subungual melanoma. Surgery 5:47, 1939
26. Pack GT, Oropeza R: Subungual melanoma. Surg Gynecol Obstet 124:571–582, 1967
27. Shah JP, Goldsmith AS: Incontinuity vs discontinuous lymph node dissection for malignant melanoma. Cancer 26:610–614, 1970
28. Stehlin JS, Clark RL: Melanoma of the extremities experience with conventional treatment and perfusion in 339 cases. Am J Surg 110:366, 1965
29. Stehlin JS, Giovanella BC, Ipolyi PD et al.: Results of hyperthermic perfusion for melanoma of the extremities. Surg Gynecol Obstet 140:339–348, 1975

CHAPTER TWENTY–THREE

MALIGNANT MELANOMA OF THE UPPER EXTREMITIES

IRVING M. ARIEL

Malignant melanoma of the upper extremities constitutes 15% of 3,305 malignant melanomas seen at the Pack Medical Group, New York City and consisted of 487 patients. Of this group, 85 patients were seen only in consultation, and 60 were referred with disseminated melanoma for which no curative therapy could be instituted. Three hundred forty-two patients were treated by the surgeons of the Pack Medical Group and are available for ten-year evaluation. Two patients were lost to follow-up and are presumed dead. Forty patients suffered from subungual melanomas but are not included in this analysis as they are considered as a separate entity (Chap. 22). Forty-four patients with melanoma of the upper extremities seen since 1967 are not included in this presentation.

CLINICAL FEATURES OF 487 PATIENTS

The clinical characteristics are presented for all 487 patients seen, but the ten-year results are given only for the 342 patients treated by us and followed for a minimum of ten years (Table 23–1).

SEX

The sex was nearly equally divided in that 51% were male and 49% were female (Fig. 23–1).

STAGING

A clinical staging was utilized. Stage I are those having a primary melanoma limited to the site of origin with lymph nodes clinically negative for evidence of metastases. Stage II were those whose lymph nodes contained metastases. Stage III were patients who had intercurrent melanoma, either melanoma cells in transit or satellitosis; and stage IV were those patients with evidence of disseminated melanoma. Inasmuch as the clinical staging was changed after histologic material became available, the stages are presented for the 342 determinate patients (Table 23–12 and Fig. 23–2).

RACE

The Caucasian group constituted most of the cases; of these, 70% had a fair complexion, 8% a dark complexion, and 19% were freckled. For 20% no record was listed on the chart. Four Negroes had melanoma, but no other races were present in this particular series.

FAMILY HISTORY

In 65% of the patients there was no evidence of any family history. In 5% of those evaluated there was a history of familial involvement by melanoma, but not necessarily at the same site, by others in the same family. In 30% of the series, the charts did not mention the presence or absence of family history (Fig. 23–3).

AGE

The largest incidence was between 30 and 60 years. Twenty-nine percent of the patients

TABLE 23-1A. Clinical characteristics of 487 Patients with Malignant Melanoma of the Upper Extremities

	Percent of Patients
Race	
White	79
Negro	0.8
Other	0
Unknown	20
Complexion	
Fair	70
Dark	8
Freckled	19
Unknown	3
Sex	
Male	51
Female	49

Age	Number	Percent
0–10	6	1
11–20	14	3
21–30	57	12
31–40	142	29
41–50	114	23
51–60	120	25
61–70	17	3
71–80	11	2
Over 80	0	0
Unknown	6	1

TABLE 23-1B. Clinical Characteristics of 487 Patients with Malignant Melanoma of the Upper Extremities

	Percent of Patients	
Family History of Melanoma		
Positive	5	
Negative	65	
Unknown	30	

History of preexisting mole	Number	Percent
Preexisting mole	367	75
Melanoma de novo	120	25

Site of Primary Melanoma	Number	Percent
Finger and hands	80	16
Arms	407	84

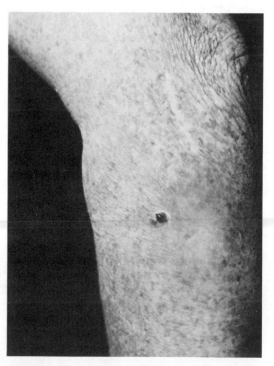

FIGURE 23-2. Small nodular melanoma of the lateral aspect of the forearm, which eventually resulted in pulmonary metastases from which the patient died.

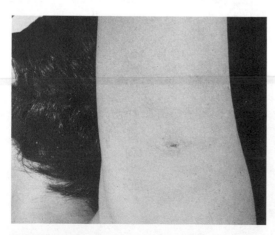

FIGURE 23-1. An inconspicuous lesion of the upper arm of a young female that proved to be a malignant melanoma with metastases to axilla.

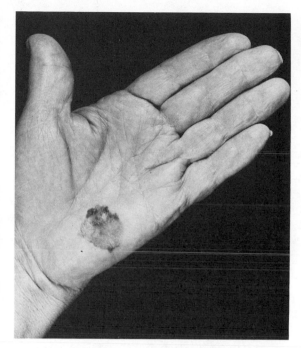

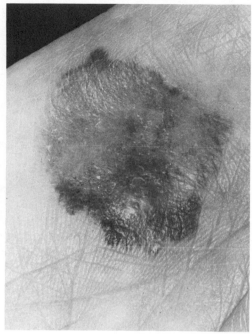

FIGURE 23-3. Left: Melanoma of the palm of the hand treated by wide local resection and skin graft. Ten years later patient remains free of evidence of melanoma. Right: Varigated appearance demon- strating color variation. Histologically this was a superficial spreading lesion. Patient's brother suf- fered from a melanoma of the trunk.

were in the fourth decade, 23% in the fifth decade, and 25% in the sixth decade. Only 17 patients (3%) were between 61 and 70 years of age, and 11 patients (2%) were between 71 and 80 years of age. Twelve percent of the patients were between 21 and 30 years, 3% between 11 and 20 years of age, and six patients (1%) were under ten years of age.

HISTORY OF PREEXISTING MOLE

Seventy-five percent of the patients gave a history of a preexisting mole that changed in character, either increasing in size or pigmen- tation, itching, ulcerating, or bleeding (Fig. 23-4). In 120 patients (25%) the melanoma ap- peared de novo, grew, became increasingly pigmented, and caused the patient to seek therapy without a history of a preexisting mole.

SITE OF PRIMARY MELANOMA

Eighty-four percent of the patients developed melanomas of the arms, and in 16% the melanoma involved the hands or fingers (Fig. 23-5). Subungual melanomas, of which there were 40, are not considered in this presentation because of their unusual clinical manifestations and behavior (Chap. 22).

SURVIVAL RATES

The total number of patients exposed to risk were 342 for the ten-year span (Table 23-2). At the end of ten years posttherapy, 216 (63%) were alive and presumably free of melanoma. Two patients were lost to follow-up and are presumed dead. Fourteen percent of the pa- tients who succumbed died between the fifth and tenth year posttherapy (30 patients).

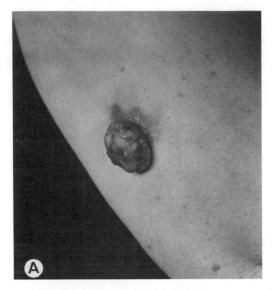
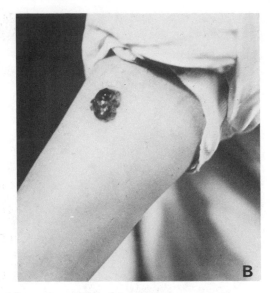

FIGURE 23–4A and B.   Clinical appearance.of nodular melanomas that developed on preexisting moles on the arms of two patients.

SEX VERSUS SURVIVAL

Of the 176 males, 108 (61%) survived ten years, almost exactly the same as the 166 females, of whom 106 (64%) survived ten years or longer (Table 23–3).

THE INFLUENCE OF AGE ON SURVIVAL

The four patients under ten years of age manifested a 100% survival, and of the ten patients between 11 and 20 years of age, the sur-

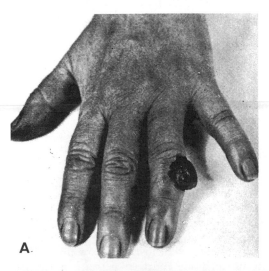
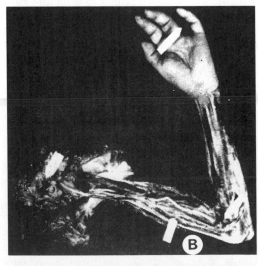

FIGURE 23–5A and B.   Melanoma of finger treated primarily by amputation of digit. Metastases to epitrochlear and axillary lymph nodes necessitated an interscapular amputation.

TABLE 23-2. Malignant Melanoma of the Upper Extremities 10-Year Survival Rate

Total number of patients	487
Indeterminate	
Number seen in consultation only	85
Patients referred with disseminated melanoma, not suitable for curative treatment	60
Determinate	
Patients available for 10-year survival analysis	342*
Number alive and free of cancer	216
Number who died during interval	126
10-year survival rate	
216/342 =	63%

*Forty patients with subungual melanoma are not considered in this presentation but are considered as a separate entity. (See Chapter 22).

vival rate was 80% (Table 23-4). Almost half of those between 21 and 30 years of age (45%) manifested a survival rate roughly equal to that of those between the 30 and 70 years of age group. Of the few patients over 71 years of age, the data are too limited to make any conclusions, but the 25% survival rate does indicate that in the aged, the malignant melanoma can be serious.

DURATION OF A PREEXISTING MOLE AND ITS INFLUENCE UPON SURVIVAL

A 33% survival rate occurred in patients whose mole was present for less than a year, which increased to 75% for those whose mole was present from one to two years (Table 23-5). If present from two to five years, the survival decreased to 37%. Above five years,

TABLE 23-3. Malignant Melanoma of the Upper Extremities. The Influence of Sex upon Survival

	Number of	10-Year Survivors	
Sex	Patients	Number	Percent
Male	176	108	61
Female	166	106	64

TABLE 23-4. Malignant Melanoma of the Upper Extremities. The Influence of Age upon Survival

	Number of	10-Year Survivors	
Age	Patients	Number	Percent
0–10	4	4	100
11–20	10	8	80
21–30	40	18	45
31–40	100	54	54
41–50	80	24	30
51–60	84	44	52
61–70	12	6	50
71–80	8	2	25
Over 80	0	—	—
Unknown	4	2	50

the survival rate was extremely good and probably indicates the fact that these moles, although present for long periods of time, had not undergone malignant transformation until a late date, and treatment after that date resulted in a high percentage of cures.

THE INFLUENCE OF THE DURATION OF CHANGES IN A MOLE UPON SURVIVAL

In 14 patients the mole changes had existed less than one month before therapy, the survival rate was 57% (Table 23-6). When the changes lasted from one to three months before therapy, the survival rate was 56%; for

TABLE 23-5. Malignant Melanoma of the Upper Extremities. The Influence of the Duration of a Preexisting Mole upon Survival

Duration	Number of	10-Year Survivors	
(Years)	Patients	Number	Percent
Under 1	6	2	33
1–2	8	6	75
2–5	16	6	37
5–10	2	2	100
10–20	20	16	80
All Life	134	66	49
Unknown	66	26	39

TABLE 23-6.   Malignant Melanoma of the Upper Extremities. The Influence of Duration of Changes in a Mole upon Survival

Duration (Months)	Number of Patients	10-Year Survivors	
		Number	Percent
Under 1	14	8	57
1–3	32	18	56
4–6	54	36	67
7–12	52	20	38
13–24	28	12	43
25–60	28	10	36
Over 60	8	6	75
Unknown	22	—	—

the 54 patients whose changes lasted from four to six months, it equalled 67%. For those over a six-month period there was a decline in survival, except for eight patients whose changes lasted over 60 months.

THE EFFECT UPON SURVIVAL OF MELANOMAS THAT APPEARED DE NOVO

In this series were 100 patients whose lesions appeared de novo (Table 23-7). Two patients were treated within one month of discovery and survived over ten years. Those who were treated with a delay of one to three months had a survival rate of 67%. The patients whose lesions were present more than

TABLE 23-7.   Malignant Melanoma of the Upper Extremities. The Influence of Duration of De Novo Lesions upon Survival

Duration (Months)	Number of Patients	10-Year Survivors	
		Number	Percent
Under 1	2	2	100
1–3	6	4	67
4–6	10	10	40
7–12	12	4	33
13–24	24	8	33
25–60	16	12	75
Over 60	10	2	20
Unknown	20	—	—

two years before they sought therapy had a 75% survival rate. The patients whose lesions were present more than five years had a survival rate of 20%. It is impossible in the group to differentiate the existence of a preexisting mole from a melanoma de novo. The data are presented as obtained from the patients.

TYPE OF SURGICAL PROCEDURE ANALYZED ACCORDING TO EFFECT UPON SURVIVAL

The effects of the treatment of the primary lesion upon survival rates are presented in Table 23-8 and Figure 23-6. The data are further broken down to determine whether there was a difference in survival in patients who were initially treated by us compared with patients who had their primary treatment elsewhere and were then referred to us for additional treatment. Of 198 patients who were originally treated at the Pack Medical Group, 82 were treated by a wide surgical excision with primary closure of the defect. Sixty-six percent of these patients survived a ten-year span, in contrast to 23% among 52 patients who had a wide resection performed elsewhere before referral to us. Among 100 patients who had a wide excision covered by a skin graft performed by us, the ten-year survival was 60% (Fig. 23-7), in contrast to 40 patients who were treated elsewhere and then referred to us for reoperation, who manifested a 30% ten-year survival. Of 14 patients who had amputation of the digit performed by us, six survived the ten-year period (43%) (Fig. 23-8); and of eight who had previous treatment elsewhere, four survived (50%). Two patients who had previous treatment elsewhere had a mid-hand amputation and they remained alive and well ten years later. Two patients treated by us had a wide surgical excision supplemented by intra-arterial chemotherapy infusion, and remained alive and free of disease ten years later. Twelve patients were treated elsewhere whose treatment was considered adequate; hence no therapy was given by us. In this group two (17%) remained alive and free of disease ten years later. It thus appears that patients who

TABLE 23-8. Malignant Melanoma of the Upper Extremities.
The Influence of Type of Surgical Procedure upon Survival

| | Patients First Seen (198) | | | Previously Treated Cases (144) | | |
| | Number of Patients | 10-Year Survivors | | Number of Patients | 10-Year Survivors | |
Type of Surgery		Number	Percent		Number	Percent
Wide excision with closure of flaps	82	54	66	52	12	23
Wide excision with skin graft	100	60	60	40	12	30
Digit amputation	14	6	43	8	4	50
Forequarter amputation	0	—	—	26	2	8
Any of the above with intra-arterial chemo-therapy perfusion	2	2	100	6	2	33
No treatment	0	—	—	12	2	17

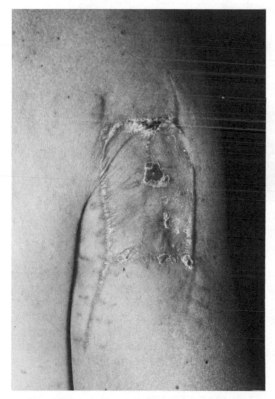

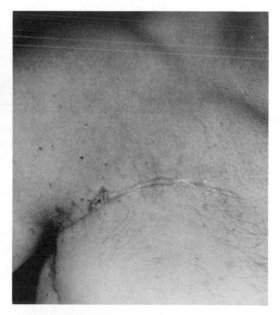

FIGURE 23-6. Left: Postoperative view of a melanoma of the posterior aspect of the arm treated by wide tridimensional resection. The scars inferior and superior to the split-thickness skin graft represent sliding flaps reducing the area to be covered by the graft. Right: Scar of axillary dissection performed with the patient lying on his back to afford adequate exposure. The patient remains free of evidence of melanoma six years later.

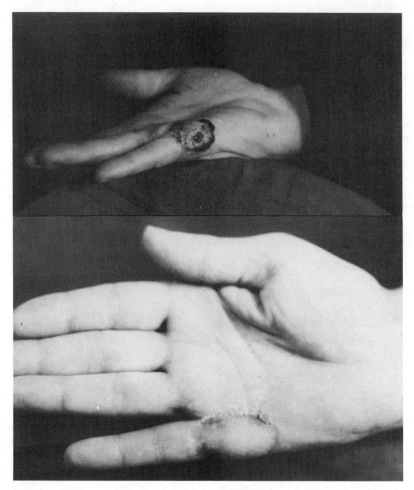

FIGURE 23-7.   Superficial melanoma at base of little finger. Because of its superficial structure it was treated by wide excision and split-thickness skin graft.

have adequate tridimensional resection of their melanomas as soon as the diagnosis is established fare better than those who have incomplete excisions to be followed at a later date by a more complete dissection.

SIZE OF LESION AND ITS EFFECT UPON SURVIVAL

Generally, the smaller the lesion, the better the prognosis (Table 23-9). Of the 80 patients whose lesions were less than 1 cm, 75% survived; this value gradually decreased as the le-

sion became larger. However, in large superficial spreading lesions one could expect a more favorable prognosis than for the infiltrating cancers. Thus six of ten patients (60%) whose lesions were over 4 cm in diameter survived over ten years.

SURFACE OF PRIMARY LESION VERSUS SURVIVAL

Of 16 patients whose primary lesion was flat, 12 (75%) survived the ten-year span; of the 100 patients who had elevated and nodular

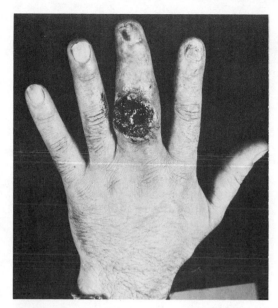

FIGURE 23-8. Large nodular ulcerating melanoma of the middle finger treated by amputation of digit and adjacent metacarpal bone. Ten-year freedom from melanoma.

primary lesions, 56 (56%) survived the ten-year span (Table 23-10). Of 44 patients with primary lesions that were elevated, ulcerated, and encrusted, 18 survived the ten-year span (41%). Of 24 patients with primary lesions that were ulcerated, encrusted, and bleeding, only two survived (8%).

HISTOLOGIC DIAGNOSIS VERSUS SURVIVAL

Ten patients were not applicable because of vague pathologic descriptions. Of ten patients diagnosed as having superficial melanomas, the ten-year survival rate was 100%, all being cured (Table 23-11). Of six patients diagnosed as having juvenile melanomas, the survival rate was 100%, each of them being cured. Of the 310 patients diagnosed as suffering from infiltrating melanoma, 192 (62%) survived a ten-year span. Six patients with amelanotic melanomas had the worst prognosis in that only two lived for a ten-year period.

TABLE 23-9. Malignant Melanoma of the Upper Extremities. The Influence of Size of the Primary Lesion upon Survival

Size (cm)	Number of Patients	10-Year Survivors	
		Number	Percent
Under 1	80	60	75
1-2	78	38	49
2.1-3	14	4	29
3.1-4	2	0	0
4.1-6	10	6	60

Note: No description of size was available for the remainder of the patients.

TABLE 23-10. Malignant Melanoma of the Upper Extremities. The Influence of the Surface of Primary Lesion upon Survival

Surface	Number of Patients	10-Year Survivors	
		Number	Percent
Flat	16	12	75
Elevated, nodular	100	56	56
Elevated, ulcerated and encrusted	44	18	41
Ulcerated, encrusted	24	2	8

Note: No description given for the remainder of the patients.

TABLE 23-11. Malignant Melanoma of the Upper Extremities. The Influence of Histologic Diagnosis upon Survival*

Histologic Diagnosis	Number of Patients	10-Year Survivors	
		Number	Percent
Superficial	10	10	100
Infiltrating	310	192	62
Juvenile	6	6	100
Hutchinson's freckle	0	0	0
Amelanotic	6	2	33

Note: 10 patients not applicable (description not adequate).
* Those instances labelled "superficial" melanoma represent Clark's classification of level II and possibly some in level III. Those labelled "infiltrating" melanoma represent Clark's levels IV and V. The slides and paraffin blocks were not available to segregate these levels. The "amelanotic" melanomas were all infiltrating (levels IV and V).

PATHOLOGIC STAGE VERSUS SURVIVAL

Sixty-four patients were diagnosed as having stage I melanoma on histologic criteria; 45 (70%) of these survived ten years or longer (Table 23-12). The 272 patients who manifested stage II melanoma had a ten-year survival of 26%; and of the six patients classified as stage III, none survived. Of the patients who presented themselves with stage IV, the average survival was one year. One patient with metastases to the lungs and one with metastases to the liver lived longer than five years. There was a 40% error in the clinical classification for 106 patients diagnosed clinically as having stage I melanoma; an elective lymph node dissection yielded 26 patients with occult metastases, and in 16 other patients metastases to axillary lymph nodes developed later.

TABLE 23-12. Malignant Melanoma of the Upper Extremities. The Influence of Pathologic Stage upon Survival

Stage	Number of Patients	10-Year Survivors	
		Number	Percent
Stage I*	64	45	70
Stage II	272	71	26
Stage III	6	0	0

* 106 patients were diagnosed clinically as stage I: an elective axillary dissection yielded 26 patients with occult metastases, and in 16 other patients axillary nodes developed later, placing the number of stage I on pathologic evaluation at 64.

Location. Of the 62 determinate patients with melanoma of the hands and fingers (excluding subungual melanomas) the ten-year survival was 60% (37 patients), slightly lower than the ten-year survival for the 280 patients with melanoma of the arms (66%). For the 173 patients with melanoma of the upper arm, the ten-year survival was 64%, almost the same as the 107 patients with melanomas of the forearm who had a ten-year survival of 68%—two of those "cured" had metastases to the olecranon nodes (Fig. 23-9).

TREATMENT OF AXILLARY LYMPH NODES

A great deal of controversy exists regarding the management of regional lymph nodes. An analysis of this series may shed light upon this problem (Figs. 23-10, 23-11, 23-12, and 23-13).

Figure 23-14 presents the effects of metastases to the lymph nodes discovered on histologic study. There were 106 patients with clinical stage I melanomas analyzed. In 55 patients an elective axillary dissection was performed for clinically negative nodes, and occult metastases were discovered in 26 patients (47%). The ten-year survival for this group was 65%. In 29 patients no metastases were discovered on routine examination of the lymph nodes and 76% of this group survived ten years or longer. Fifty-one patients were not subjected to an axillary dissection, and 16 patients (31%) developed metastases to the axillary lymph nodes later. Nine (56%) of this group survived at least ten years. Of the 35 patients who did not demonstrate metastases to lymph nodes at any time, 29 (83%) survived at least ten years.

Of those subjected to elective node dissection were 34 males and 21 females, whose primary lesions were located in the upper arm (25 patients), lower arm (18 patients) and hands and fingers (12 patients). The group subjected to therapeutic axillary dissections consisted of 25 males and 26 females. Their lesions were located in the upper arm (16 patients), lower (23 patients), and hand and fingers (12 patients).

Additional operative procedures done on a number of these patients consisted of a supraclavicular dissection in four patients, none of whom survived; and a forequarter amputation in 26 patients, two of whom survived (8%) over ten years.

SURGICAL COMPLICATIONS

Surgical complications involved in operations on these patients were relatively minimal (Fig. 23-15). Only three patients

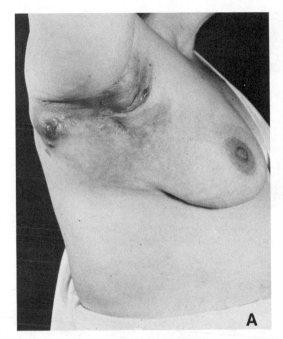

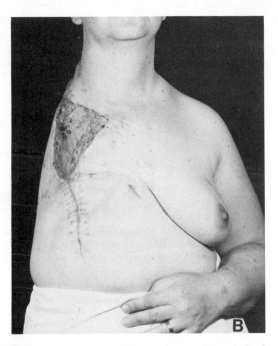

FIGURE 23-9. A: Very painful fixed metastatic melanoma of the shoulder and right breast. B: Appearance after interscapulo-mammothoracic am-putation. Excellent palliation but patient expired three years later from pulmonary metastases and metastases causing intestinal obstruction.

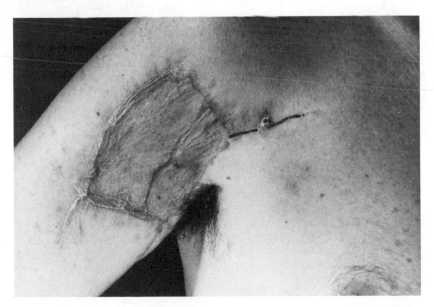

FIGURE 23-10.   Postoperative appearance after wide resection of a 1.5 cm superficial spreading melanoma closed by split-thickness skin graft; performed in conjunction with an axillary dissection. Two nodes were positive for metastatic melanoma. The patient remains well six years later.

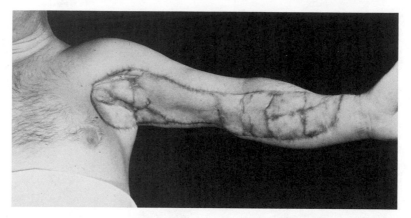

FIGURE 23-11. Resection site of primary melanoma left forearm performed in continuity with axillary dissection because of large node in axilla. Patient an achondrodiptrophic dwarf. Procedure performed due to shortness of arms.

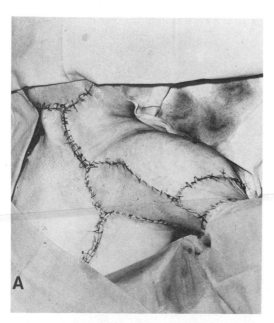

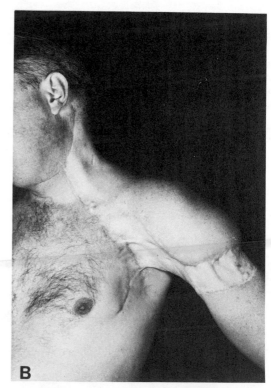

FIGURE 23-12. Melanoma of the clavicular region with metastases to the axilla and neck lymph nodes. A. Immediate postoperative appearance after a wide excision of the melanoma combined with an axillary and neck dissection. B. Appearance ten months later. Arm dysfunction was minimal. Patient was free of melanoma ten years later.

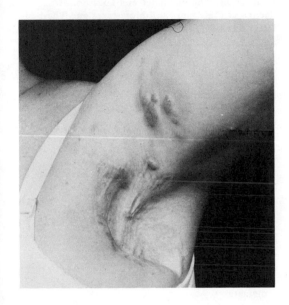

FIGURE 23-13. Satellitosis of upper arm that developed after a conservative axillary dissection.

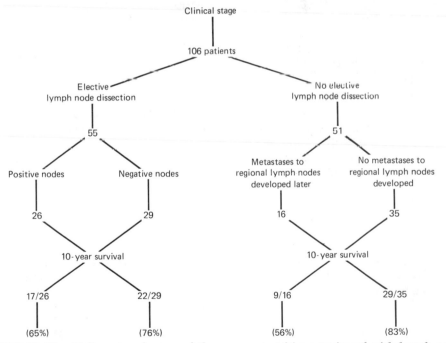

Clinical stage

106 patients

Elective
lymph node dissection

No elective
lymph node dissection

55

51

Positive nodes   Negative nodes

Metastases to
regional lymph nodes
developed later

No metastases to
regional lymph nodes
developed

26   29

16   35

10-year survival

10-year survival

17/26   22/29

9/16   29/35

(65%)   (76%)

(56%)   (83%)

FIGURE 23-14.   Malignant melanoma of the upper extremities experienced with lymph node dissection in 106 patients with clinical stage I melanoma.

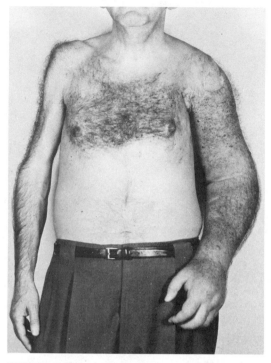

FIGURE 23-15. Severe edema and satellitosis from extensive metastases to the axilla from an infiltrating melanoma of the upper arm treated by excision and skin graft, without axillary dissection.

TABLE 23-13. Malignant Melanoma of the Upper Extremities. The Incidence and Location of Recurrent Melanoma and Metastases and Their Effect upon 5-Year Survival

Recurrent Disease	Number of Patients	5-Year Survivors Number	Percent
Local recurrence only	20	12	60
Local recurrence & metastases to regional nodes	6	3	50
In-transit recurrence	10	6	60
In-transit recurrence & regional node metastases	2	0	0
Regional nodes recurred	6	1	17
Local, regional & distant metastases	20	0	0
Distant metastases	66	2	2
Regional nodes recurred & distant metastases	4	0	0
Satellitoses	8	1	12

manifested wound infection; in five there was some necrosis of the flap; and in one patient the skin graft did not take. The data were not sufficiently accurate to measure the incidence of edema of the arm or hand, but the clinical impression is that it was minimal. Severe edema was always associated with residual or recurrent melanoma (Fig. 23-15).

THE INCIDENCE, LOCATION, AND RESULTS OF TREATING RECURRENT (METASTATIC) MELANOMA

These data are presented in terms of five-year survival, inasmuch as the results are not good, and a five-year follow-up value could be of greater significance (Table 23-13).

Of 20 patients who developed local recurrence, 12 (60%) survived five years. Six patients developed local recurrence with metastases to regional lymph nodes, and three of them survived (50%). Ten patients developed in-transit metastases, six of whom survived; and two patients developed, in addition to in-transit metastases, metastases to the regional lymph nodes and did not survive. Six patients developed a recurrent metastasis to the axillary lymph nodes after an axillary dissection had been performed, and only one of these patients survived (17%). Twenty patients developed a combination of local recurrence, regional metastases, and distant metastases, none of whom survived. Four patients developed recurrences in the regional lymph nodes and distant metastases, and none survived; 66 patients developed distant metastases, two of whom survived the five-year period.

Eight patients developed satellitoses, after an axillary dissection had been performed, and only one (12%) survived five years.

DISCUSSION

Malignant melanoma of the upper extremities was the fourth most frequent site seen by us, occurring in 15% of the 3,305 patients seen. The incidence was exceeded by melanomas of the trunk, which comprised 34%, head and neck, which comprised 23%, and the lower extremities, which comprised 20% of all patients with malignant melanoma. The incidence may vary in different institutions depending upon referral selection. Knutson et al., reporting from the Ellis Fischel State Cancer Hospital in Missouri, observed that 15.6% of 230 melanomas arose in the upper extremities, being exceeded by head and neck, which was the most frequent site, comprising 35% of their group, with the lower extremity comprising 30%, and the trunk comprising 20%.[17] McSwain et al., reporting from Vanderbilt University, observed that 24 of their 203 patients (12%) had melanomas arising in the upper extremities, the incidence there being exceeded by the head and neck, the eye, the trunk, and the lower extremity.[29] Magnus, reporting from the Cancer Registry of Norway, in which they recorded 2,866 malignant melanomas, observed 339 (12%) arising from the upper extremity.[23] In their series, twice as many females were involved with malignant melanoma of the upper extremity (230 females and 109 males). In our series, the incidence between males and females was equal.

At the Presbyterian Hospital in New York, as reported by Haagensen et al., 58 melanomas of the upper extremity were observed, of which 12 (20.4%) were subungual.[16] Das Gupta, reporting from the Abraham Lincoln School of Medicine in Chicago on 269 patients treated between 1968 and 1974, found 58 (21.5%) arising from the upper extremity.[11]

Other facets of the clinical presentation of our group were not unusual when compared with those reported by others, in that the white Caucasian group constituted almost all of our series, with only four Negroes being included. A familial history of involvement by melanoma was presented by 5% of the patients but not necessarily of the same site. The largest age incidence occurred between 30 and 60 years, with 29% being in the fourth decade, 23% in the fifth, and 25% in the sixth.

Of all patients, 75% gave a history of preexisting mole that changed in character, increasing in size or pigmentation, itching, ulceration, or bleeding.

Eighty-four percent of our patients developed the melanomas on the arms, with only 16% on the hands or fingers. Subungual melanomas, of which there were 40, are not considered in this presentation because of their unusual clinical manifestations of behavior.

INCIDENCE OF METASTASES TO LYMPH NODES

Staging. Staging depends upon the presence or absence of metastases either in transit, in the regional lymph nodes, or elsewhere. Staging should be recorded on the basis of histologic presentation as there was a 40% error between clinical staging and histologic staging of those patients listed clinically in the stage I category. One hundred and six patients were clinically diagnosed as representing stage I, but an elective axillary dissection yielded 26 patients with occult metastases. In 16 other patients in whom no axillary dissection was performed, metastases to lymph nodes developed at a later date.

Thus, of the 106 listed clinically stage I, on a histologic basis the actual number was 64 of the entire series. Including those in whom metastases were found on elective groin dissection and those who developed metastases to the regional lymph nodes later, the number of patients in stage II equalled 272 (79% of our total series). This figure is in contrast to those considered stage II when the patients were first seen, which equalled 53% of all individuals referred here with operable malignant melanoma.

At the Vanderbilt Hospital in a 1954 report, metastases were present in 75% of the patients, but in the series of 1964, metastases were present in only 38% of their patients, which included all anatomic sites. Magnus reported that 71.6% of males with melanoma of the upper extremities and 82.2% of females with melanoma of the upper extremities presented themselves with localized melanoma without metastases. This was a clinical evaluation. Haagensen et al. reported 12 of their 36 patients (33%) were found to have axillary metastases, either by prophylactic or therapeutic axillary dissection. McNeer and Das Gupta, from Memorial Hospital in New York, reported 168 patients with melanomas of the upper extremities and found metastases to the regional lymph nodes in 19.4%.[27]

Das Gupta and McNeer[12] reported before the James Ewing Society in 1963 that the dissection of the axillary lymph nodes in patients with primary melanoma of the upper extremity was performed in 118 patients of whom 83 (70.3%) revealed histologically positive nodes. They further evaluated the interval between excision of the primary tumor and clinical demonstration of metastases to regional lymph nodes and found it to be 11.15 months, the minimum being one month and the maximum 80 months. They demonstrated that 13 of 23 patients with melanoma of the finger, hand, or wrist underwent axillary dissection; nine were found to have histologic evidence of metastases to the lymph nodes (69.2%). With melanoma of the forearm, of 32 patients who underwent axillary dissection ten were found to have histologically positive lymph nodes (60.6% of the dissections demonstrated axillary metastases). They call attention to the fact that metastases to the epitrochlear lymph nodes are so rare that they question whether it should be considered.

At Columbia Presbyterian Hospital, epitrochlear nodes were invaded by squamous cell carcinoma in three instances. No mention was made of malignant melanoma. Taylor et al. stress these nodes as a site for metastases,

especially those arising from the ulnar half or the back of the hand.[43]

We have observed metastases to the epitrochlear nodes in three instances, particularly in younger patients, as the nodes undergo attrition with age.

For melanoma of the arm, of the 40 patients reported by Haagensen et al. (from the total group of 50) who underwent dissection of the regional lymph nodes, 27 (67.5%) had nodes that were positive for metastases. Of melanomas arising on the anterior shoulder, ten (71.4%) of 14 patients showed ipsilateral metastases to the cervical and/or axillary lymph nodes. Five cases demonstrated simultaneous involvement of both regional lymphatic areas, whereas in three cases metastases occurred solely in the ipsilateral/cervical lymph nodes, and in two cases in axillary lymph nodes. Thus eight (57.1%) showed involvement of ipsilateral/cervical lymph nodes at some stage of the disease.

In Taylor et al's total of 168 patients, there were only three cases of metastases to the nodes of the contralateral axilla, and two to the contralateral cervical lymph nodes. That is, only 3% of the melanomas arising in the upper extremities metastasized to the opposite side. In 18 autopsies that they performed on patients with melanoma of the upper extremities, 89% had metastases to the ipsilateral/axillary nodes and 22% to the ipsilateral/cervical nodes. Eight percent showed metastases to the contralateral axillary nodes, and 5% to the contralateral cervical lymph nodes.

Lane, Lattis, and Malm[18] from the Presbyterian Hospital in New York, made serial sections of resected metastases of lymph nodes from various sites after a so-called prophylactic lymph node dissection. They found that 42% of the patients had metastases to the lymph nodes.

These data indicate the relative frequency of metastases to the axilla in different institutions, and demonstrate the wide variations that can occur as a result of the type of patient referred to the institution, the reputation of the institution, and many other factors. They do demonstrate that a significant number of patients harboring malignant melanoma of the upper extremities do have metastases to regional axillary lymph nodes. This, of course, raises the question as to the indications for an elective axillary dissection.

RESULTS OF TREATING MELANOMAS OF THE UPPER EXTREMITIES

In our series of 487 patients observed, 145 are considered indeterminate in that 85 were referred only for consultation and were treated elsewhere and not followed up by us, and 60 patients were referred with extensive disseminated melanoma not suitable for a curative therapy. Of the 342 determinate patients who were treated by us and followed for a minimum of ten years, 216 are alive and free of evidence of melanoma, giving a ten-year survival rate of 63%. One hundred twenty-six patients have died of their melanoma, which includes two patients who were lost to follow-up and are presumed dead of melanoma.

The ten-year survival rate of 83% for patients in whom no metastases to the axilla occurred demonstrates the fact that blood-borne metastases may kill the patient even in the absence of metastases to the axillary lymph nodes.

Haagensen et al. report a five-year survival rate of 36 melanomas (exclusive of subungual melanomas) to be 47%, with 13 patients (36%) living free of melanoma from five to 19 years. Mundth et al.[31] reported a five-year survival of 43% (including subungual melanomas). McLeod, et al. reported a 76% 10-year survival for melanoma of the arm: 92.7% for those of the lower arm and 60% for those of the upper arm. Haagensen calls attention to the fact that five years is not sufficient time; of their 58 patients (including 12 with subungual melanomas) four developed metastases and died more than five years after treatment. In Mudth's series, six patients died after the five-year span posttherapy. Thirty of our patients who died from their melanomas (14%) died between the fifth and tenth year.

Charalambidis and Patterson[9] reported from Pondville Hospital on a small series of 20 cases (including subungual melanomas) where the survival rate for five years was 40%.

Magnus reported from Norway that 100 males and 230 females with melanomas of the upper extremity had a five-year relative survival rate for localized cases of malignant melanoma observed between 1953 and 1971 of 72% for males and 88% for females (interpolated from Table 23–3).

Davis, reporting from the Queensland melanoma project, has stated that their retrospective study showed that patients with melanomas of the forearm had a lower (7.3%) ten-year mortality than those with melanoma of the upper arm (40%).[13]

Milton, reporting from Australia, showed survival figures following lymph node dissection and excision of primary melanoma on the arm, and demonstrated a better survival for women, who had a 70% five-year survival, in contrast to men, who had only a 55% five-year survival (interpolated from Figure 7–2).[30]

Perzik and Baum reported a 71% five-year survival for melanoma of the arm.[37] Shah and Goldsmith reported a 63% five-year survival for 265 patients.[39] Cascinelli and colleagues reported a 60% ten-year survival of 77 patients with melanoma of the upper extremities.[8]

FACTORS INFLUENCING SURVIVAL

Various parameters were investigated to find out which influenced survival. There was no significant survival difference between the males and females in this series (61% vs 64%), although other authors have observed an improved survival among females (Milton). Age played a role in that there were four patients between zero and ten years of age, and these probably had juvenile melanomas which entity was not described at the time this study was originated. With the exception of the younger age groups, which probably contained a separate clinical entity, age did not seem to influence survival markedly. The duration of the delay before treatment in preexisting moles did influence survival in that the longer the delay, the poorer the prognosis, except for those who had moles in excess of six years, which is interpreted to mean that the mole had been quiescent and benign but had undergone malignant transformation. This was borne out by evaluating when changes had taken place in the mole before treatment was instituted, a somewhat better prognosis was indicated for those who delayed six months or less than for those who delayed longer after changes have occurred. For the patients who claimed that their lesions developed de novo, the data are not very significant as some patients stated that their new lesions lasted over 60 months, which would suggest a preexisting mole. The data are presented exactly as they were obtained from the patient and the reader is invited to draw his own conclusions. The attempt to evaluate which procedures are best for primary treatment for melanoma are so variable that no definite conclusions can be drawn, except that a better prognosis was obtained for the 198 patients who were originally treated by us than for the 144 patients who were referred to us for additional therapy. This in no way implies that our treatment was better, but does demonstrate that inadequate treatment with resultant recurrences will yield a poorer end result than a bold surgical attack upon apparently innocuous lesions that on histologic evidence demonstrate a potential malignant outlook. For those patients where the data were available, the smaller the lesion the better seemed the prognosis; those that were flat and without ulceration yielded a better prognosis than those that were elevated, nodular, ulcerated, and bled.

THE LEVEL OF INVASION

Recent studies by Clark[10] and his colleagues have definitely demonstrated that the degree of invasion of the malignant cells influences prognosis. This is expressed differently by Breslow, as to thickness which indicates growth, both exophitically and infiltratively.[7] These parameters have offered the surgeons an important landmark to help determine overall therapy (Chap. 6).

At the inception of this study, levels of invasion were not measured, and often we received only one slide, which did not permit accurate judgment of levels, inasmuch as many sections are necessary. Our pathologists listed *superficial* melanomas, which reflect Clark's level II and possibly his level III. We do not subscribe to his level III inasmuch as it is not necessarily markedly different from his level II, but represents more of a quantitative determination. Our designation of *infiltrating* melanomas represents Clark's levels IV and V. The unavailability of all the slides and all the paraffin sections to carefully evaluate the exact level precludes our separating level IV from level V, thus the infiltrating melanomas represent both levels. As important as are these designations, it should be stressed that malignant melanoma is such an unpredictable oncologic entity that complete faith should not be placed on a simple mechanistic evaluation, but studies should be continued to determine the relative incidence of the different levels in different institutions and different geographic locations.

For example, the Queensland melanoma project in Australia has a high preponderance of superficial melanomas (levels II and possibly III), whereas our series shows a marked preponderance of levels IV and V, which carry with them a worse prognosis. Investigations should continue into the immunologic factors and all other factors that determine these levels. We do not accept Clark's level I as a metastasizing malignant melanoma. These have been regarded previously by our pathologists as possibly premalignant and have been designated as active junction nevi, nevus with atypical cells, and other such designations.

All are agreed that the malignant melanoma is best treated surgically by wide local excision. Such agents as caustic escharotics, electrodissection, and other irritating local means of therapy are contraindicated. The treatment of primary melanomas by lazer beam is being explored, and there are some who claim beneficial results by radiation therapy, but this is not universally accepted.

The extent of the primary resection we consider important, as we have seen a very high incidence of local recurrences in patients who do not have a significant margin about their melanomas. Melanoma cells are mobile, they are not intimately adherent to each other, and readily break off and spread to contiguous structures. Hence a wide excision is necessary. We teach that a primary melanoma should be treated by a wide tridimensional excision and covered by skin graft. Some do not believe in dissection of the deep fascia (Olson[33]), but we do, as we have found melanoma cells resident on the fascia. The major controversy revolves about the indications for performing an elective axillary dissection in the absence of clinically manifest metastases to the axillary lymph nodes. All are agreed that an axillary dissection should be performed if metastases are clinically evident in the lymph nodes, except some, such as Ackerman and Wheat[1] who question the value of this procedure. Their opinion is shared by a few others, such as Olsen, Sandeman,[38] and Stehlin,[41] most of whom present small series, or no factual data to back up their claims.

In our series, of the 64 patients who had no evidence of metastases to the axillary lymph nodes and who did not develop them during the ten years of observation, 45 (70%) survived ten years, which value precipitously dropped to a 26% survival for the 272 patients who either presented themselves with clinical evidence of metastases to the axilla and in whom therapeutic axillary dissections were performed, or the 26 patients in whom occult metastases were discovered at the time of elective axillary dissection, or the 16 patients who developed metastases to the axilla at a later date.

Experience with 106 patients in clinical stage I reveals that where elective dissections were performed on 55 patients, 26 (47%) revealed metastases to their lymph nodes. The ten-year survival rate for this group of 26 patients was 65%. Of 29 patients who did not reveal metastases to regional lymph nodes, 22 (76%) survived the ten-year period. The lowest survival rate in this group were the 16 patients on whom no elective lymph node dissection was performed, but who later developed clinical evidence of metastases to

the nodes, nine of whom survived ten years (56%). In 35 patients in whom no elective axillary dissection was performed and who did not manifest metastases to regional lymph nodes during the ten years, 29 (83%) were presumably cured.

Gumport and Harris,[15] reporting from New York University, New York, on 64 axillary dissections over five years ago, found that those who had clinically negative nodes and microscopically negative nodes had a five-year survival rate of 60%. Those with nodes microscopically positive had an 11% five-year survival.

The W.H.O. collaborating center for evaluation of methods of diagnosis and treatment of melanoma, in their clinical trial no. 1, reported on 95 patients with melanoma of the upper extremities, and found a 74% nine-year survival where excision alone was performed, but a 60% nine-year survival when excision was accompanied by lymph node dissection.[45] The lower survival rate after regional lymph nodes were dissected suggests that the patients had a more advanced stage of their melanomas (52 patients had a lymph node dissection performed, while 43 patients had only excisions performed).

Knutson et al. favor lymph node dissection for all head and neck melanomas and for those of the upper extremities that may metastasize to the lymph nodes of the axilla. They do not favor elective lymph node dissection for melanomas of the trunk or the lower extremities.

In Mundth's series, one patient with axillary metastases survived over five years, and in the Haagenson et al. series, each of 12 patients who had axillary dissection for positive nodes (either prophylactic or therapeutic) succumbed. He states regarding the efficacy of dissection of lymph nodes:

> It leads me to recommend prophylactic dissection of axillary nodes in patients in whom they are not clinically evident because I know that they often contain metastases, which metastases surgical dissection may succeed in completely excising, and if there are no other metastases, the patient may be cured.

The tendency among several authors is to reserve axillary dissection for infiltrating melanomas (Clark's level IV & V) and not for the more superficial melanomas (Clark's levels I, II, and possibly III).

Further studies with present-day criteria, defining the different types and stages of melanomas, are needed to better establish the criteria for axillary dissection.

AMPUTATION FOR MALIGNANT MELANOMA OF THE UPPER EXTREMITIES

Interscapulo-thoracic amputation (forequarter amputation) is indicated for palliative therapy where extensive melanoma involves the upper arm and shoulder girdle. Often ulceration and infection of the tumor result in a useless swollen arm with uncontrollable, intractable pain. Although it is often a palliative procedure, the patients we have treated have often begged for the operation for relief. Prolongation of useful life has been obtained.

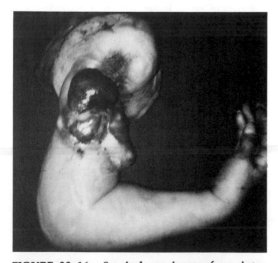

FIGURE 23–16. Surgical specimen of an interscapulo-mammothoracic amputation performed for palliation of extensive metastases to breast and axilla. Patient was better for one year and then developed generalized metastases and died.

Theoretically, treatment of melanomas of the skin of the upper limb with demonstrable involvement of the axillary nodes are best treated by excision and dissection incontinuity (Figs. 23–15 and 23–16). If this cannot be carried out, then the principle of exarticulation of the limb combined with excision of the regional lymph nodes should be performed, as claimed by Pack and McGraw.[36] Although theoretically this is the ideal procedure, it is not performed at present inasmuch as the discontinuous operation has not been shown to be as harmful as was at one time suspected.

Bowers reported nine interscapulothoracic amputations for melanoma of the upper extremity. None of his patients survived the five-year span. At times when the operation is performed, usually after multiple failures from other procedures, beneficial unexpected long-term survivals may obtain. Thus, Pack and McGraw report that of 24 patients treated for malignant melanoma by forequarter amputation, four were lost to follow-up observation, 17 died of metastatic melanoma, and three were living more than five years, and one of these for over ten years. These authors also performed an interscapulo-mammothoracic amputation, which includes a radical mastectomy combined with a quarterectomy. They reported two cases in which this was performed. Both patients received transient palliation, but eventually succumbed from widespread metastases. This operation, accordingly, should be performed only under the severest of circumstances (Fig. 23–16).

McPeak[28] and associates reported eight patients with malignant melanoma treated by interscapulo-thoracic amputation. All contained metastatic melanoma to the axilla. Two of the patients remained alive at the time of the report, one for 11 years, and the other for 13 years, thus demonstrating an unexpected long-term survival.

Turnbull, Shah, and Fortner, in 1973, reported from Memorial Hospital that two of 16 patients treated by forequarter amputation were alive and free of evidence of melanoma 11 and 18 years later, respectively.[44] Twelve patients died of widespread metastases an average of 12 months later. The interval between treatment of the primary melanoma and amputations for recurrence averaged 13 months in those who died of their disease. Only two of the 16 patients had negative axillary nodes, and they died 20 and 24 months later, respectively. They recorded two postoperative deaths, one from pulmonary embolus and the other from splenic rupture secondary to metastatic melanoma.

An opponent to these radical procedures is Ackerman, who stated:

> If if is necessry to do an interscapulo-thoracic amputation, disarticulation of the thigh, or hemi-pelvectomy in order to obtain involved lymph nodes beyond the field of the axilla or inguinal node dissection, then the melanoma is probably already beyond such indicated areas.

Experience to date with interscapulo-thoracic amputation indicates that good palliation and significant prolongation of life with suggested cures can be obtained in certain selected patients with far-advanced melanoma localized to the axilla.

AMPUTATION OF DIGITS

Inasmuch as a wide dissection cannot be obtained for melanoma of the fingers, we routinely practice amputation of the digit (and proximal metacarpal, for a better functional result) in all melanomas of the digits, including subungual melanomas (Fig. 23-17).

When an infiltrating melanoma invades the web between digits, the patient is best served by amputation of the two digits and metacarpals adjacent to the melanoma.

SUMMARY AND CONCLUSIONS

Malignant melanomas of the upper limbs, of which there were 487, constituted 15% of the 3,305 malignant melanomas seen at the Pack Medical Group in New York City, being exceeded by malignant melanoma of the trunk (34%), head and neck (23%), and the lower extremities (20%).

The majority of patients were white (79%), with a fair complexion (70%). The sexes were evenly divided (males 51%, females 49%). Most patients were between 30 and 60 years of age (78%). Five percent gave a family history of harboring malignant melanoma; 75% gave a history of the melanoma developing in a preceding mole.

The ten-year survival rate of 342 determinate patients was 63%. Fourteen percent of patients dying from melanoma died between the fifth and tenth year, indicating the need to report survival at the ten-year span.

The survival in this series was equal for the sexes (61% males, and 64% females). Age had little effect except at both extremes, where the prognosis was better.

The smaller lesions usually had a better prognosis but larger lesions of the superficial spreading type had good results (60% survival of ten patients whose lesions were over 4 cm in diameter).

Infiltrating melanomas (Clark's levels IV and V) had a survival rate of 62%. Ten patients with superficial spreading melanomas (Clark's levels II and III) and juvenile melanomas enjoyed a 100% ten-year survival. The worst prognosis was for the six patients with amelanotic melanoma, in that only two of ten patients survived 10 years or longer.

The question of elective axillary dissection where nodes are not clinically palpable (clinical stage I) remains enigmatic. Our data do not answer the question, in that among 106 patients classified as clinical stage I, elective node dissection was performed in 55 instances. Of these 55 patients 26 had had microscopic evidence of metastases and their ten-year survival was 65%. This is somewhat higher than 16 patients in whom no elective axillary dissection was performed. Among these 16, six later developed evidence of metastases and underwent therapeutic node dissection. This last group had a ten-year survival of 56%.

Radical amputation is occasionally indicated with great palliation and often prolongation of life. The indications and results are presented.

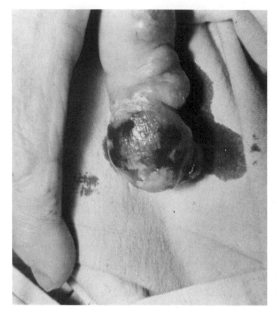

FIGURE 23-17.   Top. Melanoma of tip of thumb.
Bottom: Left—Incision for thumb amputation. Middle—Surgical technique permits good rehabilitation. Right—Surgical defect after amputation.

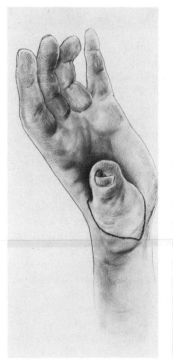

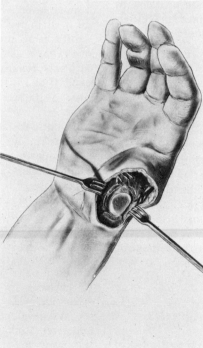

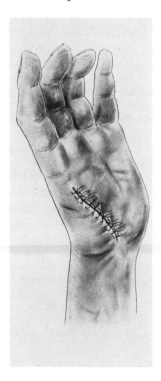

REFERENCES

1. Ackerman LL, Wheat MW: The implantation of cancer—an avoidable risk? Surg 37:347, 1955

2. Ariel IM: Tridimensional resection of malignant melanoma. Surg Gynecol Obstet 139:601, 1974

3. Attie JN, Khafif RD: Melanotic Tumors. Charles Thomas, 1964, p 135

4. Booher RJ, Pack GT: Malignant melanoma of the feet and hands. Surgery 42:1084, 1957

5. Bowers RF: Quarterectomy—Its application in malignant melanoma. Arch Surg 83:70, 1961

6. Bowers RF: Eleven years experience with quarterectomy for malignant melanoma. Arch Surg 81:752, 1960

7. Breslow A: Tumor thickness, level of invasion and node dissection in Stage I cutaneous melanoma. Ann Surg 182:572, 1975

8. Cascinelli N, Balzarini GJ, Fontana V: Long term results of surgical treatment of melanoma of the limbs. Tumori 62:233-242, 1976

9. Charalambidis PH, Patterson WB: A clinical study of 250 patients with malignant melanoma. Surg Gynecol Obstet 115:333, 1962

10. Clark WH Jr, in Bernadino EA, Mihm MC: The histogenesis and biologic behavior of primary malignant melanomas of the skin. Cancer Res 29:705, 1969

11. Das Gupta TK: Results of treatment of 269 patients with primary cutaneous melanoma: a five-year prospective study. Ann Surg 186:201, 1977

12. Das Gupta TK, McNeer G: The incidence of metastasis to accessible lymph nodes from melanoma of the trunk and extremities—its therapeutic significance. Cancer 17:897, 1964

13. Davis NC: The regional lymph nodes in malignant melanoma: Is routine excision indicated. In Ariel IM (ed): Progress in Clinical Cancer, vol 6, New York, Grune & Stratton, 1977, pp 183-194

14. Guiss LW, MacDonald I: The role of regional lymphadenectomy in treatment of melanoma. Am J Surg 104:135, 1962

15. Gumport SG, Harris MN: Results of regional lymph node dissection for melanoma. Ann Surg 179:105-108, 1974

16. Haagensen CD, Feind CR, Herter FP, et al.: The Lymphatics in Cancer. New York, WB Saunders, Co, 1972

17. Knutson CA, Hori JM, Spratt JS Jr: Melanoma. Current Problems in Surgery. Chicago, Year Book, December 1971

18. Lane N, Lattes R, Malm J: Clinicopathological correlations in a series of 117 malignant melanomas of the skin of adults. Cancer 11:1025, 1958

19. Lee JAH: The trend of mortality from primary malignant tumors of the skin. J Invest Dermatol 59:445, 1975

20. Long ER: Metastasis of squamous cell carcinoma from wrist to axilla without demonstrable intervening growth. Am J Cancer 23:797, 1935

21. Lund HZ, Kraus JM: Melanotic tumors of the skin. In Atlas of Tumor Pathology, Section I, Fascicle 3, Washington DC, Armed Forces Institute of Pathology, 1962

22. Lund RH, Ihnen M: Malignant melanoma. Clinical and pathologic analysis of 93 cases. Surgery 38:652, 1955

23. Magnus K: Incidence of malignant melanoma of the skin in Norway, 1950-1970. Cancer 32:1275-1286, 1973

24. McCune WS, Letterman GS: Malignant melanoma: 10 year results following excision and regional gland resection. Ann Surg 141:901, 1955

25. McLeod R, Davis NC, Herron JJ, et al.: A retrospective survey of 498 patients with malignant melanoma. Surg Gynecol Obstet 126:99, 1968

26. McNeer G: Malignant melanoma. Surg Gynecol Obstet 120:343, 1965

27. McNeer G, Das Gupta T: Prognosis in malignant melanoma. Surgery 56:512, 1964

28. McPeak CJ, McNeer GP, Whitely HW, Booher RJ: Amputation for melanoma of the extremity. Surgery 54:426, 1963

29. McSwain CJ, Riddel DH, Richie RF, Crocker EF: Malignant melanoma. Ann Surg 159:967-975, 1964

30. Milton GW: Malignant Melanoma of the Skin and Mucous Membrane. Sidney, Australia, Churchill-Livingstone, 1977

31. Mundth ED, Guralnick EA, Raker JW: Malignant melanoma: A clinical study of 427 cases. Ann Surg 162:15, 1965

32. Olsen G: The Malignant Melanoma of the Skin. Copenhagen, The Finsen Institute and Radium Center, 1966

33. Olsen G: Removal of fascia—Cause of more frequent metastases of malignant melanomas of the skin to regional lymph nodes. Cancer 17:1159, 1964

34. Pack GT: End results in the treatment of malignant melanoma. Surgery 46:447, 1959

35. Pack GT, Gerber DM, Scharnagel IM: End

results in the treatment of malignant melanoma: A report of 1190 cases. Ann Surg 136: 905, 1952

36. Pack GT, McGraw TA: Interscapulo-mammothoracic amputation for malignant melanoma. Arch Surg 83:694, November 1961

37. Perzik SL, Baum RK: Individualization in the management of melanoma. Am Surg 35:177-180, 1969

38. Sandeman TF: The radical treatment of enlarged lymph nodes in malignant melanoma. Am J Roentgenol 97:967, 1966

39. Shah JP, Goldsmith HS: Prognosis of malignant melanoma in relation to clinical presentation. Am J Surg 123:286–288, 1972

40. Southwick HW, Slaughter DP, et al., Role of regional node dissection in treatment of malignant melanoma. Arch Surg 85:63, 1962

41. Stehlin JS Jr: Malignant melanoma: An Appraisal. Surgery 64:1149, 1968

42. Stehlin JS Jr, Clark RL Jr, Smith JL Jr, White EC: Malignant melanoma of the extremities. Cancer 13:55, 1960

43. Taylor GW, Nathanson IT, Shaw DT: Epidermoid carcinoma of the extremities with reference to lymph node involvement. Ann Surg 113:268, 1941

44. Turnbull A, Shah J, Fortner J: Recurrent melanoma of an extremity treated by major amputation. Arch Surg 106:496, April, 1973

45. W.H.O. Collaborating Center for Evaluation of Methods of Diagnosis and Treatment of Melanoma. Clinical Trial No. 1. Data from 553 Cases. January 31, 1978. Prepared by Bufalino R

CHAPTER TWENTY–FOUR

TECHNIQUE OF AXILLARY DISSECTION FOR MALIGNANT MELANOMA *

MATTHEW N. HARRIS
AND STEPHEN L. GUMPORT

A technique for dissection of the axilla that permits excellent visualization and complete extirpation of all levels of the axillary contents is presented.

Division of the sternal segment of the pectoralis major muscle at its tendinous-insertion into the humerus and resection of the pectoralis minor muscle facilitates the exposure. Loss of the pectoralis minor muscle has no apparent clinical sequelae. The pectoralis major muscle is resutured and an excellent functional and cosmetic result is obtained provided that the innervation of the muscle is preserved. This technique affords access to the apex of the axilla without muscle retraction or arm manipulation.

Figure 24–1A shows a patient with a superficial spreading melanoma of the left forearm, invasive to level III, previously treated by wide and deep excision and split-thickness skin grafting. He is in the supine position with the arm abducted 90 degrees and draped free. A folded sheet is placed under the ipsilateral scapula to elevate the axilla. Care is taken to avoid stretching of the brachial plexus when positioning the patient. The skin incision follows the free edge of the pectoralis major muscle and extends from the area of its insertion down to the level of the nipple in the male, the upper outer quadrant of the breast in the female; an alternative incision, also depicted, may be utilized. This incision starts just below the middle third of the clavicle and

extends inferiorly and posteriorly as a gentle curve below the hair-bearing area of the axilla to the posterior axillary line. The choice of incision depends on the site of any previous biopsy to be excised.

In Figure 24–1B an anterior full-thickness flap is elevated over the pectoralis major muscle to the clavicle superiorly and to the midnipple line medially. The pectoralis major muscle fascia is not included in the flap. With sharp dissection, the thin anterior fascia of the pectoralis major muscle is removed starting superiorly and medially and continuing to the free edge of the muscle.

Figure 24–2 depicts the fascia of the pectoralis major muscle as continuous with the anterior fascia of the axilla where it forms an anterior envelope for the axillary contents (arrow).

Figure 24–3 illustrates blunt dissection, separating the clavicular and sternal fibers of the pectoralis major muscle. Several small vessels may cross this anatomically artificial separation, and they should be controlled.

Then in Figure 24–4 the sternal portion of the pectoralis major muscle is divided at its tendinous insertion into the humerus, and the muscle is retracted medially with the use of noncrushing clamps to expose the lateral axilla.

Figure 24–5 illustrates the rather firm band of fascia encountered where the pectoralis minor and the coracobrachial muscle insert into the coracoid process. This fascia is opened by sharp dissection and the underlying tongue of adipose tissue is swept inferiorly, exposing the brachial plexus and axillary vein. With

* Reprinted from Harris, MN and Gumport SL: Radical Axillary Dissection. Surg Tech Illus, 1(4): 57–65, 1976. Boston, Little, Brown and Company.

these structures plainly in view, the vein is cleared from the lateral to the medial end using sharp dissection. Vessels and nerves to the specimen are divided and ligated with 3-0 cotton sutures. White suture material is used in patients with melanoma to avoid postoperative confusion between recurrent melanoma and suture granuloma.

Figure 24-6 shows how the dissection is extended to the lateral border of the pectoralis minor muscle, which is divided between clamps at its insertion into the coracoid process. A large vessel is often located at this insertion, and care must be taken to ligate or cauterize the stump of the pectoralis minor muscle adequately at the coracoid.

Figure 24-7 illustrates the pectoralis minor muscle retracted inferiorly and medially exposing the remainder of the axillary vein and the apex of the axilla. The branches of the axillary vessels are divided and ligated to the level of the thoracoacromial vessels.

In Figure 24-8 the lateral pectoral nerve, which emerges medial to the pectoralis minor muscle, is preserved, as is the cephalic vein. The branches of the thoracoacromial vessels may be sacrificed to gain access to the apex of the axilla. The apex is cleared, with careful attention to several small vessels in this area, and the apical tissue is tagged for identification by the pathologist.

The specimen is then dissected from the chest wall, commencing at the apex of the axilla and proceeding laterally and inferiorly as shown in Figure 24-9. The fascia and the fibroadipose tissue between the pectoral muscles are removed with the specimen. The intercostobrachial nerve is sacrificed. The long thoracic and thoracodorsal nerves are preserved if there is no gross evidence of adjacent malignant disease; the thoracodorsal nerve may be sacrificed with its accompanying vessels without any major functional loss. The posteriorly directed subscapular vessels are preserved.

Figure 24-10 shows the posterior flap developed with sharp dissection. The flap thickness is just below the level of the apocrine glands of the axilla and extends posteriorly to the latissimus dorsi muscle.

Following this dissection the specimen is further dissected from the anterior serratus and subscapular muscles, remaining attached inferiorly and laterally as Figure 24-11 illustrates.

Figure 24-12 shows several large vessels being divided and ligated in the area of the upper outer quadrant of the breast. The specimen is removed.

The wound is then irrigated with copious amounts of saline solution, and hemostasis is assured. The pectoralis minor muscle is *not* resutured to the coracoid process. Muscle tissue that appears nonviable is excised. The entire pectoralis minor muscle may be removed with the specimen (Fig. 24-13A).

The sternal portion of the pectoralis major muscle is sutured to the clavicular portion close to the insertion of the latter into the humerus as shown in Fig. 24-13B. This reconstruction, which restores the axillary contour, should make use of the tendinous fibers and should be accomplished without tension using 0 or 2-0 Dexon™. Large-sized soft Hemovac™ suction catheters are placed, one under each flap (inset). These are held in position with plain catgut sutures; care is taken to avoid impingement upon any neural or vascular structure. The catheters are brought out through stab wounds and are secured firmly to the skin with sutures and umbilical tape. The wound is closed with a single layer of sutures; a light dressing is applied.

POSTOPERATIVE CARE

The suction catheters are kept in place for as long as there is drainage, usually four to six days. Careful attention is required to prevent clotting and subsequent collections under the flaps. The arm is kept abducted at 75 to 90 degrees.

Once the flaps are adherent, exercises are cautiously begun to restore full function to the arm; they are started about fourteen days postoperatively when the skin sutures are removed. The exercises prescribed are those utilized following radical mastectomy.

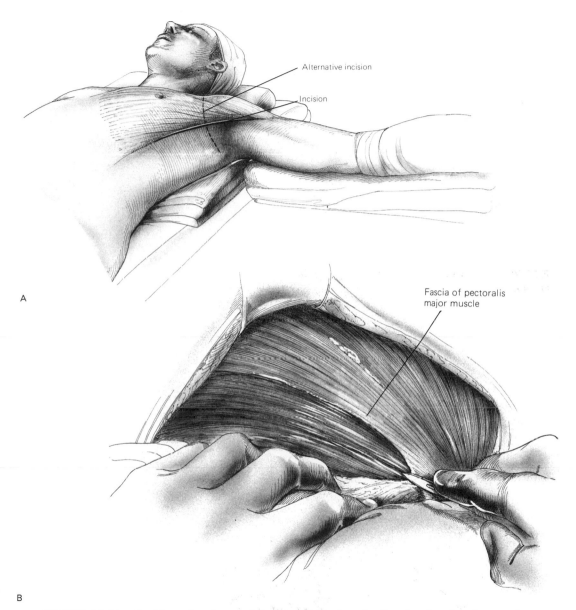

Alternative incision

Incision

A

Fascia of pectoralis
major muscle

B

FIGURE 24–1A. Position of patient and incision(s). B. Anterior flap developed and pectoral fascia removed.

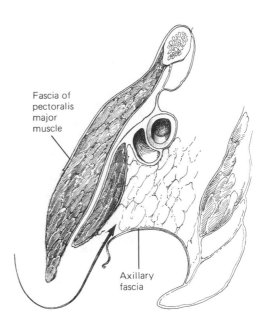

Fascia of
pectoralis
major
muscle

Axillary
fascia

FIGURE 24-2. Cross section of axilla with fascial envelope.

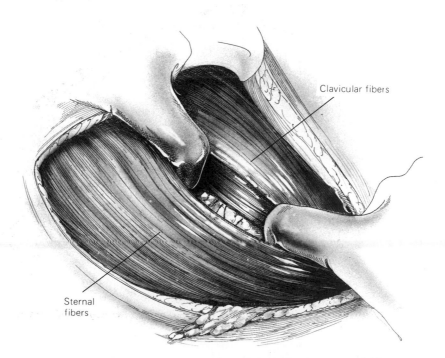

Clavicular fibers

Sternal
fibers

FIGURE 24-3.   Separation of clavicular from sternal fibers.

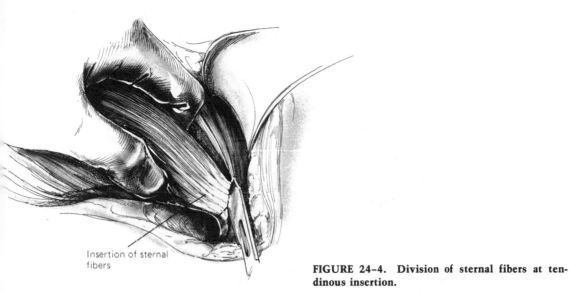

Insertion of sternal
fibers

FIGURE 24–4. Division of sternal fibers at tendinous insertion.

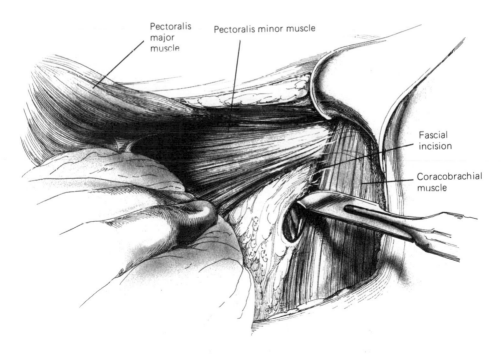

Pectoralis
major
muscle

Pectoralis minor muscle

Fascial
incision

Coracobrachial
muscle

FIGURE 24–5. Exposure of axillary vein and brachial plexus.

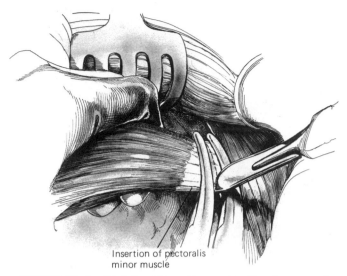

Insertion of pectoralis
minor muscle

FIGURE 24–6. Division of insertion pectoralis minor muscle.

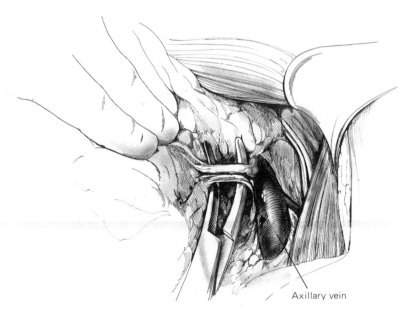

Axillary vein

FIGURE 24–7. Division of branches of axillary vessels to specimen.

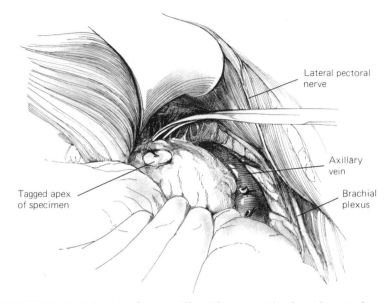

FIGURE 24-8. Clearing of apex axilla with perservation lateral pectoral nerve.

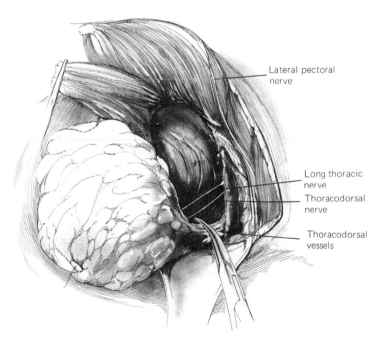

FIGURE 24-9. Specimen dissected from chest wall.

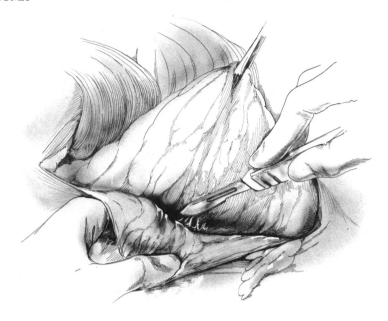

FIGURE 24-10. Developing posterior flap.

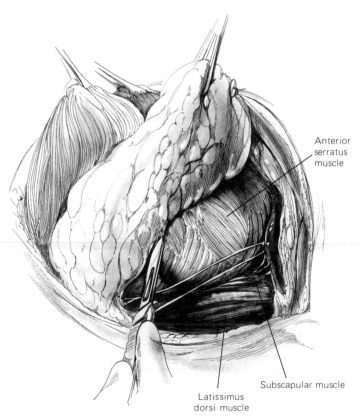

Anterior
serratus
muscle

Subscapular muscle

Latissimus
dorsi muscle

FIGURE 24-11. Clearing floor of axilla.

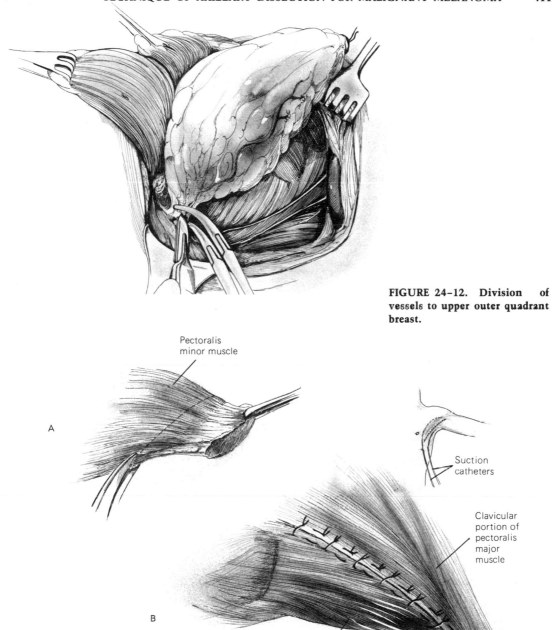

FIGURE 24-12. Division of vessels to upper outer quadrant breast.

Pectoralis minor muscle

A

Suction catheters

Clavicular portion of pectoralis major muscle

B

Sternal portion of pectoralis major muscle

FIGURE 24-13A. Resection of pectoralis minor muscle. B. Reconstruction of pectoralis major muscle and restoration axillary contour.

CHAPTER TWENTY–FIVE

MALIGNANT MELANOMA OF THE LOWER EXTREMITY

IRVING M. ARIEL

The clinical aspects of 673 patients with malignant melanoma of the lower extremity observed at the Pack Medical Group, New York City, are evaluated. Of these, 220 patients are indeterminate as 130 patients were referred for palliation, already suffering from blood-borne metastases and 90 patients were referred only for consultation, were treated elsewhere, and the results are not available for evaluation.

CLINICAL EVALUATION

LOCATION OF THE PRIMARY MELANOMA

Of the 673 patients seen, the thigh was the most frequent primary site (285 occurrences, or 42.3%). The leg was the second most frequent site (200, or 29.7%) (Fig. 25–1). There were 59 patients with malignant melanoma of the sole of the foot (8.8%) and 41 patients with malignant melanoma of the dorsum of the foot (6%). The digits exclusive of subungual melanomas comprised 4.3% of the total melanomas involving the lower extremity (29 patients), and there were 32 subungual melanomas, comprising 4.7%. In 27 patients (4.0%) the specific site of the melanoma was not listed (Table 25–1). Subungual melanomas are discussed in Chapter 22 as a distinct clinical entity.

CLINICAL STAGING

Stage I constitutes melanomas limited to the site of origin without clinical evidence of metastases to the regional lymph nodes (Fig. 25–2), stage II represents those with met-astases present in regional lymph nodes, and stage III represents those patients who have evidence of additional regional spread (Table 25–2). There were 202 patients with stage I (45%), 228 patients with stage II (50%), and 23 patients were in stage III (5%). One-hundred-thirty patients presented themselves with disseminated melanoma (stage IV) and are not considered further in this presentation, and 90 patients were seen only in consultation and are not staged. The clinical stage was changed after histologic verification.

RACE

The patients were predominantly white Caucasians, 445 patients (98%) (Table 25–3). Only five Negroes were seen (1%), and their melanomas occurred on the sole of the foot. No other groups such as Oriental or Indian were seen by us, and in three patients the racial background was not mentioned.

COMPLEXION

In 224 patients, no mention was made in the chart regarding the complexion of the patient. Of the remainder, 175 (76%) were of fair complexion, 30 patients (13%) had many freckles, and in only 24 patients (10%) the complexion was dark (Table 25–4).

FAMILY HISTORY

A history of other family members with melanoma (not necessarily at the same site) was recorded by 20 patients (4%) of the total (Table 25–5).

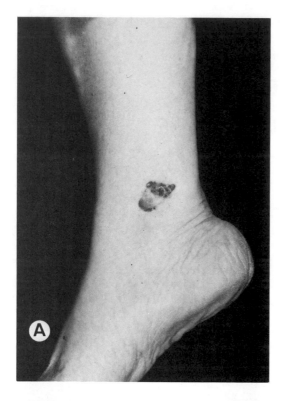

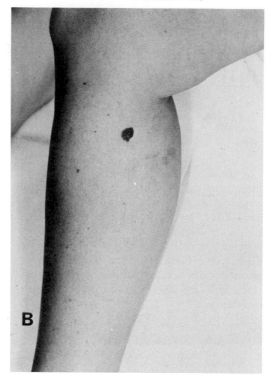

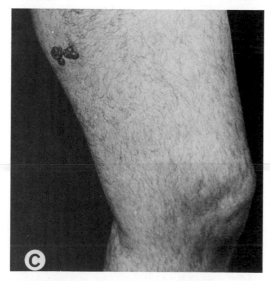

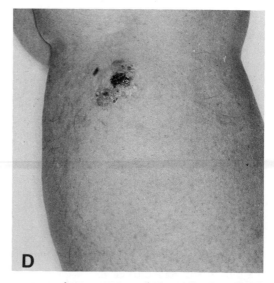

FIGURE 25-1. Examples of melanoma of the lower extremity. A. Superficial melanoma of ankle with depigmentation. B. Deeply pigmented melanoma of lower leg. C. Nodular melanoma growing in an irregular manner, presenting a clinical appearance of two separate lesions. D. Superficial melanoma with depigmentation treated by wide tridimensional excision with skin graft and in-continuity popliteal node dissection. Patient cured ten years later.

TABLE 25-1. Location of 673 Malignant Melanomas of the Lower Extremity

Location	Number	Percent
Thigh	285	42.3
Leg	200	29.7
Dorsum of foot	41	6.0
Sole of foot	59	8.8
Digits	29	4.3
Subungual	32	4.7
Not specified	27	4.0

TABLE 25-2. Initial Clinical Staging of 453 Determinate Patients with Malignant Melanoma of the Lower Extremity

Stage	Number	Percent
Stage I*	202	45
Stage II	228	50
Stage III	23	5

* Stage I was clinically staged where no histological data were available but was changed after elective groin dissection revealed occult metastases and so expressed in subsequent tables.

TABLE 25-3. Racial Characteristics of 453 Patients with Malignant Melanoma of the Lower Extremity

Race	Number	Percent
White	445	98
Negro	5	1
Other	0	0
Unknown	3	0.7

TABLE 25-4. Complexion Characteristics of 229 Patients with Malignant Melanoma of the Lower Extremity

Complexion	Number	Percent
Fair	175	76
Dark	24	10
Freckled	30	13
Unknown*	224	49

* The 224 patients whose complexions were not noted on their charts are excluded from the evaluation.

TABLE 25-5. Family History of Melanoma in 453 Patients with Malignant Melanoma of the Lower Extremity

Family History	Number	Percent
Yes	20	4
No	328	72
Unknown	105	23

AGE

There were 116 patients (26%) between 41 and 50 years and 106 (23%) between the ages of 31 and 40. Patients from 51 to 60 years of age represented 17.7%. There were considerably fewer of those both younger and older. Thus, three quarters of all the patients were between 30 and 60 years of age. There was one patient in the zero to ten-year bracket, and for four patients the age was not listed (Table 25-6).

RELATIONSHIP OF MALIGNANT MELANOMA TO PREEXISTING MOLE

A preexisting mole was noted by 337 patients. The remaining 116 patients said the melanoma appeared de novo. Of those who stated that the melanoma developed on a preexisting mole (Fig. 25-3), 111 patients said the mole had been present all their lives. In 26,

TABLE 25-6. Age of 453 Patients with Malignant Melanoma of the Lower Extremity

Age	Number	Percent
0–10 years	1	0.2
11–20 years	18	4.0
21–30 years	70	15.0
31–40 years	106	23.0
41–50 years	116	26.0
51–60 years	80	17.7
61–70 years	43	9.5
71–80 years	13	2.9
81–90 years	2	0.4
Unknown	4	0.8

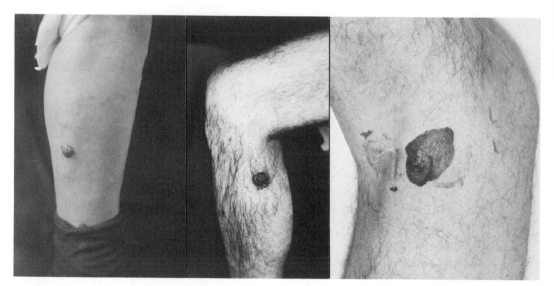

FIGURE 25-2.   Multiple views of different melanomas of the leg, which developed on preexisting moles.

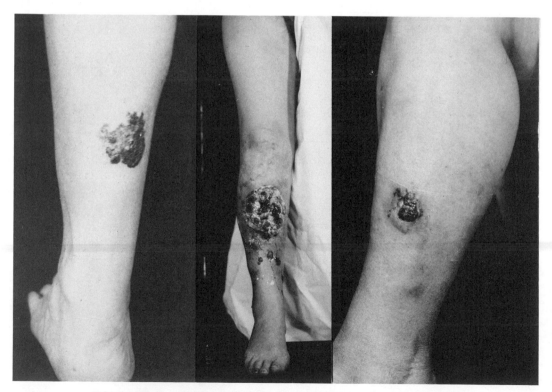

FIGURE 25-3.   Multifaceted appearance of primary melanoma of the leg.

the mole had appeared 11 to 20 years before the melanoma developed, in another 30 the mole had existed from six to ten years, and in 68 patients the mole had been present from one to five years. In 17 patients a mole had appeared and remained quiescent for a year or less before changes occurred and a biopsy revealed it to be a malignant melanoma (Table 25–12). Whether these were de novo melanomas that were quiescent for a period, or benign nevi that underwent transformation, cannot be stated (Fig. 25–4).

In 94 patients who had a history of a mole, some form of trauma, such as irritation or physical trauma, was said to have preceded the onset of changes that led to the excision of the melanoma. In 206 patients, there was no history of irritation, trauma, or other biologic feature that could be considered a possible contributory or causative factor. In 47 patients the history was not mentioned.

Among the 228 patients who estimated the length of time during which changes in the mole were observed before therapy was instituted, it was noted that in 16 the changes had occurred in less than one month, in 44 from one to three months, and in 41 from four to six months. In 64 patients the duration was between seven months and one year, in 39 patients from one to two years, and 27 patients stated that they had observed changes for two years or longer.

TREATMENT

Our policy has been to do a complete excision of the lesion where possible and paraffin study of the section by qualified pathologists in the field of malignant melanoma (Fig. 25–5).

After the diagnosis of malignant melanoma was established, a wide tridimensional exci-

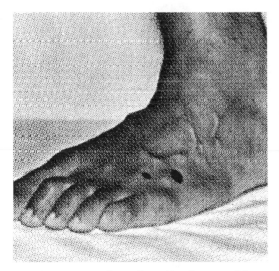

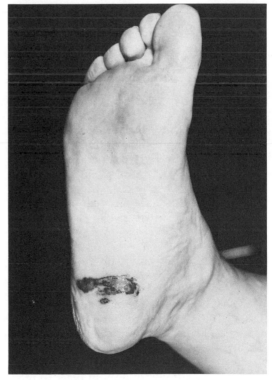

FIGURE 25–4. Left: Malignant melanoma of foot. Adjacent nevus shows clinical and microscopic evidence of growth activity. Right: Superficial spreading melanoma of the heel with invasion. Note the irregular margins, regions of depigmentation, and a satellite lesion.

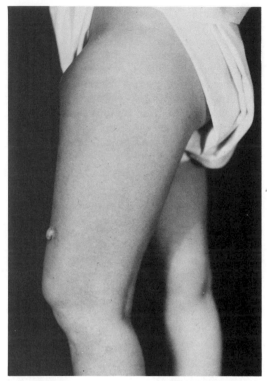

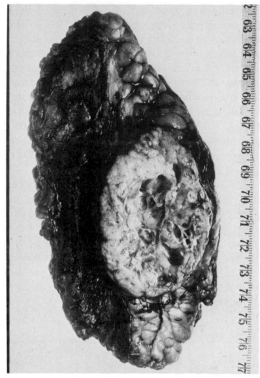

FIGURE 25–5.   Left: Amelanotic melanoma above knee treated by wide excision and groin dissection which revealed metastases in the inguinal lymph node. Right: Resected specimen showing the melanoma and the extent of the resection.

sion was performed,[3] and where possible, in continuity with a radical groin dissection. In certain instances a discontinuous operation was performed, and in other instances with specific indications, no elective groin dissection was performed. The effects of this program are evaluated (Fig. 25–6).

RESULTS OF TREATMENT

Four-hundred-fifty-three patients were treated by us and followed for a minimum of ten years (Table 25–7). All patients who died are considered as having died from melanoma regardless of the cause of death on their death certificates, and the 20 patients who were lost to follow-up are considered dead in order to present absolute figures.

TABLE 25–7. Survival of Patients with Malignant Melanoma of the Lower Extremity

	Number	Percent
Total number observed	673	
Indeterminate group	220	
Patients with blood-borne dissemination	130	
Patients seen in consultation only and not treated	90	
Determinate group	453	
Number of patients dead*	203	44.8
Number of patients alive and apparently well for 10 years or longer	250	55.2

* This includes 20 patients lost to follow-up and presumed dead and 95 patients listed as dead from other causes.

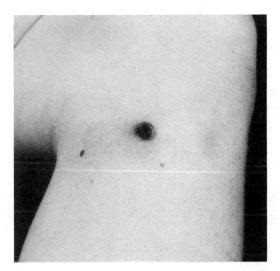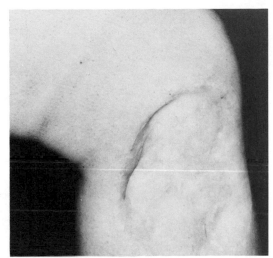

FIGURE 25-6. Left: Melanoma of lower leg. Right: Appearance two years later. Patient cured over 15 years. No groin dissection was performed.

The overall ten-year survival of the 453 patients equalled 250 patients, or 55.2% of the total group. The value would be higher if the 20 patients lost to follow-up were not considered, and if those considered dying of other causes (95 patients) were excluded from the failure group (Chart 25-1).

THE INFLUENCE OF SEX UPON SURVIVAL

Of the 152 males, 64 (42%) survived at least ten years. There were twice as many female patients, and their survival rate was significantly better (64%). This finding is in keeping with that usually ascribed to a better prognosis for females (Table 25-8).

THE INFLUENCE OF AGE UPON SURVIVAL

The one patient in the zero to ten-year bracket survived (Table 25-9). The best prognosis existed for those at both extremes of age. Of the 18 patients in the 11 to 20-year bracket, 83% survived the ten-year period, and two patients in the 81 to 90-year bracket both survived the ten-year period after treatment. This finding suggests that age, per se, should never influence the overall radical treatment necessary to treat malignant melanoma unless other contraindications exist. Of the 70 patients between 21 to 30 years of age, 60% survived ten years, and of 106 patients between 31 to 40 years of age, 73% survived. The values were roughly equal for those from 40 to 70 years of age (about 48% ten-year survival). It thus seems that the younger patients fared better than the older ones, contrary to the myth that cancers are more malignant in the younger than in the older patients.

STAGING AND ITS INFLUENCE UPON SURVIVAL

Staging in this series means that those patients who are found to have evidence of metastases in the regional lymph nodes on histologic examination are classified as stage II, and those classified as stage III are those who have local and/or in-transit satellitoses (Fig. 25-7). The ten-year survival of the 202 patients in clinical stage I was 55%, which was changed to 66% after elective groin dissection revealed occult metastases in 35 patients,

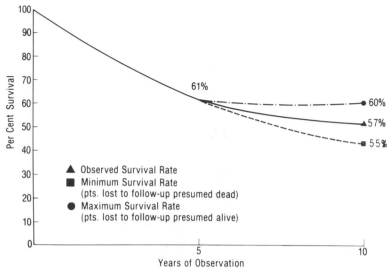

CHART 25-1. Survival of patients with malignant melanoma of the lower extremity.

that for 263 patients in pathologic stage II was 24%, with a precipitous decrease to 4% for the 23 patients in stage III (Table 25-10).

SURVIVAL OF PATIENTS WITH DE NOVO LESIONS

Of 116 patients whose melanomas arose de novo (without a history of a preexisting mole) the ten-year survival was 45.7% (Table 25-11).

Seventy-eight patients gave a history of the duration of the de novo lesion that proved to be a malignant melanoma which varied from less than one month to a period of two years. Those who delayed from one to three months had a survival rate of 61%; and of those who

delayed up to two years, 42% survived an average of ten years. The 33% ten-year survival for those who sought treatment in less than one month cannot be considered significant inasmuch as only three patients were seen who sought early treatment, and of those three only one survived.

THE EFFECT OF DURATION OF PREVIOUS MOLE UPON SURVIVAL

Patients with a history of a previous mole fared better than those whose melanoma appeared de novo 59.9% versus 45.7%. If the mole existed for less than one year (17 patients) the ten-year survival was 47%. Longer periods of the existence of a benign nevus did not seem to alter the prognosis (Table 25-12).

DURATION OF CHANGES IN MOLE VERSUS SURVIVAL

The duration of changes in the mole, such as enlargement, deeper pigmentation, ulceration, and/or pruritis, and its effect upon survival is evaluated (Table 25-13). A better prognosis

TABLE 25-8. 453 Patients with Malignant Melanoma of the Lower Extremity Analyzed According to Sex vs Survival

Sex	Number	10-Year Survivors	
		No.	%
Male	152	64	42
Female	301	193	64

TABLE 25-9. 453 Patients with Malignant Melanoma of the Lower Extremity Analyzed According to Age vs Survival

Age	Number	10-Year Survivors No.	%
0-10 years	1	1	100
11-20	18	15	83
21-30	70	42	60
31-40	106	78	73
41-50	116	50	43
51-60	80	39	49
61-70	43	20	46
71-80	13	3	23
81-90	2	2	100
91 +	0	0	0
Unknown	4	2	50

TABLE 25-10. 453 Patients with Malignant Melanoma of the Lower Extremity Analyzed According to Stage vs Survival*

Stage	Number	10-Year Survivors No.	%
Stage I	167	111	66
Stage II	263	64	24
Stage III	23	1	4

* These values differ from the data in Table 25-2 in that 35 patients listed clinically as stage I revealed occult metastases in the lymph nodes after an elective groin dissection and the classification accordingly changed.

TABLE 25-11. 116 Patients with Malignant Melanoma of the Lower Extremity Analyzed According to Appearance of Lesion De Novo vs Survival*

Time Since Appearance of Lesion De Novo	Number	10-Year Survivors No.	%
Less than 1 month	3	1	33
1-3 months	13	8	61
4-6 months	20	10	50
7-12 months	30	16	53
13-24 months	12	5	42
Unknown duration of de novo lesion	38	13	34
Total	116	53	45.7%

* 337 patients not applicable—history of previous mole.

TABLE 25-12. Duration of Preexisting Mole vs Survival in 337 Patients with Malignant Melanoma of the Lower Extremity*

Duration of Mole	Number	10-Year Survivors No.	%
Less than 1 year	17	8	47
1-5 years	68	45	66
6-10 years	30	19	63
11-20 years	26	18	69
All life	111	74	67
Unknown	85	38	45
Total	337	202	59.9%

* 116 patients not applicable (no history of mole).

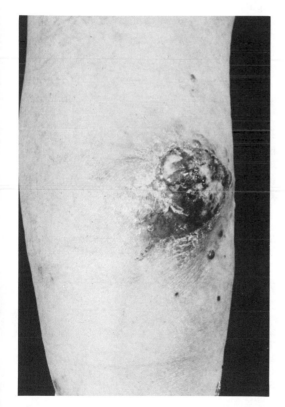

FIGURE 25-7. Fungating ulcerated melanoma of leg. Metastases were present in inguinal lymph nodes.

TABLE 25-13. 231 Patients with Malignant Melanoma of the Lower Extremity Analyzed According to Duration of Changes in Mole vs Survival

Duration of Changes	Number	10-Year Survivors	
		No.	%
Less than 1 month	16	11	69
1-3 months	44	21	48
4-6 months	41	20	49
7-12 months	64	39	61
13-24 months	39	22	56
25-60 months	16	9	56
More than 60 months	11	5	45
Unknown	106	—	—

existed for those patients who sought treatment within one month of the changes in the mole. After one month of delay the period of delay did not seem to affect the overall prognosis significantly.

HISTORY OF TRAUMA TO MOLE VERSUS SURVIVAL

Whether trauma, per se, in any way aggravated a preexisting mole to form a malignant melanoma cannot be stated (Table 25-14). Of 94 patients who claimed that trauma (a severe blow, constant irritation from a girdle, etc.) aggravated the mole, the ten-year survival was 56%. Exposure to sunlight was not considered. The ten-year survival of the 206 patients who gave no history of trauma whatsoever equalled 63%. The data are too meager to warrant any conclusion.

LOCATION OF PRIMARY MELANOMA VERSUS SURVIVAL

The best results were obtained for the 196 patients whose melanomas were located on the leg (between the knee and the foot) whose ten-year survival equalled 64% (Table 25-15). Patients with melanomas of the dorsum of the foot had an almost similar survival (57%),

TABLE 25-14. 300 Patients with Malignant Melanoma of the Lower Extremity Analyzed According to History of Trauma to Mole vs Survival*

Trauma	Number	10-Year Survivors	
		No.	%
History of trauma	94	53	56
No history of trauma	206	130	63
Unknown	37	16	43

* 116 patients not applicable (no history of mole).

which decreased to 43% when the sole of the foot was the primary site (Figs. 25-8 and 25-9), and to 36% when the digits were involved (Fig. 25-10), with the exception of the subungual melanomas, which exhibited a slightly better ten-year survival (42%). The 104 patients with melanoma of the thigh manifested a ten-year survival rate of 59%.

THE INFLUENCE OF PIGMENTATION UPON SURVIVAL

Four-hundred-thirty-eight patients presented pigmented lesions varying from pale brown to deep black. Of this group, 276 (63%) survived the ten-year span (Table 25-16). Fifteen patients were described as having amelanotic lesions, of whom four (27%) survived

TABLE 25-15. 453 Patients with Malignant Melanoma of the Lower Extremity Analyzed According to Site of Primary Tumor vs Survival

Site of Tumor	Number	10-Year Survivors	
		No.	%
Thigh	104	61	59
Leg	196	126	64
Dorsum of foot	37	21	57
Sole of foot	60	26	43
Digits	22	8	36
Subungual	26	11	42
Unknown	8	4	50

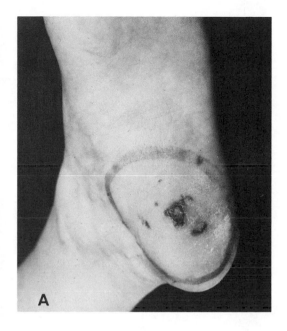

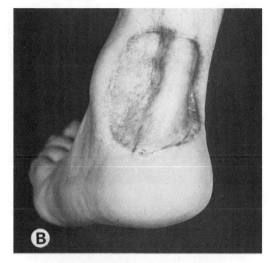

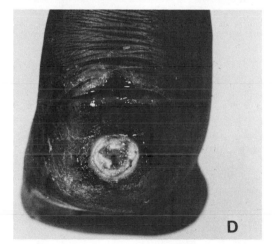

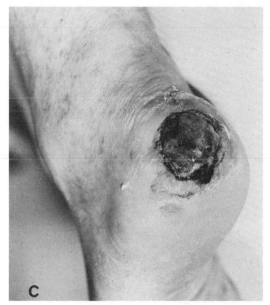

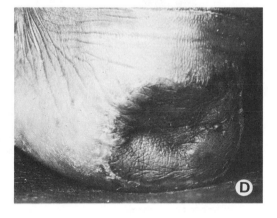

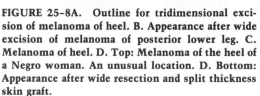

FIGURE 25-8A. Outline for tridimensional excision of melanoma of heel. B. Appearance after wide excision of melanoma of posterior lower leg. C. Melanoma of heel. D. Top: Melanoma of the heel of a Negro woman. An unusual location. D. Bottom: Appearance after wide resection and split thickness skin graft.

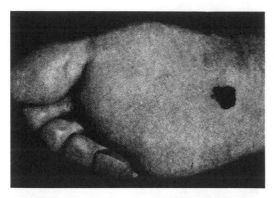

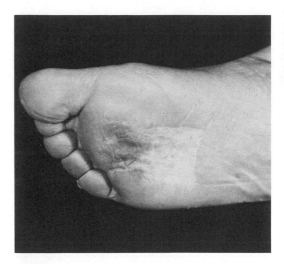

FIGURE 25-9. Left: Infiltrating melanoma of foot. Right: Appearance after excision of plantar melanoma and closure with split-thickness skin graft.

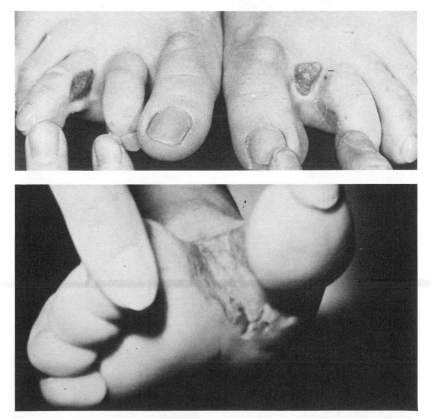

FIGURE 25-10.   Top: Papillary interdigital nevi of both feet in a young female. Bottom: Interdigital malignant melanoma of foot treated by wide excision and split-thickness skin graft. Appearance after treatment.

the ten-year span. Ten of the 15 patients with amelanotic lesions were stage II, four were stage I, and one was stage III.

THE INFLUENCE OF SIZE OF PRIMARY MELANOMA UPON SURVIVAL

Those patients with lesions of 1 cm or less had a ten-year survival of 80%, which decreased to 65% for lesions of 1 to 2 cm, and further decreased to 37% for lesions between 2 to 3 cm in size (Table 25–17). The few patients with lesions between 3 to 4 cm showed a 60% survival, which is statistically insignificant because of the small numbers. Those with lesions larger than 4 cm of which there were ten, showed only one survivor at the ten-year period.

SURFACE OF THE PRIMARY LESION VERSUS SURVIVAL

Of the 114 patients with flat, macular lesions, 70% survived the ten-year period, which decreased to 40% for the 160 patients who had elevated, lesions with smooth surface (Fig. 25–11). If the surface was ulcerated, and/or encrusted, the ten-year survival decreased to 30% (Fig. 25–12). In 40 patients with a history of bleeding, the survival rate was 20%, showing the pernicious effect of an ulcerative, bleeding lesion upon a patient with malignant melanoma (Table 25–18).

HISTOLOGIC CLASSIFICATION VERSUS SURVIVAL

Of 22 patients with superficial, spreading melanoma, the ten-year survival was 86%; of 401 patients with infiltrating melanomas, the ten-year survival rate was 55% (Fig. 25–13); the five patients with juvenile, or previously designated prepubertal melanomas had a survival rate of 80% (Table 25–19). The relationship of the classification to Clark's level of

TABLE 25–16. 453 Patients with Malignant Melanoma of the Lower Extremity Analyzed According to Color of Primary Lesion vs Survival

Color of Lesion	Number	10-Year Survivors	
		No.	%
Amelanotic	15	4	27
Pigmented	438	276	63

invasion and Breslow's thickness criteria are explained in the discussion.

The surgical management of 202 patients with clinical stage I melanoma is analyzed according to the surgical treatment of the lymph nodes in the groin (Fig. 25–14). In 102 patients an elective groin dissection was performed when there was no clinical evidence of metastases to the groin. Metastases to the groin were found in 35 (34%) of these patients (Fig. 25–15), and their ten-year survival rate was 49%. No metastases to the groin were revealed in 67 patients, and this group enjoyed a ten-year survival rate of 73%. In 59 patients who did not have an elective groin dissection, no nodes developed in the groin during the ten years of observation; these patients enjoyed a survival rate of 71%. Forty-one patients developed metastases to the nodes after treatment of the primary neoplasm without lymph node dissection, and their ten-year survival rate equalled 32%.

TABLE 25–17. 411 Patients with Malignant Melanoma of the Lower Extremity Analyzed According to Size of Primary Lesion vs Survival

Size of Lesion	Number	10-Year Survivors	
		No.	%
Less than 1 cm	122	98	80
1–2 cm	153	100	65
2.1–3 cm	121	45	37
3.1–4 cm	5	3	60
4.1–6 cm	9	1	11
More than 6 cm	1	0	—
No description	42	—	—

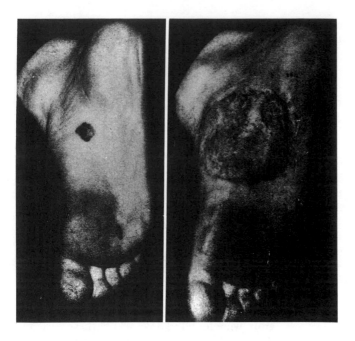

FIGURE 25–11. Melanoma of foot treated by wide excision and skin graft. (Reproduced from Booher RJ, Pack GT: Malignant melanoma of the feet and hands. Surgery 42:1084–1121, 1957, with permission of author and publisher.)

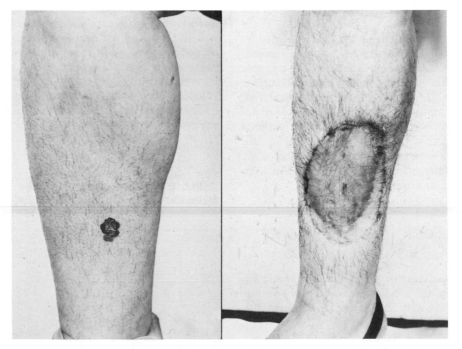

FIGURE 25–12. Left: Female, 37 years, noticed small pigmented mole on right leg for several years which grew the past three years and drained serous fluid. Right: Wound four months after closure with a large split-thickness graft. The patient is cured after ten years.

TABLE 25–18. 427 Patients with Malignant Melanoma of the Lower Extremity Analyzed According to Primary Lesion Surface vs Survival*

| Surface of Lesion | Number | 10-Year Survivors | |
		No.	%
Flat	114	80	70
Elevated	160	64	40
Ulcerated surface	153	46	30
No description	26		

* Satellitosis was seen in 26 patients: 5 survived 5 years (19%) and only 1 survived 10 years.

TABLE 25–20. Patients with Malignant Melanoma of the Lower Extremity Analyzed According to Postoperative Complications Following Surgery

Complications	Number	Percent
No complications	300	72
Edema subsequent to groin dissection	56	13
Wound infection	27	6
Skin graft failure	12	3
Flap necrosis	10	2.4
Total	414	100.0%

The fact that 41% of the patients with melanoma of the lower extremities, in whom no groin dissection was performed, did develop metastases, is significant, and the survival rate for this group was lower than when an elective dissection was performed, 32% vs 49%.

POSTOPERATIVE COMPLICATIONS

No significant complications were manifested in 300 patients. However, 56 patients (13%) demonstrated postoperative edema of a significant degree after the groin dissection; wound infections were observed in 6%; in 3% the skin graft failed to take (Table 25–20). Flap necrosis occurred in 2.4% of the patients dur-

TABLE 25–19. 428 Patients with Malignant Melanoma of the Lower Extremity Analyzed According to Histology of Lesion vs Survival

| Histology | Number | 10-Year Survivors | |
		No.	%
Superficial*	22	19	86
Infiltrating*	401	220	55
Juvenile	5	4	80
Unknown	25	—	—

* The superficial spreading melanomas represent Clark's level II (possibly his level III). The infiltrating melanomas are his levels IV and V. The unavailability of the slides precluded further subdivision.

ing the early periods of this investigation, but it was discovered that the excision of an eclipse of skin in the performance of a groin dissection prevented this complication. The charts did not contain sufficient data in 29 patients to warrant a conclusion.

TREATMENT OF RECURRENT MELANOMA

The survival of patients who developed recurrence after treatment by us is summarized in Table 25–21, and their five-year survival rates are noted because of the overall unsatisfactory results (Figs. 25–16, 25–17, 25–18). The significant survival rates of patients with a simple local recurrence, or with an in-transit recurrence, are noteworthy.

DISCUSSION

LOCATION

Of 3,305 melanomas treated by the surgeons of the Pack Medical Group, New York City, melanomas of the lower extremity were third in frequency, exceeded by melanomas of the trunk, of which there were 1,122 (33.9% of the total), and melanomas of the head and neck, of which there were 772 patients (23% of the total). Malignant melanomas of the

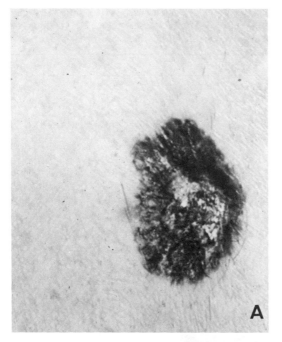

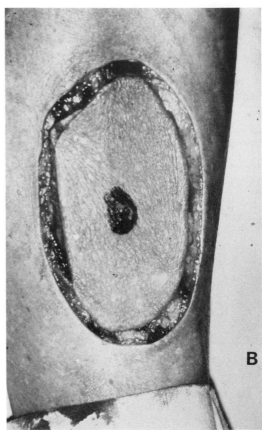

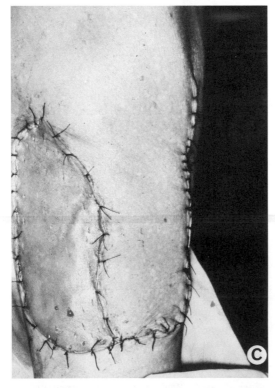

FIGURE 25–13A. Deeply infiltrating melanoma lower leg. B. Outline of wide tridimensional resection. C. Repair by transposed skin flap. Six weeks later, intra-arterial perfusion of phenylalanine mustard followed by radical groin dissection. Patient well, ten years later.

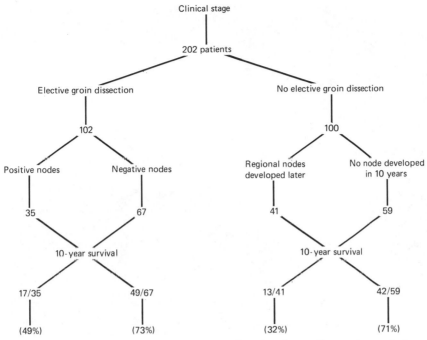

FIGURE 25-14. Shown here is the ten-year survival analyzed according to the surgical management of the groin lymph nodes of patients with clinical stage I melanoma.

TABLE 25-21. 198 Patients with Malignant Melanoma of the Lower Extremity Analyzed According to Type of Recurrent Disease vs Survival*

Type of Recurrence	Number	5-Year Survivors No.	%
Local recurrence only	27	10	37
Local recurrence & regional nodes	16	3	19
In-transit recurrence	9	5	55
Regional nodes developed	61	18	29
Regional nodes recurred	6	1	17
Local, regional, & distant metastases	16	0	—
Distant metastases	59	1	2
Local & in-transit recurrence	4	1	25

* 255 patients not applicable—no recurrent disease, or stage II or III at consult.

lower extremity, of which there were 673, comprised 20.4% of the entire group. This value is not unlike that reported by Knutson, Hori, and Spratt of the Ellis Fischel Hospital in Missouri, where they studied 230 malignant melanomas, and 68 (29.6%) arose from the lower extremity, exceeded only by those arising in the head and neck, of which there were 80 (34.8%).[15]

Knut Magnus, in a detailed study from Norway in 1977, analyzed 2,956 new cases between 1953 and 1971, and found the trunk to have the highest frequency of primary melanomas (177 patients; 40%) and the lower limb to be second (840 patients; 28%). Head and neck primaries comprised 20% of the total series, and the upper limb 11%.[19]

Das Gupta[9] reported from the Abraham Lincoln School of Medicine, Chicago, 269 patients of whom 94 (35%) presented primary melanomas involving the lower extremity.

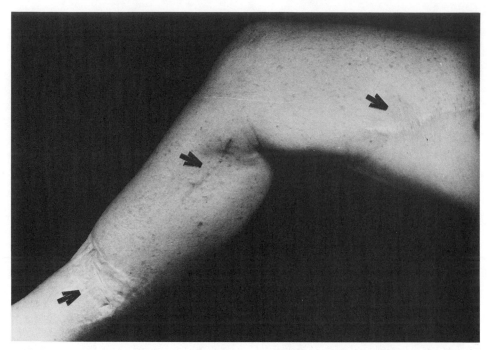

FIGURE 25-15. Infiltrating melanoma of ankle region treated by wide tridimensional resection and split-thickness skin graft and extended radical groin dissection for metastases to the lymph nodes. Four years later she developed an in-transit metastases between the site of the primary melanoma and the lower limit of the extended groin dissection. The illustration shows the site of primary melanoma (lower arrow), the lower extent of extended groin dissection, and the site of in-transit melanoma metastases in tissues at risk (upper arrows).

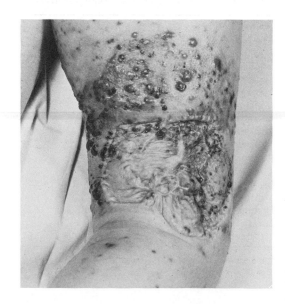

FIGURE 25-16. Extensive metastatic satellitoses after incomplete excision of the primary lesion, despite the apparently wide dissection.

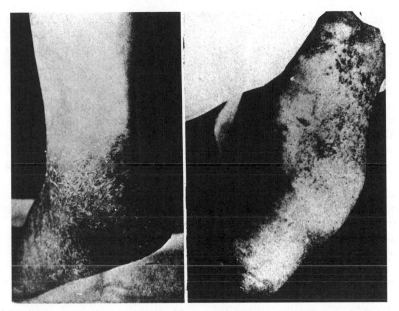

FIGURE 25–17.   Left: Recurrent melanoma of heel after incomplete local excision (elsewhere). Treated by below-knee amputation and groin dissection. Right: Extensive retrograde lymphatic metastases in the edematous stump occurred six months later.

Haagensen et al.[14] reported 98 patients with melanoma of the lower extremity seen at Presbyterian Hospital, New York City. At the same time 46 melanomas of the upper extremity and 103 melanomas of the trunk were treated.

Certain authors cite the lower extremities as the most frequent primary site, varying from one-fourth to one-third of all melanomas observed.[4,5]

At the Ninth International Pigment Cell Conference in 1975, Lee made the following statement:

There seems no doubt that the changes observed in hospital registry and mortality experience are the result of a genuine and large rise in the incidence of malignant melanoma. The sites showing the greatest changes are trunk in males and lower limb in females. The explanation of these changes must come from orderly clinical observations of cases and control subjects.[17]

The legs of women, a subject of much discussion at various levels, have shown a

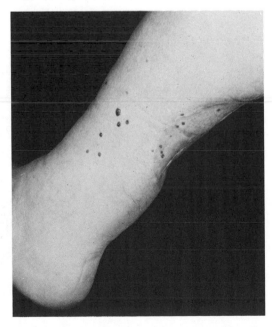

FIGURE 25–18.   Regional metastases after incomplete excision.

higher incidence of melanoma than those of men. McLeod et al. believed this to be due to the higher exposure of the skin of the legs to sunlight.[20] An interesting observation was promulgated by Bodenham[5] who attributed the sharp rise of malignant melanoma of the legs of women after the Second World War to the fact that sheer nylon stockings permitted more of the sun's ultraviolet light to reach the skin than the prewar stockings, which, although slightly less appealing, were far more protective.

In our series, the thigh and leg were the most frequent locations of the melanoma of the lower extremities, comprising 72% of the total group. There were 59 melanomas of the sole of the foot, a site singularly deficient of melanocytes. Thirty-two melanomas were subungual, but these will be considered in detail in another presentation.

Light-complexioned Caucasians comprised most of the patients harboring melanoma of the lower extremities. It is estimated that this ethnic group comprises about 11% of the population about New York, but their susceptibility to melanoma is evident by the fact that most of our patients were of this complexion. Five Negroes presented melanoma in the unpigmented regions of their feet (the soles). This feature has been noted repeatedly throughout the world.

A family history was recorded for only 4% of our group where the history was available. A familial relationship has been observed by Anderson[2] who reported 74 pedigrees with a familial history of melanoma, and believes the genetic aspects are very complicated.[2] Sutherland[29] reported 18 families in Louisiana of 1,050 patients with a familial relationship of melanoma but with a most complicated genetic explanation.[29]

RESULTS

Of the 673 patients observed, 453 patients are critically evaluated as these were the patients treated by us and followed for a minimum of ten years (Fig. 25–19). Ninety patients presented themselves for consultation only, and 130 patients were referred with disseminated melanoma and received only

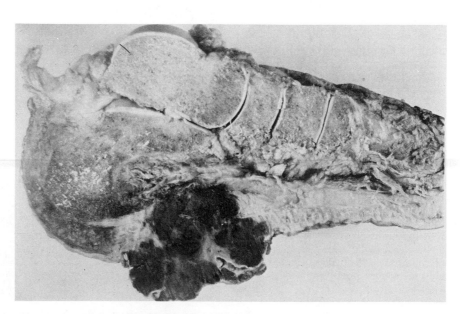

FIGURE 25–19. Malignant melanoma of the foot after amputation and dissection. Note the deep infiltration of the melanoma, demonstrating the futility of a local excision.

palliative treatment, usually with unsatisfactory results. Of the 453 patients, 20 were lost to follow-up within the ten-year period, and all of these patients are presumed dead. The absolute ten-year survival rate is 55.2%. Of the 453 patients treated and followed for a minimum of ten years, 250 were alive and well at the end of the ten-year period.

In calculating the relative ten-year results, i.e. subtracting the 20 patients lost to follow-up, the total number of patients treated and followed would be 433 patients. Of these, 95 were listed as dying from causes other than melanoma before the ten-year span, thus leaving a figure of 338 patients available for evaluation ten years after receiving treatment for malignant melanoma. Of the 338 patients, 250 are alive and well, giving a relative survival of 74%. We do not approve of this method of reporting as it does not list the total experience. Chart 25–1 presents the observed, the minimum, and the maximum survival rates, evaluating the data with different determinations.

STAGING

The staging recorded by us consists of stage I, where the melanoma is limited to the site of origin without evidence of metastases, stage II, where metastases are present in the regional lymph nodes, stage III, where there is evidence of regional spread (i.e. in-transit metastases combined with metastases to lymph nodes), and stage IV, where there is disseminated blood-borne metastases. Our data present pathologic stage II, III, and IV. In order to evaluate the reliability of clinical staging, our stage I was originally clinical staging, which was in error in 34% of the patients, as determined by discovery of metastases to lymph nodes as a result of elective groin dissection; the staging accordingly changed. An approximate 8% error occurred in noting palpable lymph nodes as metastases that proved to be lymphadenitis. Lymphography was not found useful for diagnosing metastases in doubtful cases. Pathological staging describes the presence or absence of metastases on histologic examination of the resected specimen.

Two hundred and two patients were clinically classified stage I, which changed to 167 patients after elective groin dissection demonstrated metastases to the lymph nodes in 35 patients. There were 263 patients classified stage II on histologic evidence, and there were 23 patients in stage III (5%). Stage IV indicates distant dissemination of the metastases, but this category is not included in this discussion inasmuch as the 130 patients referred received only palliative therapy without noteworthy results regarding longevity.

RELATIONSHIP OF BENIGN MOLES UNDERGOING MALIGNANT TRANSFORMATION

The relationship of a benign mole undergoing malignant transformation has been a rather controversial question. There were 337 of our patients who complained of a preexisting mole, and the remaining 166 gave a history of the melanoma appearing de novo. It was sometimes difficult to determine from the history which melanomas arose de novo, especially after they had been present for a prolonged period, and to differentiate those from the history given by a patient of a mole having been present for a relatively short time that proved to be a malignant melanoma. There were 94 patients who reported that some form of trauma, such as irritation from a garter belt, or repeated physical trauma, preceded the onset of changes that led to excision of the melanoma. It is not possible from the data on hand to attribute any malignant transformation to trauma, per se. Other forms of trauma such as electrolysis, irradiation, caustic pastes, endocrine factors such as pregnancy or endocrine abnormalities such as xeroderma pigmentosa, were not elicited from our patients.

Sunlight has been considered a carcinogen or cocarcinogen in the production of melanomas. Inasmuch as many of these patients had their limbs exposed to sunlight, this could be a factor, although our data do not warrant any conclusions.

TREATMENT OF MELANOMA OF THE LOWER EXTREMITY

It is agreed that surgical resection is the best method of treating malignant melanoma. The recent classifications by Clark, and independently by Breslow, have added some objective boundaries that help determine the extent of surgery that should be accomplished. All agree that a wide resection of the primary melanoma is indicated after the histologic diagnosis has been confirmed by a competent pathologist skilled in the pathology of malignant melanoma. All are further agreed that if metastases are evident in the inguinal region, a groin dissection should be performed.

Controversy exists as to whether an elective groin dissection should be performed, i.e. a groin dissection in the absence of clinical palpable lymph nodes. Subfactors in this decision are questions as to whether the groin dissection should be a superficial groin dissection that includes the femoral and inguinal lymph nodes, or whether it should be a radical groin dissection that extends into the retroperitoneal space and would include Cloquet's node, the iliac nodes, and the obturator lymph nodes. In addition, there is no unanimity of opinion as to whether a discontinuous groin dissection is in any way inferior to one done in continuity. Our data attempt to answer some of these questions (Fig. 25–20).

It has been the policy of the surgeons of our group to perform a radical groin dissection wherever possible. In the past, before the histologic criteria predicting prognosis was available, this was performed on most patients.

Of the 453 determinate patients, 203 patients are dead of their melanomas. (This includes 20 patients lost to follow-up and considered dead of melanoma. It also includes patients whose death certificates attributed death to other causes inasmuch as one can never be absolutely certain that the melanoma was not present and did not contribute to the death. There were 250 patients (55.2%) alive and apparently free of melanoma for ten years or longer. The need for tabulating end results for malignant melanoma at the ten-year period

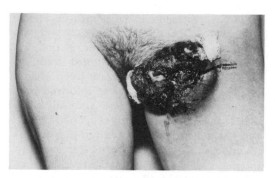

FIGURE 25–20. Exfoliating, ulcerated, infected metastases from a primary melanoma of the foot. An elective groin dissection might have prevented the dissemination. Excision of metastases when they present clinically could avoid the exophytic, ominous, clinically intolerable consequences. Palliative hemipelvectomy performed.

is emphasized by the fact that 22 patients who succumbed (11%) died between the five- and ten-year period. This value is similar to that of Haagensen et al. who state that 53 of their 98 patients survived for five years after treatment, but eight of the 53 died of melanoma after the five-year period. Others have commented also on the futility of considering a patient cured after five years, inasmuch as delayed evidence of recurrences or metastases frequently occur after the five-year span, and for that matter, many years after primary treatment. One of our patients whose melanoma of the ankle was removed remained asymptomatic for 27 years after treatment before regional and hematogenic spread occurred.

SURVIVAL OF DE NOVO MELANOMAS COMPARED WITH MELANOMAS ARISING FROM PREEXISTING NEVI

It is difficult sometimes to determine which melanomas arose de novo, especially when the patient stated that the melanoma had been present for a prolonged period, and which arose from a preexisting nevus, especially if the nevus had been observed for a relatively short period within one year. Histories as obtained from patients revealed that 116 patients believed their melanomas arose de novo; these patients had a ten-year survival rate of 45.7%. It further appeared that the delay after the observation of the nevus seemed to exert a detrimental effect upon survival. A 47% ten-year survival was obtained for the 17 patients whose mole existed less than a year. Those who delayed for less than one month had a ten-year survival rate of 61%, and those who delayed up to two years had a ten-year survival rate of 42%. For those with a previous mole that existed less than a year, the ten-year survival rate equalled 47%. Longer existence of the benign nevus did not seem to alter the prognosis. However, when changes occurred in the mole, there was a better prognosis for those who sought treatment within one month after changes occurred. Our data do not permit any conclusive evidence regarding the effects of trauma, such as constant irritation, upon the survival rate.

Pack believed that all melanomas arise from benign moles, often invisible to the naked eye.[24]

Five of our patients had multiple primary melanomas, which did not seem to affect prognosis.[6]

THE EFFECT OF LOCATION OF PRIMARY UPON SURVIVAL

The location of the primary melanoma did exert an effect upon survival, and the best survival obtained for ten years was for the 196 patients with melanoma located on the leg between the knee and the foot, who manifested a ten-year survival of 64%. The 104 patients with melanoma of the thigh had a ten-year survival rate of 59% (61/104). Those with melanomas of the foot and digits showed a lower ten-year survival rate, varying from 36% to 57% (Table 25–15).

THE EFFECT OF PIGMENTATION UPON SURVIVAL

The effects of pigmentation upon survival reveal a 27% ten-year survival rate for 15 pa-

tients having amelanotic melanomas, demonstrating that the amelanotic melanomas have a somewhat poorer survival rate. This is in accord with the study of Shah, from Memorial Hospital in New York, who also demonstrated a poorer survival for patients with amelanotic melanomas from various sites.[27] His five-year survival for patients with stage I amelanotic melanoma was 71%, which compares with that for patients with pigmented melanoma. However, for patients in stage II the five-year survival was 15%, in contrast to 42% five-year survival for stage II patient with pigmented melanomas.

INFLUENCE OF SIZE OF PRIMARY MELANOMA UPON SURVIVAL

The smaller the lesion, as a rule, the better the prognosis. Those patients with 1 cm lesions or less had a ten-year survival rate of 80%, which decreased to 65% for those with lesions of 1 to 2 cm. None of those with lesions over 4 cm, of which there were ten, survived after ten years.

SURFACE OF THE MELANOMA AND ITS EFFECT UPON SURVIVAL

The nature of the surface of the melanoma affected survival. The 114 patients with flat macular lesions manifested a ten-year survival rate of 70%, which decreased to 40% for 160 patients with elevated nodular lesions and smooth surfaces. If the surfaces were encrusted, the ten-year survival rate decreased to 30%, and of 40 patients with a history of bleeding the survival rate was 20%.

HISTOLOGIC CLASSIFICATION AND ITS EFFECT UPON SURVIVAL

The histologic classification determining the superficial spreading and the infiltrating lesions showed that of 22 patients with superficial spreading melanomas the ten-year survival rate was 86%, and for the 401 patients with infiltrating melanomas the survival rate was 55%.

In this retrospective study we do not include Clark's level I; which we do not consider a metastasizing malignant melanoma. Those authors who do include this category could beneficially influence the end results. Our superficial melanomas are usually Clark's level II and possibly III. His level III category does not seem to be a distinct entity, but rather a quantitative determination. Our infiltrating melanomas are Clark's level IV and V. The slides were not available to subdivide these levels nor to determine the thickness as described by Breslow.

Our data indicate that of 263 patients with metastases to the groin, in whom a radical groin dissection was performed, that 64 patients (24%) survived.

Haagensen et al.[14] reported 17 patients on whom a therapeutic groin dissection was performed, of whom 13 manifested metastases to the groin and 8% survived a ten-year period.

Our data indicate that of 202 patients who did not have clinical evidence of metastases to the groin, an elective groin dissection was performed in 102 and metastases to lymph nodes were found in 35 (34%). There were 67 patients who did not manifest any metastases. Of the 35 with occult metastases discovered at the time of operation, 17 (49%) survived ten years. In 100 patients no elective groin dissection was performed, and 41 of these patients later developed metastases to the lymph nodes, and 13 of these (32%) survived the ten-year period. The difference between the 49% ten-year survival of patients in whom micrometastases were discovered during an elective procedure, in contrast to the 32% ten-year survival for the 41 patients whose therapeutic groin dissection was performed after nodes became clinically evident, prove the advisability of the elective groin dissection in this series.

Haagensen et al. reported 98 patients of whom 69 had an elective groin dissection. Metastases were found in the nodes of 15 of these patients (22%). The five-year survival rate of these 15 patients was 47%. They stated: "Our series of cases of melanoma of the lower extremity provide solid evidence of the value of lymph node dissection, not only prophylactically, but also in patients who have involved but not necessarily enlarged inguinal nodes on admission."

Mundth et al.[23] reported 83 patients on whom an elective groin dissection was performed. Metastases to the inguinal nodes were present in 52, and 25% of these patients survived five years or longer.

Magnus show an age-standardized five-year relative survival rate for localized cases of malignant melanoma of the skin, in Norway: For the lower limb exclusive of the foot the males showed a 60% five-year survival and the females 80%; for the foot, the males showed 58% and the females 75%.[19]

In a study performed by the W.H.O. melanoma group[31] to evaluate the efficacy of elective lymph node dissection a combined randomized prospective therapeutic trial was conducted from September, 1967 to January, 1974, involving 17 cancer institutes in 12 countries, which included three from the USSR, two from Italy, three from Poland, and one each from Holland, Brazil, Peru, France, Belgium, Norway, Bulgaria, Czechoslovakia, and Hungary. This ambitious effort to determine the efficacy of immediate node dissection for stage I melanomas of the limb is commendable. It is regrettable, however, that more representative cancer institutes from the western hemisphere were not included, inasmuch as the possibility exists that different populations may harbor melanomas that behave differently from an immunologic standpoint. For example, the largest percentage of melanomas seen in the Queensland melanoma project in Australia is by far the superficial spreading melanoma, whereas the vast majority of melanomas seen by the Pack Medical Group were infiltrating melanomas.

Furthermore, they limited their selection of cases for lower limb melanomas to include only those that originated below the horizontal line dividing the second third from the distal third of the thigh, and the upper limb melanomas into the distal half of the arm and in the forearm and hand. No mention was made as to whether subungual melanomas were included.

Evaluation was performed with randomization being conducted within each of the hospitals, and the pathologic material critically reviewed by expert pathologists well-versed in the study of malignant melanomas. The survivals, according to Clark's levels, were evaluated for levels III and IV only, because cases classified as level I, II, or V were too few (12 cases for level I and II, and 22 for level V). The conclusion was that the actuarial survival rates for levels III and IV were comparable between the two treatment groups. They further conclude that with Breslow's measurements of thickness, immediate lymph node dissection did not achieve better results than dissection "on request." Their conclusion is that:

> In Stage I melanoma of the limbs, delayed dissection of lymph nodes, i.e., performed at the time of the appearance of regional metastases, is as effective in the control of disease as immediate dissection. Since the proportion of positive nodes ranged from 20% to 25%, the wait-and-see policy avoids unnecessary postoperative complications in three quarters of the patients for whom 'prophylactic' dissection would result in negative histologic findings in regional nodes. Delayed dissection is advisable as long as the patient can be kept under strict clinical control.

They make no attempt to determine the results of those melanomas of the lower limb subjacent to the lymph-node-bearing region. Of their patients treated with elective lymph node dissection, 19.7% demonstrated occult metastases, whereas in our series of melanomas of the lower extremity, 76 of 202 patients in clinical stage I had occult metastases. (Of 102 patients, 35 had occult metastases discovered after an elective groin dissection, and 41 of 100 patients in whom no dissection was performed developed metastases to the nodes later.) In their series, 24.2% with excision of the primary melanoma alone

had regional lymph nodes develop, contrast to our series where 46% developed metastases when no elective groin dissection was performed.

Their study evaluates the five-year results, and our data demonstrate an approximate 10% demise from melanoma between the fifth and tenth year. (At the International Union Against Cancer meeting in Buenos Aires in November, 1978, Dr. Veronesi commented that the ten-year results are similar to the published five-year end results.)

This laudable study should be continued as it might reveal certain subtle causes for the unpredictable behavior of melanomas.

Goldsmith, Shah, and Kim[11] analyzed records of 1,552 patients seen at Memorial Hospital from January 1, 1950 to January 15, 1965. Of this group, 707 patients were placed in clinical stage I, and 537 in clinical stage II. Of the entire group where no metastases were discerned, the five-year survival rate in stage I was 85% (208/246). Fifty patients originally classified as clinical stage I were found to harbor microscopic evidence of malignant melanoma in their exicised lymph nodes. This group was then placed in pathological stage II with a five-year survival rate of 48% (25/50).

These authors state that the five-year survival rate should not be considered the true index of control of the disease, as progressive mortality from melanoma occurs over the years. The ratio of survival rates between pathologic stage I and stage II at the five-year level is approximately 2 to 1 (80%: 39%). At 15 years the ratio between these two groups changes to approximately 3 to 1 (53%: 15%).

Microscopic foci of melanoma were found in their clinical stage I in 48% of the patients (24/50), and of patients who did not have an elective node dissection 52% (43/83) later developed metastases. They further state, "Though these two groups are dissimilar in size, their survival rates are comparable and would raise the question for justification of a routine lymph node dissection."

There was a 10% variation in the overall survival rates in clinical stage I patients who had lymph node dissection (78%; 232/296) as compared with those who did not (68%; 280/411). They believe that the 10% improvement in survival in a large series of patients is a significant figure and should not be minimized.

They further state that if one elects not to perform a lymph node dissection for nonpalpable lymph nodes, one must accept the fact that a sizable proportion of the patients of this group will have histologic foci of melanoma in their retained lymph nodes; in their series, 17% (50/296). They state:

> Electing to permit one out of every five or six patients to retain lymph nodes that harbor microscopic melanoma is a decision that is difficult to justify.

Among the 411 patients who did not have a routine lymph node dissection for clinically negative lymph nodes, 82 developed local recurrences of their melanomas, and although they did not develop palpable nodes at the time of the local recurrence, 35 underwent a routine lymph node dissection in addition to the wide excision of their recurrent melanoma. Of these 35 patients, nine (26%) were found to have microscopic evidence of melanoma in their excised lymph nodes. Goldsmith et al. conclude that this factor indicates that if a melanoma recurs locally, the chances of finding microscopic melanoma in the nonpalpable lymph nodes are increased. They further found a lower incidence of recurrent disease in patients treated by routine lymph node dissection for palpable regional nodes. Recurrent melanoma was developed by 52% (212/411) of patients not subjected to routine lymph node dissection, as opposed to only 19% (54/296) of patients subjected to a routine lymph node dissection.

It was also observed by these authors that patients who went from clinical stage I directly to stage IV due to blood-borne metastases were comparable regardless of whether a lymph node dissection was or was not performed (10% vs 12%).

Goldsmith, Shah, and Kim conclude:

The findings of this study have permitted us to conclude that the best form of treatment for patients with malignant melanoma is a wide excision of the primary lesion in association with a routine lymph node dissection, regardless of the clinical stages of the lymph node.

From 1949 through December, 1971, more than 800 patients with melanoma were reported by Gumport and Harris in 1974, and 306 regional lymph node dissections were performed.[12] Only 10% of the patients were alive and well five or more years after their lymphadenectomy when they were clinically and microscopically involved by metastases. The authors believe that this supports the impression that there is a hazard in waiting for these nodes to become grossly positive before removing them.

Gumport and Meyer in 1959 reviewed 126 cases treated over five years ago at the New York University Medical Center, and concluded that the best results were obtained when an elective lymph node dissection was performed in addition to a wide and deep excision of the primary site of the lesion.[13]

Lane, Lattes, and Malm, in 1958, reported from the Presbyterian Hospital in New York that 42% of the patients were found to have metastases to the lymph nodes after a so-called "prophylactic lymph node dissection."[16] Serial sections were performed and give a far more accurate evaluation than when randomized specimens are performed.

Wanebo, Woodruff, and Fortner,[32] in their recent report from Memorial Hospital, New York, regarding the level of invasion of the primary melanoma and the evidence of metastases to the lymph nodes, propose drawing the following conclusions:

1. A correlation exists between the measured mean depth of invasion of primary melanoma and Clark's level; combining these two techniques offers greater prognostic information than using either alone. Microstaging by depth of invasion shows a much higher correlation to clinical course than that found by histologic typing of primary tumors as nodular

melanoma or superficial spreading melanoma.

2. There is a correlation between the depth of invasion by Clark's levels and the incidence of lymph node metastases in patients with stage I melanoma who have elective node dissection. The incidence of nodal metastases is 4% for level II, 7% for level III, 25% for level IV, and 70% for level V.

3. There is a correlation between Clark's level of invasion and survival after surgery. The five-year cure rate was 100% for level II, 88% for level III, 66% for level IV, and 15% for level V.

4. The presence of nodal metastases augurs a much worse prognosis than Clark's level per se. In patients with level IV melanomas, the five-year cure rate was 82% in patients with negative lymph nodes, and 27% in those with nodal metastases following elective node dissection.

5. Use of the measured depth of invasion provides significant clinicopathologic information regarding the incidence of nodal metastases at elective node dissection and survival. The incidence of nodal metastases at elective node dissection was 5% to 9% for primary melanoma showing 0.6 to 2.0 mm of invasion, 22% for melanoma measuring 2.1 to 3.0 mm, and 39% for melanomas invading beyond 3.0 mm. The five-year cure rate was 100% for melanoma measuring 1.0 mm or less (one patient died at 71 months from a melanoma invading 0.6 mm), 83% for melanoma invading 1.1 to 2.0 mm, 58% for lesions mesuring 2.1 to 3.0 mm, and 55% for melanoma invading over 3.0 mm.

6. The measured depth of microinvasion adds prognostic insight to each Clark's level. The minimal invasion at which nodal metastases occurred was 0.6 mm for level II, 0.9 mm at level III, 1.5 mm at level IV, and 4.4 mm at level V. The minimum level of invasion related to five years' failure from disease was 1.1 mm for level III, 1.5 mm for level IV, and over 4 mm for level V.

7. The microstage technique serves as a useful standard with which to compare results of different surgical techniques. In our series of extremity melanomas only, there was no ap-

parent difference between local excision and lymphadenectomy for level II. At level III and level IV melanoma, lymphadenectomy gave higher cure rates than wide excision only at both the five- and nine-year levels after surgery. These results were statistically significant only for patients with level III, however.

8. The microstage technique combining Clark's levels and the measured depth of invasion is useful as a prognostic index and as a standard guide to treatment for primary melanoma of the extremities.

Elias and Didolkar, from the Roswell Park Memorial Institute, evaluated 248 patients who were treated between January 1965 and December, 1969.[10] Of 188 patients, 96 (51%) did not require lymphadenectomy at any time during the course of disease, which indicates that 49% did develop metastases to the lymph nodes. Local recurrences were four times more common in those patients treated by local excision only, but satellitosis was more common in those treated initially by lymphadenectomy. When their survival data were correlated with the level of invasion, there was a strong statistical correlation, and an indication of the significantly poorer prognosis for those patients having Clark's level IV and V compared with those having levels II and III. The level of invasion also correlated with the incidence of metastases to the lymph nodes and the presence of tumor cells in the lymphatics or blood vessels at the site of the primary lesion. In their study, females had a better prognosis. The level of invasion was found to be equally distributed among the males and females.

AMPUTATION FOR MELANOMA OF THE EXTREMITY

McPeak and his colleagues, in 1963, analyzed the results of 54 patients with malignant melanoma of the extremities who were subjected to a major amputation for their malignant melanomas.[21]

Earlier studies at Memorial Hospital by Pack, Gerber, and Scharnagel, from 1917 to 1950, reported 16 patients who had an amputation for melanoma with a 31.2% five-year survival (Fig. 25–20).[25] In the series reported by McPeak et al., 54 patients subjected to amputation had a similar five-year survival rate, namely 33.3% survival rate.[21] There was a preponderance of females: 17 males and 28 females. The average age of all patients was 47 years. They call attention to the fact that the plantar surface of the foot, which comprises a small skin area, was the primary site in 18 of their 46 melanomas of the lower extremity (39%). Metastases to the lymph nodes were present in 12 of the 16 patients cured by major amputation of the lower extremity. Most of the lower extremity amputations were hip-joint disarticulations, 25 in all. Ten patients remained free of disease for over five years. Although there appeared to be little difference in the clinical background of the survivors and the failures, microscopic analysis of the lymph nodes were of definite prognostic value. There were no positive lymph nodes above the femoral area in any of the survivors. Every patient with positive iliac nodes died as a result of a disease.

Thus amputations for extensive malignant melanoma that were considered uncurable by any means except a major amputation showed a significant prolongation of life.

Turnbull, Shah, and Fortner[30] reported 60 patients with recurrent melanoma treated by major amputation between 1950 and 1964. Of these, 12 (21%) were free of cancer an average of 13 years later, including two patients who had forequarter amputations and two others who had hemipelvectomy. Eight of the survivors underwent hip disarticulation. There were three postoperative deaths, one from pulmonary embolism, one from splenic rupture because of metastatic melanoma, and one from sepsis.

These authors state that amputation appears indicated when recurrent disease is extensive, or when regional perfusion or other conservative measures have failed. They feel encouraged that one out of five such desperately ill patients can be salvaged by these radical treatments.

Of the 20 patients treated by hip-joint disarticulation, eight were free of melanoma an average of 11 years (5–20 years). One patient subsequently died of uterine cancer years later.

Of the 24 patients undergoing hemipelvectomy, two were free of disease six and one-half and nine years later, respectively. One of the survivors had metastases to the femoral lymph nodes, one died postoperatively from sepsis, 21 died from widespread melanoma an average of 20 months after amputation. The disease-free interval of those who died ranged from three months to 16 years.

Miller in 1977 reported his experience with 126 hemipelvectomies, of which 18 were for patients suffering from advanced melanoma.[22] Three patients (17.6%) survived five years or longer.

Thus, in advanced cases, major amputation has offered palliation and often prolongation of life. Careful clinical judgment must be exercised in this decision (Fig. 25–21).

SUMMARY AND CONCLUSIONS

Malignant melanomas of the lower extremities comprised 20.4% (673 patients) of the 3,305 melanomas studied by the surgeons of the Pack Medical Group, New York City.

Females comprised 66% of the patients (453 individuals), and males comprised (34%).

The thigh was the most frequent site, comprising 42.3% of the 453 determinate patients; the leg was the second most frequent site comprising 29.7%. Thirty-two patients (4.7%) presented subungual melanomas.

Two hundred and two patients (45%) presented stage I melanomas; 228 patients (50%) were classified histologically as stage II; with 23 patients (5%) being in the stage III classification. If the patient was clinically staged where no histologic date were available, it was changed after elective groin dissection revealed occult metastases. Stages II and III were staged on histologic criteria.

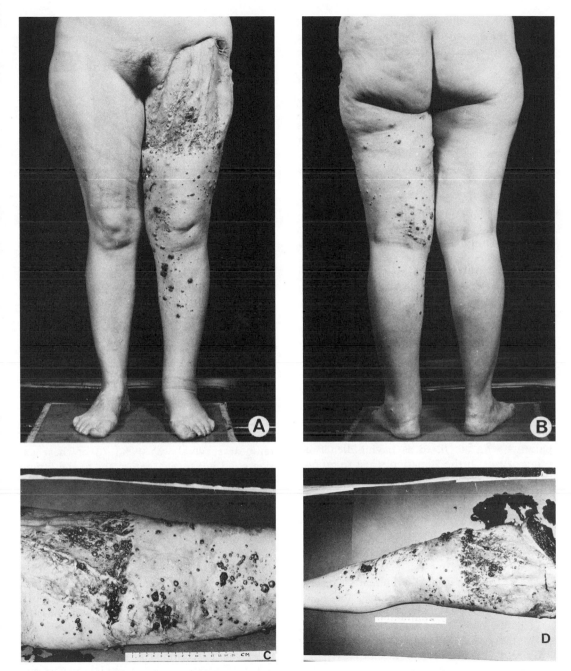

FIGURE 25-21. Retrograde lymphatic spread of extensive melanoma of thigh incompletely excised necessitating a palliative high joint dissection. Patient expired from widespread metastases three years later. A. Anterior view showing site of original excision and skin graft. B. Posterior view showing retrograde spread along course of lymphatics. C. Close-up view demonstrating the nature of the lesion. D. Surgical specimen following hip joint disarticulation.

Twenty patients (4%) revealed a history of other members of the family also suffering from melanoma (not necessarily of the same site).

Patients in the fourth decade were the most numerous, comprising 26% of the total, seconded by those in the 31 to 40 year bracket, comprising 23% of the total. The curve goes steadily downward in both directions, younger and older from these decades.

A preexisting mole was complained of by 337 patients, whereas 116 patients gave a history of a melanoma appearing de novo. Almost 100% of our patients were Caucasians, with light complexion. Only five patients (1%) were Negroid, with their melanomas appearing in nonpigmented regions.

Our treatment policy consisted of a conservative excision of the lesion for paraffin study by a qualified pathologist, and if the diagnosis of malignant melanoma was established, we performed a wide tridimensional resection with the defect covered by skin graft and, where feasible, a radical groin dissection.

The absolute ten-year survival rate of the 453 patients was 55.2% (250 patients). Two hundred and three patients (44.8%) are listed as dead. This value includes the 20 patients lost to follow-up and presumed dead, and 95 patients who are listed as having died from other causes. If the 20 patients lost to follow-up are considered indeterminate, and the 95 patients whose death certificates listed other diseases as the cause of death are not included, then 98 patients would have died of their malignant melanoma of the 338 patients treated and available for analysis. This would provide a relative ten-year survival rate of 74%. We do not favor this method of recording, inasmuch as total experience should be presented.

Females had a markedly better survival (64%) than males (42%). Age did not appear to influence survival except at both extremes (youngest and oldest).

Staging played a most significant part in determining prognoses. In 167 patients classified as stage I the ten-year survival rate was 66%, which dropped precipitously for the 263 patients in stage II to 24%. Of the 23 patients classified as stage III, only one (4%) survived ten years.

Patients with a history of a mole undergoing malignant transformation, of which there were 337, revealed a somewhat better prognosis (59.9% ten-year survival) than did the 116 patients who believed the melanoma arose de novo, of whom 45.7% survived the ten-year span.

The location of the melanoma did seem to affect prognosis significantly. The best results were for the 196 patients with melanoma involving the leg (between the knee and the ankle) who had a 64% ten-year survival. Those of the thigh, of whom there were 104 patients, had a ten-year survival of 59%. The lowest values were those for the sole of the foot (43%), the subungual melanomas (42%), and the digits (36%).

Fifteen patients presented amelanotic melanomas, with a ten-year survival of 27%, in contrast to the 438 patients whose ten-year survival equalled 63%.

The management of the 202 patients with clinical stage I melanomas consisted of an elective groin dissection for 102 patients, which revealed occult metastases to the lymph nodes in 35 of these individuals; their ten-year survival was 49%; 73 of these patients did not reveal metastases to the lymph nodes, and their ten-year survival was 73%. In 100 patients no elective groin dissection was performed, but 41 of these patients did develop metastases to the inguinal lymph nodes at a later date, and their ten-year survival rate was 32%, somewhat lower than the 48% who had positive nodes discovered on elective groin dissection. Although an unnecessary operation was performed on 62% of the patients with clinically negative nodes, the increased survival of the 17% of the patients who did reveal occult metastases would suggest that an elective groin dissection is an indicated procedure in patients with malignant melanomas of the lower extremities, especially those with infiltrating melanomas. All but 7% of the patients in this analysis presented with infiltrating melanomas.

There was an 11% mortality between the fifth and tenth year for patients dying from melanoma. This indicates that the ten-year survival rate should be the period for which end results are tabulated, rather than the five-year period.

REFERENCES

1. Allen AC, Spitz S: Malignant melanomas, a clinicopathologic analysis of the criteria for diagnosis and prognosis. Cancer 6:1–45, 1953
2. Anderson PE: Clinical characteristics of the genetic variety of cutaneous melanoma in man. Cancer 21:721–725, 1971
3. Ariel IM: Tridimensional resection of malignant melanoma. Surg Gynecol Obstet 139:601, 1974
4. Attie JN, Khafif RD: Melanotic tumors. Charles Thomas, Springfield Ill, 1964, p 135
5. Bodenham DC: A study of 650 observed malignant melanomas in the south-west region. Ann R Coll Surg Engl 43:218–239, 1968
6. Booher RJ: Recognition and treatment of melanoma. Surg Clin North Am 49:389–405, 1969
7. Breslow A: Tumor thickness, level of invasion and node dissection in Stage I cutaneous melanoma. Ann Surg 182:572–575, 1975
8. Clark WH Jr, From L, Bernardino EA, Mihm MC: The histogenesis and biologic behavior of primary human malignant melanomas of the skin. Cancer Res 29:705–727, 1969
9. Das Gupta TK: Results of treatment of 269 patients with primary cutaneous melanoma: A five-year prospective study. Ann Surg 186–201, 1977
10. Elias EG, Didolkar NS, Goel IP, et al.: A clinical pathologic study of prognostic factors in cutaneous malignant melanoma. Surg Gynecol Obstet 144:327–334, 1977
11. Goldsmith HS, Shah JP, Kim DD: Prognostic significance of lymph node dissection in the treatment of malignant melanoma. Cancer 26:3, Sept 1970, pp 606–609
12. Gumport SL, Harris MN: Results of regional lymph node dissection for melanoma. Ann Surg 179:105–108, 1974
13. Gumport SL, Meyer HW: Treatment of one hundred and twenty six cases of malignant melanoma: Long term results. Ann Surg 150:989, 1959
14. Haagensen LD, Feind CR, Herter FP, et al.: The Lymphatics in Cancer. Philadelphia, WB Saunders Co, 1972, pp 470–483.
15. Knutson CO, Hori JM, Spratt JS Jr: Melanoma: Current Problems in Surgery. Year Book Medical Publishers, Dec 1971, vol 7, pp 171–172
16. Lane N, Lattes R, Malm J: Clinicopathological correlations in a series of 117 malignant melanomas of the skin of adults. Cancer 11:1025–1043, 1958
17. Lee JAH: The current rapid increase in mortality from malignant melanoma in developed societies. Pig Cell 2:414–420, Karger, Basel, 1976
18. Lee JAH: The trend of mortality from primary malignant tumors of the skin. J Invest Dermatol 59:445–448, 1975
19. Magnus K: Prognosis in malignant melanoma of the skin, significance of stage of disease, anatomical site, sex, age, and period of diagnosis. Cancer 40:389–397, 1977
20. McLeod GR, Beardmore GL, Little JH, et al.: Results of treatment of 361 patients with malignant melanoma in Queensland. Med J Aust 1:1211–1216, 1971
21. McPeak CJ, McNeer GP, Whiteley HW, Booher RJ: Amputation for melanoma of the extremity. Surgery 54:3, Sept 1963, pp 427–431
22. Miller TR: Hemipelvectomy in lower extremity tumors. Orthop Clin North Am 8:4, 903–919, Oct 1977
23. Mundth ED, Guralnick EA, Baker JW: Malignant melanoma: A clinical study of 427 cases. Ann Surg 162:15–27, 1965
24. Pack GT: The pigmented mole and the malignant melanoma. CA 12:11–26, 1962
25. Pack GT, Gerber DM, Scharnagel IM: End results in the treatment of malignant melanoma; a report of 1190 cases. Ann Surg 136:905–911, 1952
26. Pack GT, Oropeza R: Subungual melanoma. Surg Gynecol Obstet 124:571–582, 1967
27. Shah JP: Amelanotic melanoma. In Ariel IM: Progress in Clinical Cancer, vol 6. Grune & Stratton, New York, 1975, pp 195–197
28. Spitz S: Melanomas of childhood. Am J Path 25:591–609, 1948
29. Sutherland EM, Klopfer HW, Mansell PW, and Krementz ET: Familial melanoma, in Proceedings of the IX International Pigment Cell Conference, Houston, 1975, p 60

30. Turnbull A, Shah J, Fortner J: Recurrent melanoma of an extremity treated by major amputation. Arch Surg 106:496–498, April 1973.

31. Veronesi U, Adamus J, Bandiera DC, et al.: Inefficacy of immediate node dissection in Stage I melanoma of the limbs. N Engl J Med 297:627–630, 1977

32. Wanebo HJ, Woodruff J, Fortner JG: Malignant melanoma of the extremities: A clinicopathologic study using levels of invasion (microstage). Cancer 35:3, March 1975, p 675

PRINCIPLES OF THE SURGICAL TREATMENT OF MALIGNANT MELANOMA

IRVING M. ARIEL

TRIDIMENSIONAL RESECTION OF THE PRIMARY MELANOMA

When a cutaneous lesion is suspect of being a malignant melanoma and if not too large, a total conservative tridimensional excision of the lesion should be performed (Fig. 26-1). When a diagnosis of malignant melanoma has been established the best treatment is a wide tridimensional resection of the tumor. An area of ± 5 cm about the tumor should be excised except in certain instances of small superficial lesions. Melanoma cells are only loosely attached to each other with practically little or no cohesiveness. The "breakaway" of melanoma cells to the surrounding tissue can occur. Approximately 10% of all our patients have evidence of local recurrence strongly indicating inadequate excision. The extent of the excision is often determined by the anatomy of the tissue hosting the tumor.

Figure 26-2 (top) describes the surgical technique for a tridimensional excision with closure by sliding flaps. Figure 26-2 (bottom) depicts the surgical defects of the extremities, which should be closed by split-thickness skin graft.

DISSECTION IN CONTINUITY

Resection of the primary cancer in continuity with the intervening lymphatics and the regional eschelon of lymph nodes that drain the site and often harbor metastatic cancer is the principle underlying most cancer operation. It is the principle of such operations as the Halsted radical mastectomy for breast cancer, the Wertheim radical hysterectomy for uterine cancer, the Miles' abdominoperineal rectal resection for rectal cancer, and others (Fig. 26-3).

Pringle[12] is credited with advocating the principle of "en bloc" dissection for malignant melanoma in 1908, one year after Handley[6] had described the spread of cancer cells through the lymphatics within certain facial planes to the neighboring lymph nodes.

Just 50 years before Pemberton[11] had advocated a wide excision of the lesion, surrounding skin, and all integument between the underlying skin to the underlying muscle. He did perform one groin dissection but did not advocate dissection in continuity.

Pack has been a foremost advocate of "dissection in continuity" and has devised many surgical procedures, promulgated by the anatomic location of the melanoma and the lymphatic circulation draining that site. Some of the examples shown here represent unpublished examples of such procedures performed by the late Dr. George T. Pack (with permission of the executors of his estate (Figs. 26-4 through 26-10).

THE EXTENDED RADICAL GROIN DISSECTION

INTRODUCTION

The successful treatment of malignant tumors that metastasize to the groin depends upon complete removal of the primary neoplasm and associated lymph nodes. The procedure of groin dissection has varied in its

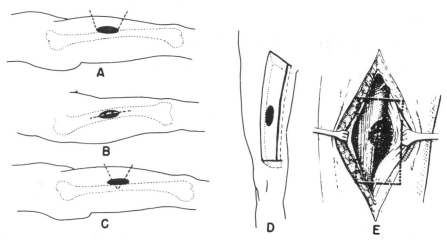

FIGURE 26-1.   Technique for excision of a lesion suspect of a beginning malignant melanoma, for histologic diagnosis and evaluation. A, B, and C show incorrect methods. A: Two-dimensional excision of limited scope. B: The superficial portion is not adequately excised. C: The often-performed triangular excision does not remove tumor in the depth. D and E: The correct procedures, tridimensional in scope, supply the pathologist with tissue surrounding the melanoma and permit the evaluation of the depth of invasion and the thickness of the tumor.

degree of radicality. Basset[3] described a technique of groin dissection in which the inguinal ligament was split to enable a conjoined surgical removal of iliac and inguinal lymph nodes. The Basset procedure was later modified by Taussig[15] by the inclusion of the hypogastric nodes. The radical groin dissection has, since that time, become standardized with the removal of the inguinal, iliac, obturator, and hypogastric lymph nodes. This has been summarized in detail.[9]

INDICATIONS

Groin dissections are performed for metastatic melanomas that occur in the skin of the lower extremity, the female and male genitals, the perineum, perianal zone, gluteal region, and the infraumbilical segment of the abdominal wall. Malignant tumors of the umbilicus, the infraumbilical or midabdominal skin, the skin of the anus and scrotum, the perianal zone, and the female genitals all are capable of metastasizing to either the right or the left group of groin nodes, or to both groups.

The basic postulates for successful groin dissection are: the primary malignant tumor should be controlled or controllable; there should be no clinical evidence of blood stream metastases; the lymph stream must be centralward, with no evidence of blockage and retrograde extension; it should be technically possible to excise all of the lymph nodes involved, or suspected of becoming involved, in the immediate neighborhood; there must be some possibility of interruption of the lymphatic spread of the malignant disease by an excision of these nodes; and there certainly should be evidence that the malignant tumor has metastasized only to the regional group of nodes to be attacked in the groin dissection. The question of elective groin dissection (when the nodes are not clinically palpable) remains problematical.

If the primary malignant neoplasm is in the vicinity of the groin, an all-encompassing en

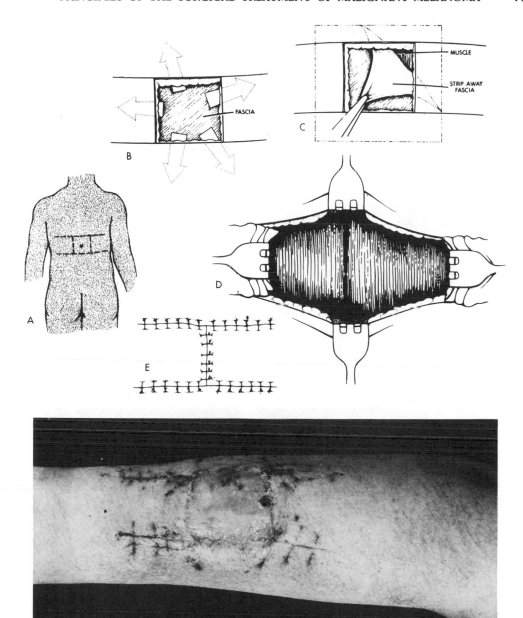

FIGURE 26-2. Top: The surgical technique for a tridimensional excision with closure by sliding flaps. Bottom: Illustration of a resected site repaired with a split-thickness skin graft. The healed incisions about the graft represent flaps of skin dissected to permit a wide resection of underlying tissue and by approximation limiting the amount of graft needed. (Top figure from Ariel IM: Tridimensional resection of primary malignant melanoma. Surg Gynecol Obstet 139: 601–603, 1974 by permission of Surgery, Gynecology, & Obstetrics.)

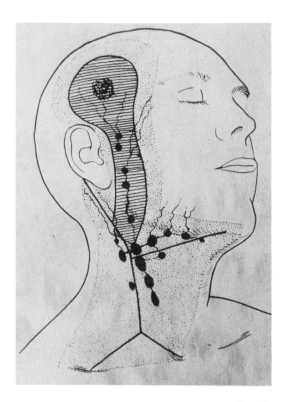

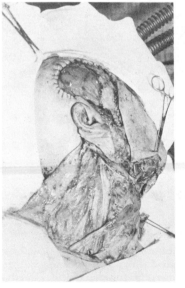

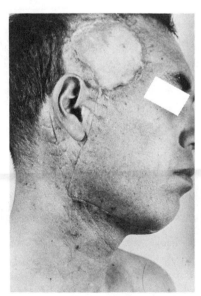

FIGURE 26–3.   Top: Drawing of surgical plan to excise in continuity a melanoma of the scalp combined with a radical neck dissection. Bottom Left: Operative photo showing extent of dissection. Bottom Right: Two weeks later, healing of neck dissection and complete take of split-thickness skin graft to scalp.

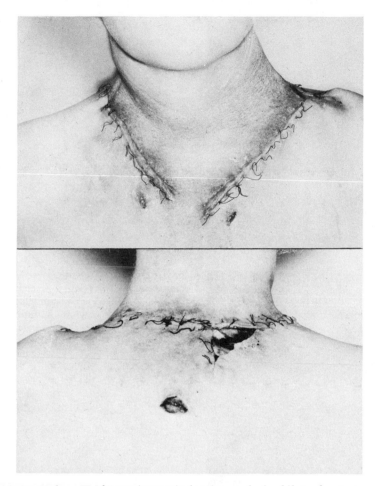

FIGURE 26-4. Melanoma of posterior cervical region producing bilateral metastases to cervical lymph node. Top: Anterior view showing bilateral incision. Bottom: Posterior view demonstrating site of excision of primary melanoma.

bloc resection of the primary malignant tumor, the intervening lymphatic vessels, and the lymph nodes of the groin is indicated.

The proper management of a melanoma distant from the primary echelon of lymph nodes draining the site of the malignant tumor remains an enigma. Many surgeons perform a discontinuous operation, that is, removal of the primary melanoma and the performance of a groin dissection as repeated procedures. This practice ignores the lymphatic vessels intervening between the resected tissues in which melanoma cells may be present.

Different procedures have been advocated to cope with the surgical deficiency that exists in the performance of the discontinuous operation. These include perfusion of the extremity with cancer chemotherapeutic drugs; infusion of the extremity with cancer chemotherapeutic drugs, and the endolymphatic administration of radioactive isotopes.

Pack and Rekers, on the other hand, favor radical amputation of the extremity with active malignant tumors of the feet and metastases to the femoral and inguinal lymph nodes.[9] They stated,

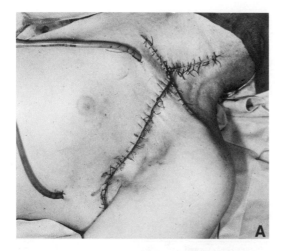

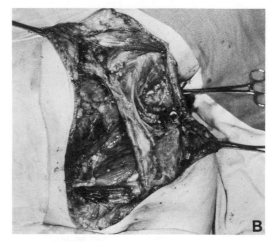

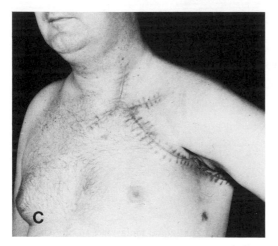

FIGURE 26–5.   Melanoma of skin over left clavicle treated by resection of primary melanoma with combined axillary and supraclavicular dissection and resection of clavicle. A. Immediate postoperative incision. B. Appearance of clavicular bed during operation. C. Wound site three weeks postoperation.

The proper way of handling, for example, melanoma of the foot metastatic to the groin is still an enigma . . . . In the absence of clinical evidence of suspicious lymph nodes in the groin, the primary cancer of the distal extremity is excised with skin grafting, or a digit is amputated, depending upon the location of the neoplasm. Groin dissection is not done electively when it cannot be done in continuity. The patient is kept under close and frequent observation. If an enlarging node in the groin is discovered, it is removed for microscopic study; if metastases are found, the leg is removed by hip joint disarticulation with deep iliac nodal dissection. It has been our belief, substantiated by personal experience, that

the lymph nodes in the groin should remain to exercise their function as catchment basins or filters for malignant cells which may be metastasizing at the time the primary cancer is removed. . . . . In patients who concurrently have active skin cancers of the feet or lower legs and proved metastases in femoral and inguinal lymph nodes, the hip joint disarticulation with deep iliac nodal dissection is done as the primary operation. It is most unlikely for any cancer as highly malignant as a melanoma to spread all the way from the foot to the groin, through the myriad of lymphatics and their sluggish circulation, without some of the cancer cells becoming lodged en route in the tiny nodes intercalated along these pathways. A

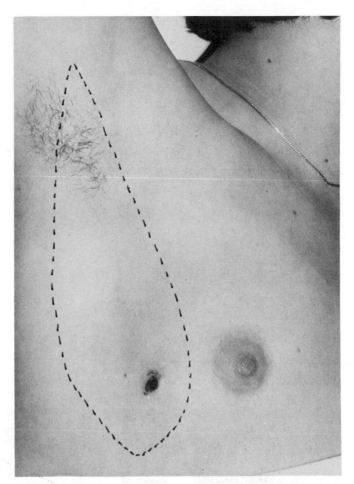

FIGURE 26-6. Melanoma lateral to breast: excision and dissection in continuity with axillary dissection.

few long-term cures, however, in patients with the extremity preserved, attest to this possibility; but the chances are so few that we have no compunctions in advising and practicing the sacrifice of the extremity.

Many patients refuse amputation and, though the described hypothesis is logical, the practice of amputation is seldom indicated and performed only in cases of patients with fixed, locally inoperable melanomas.

Inasmuch as the lymphatics of the lower extremities drain into the lymph nodes of the groin by way of a chain of lymphatic vessels that are located in the medical aspect of the thigh, an extension of the classic groin dissection will permit removal of a large segment of the lymphatic vessels and minimize the risk of endolymphatic cancer cells. If the classic groin dissection should be extended inferiorly to the region known as the popliteal space, approximately 50% of the intervening lymphatic vessels will, therefore, be excised.

Lymphatic Vessels of the Lower Extremity. The lymphatic trunks of the lower extremities usually follow the course of the greater

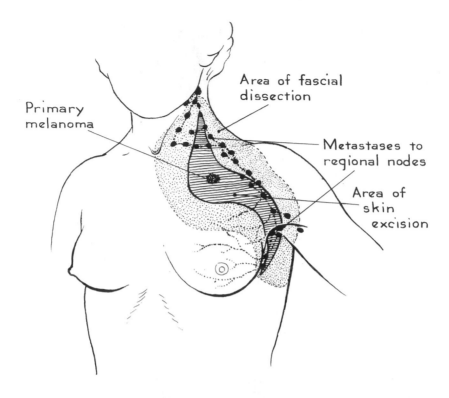

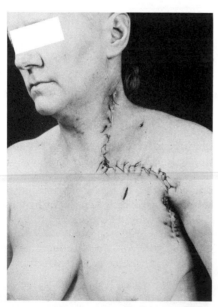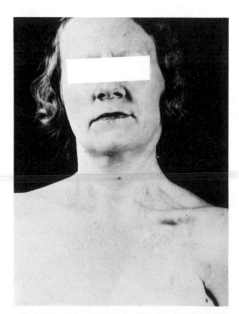

FIGURE 26–7. Top: Illustration of the planned skin incision and scope of fascial and regional lymph node dissection for a melanoma of the anterior pectoral region metastatic to axillary and supraclavicular nodes. Bottom: Immediate and delayed operative appearance.

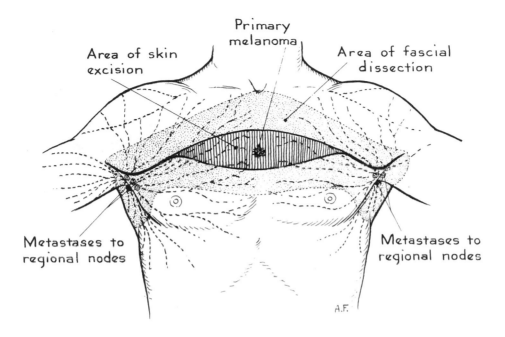

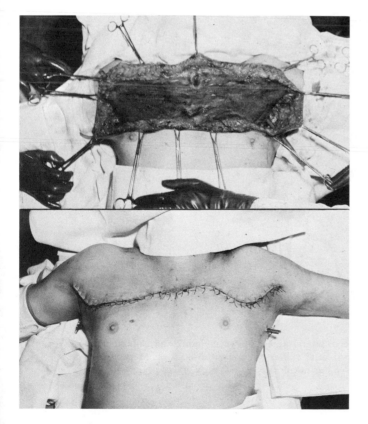

FIGURE 26-8. Top: Illustration of the length of incision, the comparative amount of skin and fascia removed, and the general scope of the operation for excision and dissection in continuity, of a melanoma of the anterior midline of the thoracic skin. Middle: Photo at operation to show development of skin flaps, plan of incision, scope of fascial removal, and bilateral axillary dissection in continuity. Bottom: Primary wound closure.

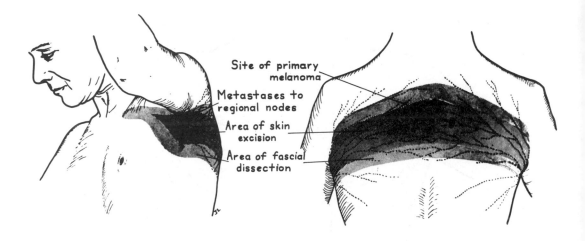

FIGURE 26–9. Melanoma slightly to right of midline of skin of posterior thoracic wall. Scope of skin and underlying tissue to be excised combined with a right radical axillary dissection.

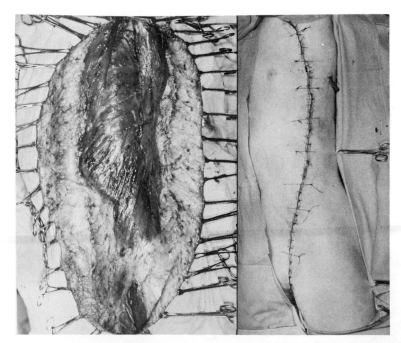

FIGURE 26–10. Melanoma of skin of lateral aspect between thorax and abdomen, treated by wide excision combined with an ipsilateral axillary and groin dissection. Metastases were encountered in the axillary lymph nodes but not in the groin lymph nodes.

saphenous vein—vena saphena magna system (Figs. 26-11 and 26-12). The lymphatic vessels vary from 0.25 to 1 mm in diameter, usually retaining their caliber as they ascend toward the inguinal region and usually following a straight course to end abruptly. If a contrast medium is injected into a lymphatic vessel on the dorsum of the foot, the lymphatic vessels of the lower extremity are visualized as one or more trunks coursing proximally along the *anteromedial* aspect of the leg, converging toward the knee, then

ascending, and dividing into 12 to 16 divisions as they enter the superficial inguinal lymph nodes. If the opaque material is injected into a lymphatic vessel along the lateral aspect of the foot, the lymphatic vessels are seen to course proximally toward the popliteal fossa— saphena parva system—where one or two popliteal nodes are usually found. The latter are found routinely in dogs, whereas in man they are absent in a significant number of patients. The lymphatic vessels continue to course proximally to the deep lymphatic chain

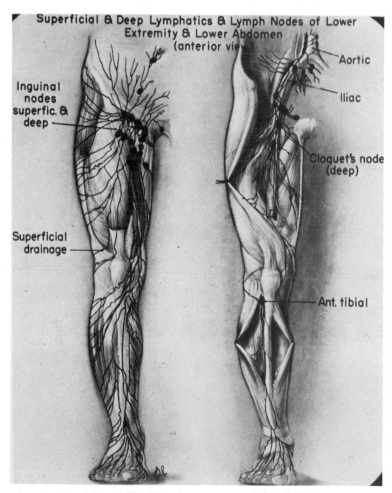

FIGURE 26-11. Superficial and deep lymphatics and lymph nodes of the lower extremity and lower abdomen (anterior aspect).

and terminate in the superficial inguinal vessels, which course to the thigh and extend mesially to enter the groin in juxtaposition to the femoral vessels (Fig. 26–13).

Inguinal and Iliac Lymph Nodes. Normally, there are from four to ten inguinal nodes, both superficial and deep, presenting a variable pattern. Efforts to divide this group into subgroups based on a relationship to the greater saphenous vein are believed to be of no practical use in clinical roentgenographic diagnoses.

As originally described by Rouvière,[13] the efferent lymphatic vessels from the inguinal nodes continue proximally to the external iliac chain of nodes to divide into three chains: a lateral chain located lateral to the external iliac artery (one to four nodes), a middle group that lies on the posterior surface of the external iliac vein (two to four nodes), and a medial group (three to four nodes) situated posterior to the external iliac vein usually in juxtaposition to the lateral pelvic wall. The obturator node is considered a part of the medial group of the external iliac chain of nodes and is found

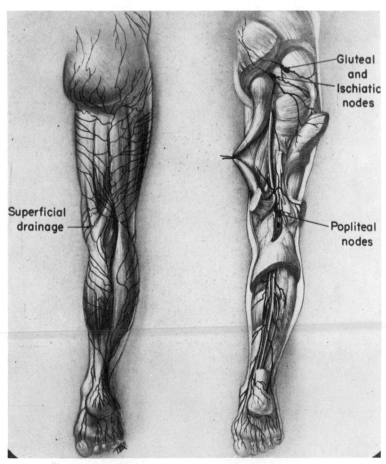

FIGURE 26–12. Superficial and deep lymphatics and lymph nodes of the lower extremity (posterior aspect).

roentgenographically related; it may either lie in direct continuity with the remainder of the medial chain or be situated somewhat distant as a solitary node within the obturator fossa, usually between the external iliac vein and the obturator nerve and vessels.

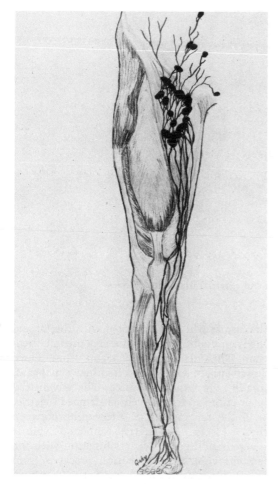

FIGURE 26–13. Diagrammatic view of lymphatics of lower extremity demonstrating that all lymphatics below the knee extend to the groin in the medial aspect of the thigh.*

* Figures 26–13, 26–17, 26–18, and 26–20 are reproduced from Ariel IM: The extended radical groin dissection for melanoma of the lower extremity. Surg Gynec Obstet, 132:116, 1971 by permission of Surgery, Gynecology & Obstetrics.

Continuing proximally, the common iliac chain, four to 12 nodes lying in close relationship to the common iliac artery and vein, subdivides into the hypogastric nodes, two to eight in number, and courses along the hypogastric artery (Fig. 26–14). From the common iliac nodes, several trunks course craniad along the aorta and inferior vena cava to form the abdominoaortic lymph node group, 25 to 45 nodes (Fig. 26–15).

EFFECTS OF A DISCONTINUOUS OPERATION ALTERING LYMPHATIC DYNAMICS AND ITS EFFECT ON TRANSPORT OF MELANOMA CELLS

The performance of a discontinuous operation with transection of the lymph nodes only in the groin will result in a decrease in the flow of lymph with the production of a stagnant state. If such a situation has occurred, the possibility of cells in-transit to be trapped and to grow in these deep lymphatics becomes enhanced. The removal of a large portion of lymphatic vessels leading to the lymph nodes of the groin will tend to minimize the hazards regarding transport of melanoma of the incomplete operation and remove increased sites at risk of harboring melanoma (Chap 12).

Technique of Extended Radical Groin Dissection. The patient is placed upon the operating table with the corresponding thigh slightly abducted and externally rotated, the knee being slightly flexed over a small sandbag. In the male, the scrotal sac superficially is sutured over the genitals to the opposite groin to withdraw the genitals from the operative field.

The skin incision differs from those previously described by Taussig and Basset, inasmuch as it entails the removal of a wide ellipse. The motives for removal of the skin are that it lessens the possibilities of any local skin recurrence, it avoids the almost inevitable sloughing of the skin that follows wide fascial dissection, and it aids in wound

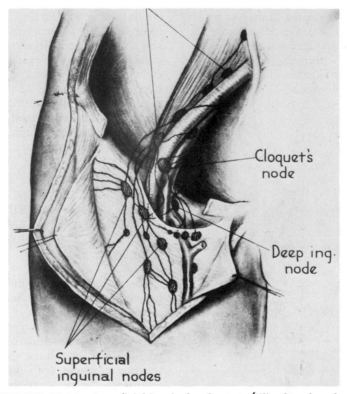

Cloquet's node

Deep ing. node

Superficial inguinal nodes

FIGURE 26–14.   Superficial inguinal and external iliac lymph nodes.

healing. The upper extremity of the incision is located two inches above and one inch medial to the anterior surface of the iliac spine. From this point, it sweeps downward in a wide ellipse and then in a medial direction over the inguinal region and the femoral trigone to terminate at its lower extremity at the medial border of the popliteal space (Fig. 26–16). After the skin edges have been defined by the scalpel, sterile towels are applied to the lateral edges of the wound by means of numerous tenacula, which are helpful in facilitating subsequent dissection of the fat and fascia from the skin.

With the tenacula elevated, the subcutaneous fat is dissected widely in all directions until the entire thigh, the inguinal region, and the lower part of the abdominal wall over the iliac quadrant have been denuded of skin. The dissection then continues deep to the underlying muscles (Fig. 26–17), through the fascia, which is dissected with the fat and the lymphoid tissues en bloc in a medial direction. This dissection is begun from above downward to expose the inguinal canal and, finally, the femoral vessels. The adventitial layer of the artery and vein is stripped together with the fat and fascia intervening between these vessels. The internal saphenous vein is severed and ligated near its junction with the femoral vein. The dissection proceeds from above downward, all of the fascia being removed from the muscles of the anterior aspect of the thigh sartorius, iliacus, pectineus, adductor brevis, and rectus femoris. The sartorius muscle is retracted as the dissection proceeds down through Hunter's canal. The internal saphenous vein again is severed and ligated where it enters the operative field overlying the middle segment of the sartorius muscle. This bulk of tissue then is removed, and the first stage of the groin dissection is

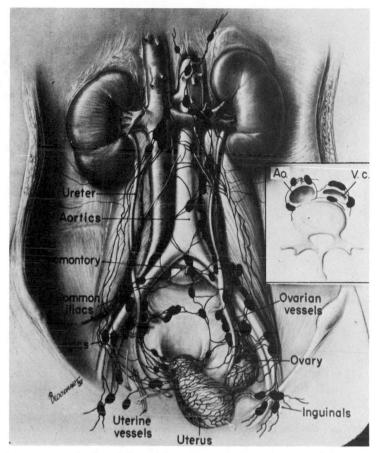

FIGURE 26–15. Lymphatics of the pelvic, aorta, and inguinal regions (laboratory exposure).

complete. Upon completion of this phase of the operation, the superficial lymph nodes of the groin, the areolar tissue and fat, the fascia, and the lymphatic vessels have been removed, and the muscles of the anteromedial aspect of the thigh from Poupart's ligament to the medial aspect of the popliteal space have been laid bare (Fig. 26–18).

The sartorius muscle sometimes is sutured slightly medially in an attempt to obliterate the dead space of Scarpa's triangle and to protect the femoral vessels more adequately. All bleeding vessels are tied with silk ligatures, a practice that has greatly lessened the amount of serous discharge. If the tumor is fungating through the skin or a radiation ulcer is present, catgut ligatures are used, and drainage is established through a standard incision placed in the most dependent portion of the wound on its medial aspect. The skin is usually closed with interrupted silk sutures. Continuous suction through a small sump drain during the immediate postoperative period prevents an accumulation of lymph and serum in the wound.

The second step is then carried out in the routine manner by excising Poupart's ligament and removing the deep iliac nodes, including Cloquet's and the obturator nodes (Fig. 26–19).

Results. In a series of 25 patients treated by this technique, there have been no untoward complications. Wound healing has occurred

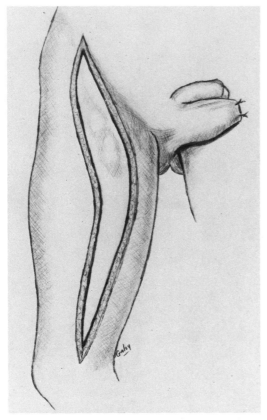

FIGURE 26–16. Incision for extended radical groin dissection.

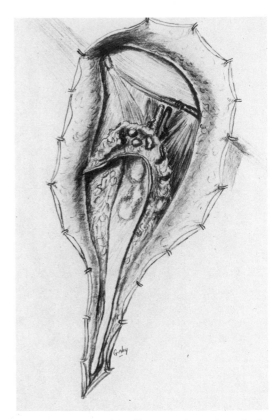

FIGURE 26–17. Skin flaps are formed, and the dissection is continued deep to the underlying muscles.

per primum with no complications. Most of these patients suffer a slight amount of lymphedema of the lower extremity, and in only one of them was it considered more severe than from the classic conventional groin dissection. The data do not permit including ten-year results and whether these results are better than those obtained by the orthodox groin dissection.

Summary. A surgical technique has been used in 25 patients with malignant tumors of the lower extremities, whereby a large number of lymphatic vessels are removed in combination with a groin dissection. This procedure is considered particularly important in patients with a malignant melanoma when a discontinuous operation must be performed. The removal of approximately 50% of the lym-

phatic vessels reduce the hazards that can result from a discontinuous operation. The presence of melanoma within a lymphatic vessel is demonstrated in Figure 26–20.

THE TECHNIQUE OF CONSERVATIVE HEMIPELVECTOMY (WITH PARTIAL RESECTION OF THE INNOMINATE BONE)

INTRODUCTION

Major amputations of the lower extremities have been adequately described.[58] The conservative hemipelvectomy has been developed relatively recently and consists of partial resection of the innominate bone with amputation of the subjacent extremity. It is more radical than a hip-joint disarticulation but more conservative than the orthodox hemipelvectomy (interilioabdominal amputation). It was first described in 1960 by Charles Sherman[14] and developed by Caceras and Sherman.[4] A graphic description of this useful operation has been published by Ariel and Shah.[2]

DEFINITION

The conservative hemipelvectomy consists of that operation where the extremity and parts of the innominate bone (pubes and ischium) are resected en bloc. In contrast to the orthodox hemipelvectomy, whereby the entire innominate bone is removed by means of transecting the sacral iliac synchondrosis, in the conservative hemipelvectomy the synchondrosis is left intact and the ilium inviolate. This is accomplished by severing the ilium from the subjacent innominate bone through the sciatic notch.

INDICATIONS

The conservative hemipelvectomy has proved beneficial and at times curative in those instances where a melanoma metastasizes, is locally inoperable, is in approximation to the hip joint, and where a hip joint

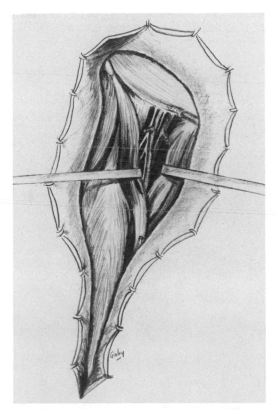

FIGURE 26-18. The superficial dissection has been completed. The superficial lymph nodes of the groin, areolar tissue and fat, fascia, and lymphatic vessels have been removed, and the muscles of the anteromedial aspect of the popliteal space have been laid bare.

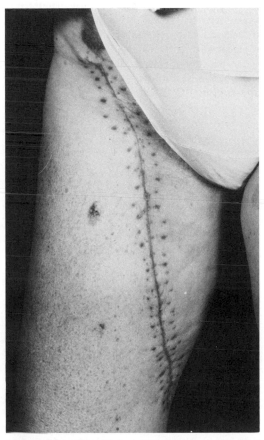

FIGURE 26-19. Clinical appearance of radical groin dissection.

disarticulation might prove too conservative. Specifically for these melanomas, where amputation is indicated and where a deep lymph node dissection is considered necessary in conjunction with the amputation, the conservative hemipelvectomy removes the involved chain of lymph nodes en bloc with the subjacent extremity.

PRINCIPLES OF OPERATION

The techniques permit performing the entire resection without turning the patient. By the complete draping of the involved extremity, the posterior dissection can be done by manipulating the lower extremity to afford the necessary exposure. The operation takes from 1 to 1½ hours, and has been found to be far less traumatic than a hip joint disarticulation inasmuch as fewer muscles are actually transected. Approximately 1 liter of blood replacement is necessary. There has been no recorded postoperative death from this procedure. We have observed no bladder or bowel dysfunction. One patient who had the common iliac artery transected rather than the external iliac artery, suffered from necrosis of the posterior wound, which was repaired by split-thickness graft. One patient suffered from severe pain at the site of the severed sciatic nerve, which was believed to be an amputation neuroma and was treated by the injection of alcohol, causing the pain to completely subside. The operation leaves the patients with good balance, unlike an orthodox hemipelvectomy. One of our patients has become an expert amputee skiier and another, whose favorite sport is golf, states that his only limitation is that instead of having a full swing, he now has a three-quarters swing.

The iliac bone has proved to be stable and supports a prosthesis without any difficulty.

A five-year survival of 50% (four of eight patients) has been obtained by the performance of the conservative hemipelvectomy.

TECHNIQUE OF OPERATION

The patient lies on his back with the involved side elevated and the extremity slightly

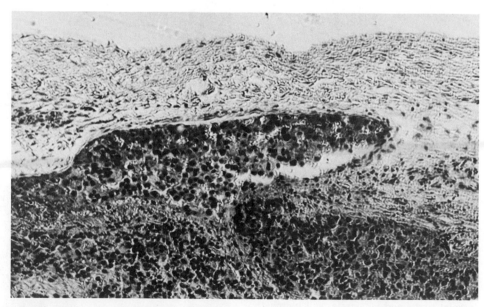

FIGURE 26–20. Photomicrograph demonstrates malignant melanoma within a lymphatic vessel. Hematoxylin and eosin, × 64.

abducted and flexed. The anterior incision is made first, parallel to the inguinal ligaments, approximately 2 cm superior to the ligament. The incision extends from the symphysis pubis cephalid to a point approximately at the junction of the lower two-thirds of the outer border of the ilium and the upper one-third of the ilium. Skin flaps can then be developed to help expose the deeper structures and expose the anterior superior spine where indicated. (It is not good policy to have the incision extend to the anterior superior spine as with the orthodox hemipelvectomy because of poor healing of this region.) It has been found useful to add a horizontal component to the lower pole of the incision, extending from the symphysis pubis to the opposite pubes. This facilitates the identification and transection of the symphysis at a later stage of the operation (Fig. 26-21). The posterior incision is delayed until the anterior dissection is completed.

The anterior abdominal muscles are then transected to the peritoneum. The spermatic cord in males is then identified and retracted (Fig. 26-22). The retroperitoneal space is then entered by retracting the peritoneum with a wide Deever retractor. The ureter and bladder are retracted medially. The external iliac artery vein, femoral nerve, and lymph nodes are thus exposed. The external iliac artery is transected and ligated with number 00 silk sutures; the same is accomplished for the external iliac vein and for the femoral nerve. Any lymph nodes that might be superior to the line of resection are dissected starting at the bifurcation of the aorta and extending distally (Fig. 26-23). The insert demonstrates the vessels and nerves transected and the lymph nodes, including the common iliac lymph nodes having been resected from above inferiorly. Figure 26-24 illustrates preparation for transection of the iliopsoas muscle which is accomplished by placing two fingers between the posterior portion of the iliopsoas muscle and the bone. The left hand is separating the iliopsoas from the pelvic bone and the right hand extends posterior to the pelvic bone between the Gluteus minimus and the pelvic bone, thus exposing and freeing the sciatic notch. The iliopsoas muscle is then transected. Figure

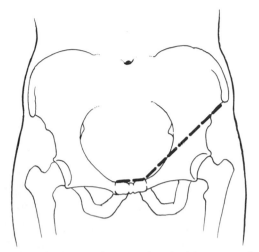

FIGURE 26-21. The anterior incision extends from the symphysis pubis proximal and lateral toward the upper portion of the ilium.*

26-25 shows the transection of the ischium from the ilium. The Gigli saw has been passed through the sciatic notch after the anterior musculature has been transected and the posterior musculature freed. The insert shows the usual line of resection with the resection carried out through the sciatic notch. The symphysis pubis is next skeletonized and the Gigli saw is passed beneath the symphasis and transected (Fig. 26-26). It is important to make certain that the symphysis is the anatomic site for the resection. If the symphysis is missed and the transected is made through one or the other pubic bones, the sawing is much more difficult and bleeding more profuse. The horizontal incision as shown in Figure 26-21 facilitates the exposure of the symphysis pubis. Figure 26-27 demonstrates the anterior view of the transected symphysis pubis and ischium from the ilium. The abductor muscle is severed at its medial border, which permits better resection of the extremities at the completion of the

* Figures 26-21 through 26-30 are reproduced from Ariel IM, Shah JP: The conservative hemipelvectomy Surg Gynec Obstet, 144:406–413, 1977 by permission of Surgery, Gynecology & Obstetrics.

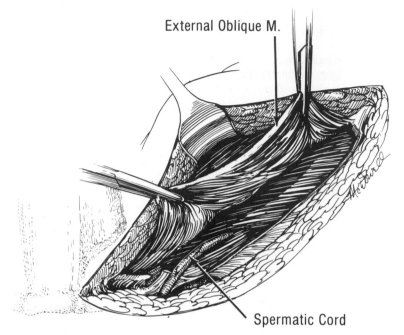

External Oblique M.

Spermatic Cord

FIGURE 26–22.   The anterior abdominal muscles are transected.

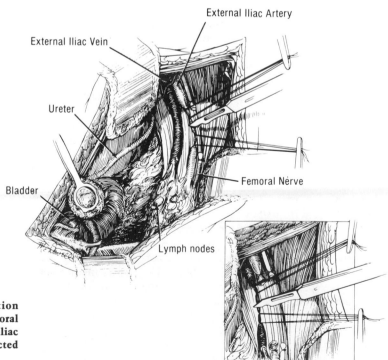

External Iliac Artery

External Iliac Vein

Ureter

Bladder

Femoral Nerve

Lymph nodes

FIGURE 26–23.   Transection of the iliac vessels and femoral nerve. The inset shows the iliac lymph nodes being dissected from above inferiorly.

Iliopsoas M.

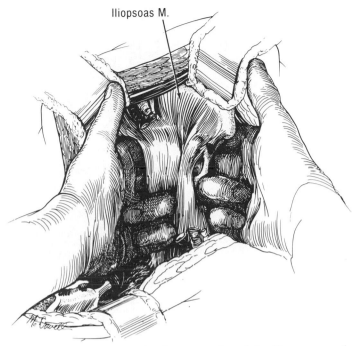

FIGURE 26–24.   Preparation for transection of the iliopsoas muscle.

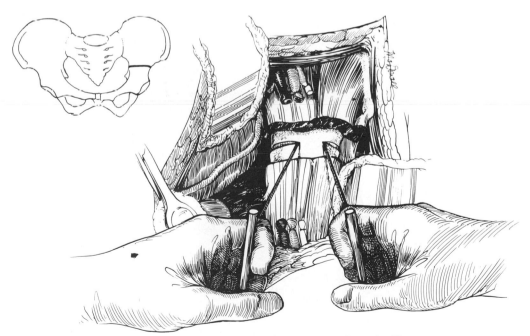

FIGURE 26–25.   Transection of the ischium from the ilium.

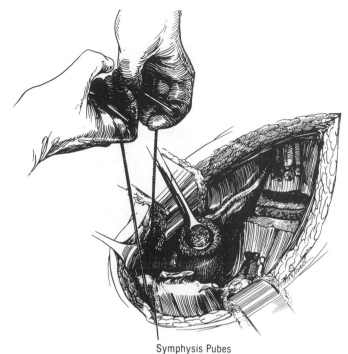

FIGURE 26–26.   The symphyis pubis is skeletonized and transected.

Symphysis Pubes

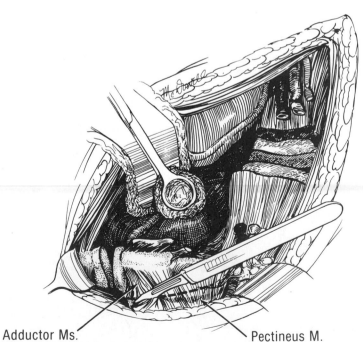

Adductor Ms.   Pectineus M.

FIGURE 26–27.   The anterior view of the transected symphysis pubis and separated ischium from the ilium.

posterior resection. Figure 26–28 illustrates the posterior incision which continues near the distal crease below the buttock extending medially to meet the anterior incision at the level of the symphysis pubis. The gluteal muscles are then transected as shown in Figure 26–29. The glutei muscles can be transected near its insertion (if there are no contraindications) to assist in the fitting of the prosthesis. The inferior gluteal artery and vein are transected and doubly ligated with silk sutures. The sacrotuberous ligament is divided, after which the sciatic nerve, which is taut and holds the extremity in position, is transected, severing the lower extremity, pubes, and ischium from the body. The muscles are approximated in the closure with interrupted Chromicized-0 catgut and the skin closed with interrupted 3-zero and 2-zero silk sutures. Two large hemovacs are left in situ for drainage purposes. Figure 26–30 illustrates the completed operation and demonstrates the

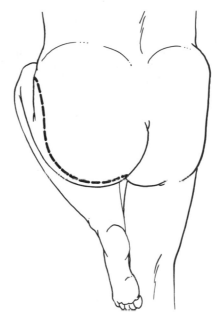

FIGURE 26-28. Posterior incision.

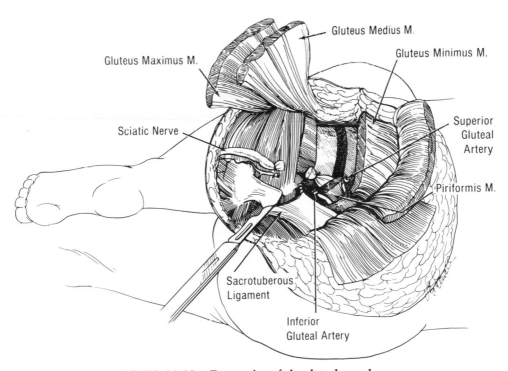

FIGURE 26-29. Transection of the gluteal muscles.

defect, which is not dissimilar from that accomplished from a hip-joint disarticulation. The operation has been performed for eight patients with fixed melanomas of the groin. Four are alive and apparently free of melanoma five years after the operation (Fig. 26–31).

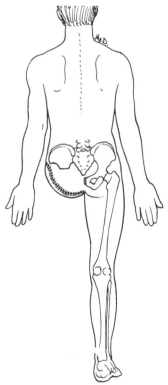

FIGURE 26–30. The completed conservative hemipelvectomy.

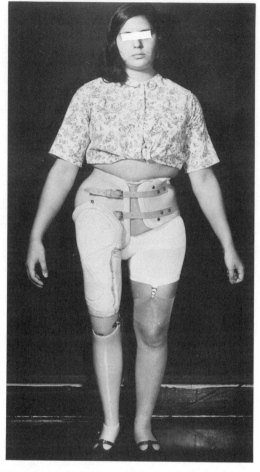

FIGURE 26–31. Photograph of 15-year-old girl who underwent a conservative hemipelvectomy.

REFERENCES

1. Ariel IM: The extended radical groin dissection for melanomas of the lower extremity. Surg Gynecol Obstet 132:116, 1971
2. Ariel IM, Shah JP: The conservative hemipelvectomy. Surg Gynecol Obstet 144:406, 1977
3. Basset A: Traitement chirurgical opératoire de l' épithélioma primitif du clitoris; indications, techniques, résultats. Rev Chir 46:546, 1912
4. Caceres E, Sherman CD Jr: Conservative hemipelvectomy. Treat Cancer Allied Dis 7:303, 1964
5. Coley BL, Higinbotham NL: Management of malignant diseases in the neighborhood of the hip. Surg Gynecol Obstet 99:727, 1954
6. Handley WS: The pathology of melanotic growths in relation to their operative treatment. Lancet 6:1927, 1907
7. Herman PG, Benninghoff D, Schwartz S: A physiologic approach to lymph flow in lymphography. Am J Roentgen 91:1207, 1964
8. Pack GT, Ariel IM: Tumors of the Soft Somatic Tissues: A Clinical Treatise. New York, Paul B Hoeber Inc, 1958
9. Pack GT, Rekers P: Radical groin dissection, In

Cooper P (ed): The Craft of Surgery. Boston, Little Brown, 1964

10. Pack GT, Rekers P: The management of malignant tumors in the groin. Am J Surg 56:545, 1942
11. Pemberton O: Observations on the history, pathology and treatment of cancerous diseases, London, Churchill, 1858, vol 8
12. Pringle JH: Operation in melanotic tumors of the skin. Edinburgh Med J 23:496, 1908
13. Rouvière H: Anatomy of the human lymphatic system. Ann Arbor, Edward Bros, 1938
14. Sherman CD Jr, Duthie RB: Modified hemipelvectomy. Cancer 13:51, 1960
15. Taussig FJ: Primary cancer of vulva, vagina and female urethra: Five year results. Surg Gynec Obstet 60:477–478, 1935

CHAPTER TWENTY–SEVEN

MALIGNANT MELANOMA OF THE GASTROINTESTINAL TRACT

RUBEN OROPEZA AND
RAJENDRA M. AGRAWAL

With the exception of melanomas of the anal canal and some from the esophagus, most melanomas of the gastrointestinal tract have to be considered metastatic. The fact that malignant melanomas may produce catastrophic symptoms due to intestinal obstruction, bleeding, perforation, intusception, and that proper treatment may be rewarding demands a separate chapter be devoted to melanoma to this subject.

In a 35-year experience at the Pack Medical Group, New York City, 22 primary melanomas of the gastrointestinal tract were encountered among 3,305 melanomas, placing the incidence at 0.07%.

MELANOMA OF THE ESOPHAGUS

Primary malignant melanoma of the esophagus is rare. Only 31 cases have been reported, and only one primary case was found at the Pack Medical Group. Metastasis of malignant melanoma to the esophagus is also very rare. There was a 4% incidence of metastatic melanoma in the esophagus in a series of 100 autopsies of melanoma patients reported by Das Gupta and Brasfield.[11]

ETIOLOGY

The origin of melanoma of the esophagus is controversial. Traditionally, the esophageal epithelium was considered devoid of melanoblasts.[5,15,41] Stout and Lattes[37] stated:

We do not wish to deny that malignant melanoma can be primary in the esophagus. We simply regard the published evidence as unconvincing. If it could be demonstrated that melanoblasts occur in the esophagus or that benign pigmented nevi occur there, we would not further question the occurrence of primary malignant melanoma.

In 1963, De La Pava, et al.[14] reported that in four out of 100 esophagi, typical melanoblasts with melanin granules and dendrites were found in the basal layer of the mucosa in the upper third of the esophagus in two cases and in the middle third of the esophagus in two cases.

In 1949 and through 1953, Allen and Spitz[1,2] developed histologic criteria for primary malignant melanoma in which they emphasized the presence of functional nevus changes at the periphery of the lesion. After a review of 934 cases of melanoma, they broadened the concept of functional changes as an essential criterion to include visceral melanomas, wherever they may arise. A rapidly growing and expanding tumor may destroy adjacent functional change. However, criteria established by Allen is generally accepted. Only half of the reported cases meet their criteria.

Four cases have been described in which malignant melanomas developed in the presence of melanosis of the esophagus, and in one case reported by Piccone et al.[31] melanosis was present throughout the esophagus. The absence of melanosis in most primary malignant melanomas of the esophagus indicates that the tumor more commonly originated in some other way. One can speculate an origin from some of the few normally occurring melanoblasts, metaplasia of normal esophageal basal epithelial cells in patients where there was ectopic melanoblast-containing epithelium included within the esophagus during development.

PATHOLOGICAL APPEARANCES

Primary malignant melanomas of the esophagus are large, fleshy, pedunculated and polypoid or lobulated tumors. They may be pigmented or nonpigmented. Superficial ulceration is often present, which may cause considerable hemorrhage.

Ideally the diagnosis of a primary esophageal malignant melanoma should be based on the following criteria, as suggested by Raven and Dawson.[33]

1. The tumor should have the characteristic structure of a melanoma and contain pigment that is demonstrable as melanin by appropriate staining techniques.

2. It should arise from an area of functional change in squamous epithelium.[1,2]

3. The adjacent epithelium should also show functional changes with the presence of cells containing melanin pigment. In practice the epithelium over the tumor is often ulcerated and a direct origin from functional epithelium may not be detectable. Raven and Dawson[33] therefore feel that if either two or three criteria are fulfilled, the tumor may be regarded as primary.

CLINICAL FEATURES

Age and Sex. The patients ages range from seven to 77 years old. The youngest one and the only child was a boy of seven reported by Basque et al.[4] Out of 31 cases reported, the average age of 19 males was 57 years and 12 females was 60 years. There is no significant difference in sex ratio.

Symptoms. The most common symptoms are progressive dysphagia for solid foods and a feeling of fullness and discomfort or even postprandial chest pain of mild and inconstant nature; hematemesis may be present. In addition, there are frequently malaise, nausea, flatulence, and a loss of strength and weight. Some patients have cough, hoarseness, and orthopnea.

Signs. Physical signs of the disease apart from those of recent weight loss are generally absent. Very occasionally adenopathy in the neck or occult blood in the stool may be present.

DIAGNOSIS

In addition to radiological studies of the esophagus, endoscopy and biopsy of the lesion are necessary for the establishing the diagnosis.

RADIOLOGICAL APPEARANCES

Most of the tumors are polypoid and bulky, and are associated with ulceration. A short pedicle is often present. A significant degree of obstruction is common. Most common locations of the tumor are middle and lower thirds of the esophagus.

ENDOSCOPY AND BIOPSY

Endoscopy usually reveals a bulky, polypoid, irregularly pigmented or nonpigmented lesion projecting into the lumen of the esophagus. Biopsy is mandatory to confirm the diagnosis.

TREATMENT AND PROGNOSIS

The usual treatment is partial esophagectomy and restoration of the gastrointestinal tract. Continuing radiation has been used in one patient without discernible benefits. Due to rapid generalized metastases with a fulminating course, in most patients only symptomatic treatment is indicated.

Prognosis is always grave with widespread metastasis. Most patients die within six months but there has been one six-year survivor following surgical resection.

MELANOMA OF THE STOMACH

Laennec (1856) first described melanoma in man as a separate clinical entity.[28] Since then, many have reported metastatic spread to the stomach, frequently found during autopsy. Das Gupta and Brasfield[10,11] reported stomach metastases in 2% of 100 autopsies of malignant melanoma. Goldstein et al.[18] had seen involvement of the stomach in sixteen patients in 67 postmortems for melanoma patients. Very few cases were diagnosed during life.[7] A possible primary origin that could be from Meissner's plexus of the gastric submucosa has been published, but this was not substantiated by Chandler and Jones.

CLINICAL FEATURES

Metastatic melanoma of the stomach usually presents with hematemesis and anemia. The patients were often operated upon under the suspicion of a bleeding ulcer, and diagnosis was established only after exploration. Other symptoms are: anorexia, nausea, vomiting and weight loss; epigastric pain may be the presenting symptom. Postprandial bloating, pain, melena and obstruction have been noted. The gastric symptoms may be overshadowed by those due to metastases elsewhere. Ascites is commonly found in association with melanoma of the gastrointestinal tract.

Age. The ages vary from 24 to 80 years. Metastasis to the stomach may take from three months to nine years to appear from the initial presentation of the primary lesion.

DIAGNOSIS

In a patient known to have had a primary melanoma who presents with symptoms related to the gastrointestinal tract, metastasis to the stomach or intestine should be considered and diagnosis established by radiographic study, endoscopy, and biopsy.

The majority of secondary melanomas of the stomach occur in the body and fundus. The lesser curvature is an uncommon site. The lesions may appear as single or multiple polyps, or as a sessile mass projecting from the mucosa, or it may present as a single or multiple ulcerations. Intramural nodules are by far the most commonly encountered melanoma in the stomach,[18] which have the tendency for umbilicated ulceration at the tip, resulting in a central radiopaque area of the "target sign" or "bull's eye sign" which is a characteristic roentgenologic picture.

Recently, Goldstein et al.[18] emphasized the importance of routine double contrast examination of the stomach. By this technique three solitary submucosal metastatic foci were detected. In the same series, in two instances, gastric tumors also had a large extragastric component. Extrinsic pressure on the stomach usually occurs from extragastric metastases.

Endoscopic examination is usually diagnostic. Multiple biopsies confirm the diagnosis.

Exfoliative cytology is often secondary to establishing the diagnosis, using Papanicolaou's stain. Melanin in urine is negative most of the time.

TREATMENT AND PROGNOSIS

The disease is usually extensive by the time diagnosis is established, and the management should be conservative. Before any attempt is made to do a partial or total gastrectomy, the presence and/or extent of the disease to the small bowel should be determined, as the incidence to the small bowel is high. The results reported with any type of treatment are very discouraging. We have had a patient surviving over five years after total gastrectomy from metastatic melanoma from the right arm. The primary was removed five years before the metastases occurred. And a three-year survivor after total gastrectomy for metastatic melanoma, primary in the eye was obtained (Fig. 27–1). Palliative resection is indicated when the main or only site of metastasis is the stomach or when there is an acute catastrophe, such as acute hemorrhage or perforation, even in the presence of extensive metastasis. Five such cases seen at the Pack Medical Group were benefited.

MELANOMA OF THE GALLBLADDER

We must consider reported melanomas of the gallbladder metastatic until proven otherwise. The fact that the primary site is not found does not mean that there is no cutaneous origin, since melanomas are notoriously known to have "spontaneous involution." In no patient of the Pack Medical Group was a verified case of primary melanoma of the gallbladder found. In those cases that presented with symptoms of either cholecystitis-like pain or obstructive jaundice, a primary melanoma has been previously removed. Lesions in the pancreas were also metastatic.

MELANOMA OF THE DUODENUM, SMALL BOWEL, AND COLON

Localized melanoma of the duodenum, small bowel, and colon is rare; less than 50 cases have been reported in the world literature. On the other hand, small bowel is a common site of metastases in autopsies of patients with malignant melanoma. In a series of 100 autopsies[8] with malignant melanoma patients, small bowel lesions were demonstrated in 58% of the patients (Fig. 27–2).[11,18] In 1952, Willis[42] reviewed 135 reported cases of tumor metastases to the small bowel and, of these, malignant melanomas (45 cases) were the most common. Van der Veer and Kellert[41] did the first resection of melanoma of the intestine in 1917. By 1925, there were 25 cases

of melanomas of the small intestines reported, and nine of these were thought to be primary because no other lesion was found, whereas 16 cases were known to be metastatic.[14]

A number of reports suggested that intestinal melanomas may on occasion be a primary lesion.[6,13] The possibility of multifocal, submucosal, polypoid, primary melanomas throughout the intestinal tract is remote and demands further proof.

CLINICAL FEATURES

Symptoms and Signs. Small bowel metastases are known to produce both obstructive symptoms, due to intussusception, which may be intermittent and show bleeding, and due to superficial ulceration of a polypoid lesion. Intussusception of the jejunal, ileoileal, or ileocecal types are the major causes of obstruction. However, there have been instances of sizable metastases in the region of the intestine without any conclusive clinical signs of obstruction. These intestinal metastases rarely become large enough to be palpable. Intestinal bleeding is common and usually an early manifestation. The bleeding is usually slow and steady, and is secondary to the more dramatic and acute problem of intestinal obstruction or intussusception.

Willibanks and Fogelman[40] reported 18 cases of melanoma of the small and large intestine. They indicated that intestinal melanomas may occur in two distinct clinicopathological types with important therapeutic and prognostic differences. More commonly, melanoma presents as intestinal obstruction due to intussusception of multiple, melanotic, polypoid submucosal and mucosal metastatic lesions. Less commonly, it presents as a solitary infiltrative melanotic lesion with hemorrhage or obstruction. The survival rate in solitary tumors is better. In one of the authors' cases a melanoma of the back had been removed 16 years previously, and ten years later a "second" primary melanoma of the shoulder was excised with a metastasis to the right axilla. He has had two episodes of in-

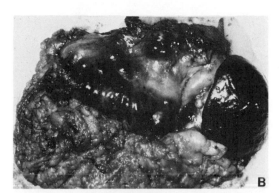

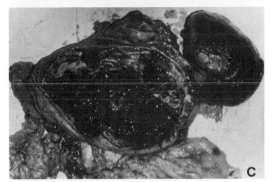

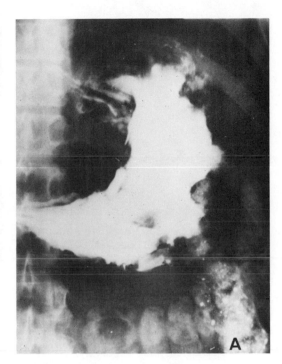

FIGURE 27-1A: A preoperative x-ray of the stomach demonstrating large defects of the fundus and body of the stomach. B: Operative specimen of the same patient: Total gastrectomy, splenectomy, and removal of tail of the pancreas to remove the tumor en bloc. C: Same specimen demonstrating large and bulky fungating melanomas of the stomach. Oropeza R: Melanomas of special sites. In Andrade et al.: Cancer of the Skin. Philadelphia, WB Saunders Co., 1976, p 974. With permission.

tussusception treated by small bowel resection followed by immunochemotherapy, and he has remained well for the past six years.

Radiological Appearance. The tumor usually produces an enlarging pedunculated mass projecting into the bowel lumen, but rarely as an annular constriction. The mucosa often overlies the lesion. The muscularis may be secondarily involved. If the lesion is ulcerative, there may be multiple oval or round filling defects with a central collection of barium, the so-called "bull's eye" lesions or target lesions. The target appearance occurs much less frequently than in the stomach and duodenum.

Urine. The patient with malignant melanoma may develop melanuria in a small number of cases.

PROGNOSIS

The course of malignant melanoma is unpredictable. The metastatic involvement of the gastrointestinal tract is usually a reflection of widespread metastases and a poor prognosis. The majority of patients die within one year. McNeer and Das Gupta reported 99% mortality within one year of the first clinical evidence of visceral metastases, although long survivals have been observed from time to

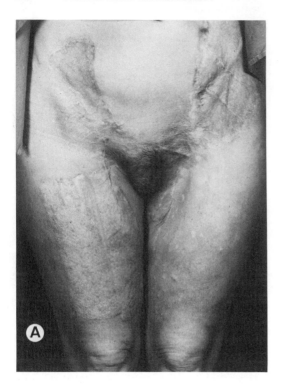

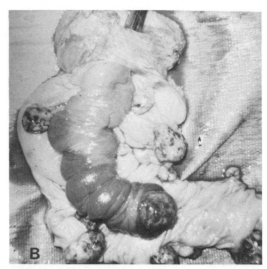

FIGURE 27–2A: A 48-year-old female patient with spontaneous involution of satellites of buttocks and thigh, showing leukoderma acquisitum centrifugum. B: Same patient presenting with an acute intussusception of the terminal ileum into the ascending colon. Specimen demonstrative of many polypoid melanomas in small and large bowel.

time.[28] Single polyploid lesions in general have longer survival rates than the multiple polypoid lesions.[40]

TREATMENT

Surgical intervention is required of patients presenting evidence of intestinal bleeding or obstruction due to intussusception of polypoid lesion. When the multiple polypoid lesions are present, resection of all the tumor-bearing areas, if possible, is desirable. Solitary infiltrative lesions on the other hand may involve more mesentery than is grossly discernible and, hence, resection should include a generous wedge of mesentery (Fig. 27–3).[26,40]

In many patients x-rays will not reveal metastatic lesions. Therapy should not be withheld because of lack of radiologic evidence. The management of such a clinical picture is essentially conservative, but it is important that if obstruction is present, it should be relieved. Segmental resection of the intestine with an end-to-end anastomosis or a simple bypass procedure is sometimes the treatment of choice. Segmental resection has not appreciably increased survival time in most patients. It is too early to assess the role of chemotherapy and immunotherapy in the management of metastatic malignant melanoma.

MELANOMA OF THE ANORECTUM

Anorectal melanomas are uncommon;[28] however, if one considers the size of the anal canal per square inch in proportion with the rest of the skin of the body, there is little difference in the relative incidence. Melanomas of the anus comprise about 0.25% to 1.25% of all

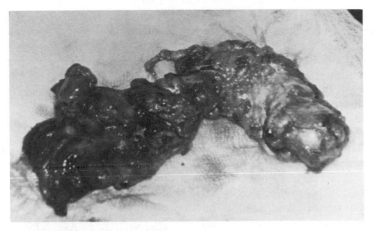

FIGURE 27–3. A 48-year-old primary melanoma of back removed 16 years before. An acute abdomen due to intussusception in two occasions. Patient living and well for four years after without evidence of melanoma.

malignant tumors of this region (Table 27–1). There is about one melanoma for every eight squamous cell carcinomas of the anus, and for every 250 adenocarcinomas of the rectum.[25,26,27,28]

Since the first report of a case of malignant melanoma of the anus by Moore in 1857, quoted by Pack and Oropeza,[28] about 200 cases have been reported. Of these, 17 cases have involved the rectal ampulla or the rectosigmoid colon without evidence of a melanotic lesion of the anus and anal canal; these cases are controversial as to the site of origin because they can originate in the area of transitional anorectal epithelium and are difficult to prove one way or the other.

Primary melanoma of the anal canal is well documented, but the validity of primary melanoma of the rectum is controversial. A lack of definition of accurate boundaries of the anal canal has promoted a barren controversy concerning the origin and location of melanoma of the anorectum. Mason and Helwig[24] believe that the melanomas that appear to begin in the mucosa of the rectum above the anus actually represent a form of submucosal spread proximally with a small primary lesion in the anorectum.

ANATOMY OF THE ANORECTUM

The lower anal canal is lined by squamous mucous membrane, and Hilton's line is represented by its junction with the anal skin. The adult pecten extends for 8 mm to 15 mm above this line. Melanin is present throughout the extent of the pecten, but gradually diminishes in amount from below up and is no longer present a short distance below the valves. The pecten ends at the anal valve, above which lies the transitional zone, covering the sinuses of Morgagni. There is a 3 mm to 11 mm zone of columns and si-

TABLE 27–1. Malignant Melanotic Tumors of the Anal Canal: Clinical Features

Total number of patients	20
Age (years)	
Youngest	34
Oldest	73
Mean	53.5
Primary (untreated patients)	8
Secondary (treated patients)	12
Metastasis to lymph nodes	6

nuses of Morgagni interposed between the rectal mucosa and the anal mucosa. This zone is lined by transitional or stratified columnar epithelium that bears islands of stratified squamous epithelium, but the transitional epithelium is not present on the surface of the columns of Morgagni. The transitional epithelium extends cephalad to the apex of the columns of Morgagni, where they form the "dentate line." This junction is complicated by two types of epithelium often with overlapping histologic characteristics. Mason and Helwig[24] concluded that, first, there is no histologic anorectal junction and, second, no histologic distinction can be made between tumors of rectum and anus when both arise from the columnar mucin-secreting epithelium.

The anal canal commences at the level of the levatores ani muscles and this site corresponds to the palpable anorectal ring, thus the cephalad portion of the anal canal is lined for 4 mm to 16 mm by mucosa of rectal type. Morson and Volkstadt[25] have suggested that these melanomas are the result of metaplasia or heterotopia, so the issue remains controversial. Thus, only a few instances of rectal melanoma that can meet the above criteria can be found in the literature.

MATERIAL

Twenty patients with melanoma of the anal canal were studied by Pack and Oropeza.[28] Because of their location in a region that is infrequently inspected minutely, melanomas of the anal canal, like melanomas of the genitalia,[29] are frequently overlooked. The chief symptoms are itching and bleeding, which are also common symptoms of such benign conditions as hemorrhoids and anal fistulas (Table 27-2). This similarity may mask the true disease and delay treatment. Of the twenty patients, fourteen (70%) had melanomas that originated in the anal canal, and the remaining six patients (30%) had lesions that originated in the anocutaneous junction.

TABLE 27-2. Malignant Melanoma Tumors of the Anal Canal: Initial Symptoms

Initial Symptoms	Number of Patients
Bleeding	9
Mass noted by patient	4
Pain	3
Itching	1
Other or unknown	3
Total	20

CLINICAL DIAGNOSIS

Pigmented nevi are seldom encountered or recognized in the anal canal. An accurate clinial diagnosis of melanoma is rarely made at the first examination, because it is not suspected. The final diagnosis is made by the pathologist, usually unexpectedly after the removal of what appeared to be hemorrhoidal tissue, anal tags, or polyps. Any pigmented lesion of the anal canal should be considered melanoma until proven otherwise under careful microscopic examination.

In amelanotic lesions the differential diagnosis will be between such benign conditions as hemorrhoids, fissures, anal tags, cysts, papillomas, and dermatitis. The chief malignant lesion in this region is the epidermoid carcinoma (Fig. 27-4). If the lesion is extensive and involves a great portion of the anal canal, it most probably will be an epidermoid carcinoma. Because of the polypoid appearance of melanomas, as compared with epidermoid carcinoma, patients often noted the appearance of a mass in the rectal outlet (often mistaken for thrombosed hemorrhoids), before seeking medical advice.

CLINICAL FEATURES

Age. It has been reported to have its onset at age 22, but the ages may vary from 22 to 85 years with most of the patients between 50 and 60 years; not different from other melanomas (see Table 27-1). One patient was

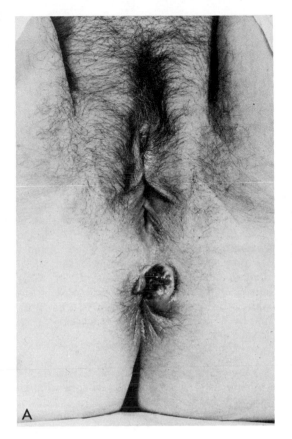

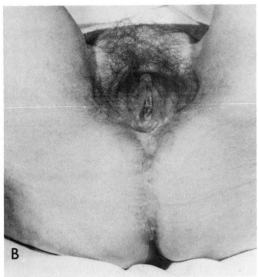

FIGURE 27-4A and B. Melanoma of the anus amelanotic in most of its surface, resembling an epidermoid carcinoma. Patient treated with an abdominoperineal resection and bilateral groin dissection.

pregnant at the time the melanoma became evident.

Sex. According to Morson et al., there are no differences in occurrence due to sex. However, in our series,[28] the ratio to women and men was 3:1, a disparity attributable to the fact that this was a relatively small series.

Race. As with other melanomas, most of the patients who contract the disease are Caucasian with sandy hair, blue eyes, and fair skin. Only five cases of melanoma of anorectum has been reported in blacks.[25] Only one case was a true primary melanoma of the rectum; while the remainder were of the anal canal. One man was described as a Latin American and one as a Puerto Rican. Only a few cases have been reported in the Asiatic In-

dian literature. In addition, one case has been noted in a Turk.[28]

Signs and Symptoms. The most common symptom (50%) is rectal bleeding, which may be spontaneous or associated with defecation. The other symptoms, in order of occurrence, are mass, pain, loss of weight, pruritis, and constipation or change in bowel habits. (See Table 27-2.) Pain evolves from frequent involvement of the anal sphincters. Rarely the disease manifests as an inguinal mass caused by a cryptic primary tumor with symptoms or signs indicating advanced disease.

The duration of the symptoms ranged from less than one month to 48 months with an average time of 8.1 months. In our series, nine patients (45%) had symptoms for three months or less. None of our patients described a history of any presence of a longstanding mole, and this hardly is surprising because of the inaccessibility of this region to inspection. None of these patients reported a family history of melanoma.

Pathology and Gross Appearance. Grossly, the tumor is polypoid and rarely ulcerated. The ulceration usually results from trauma of defecation and/or from surgical removal of lesions misdiagnosed as hemorrhoids. The size ranges from that of a small miliary nodule to the size of an orange. Generally the tumor is a single lesion but may be multiple. There might be satellites (Fig. 27–5) rather than multiple primaries. Most of the lesions (30 to 50%) are amelanotic.[28]

Histological Appearance. Anorectal melanomas are cellular and anaplastic. The cells are often polygonal and sometimes purely spindle. Rarely two types of cells are approximately equal in numbers—a mixed type. Multinucleated and polymorphous giant cells are common in melanomas; they are exceptional when found in cases of rectal adenocarcinoma and squamous cell carcinoma.

Junctional changes have been demonstrated in the anal squamous mucous membrane in 20% to 40% of the cases. The presence of melanocytes in normal rectal mucosa has not been accepted. In our opinion, these findings negate a rectal origin and favor an anal origin of anorectal melanoma.

The microstaging of Clark and Breslow for melanomas of the skin has no practical value in melanomas of the anal canal, because of the advanced stage of the disease when the clinical diagnosis is made and the few cases seen with this malignancy.

SPREAD OF ANORECTAL MELANOMA

Direct Spread. The tumor spreads upwards in the submucous plane of the rectus and pro-

duces submucous satellites and polyps (Fig. 27–5A).

Direct spread can occur to the perianorectal area, but it is rare. The reason why this is rare is probably due to the fact that the rectal fascia acts as a protective layer.

Lymphatic Spread. Lymphatic spread occurs mainly in three sites: along the superior hemorrhoidal vessels, lateral to the iliac and obturator lymph nodes, and via the perianal lymphatics to the medial superficial inguinal lymph nodes. Positive inguinal lymph nodes are less frequent in melanoma (14%) than in epidermoid carcinoma (42%) (Fig. 27–5B and C). On the contrary, positive mesenteric nodes are more frequent in melanomas (33% to 38%) than in epidermoid carcinoma (15%). Early spread apparently had been provoked by incomplete local excision and trauma from repeated defecation and infection. (Fig. 27–6).[26]

Venous Spread. The rich vascularization of melanomas, and the possible embolization by way of branches of the portal vein or inferior vena cava, explains the early spread of melanoma to the liver, which is the most frequent cause of death.

TREATMENT

The stage of the disease seems to be the most important factor affecting prognosis. The extent of the operation seems of little value in the final outcome of these patients treated by simple excision of the anal canal (Table 27–3).

CONSERVATIVE SURGERY

All nevi of the anal canal and anal region should be excised prophylactically and the specimen sent for microscopic diagnosis. If the excised lesion proves to be a melanoma, abdominoperineal resection of the rectum with

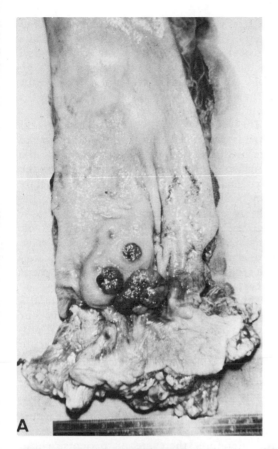

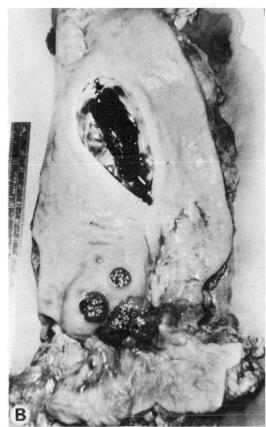

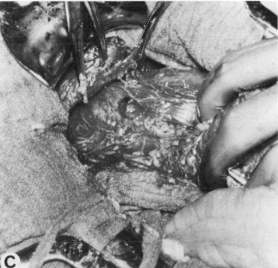

FIGURE 27-5A. Polypoid melanoma of the anorectal junction with satellites on the rectal mucosa. B. Same patient: Incision through rectal mucosa reveals metastasis on retrorectal lymph nodes. C. Metastasis to mesenteric lymph nodes seen at the time of an abdominal operation in the same patient.

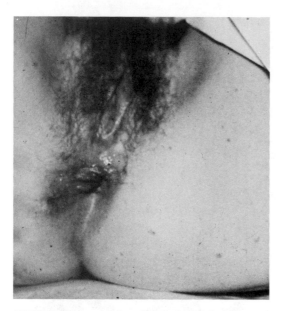

FIGURE 27-6. Anal melanoma with local spread following biopsy of the perianal skin.

TABLE 27-3. Malignant Melanoma Tumors of the Anal Canal: Previous Treatment

Initial Treatment	Number of Patients
None	2
Wedge excision or limited biopsy	1
Biopsy (type unstated)	3
Limited excision with local recurrence	6
Limited excision without local recurrence	5
Adequate excision without local recurrence	1
Desiccation and/or administration of caustics and local recurrence	2
Abdominoperineal resection	0
Totals	20

bilateral groin dissection is the theoretic treatment of choice. Whenever possible one should consider a less radical procedure, as the radical operation has proven to be ineffective to control most melanomas, especially if the pathologist demonstrates no invasion to the deep portion of the dermis.[28]

The prognosis for melanoma of the anal canal is influenced only slightly by the type of treatment regardless of the stage of the neoplasm; few patients' melanomas of the anal canal are diagnosed early enough before they become invasive and metastasize.

More often a palliative result is the most that one can expect (Tables 27-4 and 27-5). This highly malignant lesion will usually have extended beyond the confines of the pelvis and the regional nodes at the time that treatment is begun.

The medical literature reveals about 107 cases with long-term follow-up. Seventy-four patients were treated by radical surgical procedures. Five survived 60 months or more postoperatively. One of Pack and Oropeza's 20 patients lived longer than ten years (Fig. 27-7). The earliest case was reported by Esmarch in 1875 as alive and well 132 months postoperatively.[28] Of the 69 non-five-year survivors treated by radical surgery, as reported in the literature, there are 38 patients whose follow-up survival periods are reported, and average 12.1 months postoperatively. Similarly, 25 non-five-year survivors treated by local excision have a mean survival time of 16.4 months.

It is evident that melanoma of the anus is highly malignant and that treatment has little effect on the final outcome. Nevertheless, surgical extirpation of the primary lesion should be carried out in the hope of obtaining the rare cure and to prevent obstruction or bleeding. Pack and Oropeza,[28] in advocating abdominoperineal resection with bilateral groin dissection, the theoretic optimal form of treatment, state: "Its curative value is unpredictable and the likelihood of failure is great." For those rare cases that are perianal rather than located in the anal canal, a less radical operation is justified.

TABLE 27-4. Melanoma of the Anal Canal: Five-Year End Results According to Clinical Stages (1930 to 1965)

Stage	Condition on admission	Total	Living NED	Of melanoma	Other causes	Not treated or lost to observation	5 yrs. not elapsed
I A	Primary melanoma not treated or recent biopsy only	5	1	3		1	
B	Melanoma locally recurrent after improper treatment	8		3	2	1	2
II A	Primary melanoma not treated; lymph-node metastasis	2		1		1	
B	Primary melanoma controlled; lymph-node metastasis	1				1	
C	Recurrent primary melanoma; lymph-node metastasis	2		1	1		
III	Distant metastasis or disease advanced locally	2	—	—	1	1*	—
	Total	20	1	8	4	5	2

* Treated but lost to observation.

TABLE 27-5. Melanoma of the Anal Canal: Five-Year Survival Rate According to Type of Treatment (1930 to 1965)

Stage	Treatment	Total	Living, NED	Of melanoma	Other causes	Lost to observation	5 yrs. not elapsed
I	No treatment	2				2	
	Wide excision with unilateral groin dissection	2					2
	Abdominoperineal resection	3		3			
	Abdominoperineal resection with bilateral groin dissection	6	1	3	2		
II	No treatment	2				2	
	Wide excision with bilateral groin dissection	1		1			
	Abdominoperineal resection with bilateral groin dissection	2		1	1		
III	No treatment; exploratory laparotomy only	1				1	
	Unilateral groin dissection	1	—	—	1	—	—
	Total	20	1	8	4	5	2

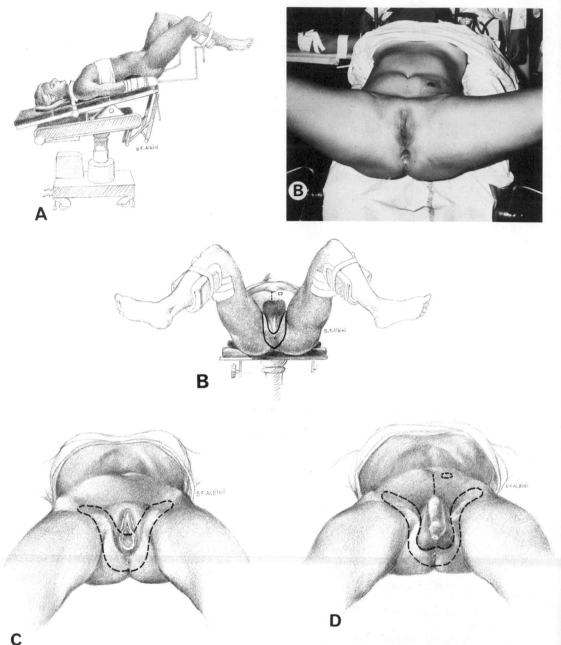

C

FIGURE 27–7A. Position of patient for synchronous two-team abdominoperineal resection and groin dissection. B. Perineal exposure (actual patient and sketch) for surgical team doing the perineal dissection. C. Scope of inguinoperineal incision in women. D. Scope of inguinoperineal incision in men. E. Transverse low abdominal incision for abdominal part of the rectal resection. F. Schematic outline of the lymph node dissection. G. Scope of pelvic and perineal resection. (From Pack GT and Oropeza R: A comparative study of melanomas and epidermoid carcinomas of the anal canal: a review of 20 melanomas and 29 epidermoid carcinomas 1930–1965. Dis Colon Rectum 10(3): 161, 1967.) **See facing page for Figs. 27–7E–H.**

FIGURES 27 E–H Cont.

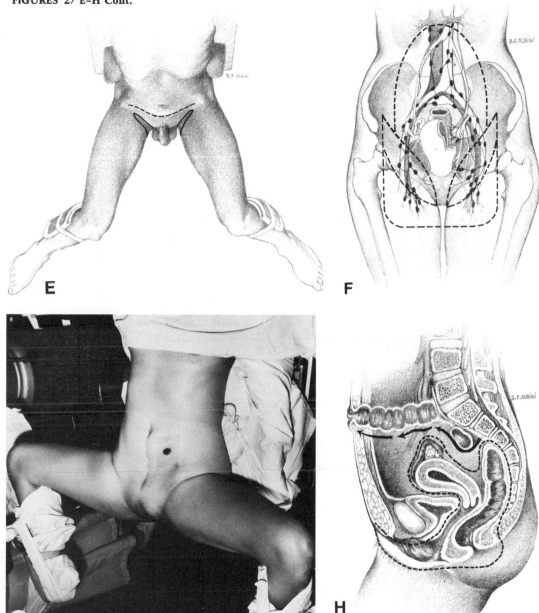

REFERENCES

1. Allen AC, Spitz S: Histogenesis and clinico-pathologic correlation of nevi and malignant melanomas: Current status. Arch Dermatol 69:150, 1954
2. Allen AC, Spitz S: Malignant melanoma: A clinicopathological analysis of the criteria for diagnosis and prognosis. Cancer 6:1, 1953
3. Alexander RM, Cone LA: Malignant melanoma of the rectal ampulla. Dis Colon Rectum 20:53, 1977
4. Basque GJ, Boline JE, Holyoke JB: Malignant melanoma of the esophagus: First reported case in a child. Am J Clin Pathol 53:609, 1970
5. Becker SW: Melanin pigmentation: A systematic study of the pigment of human skin and upper mucous membrane with special consideration of pigmented dendrite cells. Arch Dermatol Syphilol 16:259, 1927
6. Beeman JAP, Menne FR: Multiple primary melanomas of the small intestine. Am J Dig Dis 3:786, 1936
7. Booth JB: Malignant melanoma of the stomach. Report of a case presenting as an acute perforation and review of the literature. Br J Surg 52:262, 1965
8. Chandler AB, Jones GF: Malignant melanoma of the gastrointestinal tract. Am Surg 17:719, 1951
9. Chulani HL: Anal malignant melanoma. Dis Colon Rectum 20:6–517, 1977
10. Das Gupta TK, Brasfield RD: Metastatic melanoma: A clinicopathological study. Cancer 17:1323, 1964
11. Das Gupta TK, Brasfield RD: Metastatic melanoma of the gastrointestinal tract. Arch Surg 88:969, 1964
12. Das Gupta TK, Brasfield RD, Paglia MA: Primary melanomas in unusual sites. Surg Gynecol Obstet 128:841, 1969
13. De Castro CA, Dockerty MB, Mayo CW: Metastatic tumors of the small intestine. Surg Gynecol Obstet 105:159, 1957
14. De La Pava S, Nigogosyan G, Pickran JW, Cabrera A: Melanosis of the esophagus. Cancer 16:48, 1963
15. Fleming PE, Van der Merme SB: A case of primary malignant melanoma of the esophagus. Br J Surg 46:121, 1958
16. Frable WJ, Kay S, Schatzki P: Primary malignant melanoma of the esophagus: An electron microscopic study. Am J Clin Pathol 58:659, 1972
17. Garfinkle JM, Cahan WG: Primary melanocarcinoma of the esophagus. First histologically proved case. Cancer 5:921, 1952
18. Goldstein HM, Beydoun, MT, Dodd GD: Radiologic spectrum of melanoma metastatic to gastrointestinal tract. Am J Roentgenol 129:605, 1977
19. Goldman SL, Pollak EW, Wolfman EF: Gastric ulcer. An unusual presentation of malignant melanoma. JAMA 237:52, 1977
20. Hambrick E, Abcarian H, Smith D, Keller F: Malignant melanoma of the rectum in a Negro man. A case report and review of the literature. Dis Colon Rectum 17:360, 1974
21. Johnson EP: The development of the mucous membrane of the esophagus, stomach and small intestine in the human embryo. J Anat 10:251, 1910
22. Keeley JL, Rooney JA, Guzauskas AC, Brynjolfsson G: Primary malignant melanoma of the esophagus. Surgery 42:607, 1957
23. Klein A: Malignant melanoma of the anus. Report of 10 cases. Pol Med J 7:1113, 1968
24. Mason JK, Helwig EB: Anorectal melanoma. Cancer 19:39, 1966
25. Morson BC, Volkstadt H: Malignant melanoma of the anal canal. J Clin Pathol 16:126, 1963
26. Oropeza R: Melanomas of special sites in Andrade et al.: Cancer of the Skin. Philadelphia, WB Saunders Co, 1976, p 974
27. Pack GT, Martins FG: Treatment of anorectal malignant melanomas. Dis Colon Rectum 3:15, 1960
28. Pack GT, Oropeza R: A comparative study of melanoma and epidermoid carcinomas of the anal canal: a review of 20 melanomas and 29 epidermoid carcinomas (1930–1965). Dis Colon Rectum 10:161, 1967b
29. Pack GT, Oropeza R: A comparative study of melanomas and epidermoid carcinomas of the vulva: A review of 44 melanomas and 58 epidermoid carcinomas (1930–1965). Rev Surg 24:305, 1967c
30. Palma F: Malignant melanoma of the anus and rectum. Am J Proctol 21:271, 1970
31. Piccone VA, Klopstock R, LeVeen HH, Sika J: Primary malignant melanoma of the esophagus associated with melanosis of the entire esophagus. J Thorac Cardiovasc Surg 59:864, 1970
32. Pomeranz AA, Garlock JH: Primary melanocarcinoma of the esophagus. Ann Surg 142:296, 1955

33. Raven RW, Dawson I: Malignant melanoma of the esophagus. Br J Surg 51:551, 1964

34. Thomson H: A case of melanotic sarcoma with secondary growths of unusual size in the small intestine. Trans path Soc (London) 50:237, 1899

35. Sinclair DM, Hannah G, McLaughlin IS, et al.: Malignant melanoma of the anal canal. Br J Surg 57:808, 1970

36. Smith JL Jr, Stehlin JJ Jr: Spontaneous regression of primary malignant melanomas with regional metastasis. Cancer 18:1399, 1965

37. Stout AP, Lattes R: Tumors of the esophagus. In Atlas of Tumor Pathology. Washington DC, Armed Forces Institute of Pathology, 1957

38. Schrodt GR: Melanosis coli. A study with the electron microscope. Dis Colon Rectum 6:277, 1963

39. Treves F: Intestinal Obstruction. New revised ed: Varieties with their Pathology, Diagnosis, and Treatment. New York, William Wood and Co, 1899, p 268

40. Willibanks OL, Fogelman MJ: Gastrointestinal melanosarcoma. Am J Surg 120:602, 1970

41. Van der Veer EA, Kellert E: Melanotic sarcoma of the small intestine. Report of a case. NY J Med 17:335, 1917

42. Willis RA: The Spread of Tumors in the Human Body, ed 2. London, Butterworths, 1952, p 212

43. Zimmerman MJ: Sigmoidoscopy finding in melanosis coli. Report of an illustrative case. Gastrointest Endosc 15:56, 1968

CHAPTER TWENTY–EIGHT

MALIGNANT MELANOMA OF THE FEMALE GENITAL SYSTEM

IRVING M. ARIEL

Most melanomas of the genitalia arise from the mucous membrane surface areas, especially the labia minora and the clitoris. The mucous membrane is known to be the seat of melanocytes in many instances. Although the occurrence of the melanocyte in the vagina has been debated, that they do occur has been well documented and established.

Of the 3,305 melanomas in our series, 3% involved the female genital tract. This corresponds with the actual extent of skin of the external female genitalia, which represents 1% to 2% of the total skin area. This demonstrates no specific susceptibility nor immune factor for this site to develop melanoma.

At the Pack Medical Group, 45 melanomas of the vulva and three of the vagina were treated (Fig. 28–1). None arising from the urethra, cervix, or endometrium were observed by us. A large number of melanomas of the ovary were encountered but these were considered metastatic.

VULVAR MELANOMA

Nevi of the vulva represent 0.1% of all nevi afflicting the skin of the female.[43] Practically all vulvar nevi are junctional.[4] Melanoma of the vulva is exceeded in incidence by squamous carcinoma and accounts for approximately 10% of all cancers of this site.

Hewett[23] is credited with the original description of melanoma of the vulva in 1861. Since then approximately 376 melanomas of the vulva have been reported (Table 28–1). Thirty-eight instances of vulvar melanoma,

reported by Pack and Oropeza, were seen between 1930 and 1965. Between 1965 and 1975, seven additional vulvar melanomas were encountered, bringing the total number of vulvar melanomas treated by us to 45 (Figs. 28–2 through 28–4).

CLINICAL FEATURES OF VULVAR MELANOMA

Age. The mean age of the 41 patients reported by Pack and Oropeza was 56 years, the youngest being 15 years and the oldest 84 years. Among the seven patients seen since 1965, the average age was similar, 55 years, and varied between 20 and 65 years (Fig. 28–5). Six patients under 30 years of age indicate that the younger female after adolescence can be a candidate for developing malignant melanoma. No vulvar melanomas were observed before puberty.

Complexion. All of our 45 patients were Caucasians. Thirty-two were blondes, seven were redheads, six had brown hair. There were no Negroes nor Orientals.

Symptoms. The primary symptom was bleeding, which occurred in 38% of the patients (Tables 28–2 and 28–3). Pruritis was the complaint in 27%, and both bleeding and puritis in three patients (7%). Four patients stated that they had a mole in the region of the vulva, which they noted by squatting and looking in a mirror. The mole changed in size, becoming larger and, in one patient, more deeply

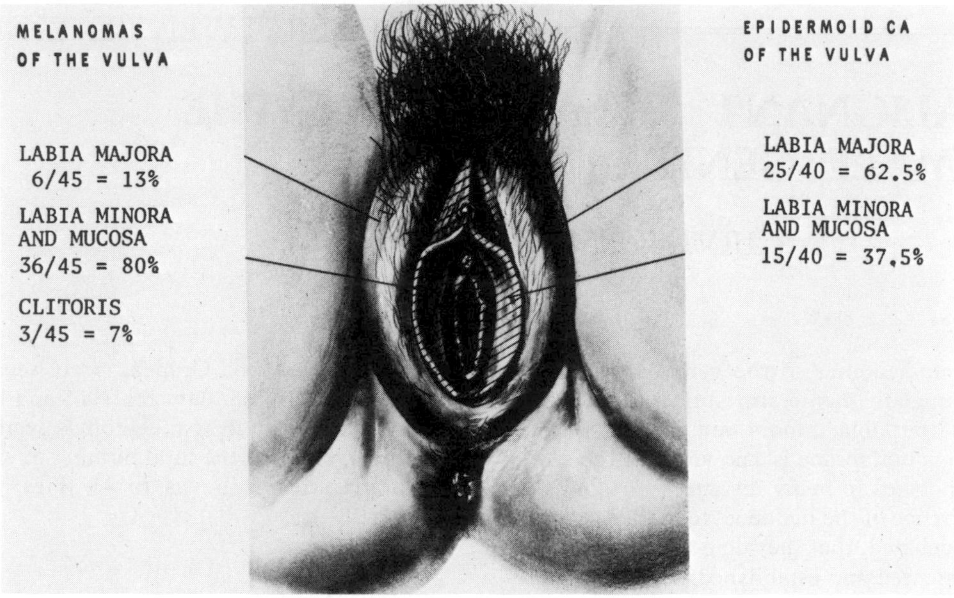

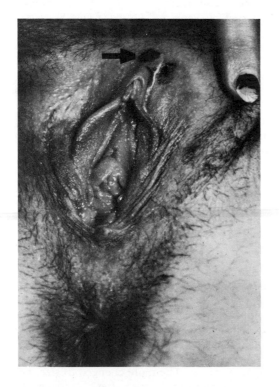

MELANOMAS
OF THE VULVA

LABIA MAJORA
6/45 = 13%

LABIA MINORA
AND MUCOSA
36/45 = 80%

CLITORIS
3/45 = 7%

EPIDERMOID CA
OF THE VULVA

LABIA MAJORA
25/40 = 62.5%

LABIA MINORA
AND MUCOSA
15/40 = 37.5%

FIGURE 28-1. Anatomic distribution of melanomas and epidermoid carcinomas of the vulva in the author's series.

FIGURE 28-2. Melanoma above prepuce; cryptic and discovered only after metastasis to groin lymph nodes made necessary a careful search for the primary lesion.*

* Figures 28-2, 28-3, 28-7, 28-9A-E are reproduced from Pack GT, Oropeza R: A comparative study of melanomas and epidermoid carcinomas of the vulva: A review of 44 melanomas and 58 epidermoid carcinomas (1930-1965). Rev Surg 24(5): 305-324, 1967 with permission.

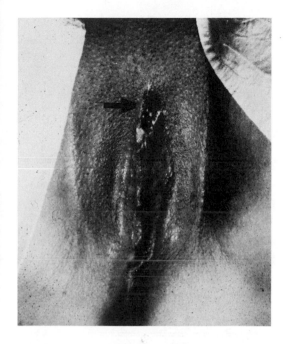

FIGURE 28-3. Melanoma of the clitoral prepuce causing bleeding and discomfort.

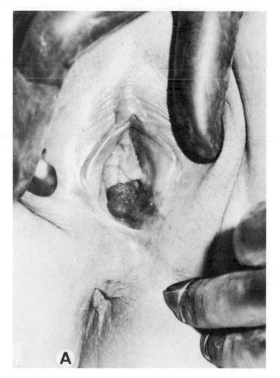

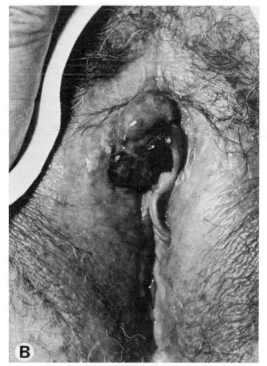

FIGURE 28-4A. Melanoma of the fourchette and extrahymenal mucosa. B. Bulky melanoma of the clitoris.

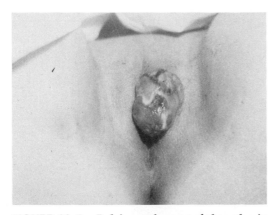

FIGURE 28-5. Bulging melanoma of the vulva in a 15-year-old girl. No response to irradiation as shown. Radical vulvectomy and groin dissection was eventually unsuccessful. Patient died 3 years later from local recurrence and dissemination.

pigmented. These changes caused the patient to seek medical advice. Eight lesions were detected by a physician on a routine physical examination, the patient having no idea that she suffered from a malignant form of cancer. Eleven patients presented themselves with a mass in the groin. In four (9%) the groin mass was associated with a subjective symptom of a vulvar lesion, whereas in seven patients the mass was present in the groin but the patient was not aware of a lesion in the region of her vulva (Fig. 28-2). In six patients there was no history detailed on the chart to permit evaluation. These data are not mutually exclusive.

Most lesions occurred in the labia minora (80%); fewer involved the labia majora (13%) and the clitoris (7%).

CLINICAL FEATURES OF MELANOMA OF THE VULVA

The majority of the malignant melanomas of the vulva were brown to black with various shades of pigmentation. The lesions were usually flat, occasionally nodular. They had a tendency to spread in a serpiginous manner extending peripherally throughout the entire circumference. On occasion, satellites were noted adjacent to the main melanoma. Often

TABLE 28-1. Reported Series of Vulvar Melanoma

Author	Year	No. Cases
Kehrer	1927	83
Ahumada	1953	48
Symmonds et al.	1960	19
Janovski et al.	1962	23
Das Gupta and D'Urso	1964	23
Pack and Oropeza	1966	38*
Yacket et al.	1970	20†
Cascinelli et al.	1970	14
Morrow and Rutledge	1972	39**
Fenn and Abell	1973	9
Ragni and Rabon	1974	6
Ariel	1978	45††
Chung et al.	1978	24
Karlen et al.	1978	23
Total		414
Less 38 cases reported by Pack & by Oropeza		−38
Total		376

* Excludes 3 vaginal melanomas.
† Excludes 9 cases previously reported by Symmonds and 2 cases of melanoma metastatic to the vulva.
** Excludes 1 case of melanoma metastatic to the vulva.
†† Includes 38 cases previously reported by Pack and Oropeza.
Reproduced with additions from Morrow CP, DiSaia PJ: Malignant melanoma of the female genitalia: A clinical analysis. Obstet Gynecol Surv 31:4, 1976, with permission of the authors and The Williams and Wilkins Co., Baltimore.

TABLE 28-2. Symptoms of 45 Vulvar Melanomas Pack Medical Group

Symptoms	Number	Percent
Bleeding	17	38
Pruritis	12	27
Bleeding and pruritis	3	7
Vulvar burning	0	0
Change in preexisting mole	4	9
Detected by physician	8	18
Mass in groin		
Associated with a known vulvar lesion	4	9
Without known vulvar lesion	7	15
Not stated	6	13

TABLE 28-3. Location of 45 Melanomas of the Vulva Pack Medical Group

Location	Number	Percent
Labia minora	36	80
Labia majora	6	13
Clitoris	3	7

an inflammatory reaction was noted surrounding the melanoma, producing an erythematous collar. The melanomas tend to spread superficially. Those invading the anterior vulvar region may involve the urethra and extend into the vagina. Metastases to the inguinal nodes were present in 30% of the patients (Figs. 28-6 and 28-7).

SURGICAL MANAGEMENT OF MALIGNANT MELANOMA OF THE VULVA

Any pigmented lesion in the region of the vulva or the skin adjacent to the labia should be locally excised for histologic evaluation. If diagnosed positive for malignant melanoma, the best treatment is radical vulvectomy with bilateral groin dissection including a generous portion of the surrounding skin, especially of the mons veneris. A wide removal of the skin, subcutaneous fat, and fascia and lymph nodes must be done with transsection of the Poupart's ligament and a resection of the deep iliac and obturator nodes (Fig. 28-8). The following structures are visualized prior to skin closure: the ischial cavernous muscle, bulbo cavernosis muscle, triangular ligament, superficial transverse perineal muscle, crest of the pubes, ilioinguinal ligament, aponeuroses of the external oblique muscles, and all the vessels and structures of Scarpas triangles (Fig. 28-9).

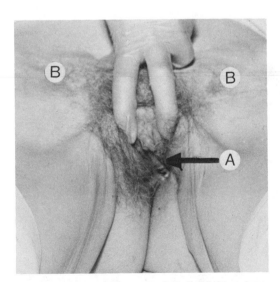

FIGURE 28-6. Melanoma of the left labia minora with clinically palpable bilateral inguinal metastasis. A—primary melanoma. B—metastases to regional lymph nodes.

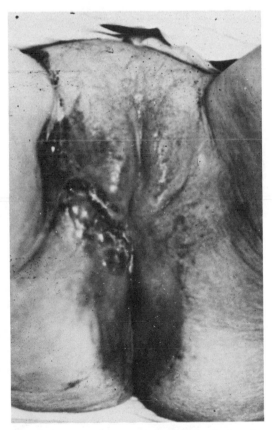

FIGURE 28-7. Advanced inoperable vulvar melanoma with extensive local and regional spread.

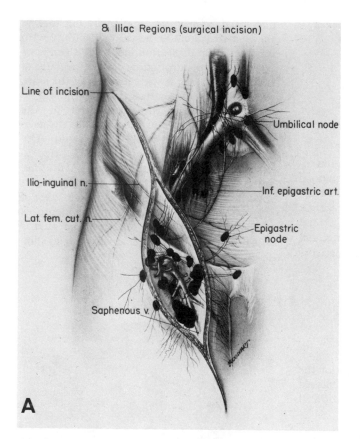

& Iliac Regions (surgical incision)

Line of incision

Ilio-inguinal n.

Lat. fem. cut. n.

Saphenous v.

Umbilical node

Inf. epigastric art.

Epigastric node

A

FIGURE 28–8A and B. Lymphatics of the vulvar structures.

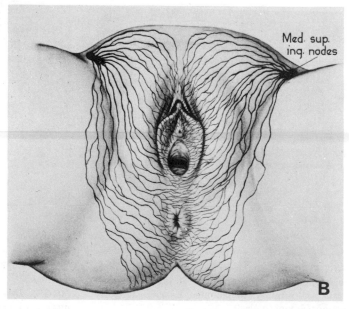

Med. sup. inq. nodes

B

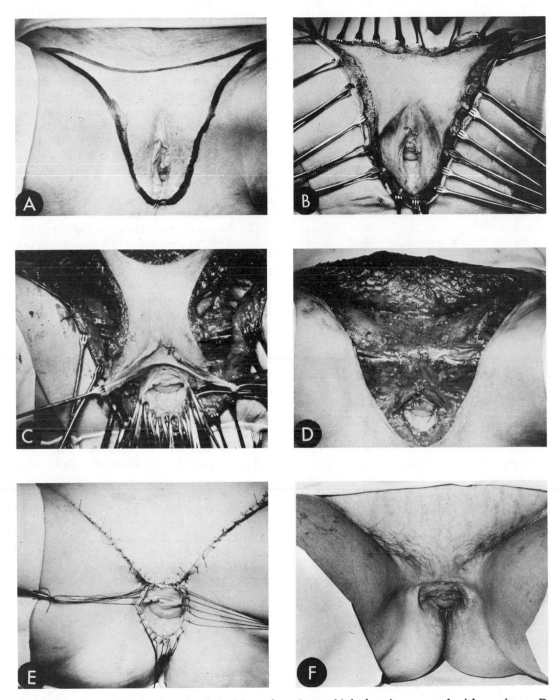

FIGURE 29-9A. Outline of regional incision of radical vulvectomy. B. Preliminary incision; clamps for traction to permit wide development of skin flaps. C. Dissection below fascia; muscles exposed. Outer third of vagina removed with specimen. D. Resultant wound. Bilateral groin dissection and removal of mons veneris. E. Wound closure. F. Final postoperative result.

It may be useful to utilize two teams in performing this extended operation. One team may perform the vulvectomy while another team performs one side of the groin dissection. At the completion of the vulvectomy the first team can then perform the opposite lymphadenectomy (Fig. 28–9).

If the vagina or urethra are involved, it is considered essential to perform a radical resection. A simple removal of the clitoris or a portion of the vagina or the terminal portion of the urethra practically never suffices. With involvement of the urethra or bladder, an anterior pelvic exenteration should be accomplished (Fig. 28–9). If a posterior lesion involves the rectum, a posterior pelvic exenteration should be performed.

RADIATION THERAPY FOR VULVAR CANCER

Radiation therapy was used by us during the early years. The moist skin of the vulva, and often the atrophy of the skin and the mucosa of postmenopausal women, do not permit large doses of irradiation without producing radiation necrosis and fibrosis. No cures were obtained from radiation therapy and this form of therapy for cure has been abandoned.

RESULTS

Pack and Oropeza reported a 35% five-year survival, but three of their patients who were alive with disease at the time of their report have succumbed (Table 28–4). An additional three patients died after the five-year period. They recorded 20 patients who were eligible for five-year survival. Since then 38 have become eligible for five-year survival. Twelve patients are alive and free of melanoma, placing the survival rate at 31.6%; not significantly different from their reported 35% five-year survival rate (Fig. 28–10).

Of the seven patients recorded after the previous report, five had lesions located in the labia minora, one in the labia majora, and one involving the clitoris.

Treatment consisted of radical vulvectomy with bilateral groin dissection in five patients; three of whom are alive and free of melanoma after a five-year period. One patient's treatment consisted of a radical vulvectomy and unilateral groin dissection involving the ipsilateral side, because she refused a bilateral groin dissection. The opposite side was treated with the endolymphatic administration of radioactive isotopes, and she remains alive and free of disease eight years after therapy.

Morrow and DiSaia[34] culled the literature and recorded 132 instances of vulvar mel-

TABLE 28–4.   Vulvar Melanoma 5–Year Survival

	Total Cases	Recurrent	Meta- static to Vulva	Total Fresh Cases	Eligible 5-year Survival	Alive 5 years	% 5-Year Survival
Das Gupta and D'Urso	23	0	0	23	23	7	30
Pack and Oropeza*	41	10	0	31†	20	7	35
Yackel et al.	31	2	2	27	20**	7	35
Morrow and Rutledge	40	9	1	30	14	7	50
Total	135	21	3	110	77	28	36.4

* Three patients died after the 5-year period.
† Includes 3 vaginal melanomas.
** Excludes 1 case metastatic to vulva.
Reproduced with changes from Morrow CP, DiSaia PJ: Malignant melanoma of the female genitalia: A clinical analysis. Obstet Gynecol Surv 31:4, 1976, with permission of the authors and The Williams and Wilkins Co., Baltimore.

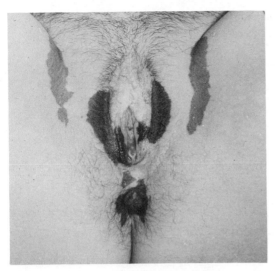

FIGURE 28–10. Benign perineal melanoses; observed for changes but otherwise untreated.

anoma of which 21 were recurrent, and three were metastatic to the vulva. In their report, 77 were eligible for the five-year survival analysis. Twenty-eight patients (36.4%) were alive five years after treatment. These authors call attention to the fact that of 95 potentially curable patients, only 72 (76%) received optimal therapy. They record three patients who developed recurrent melanomas more than five years after treatment. Two of these had only a vulvectomy as the primary therapy, and a third had occult metastasis with clinically negative pelvic nodes. Recurrences in these patients developed between five and one-half and ten years posttreatment, emphasizing the fact that the five-year freedom from melanoma is no absolute criterion for cure.

In the series at the Pack Medical Group, six patients developed either recurrences or metastases between the five- and ten-year period, all of whom eventually died from their melanomas.

Fenn and Abell[20] recorded a recurrence of vulvar melanoma 12 years after the initial treatment, with death ensuing five years after the recurrence.

At the M.D. Anderson Hospital, six of eight patients (75%) in stages I and II (Figo staging) survived five years, while only one of six patients in stages III and IV survived five years.[35]

Metastases to Groin Nodes and the Effect of Prognosis. A survival of 56.1% is recorded in patients where the nodes were free of metastases, which value declines to 14.3% when metastases are present in the groin nodes on histologic examination of resected lymph nodes.[35] Morrow and Rutledge record 2.2% occult metastases in the nodes of 45 patients, and Das Gupta and D'Urso[14] record 29.4% in 17 patients subjected to elective groin dissection. The series at the Pack Medical Group averaged 32% metastases to lymph nodes (Table 28–5).

Influence of the Size of Melanoma on Survival. In contrast to many cancers, the size of the primary melanoma did not seem to have an adverse effect on the prognosis, as noted by the Pack Medical Group, the M.D. Anderson Hospital, and the Mayo Clinic (Fig. 28–10). This resulted because most of those melanomas are superficial spreading tumors, and focus upon the need for a wide resection of the surrounding integument as part of the radical vulvectomy. An adverse prognosis is related to the presence of satellites, metastases to the regional lymph nodes, the extension of the melanoma to involve the urethra or the vagina, which involvement has often resulted in inadequate resection in the past. Once distant metastases have occurred, nothing can effect a cure.

MELANOMA OF THE VAGINA

Primary melanomas of the vagina are rare. In earlier literature their existence was doubted.[40] It is established that melanocytes do exist within the mucous membrane throughout the body, including the vagina. A classic example is that of Nicholson[37] who, in 1936, reported an instance of "epidermal heteromorphosis": a 1 cm area in the upper

TABLE 28-5.   Vulvar Melanoma: Survival Related to Metastases to Regional Lymph Node

	No. Cases	Groin Nodes			
		Total Pos.	Clin. Pos.	Occult Pos.	No. Bilat.
Das Gupta and D'Urso	23	13	8/23	5/17	1/12
Pack and Oropeza	28	13	—	—	—
Yackel et al.	27	7	—	—	—
Morrow and Rutledge	30	6	5/30	1/45	4/5
	108	39	13/53	6/62	5/17

	5-Year Survival			
	Pos. Nodes	%	Neg. Nodes	%
Das Gupta and D'Urso	1/12	8.3	6/11	54.5
Pack and Oropeza	3/11	27.3	4/5	80.0
Yackel et al.	0/7	0	7/16	43.7
Morrow and Rutledge	1/5	20.0	6/9	66.7
	5/35	14.3	23/41	56.1

Reproduced with changes from Morrow CP, DiSaia PJ: Malignant melanoma of the female genitalia: A clinical analysis. Obstet Gynecol Surv 31:4, 1976, with permission of the authors and The Williams and Wilkins Co., Baltimore.

vagina that contained two pigmented nevi within other epidermal structures. Norris and Taylor[39] reported two benign pigmented lesions of the vagina not associated with epidermal structures. Batsakis and Dito[9] demonstrated melanin pigment in 1 of 100 vaginal surgical specimens. Nigogosyan[38] found melanocytes in 3 of 100 vaginas from autopsy specimens. Junctional changes of the vaginal membrane adjacent to vaginal melanoma have been established.[4,18]

INCIDENCE OF MELANOMA OF THE VAGINA

At the Pack Medical Group, three malignant melanomas primary in the vagina were encountered in a total of 3,305 cases (Table 28-6). At the Armed Forces Institute in Pathology, only three vaginal melanomas were listed per 1,000 cutaneous melanomas. At the Mayo Clinic, from 1945 to 1960, only one malignant melanoma was encountered of 37 primary invasive cancers of the vagina. Morrow and DiSaia have tabulated 80 primary melanomas of the vagina recorded to 1974.

In 1978, Masubuchi et al.[31] reported four new instances of melanoma while Jentys et al.[24] reported seven patients and Deutsch et al.[17] reported five patients.

CLINICAL DATA REGARDING VAGINAL MELANOMA

The average age recorded was 55 years, varying from 22 to 80 years. The women were usually postmenopausal, and all were Caucasians. (Table 28-7).

The symptoms consisted essentially of vaginal bleeding or discharge. There were some complaints of a lump and pain, and a few of dysuria, nausea, and vomiting. Only one patient was asymptomatic. The duration of symptoms before treatment varied from a few weeks to one year, with an average of three months (Table 28-8).

TABLE 28-6. Incidence of Recorded Melanoma of the Vagina

Author	Year	No. Cases
Mino et al.	1948	15*
Ahumada	1953	7
Hauschild	1956	4
Freund et al.	1959	11
Mullaney	1961	3
Ehrmann et al.	1962	6
Stark	1963	1
Beyer and Chicano-Marcos	1965	2
Sesai and Cavanagh	1966	2
Koenig	1966	5
Collantes et al.	1967	9
Laufe and Bernstein	1971	3
Linthicum	1971	1
Daw	1972	3
Fenn and Abell	1973	2
Garcia-Valdecasas et al.	1974	1
Ragni and Rabor	1974	5
Ariel	1975	3
Total		83

* Excludes 3 cases considered cervical or vulvar in origin. Reproduced with additions from Morrow CP, DiSaia PJ: Malignant melanoma of the female genitalia: A clinical analysis. Obstet Gynecol Surv 31:4, 1976, with permission of the authors and The Williams and Wilkins Co., Baltimore.

PATHOLOGY OF MELANOMA OF THE VAGINA

Melanomas of the vagina may arise anywhere in the vaginal canal, but have a predilection for the lower half of the anterior surface. They may be small, pedunculated, and fungating, with ulceration and necrosis present. They may exist as a small polypoid lesion or fill the entire vagina. They vary in color from reddish brown to dense black. Six percent are amelanotic. Approximately 20% will have distant metastases when first seen.

RESULTS

Of the two patients reported by Ariel,[6,7] one was cured, with no evidence of recurrence, when she died from heart disease seven years

TABLE 28-7. Clinical Data Pertaining to Vaginal Melanoma Ages of Reported Cases

Age	No. Cases	Percent Total
20–29	2	4.1
30–39	4	8.2
40–49	11	22.6
50–59	13	26.6
60–69	11	22.6
70–79	7	14.3
80+	1	2.0
Total Cases	49	100.0

Reproduced with additions from Morrow CP, DiSaia PJ: Malignant melanoma of the female genitalia: A clinical analysis. Obstet Gynecol Surv 31:4, 1976, with permission of the authors and The Williams and Wilkins Co., Baltimore.

after treatment of her melanoma. The second was presumed cured, but died from metastases of a breast cancer to the liver seven years after treatment of her melanoma. Autopsy revealed local recurrence of the melanoma. Mino, Mino and Livingstone[32] reported a 28-year-old woman with a 2 cm melanoma of the lower vagina, which was treated by a wide surgical resection followed two and one half years later by a radical vulvectomy, partial vaginectomy, and bilateral groin dissection because of local recurrences, and she survives. A report of a 50-year-old woman with an ulcerated 2.5 cm lesion of the lower third of the anterior vagina was made by Casas et al.;[11] she received a radium implant for the local lesion plus a bilateral lymphadenectomy, which revealed metastases to the lymph nodes. This was followed by postoperative irradiation. Five years later a recurrence in the vagina and vulva was treated by radical surgery and the patient remains alive six years posttherapy.

TREATMENT

The best treatment for vaginal melanoma is radical surgery. Ehrmann and colleagues[18] examined the entire vagina of a patient who had only an 8 mm melanoma and found multiple foci of melanoma arising from large areas of

TABLE 28–8.   Clinical Data Pertaining to Vaginal Melanoma

Presenting Symptoms*	No. Cases	% Cases
Vaginal bleeding	29	64.5
Vaginal discharge (bloodstained in 6)	14	31.2
Lump	8	17.8
Pain (abdominal, pelvic, vaginal)	5	11.5
Dysuria	2	4.4
Nausea and vomiting	1	2.2
Asymptomatic	1	2.2

* Based on 45 cases. Some patients had more than one symptom.
Reproduced with additions from Morrow CP, DiSaia PJ: Malignant melanoma of the female genitalia: A clinical anlaysis. Obstet Gynecol Surv 31:4, 1976, with permission of the authors and The Williams and Wilkins Co., Baltimore.

junctional activity that involved most of the vaginal mucosa. Thus a radical hysterectomy and vaginectomy for lesions involving the upper third of the vagina is indicated (Fig. 28–11). For those involving the mid- and lower third of the vagina, a radical hysterectomy, vaginectomy, and ilio-inguinal node dissection is the preferred method of treatment (Fig. 28–12). In view of the fact that the upper third of the vagina may drain directly into the iliac and obturator nodes of both sides, it is preferable that the bilateral groin dissection be performed for upper vaginal melanomas also.

Anterior or posterior exenteration should be done if the cancer extends to the bladder or the rectum in the absence of distant metastases. Partial resection is unsafe. If a patient is unsuited for surgery due to medical reasons or refuses surgery, radiation can be useful. Although melanoma is a radioresistant lesion, it is radio-responsive and palliation can be obtained.

MELANOMA OF THE FEMALE URETHRA

Melanoma of the female urethra is extremely rare. Only about 40 instances have been reported. The rarity is emphasized by studies from the Mayo Clinic by Long et al.[29] where 77 patients had malignant lesions of the urethra among 700,000 female admissions; and of these there were only three primary

malignant melanomas, a ratio of 25 carcinomas to 1 melanoma. Morrow and DiSaia credit Reed[46] for reporting the first urethral melanoma in 1896. The average age was 64 years, varying from 32 to 80 years. Taylor and Tuttle[52] reported one case in a Negro woman, and Upton[53] reported one case in a pregnant female.

Rabon[45] recorded the only instance of a melanoma developing in an urethral caruncle. No primary urethral melanoma was found in the Pack Medical Group series.

Morrow and DiSaia report only five survivors in the literature. Two of these patients had recurrences before the five-year interval and both succumbed. An exciting case report is that of Das Gupta and Grabstald[15] concerning a patient who presented herself with an urethral melanoma and liver metastases and who has survived a five-year period without treatment.

Of the 42 patients whose treatment was recorded, Morrow and DiSaia state that in only ten could the treatment be commensurate with current standards of therapy, that is, a minimum of a wide local excision and regional node dissection. They indicate that two of the ten cases receiving radical surgery did so only after recurrences developed following local excisions. They further state that of the three patients who are five-year survivors, one received no therapy and two were subjected to radical surgery.

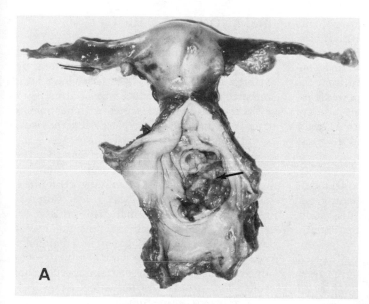

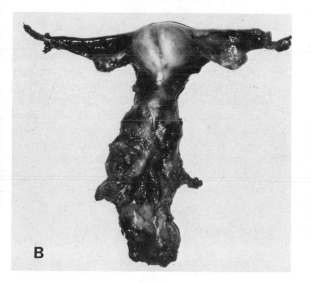

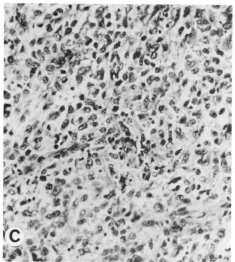

FIGURE 28-11. Vaginectomy and hysterectomy for vaginal melanoma. Patient cured; died 6 years later from heart disease. Autopsy showed absence of melanoma. A. Anterior view. B. Posterior view. C. Low power photomicrographic.

MELANOMA OF THE CERVIX

Melanoma of the cervix is also extremely rare, only 15 patients having been reported (Fig. 28-13). Simmons[48] in 1956 stated that melanomas of the vagina and cervix were always secondary to vulvar melanomas. Cid[13] reported that 3.5% of the cervixes harbored melanin-containing cells. Goldman and Friedman[21] reported three instances of melanotic nevi occurring in the uterine cervical stump. Associated junctional changes demonstrating the primary status of cervical malignant melanoma have been described.[1,25,49,54]

Treatment has varied from simple excision of the melanoma to radical hysterectomy.

Morrow and DiSaia reported only two patients living more than three years after diagnosis. One patient[52] lived 13 years after vaginal hysterectomy, although she suffered numerous recurrences and finally died from the melanoma. Jones et al. in 1971 reported a patient who remained free from cancer for five years but who suffered a recurrence 11 years postradical hysterectomy and died 13 years later. There has been no cure of a cervical melanoma by local excision.

The treatment for cervical melanoma should consist of radical hysterectomy and vaginectomy with bilateral groin dissection. Only three patients have had this treatment.

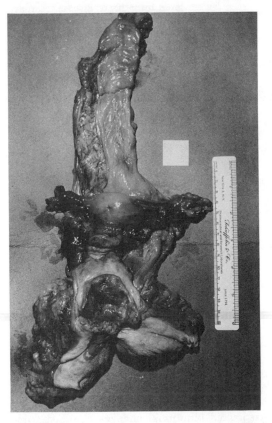

FIGURE 28–12. Surgical specimen of radical vaginectomy, hysterectomy, and bilateral vaginectomy for vaginal melanoma. Patient expired two and one-half years later from disseminated melanoma.

MELANOMA OF THE UTERUS

The first documented case of malignant melanoma of the uterus was reported by Schultz in 1957.[47] Only four cases have been reported, all affecting older women from 53 to 80 years of age who presented with postmenopausal vaginal bleeding. No patient has survived; the longest survival was one year.

An interesting feature is the fact that the melanoma, although containing abundant melanin, can consist of varying structures. Several authors described three different tissues involved in the malignant process: (1) endometrial adenocarcinoma, (2) solid areas of undifferentiated, nonpigmented malignant neoplasias, and (3) areas with irregular spaces lined by large melanin-containing epithelial cells. The stroma was not sarcomatous.[22a,47] One reported case contained areas of embryonic cartilage.[47]

A tumor reported by Cantaboni and Sabbioni[10] also contained gland-like structures. These cases could be mixed mesodermal tumors (malignant teratomas); and there is also a striking similarity to the retinal anlage (melanotic prognoma) tumor. The origin of these melanocytes is difficult to determine inasmuch as melanocytes have not been identified in the uterus, although Babes[8] has reported melanin in an endometrial polyp, which he suggests showed evidence of melanocyte activity.

MELANOMA OF THE OVARY

Primary melanomas of the ovary are so rare as to be oncologic curiosities. There have been only about 13 reported cases in the world literature that can be considered primary ovarian melanomas. The proclivity of many cancers, including melanomas, to metastasize to the ovaries precludes accepting many reports of primary ovarian melanomas. Another consideration is the fact that metastases may present many years after treatment of the primary lesion. For instance, Dawson[16] reported a metastatic ovarian

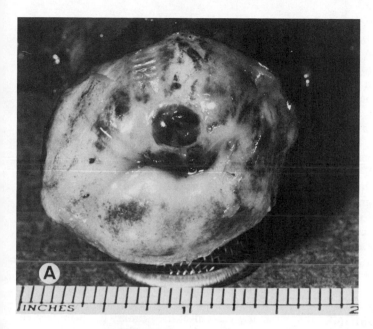

FIGURE 28-13A. Melanoma of cervix. B. Same, with intracervical spread. Whether this is a primary cervical melanoma or spread from a vulvar melanoma is unknown.

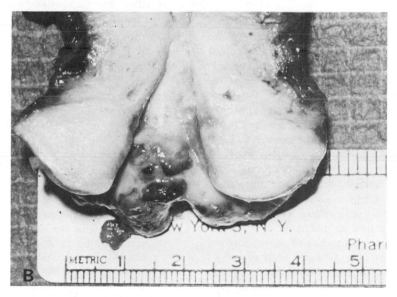

melanoma presenting 14 years after a primary melanoma of the choroid had been resected. Thiery and Willighagen[51] report a very long latent period before metastatic ovarian melanomas presented themselves. Often the primary tumor site may be unknown.

Another intriguing factor is the observation that ovarian melanomas may exist as part of a teratoid lesion. Inasmuch as the ovary does not contain melanocytes, per se, the identification of teratoid elements associated with ovarian melanoma aids in accepting ovarian melanoma as a primary tumor.[30,41] Of the 13 reported primary ovarian melanomas, six were associated with teratomas. A malignant ovarian melanoma similar histologically to the retinal anlage tumor has been reported.[22]

Benign melanotic tumors in the ovary have been reported. In one instance, a huge cyst contained melanocytes;[3] one was reportedly associated with melanuria.[50] A case of mucinous cystoma of the ovary with a melanotic deposit on the wall[50] has been recorded. Anderson and McDicken[5] published an instance of a benign melanotic ovarian tumor believed to be of neurectodermal origin and not of neurocrest origin, because the melanin-containing cells resembled retinal pigment cells more than melanocytes.

SUMMARY AND CONCLUSIONS

1. Malignant melanomas may affect the vulva, vagina, cervix, uterus, and ovaries. The oncogenesis of these tumors, and the origin of the melanocytes from which melanomas arise, are intriguing subjects that have been investigated extensively.

2. Melanomas of the genital tract comprise 3% of all melanomas afflicting females.

3. Forty-five melanomas of the vulva (1.5% of all melanomas) were treated by us; most by a radical vulvectomy and bilateral groin dissection. Thirty-two percent had metastases to the regional lymph nodes: The five-year survival is 31.6%. Indications for the various surgical procedures are discussed.

4. Malignant melanomas of the vagina are extremely rare; only 80 have been recorded; three have been treated by us. A total vaginectomy and hysterectomy of the Wertheim type and bilateral radical groin dissection is the treatment of choice. If the bladder or rectum are involved, an anterior or posterior pelvic exenteration is indicated. Cures are very rare. One patient of the three treated by us was cured, but the two others developed delayed metastases and local recurrences and died.

5. Melanomas of the female urethra are extremely rare, with only about 40 cases having been reported. Only five survivors have been reported.

6. Melanomas of the cervix present an unique oncologic entity, with only 15 patients having been reported in the literature. There have been no cures. A number of patients have lived many years before recurrences and/or metastases occurred, causing the patients to succumb.

7. There have been only four cases reported of primary melanomas of the uterus, all of which caused death within one year.

8. Melanomas of the ovary present a fascinating entity in cancer nosology in that 6 of 13 ovarian melanomas have occurred within teratomas. The exact number of true primary ovarian melanomas is unknown, inasmuch as many malignant melanomas from other sites will metastasize to the ovary, sometimes many years after the primary has been treated, or at times from an unknown primary site. Radical panhysterectomy and omentectomy is the treatment of choice. Whether any absolute cures of malignant melanoma of the ovary have been obtained is doubtful.

REFERENCES

1. Abell MR: Primary melanoblastoma of the uterine cervix. Am J Clin Pathol 36:248, 1961
2. Ackerman LV: Malignant melanoma of the skin. Am J Clin Pathol 18:602, 1948
3. Afonso JF, Martin GM, Nisco FS, de Alvarez RR: Melanogenic ovarian tumors. Am J Obstet Gynecol 84:667, 1962
4. Allen AC, Spitz S: Malignant melanoma. A clinicopathological analysis of the criteria for diagnosis and prognosis. Cancer. 61:1, 1953
5. Anderson MC, McDicken IW: Melanotic cyst of the ovary. J Obstet Gynecol Brit Common 78:1047, 1971
6. Ariel IM: Five-year cure of a primary malignant melanoma of the vagina by local radioactive isotope therapy. Am J Obstet Gynecol 82:405, 1961
7. Ariel IM: Malignant melanoma of the vagina. Obstet Gynecol 17:222, 1961

8. Babes A: Cellules pigmentaires rameuses dans un polype de la muqueuse uterine. Ann Anat Pathol 4:373, 1927

9. Batsakis JG, Dito WR: Primary malignant melanoma of the vagina. Obstet Gynecol 20:109, 1962

10. Cantaboni A, Sabbioni D: Contributo allo studio di melanomi a sede rara e controversa: tumore "melanotico" dell utero. Bull Soc Ital Pat 9:15 (fasc 1), 1965–66

11. Casas PF, Picena J, Garcia CG: Malignant melanoma of the vagina. Surg Gynecol Obstet 94:159, 1952

12. Chung AF, Woodruff JM, Lewis JL Jr: Malignant melanoma of the vulva: a report of 44 cases. Obstet Gynecol 45:6, June 1975

13. Cid JM: La pigmentation mélanique de l'endocervix. Ann Anat Pathol 4:617, 1959

14. Das Gupta T, D'Urso J: Melanoma of female genitalia. Surg Gynecol Obstet 119:1074, 1964

15. Das Gupta T, Grabstald H: Melanoma of the genitourinary tract. J. Urol 93:607, 1965

16. Dawson HGW: Melanotic sarcoma of choroid and ovary. Br Med J 2:757, 1922

17. Deutsch M, Fried AB, Parsons JA, Sartiano G: Primary malignant melanoma of the vagina. Oncology 30:509–516, 1974

18. Ehrmann RL, Younge PA, Lerch VL: The exfoliative cytology and histogenesis of an early primary malignant melanoma of the vagina. Acta Cytol 6:245, 1962

19. El-Minawi MF, Hori JM: Malignant melanoma in bilateral dermoid cysts of the ovary. Int J Gynaecol Obstet 11:218, 1973

20. Fenn ME, Abell MR: Melanomas of vulva and vagina. Obstet Gynecol 41:902, 1973

21. Goldman RL, Friedman NB: Blue nevus of the uterine cervix. Cancer 20:210, 1967

22. Hameed K, Burslem MRG: A melanotic ovarian neoplasm resembling the "retinal anlage" tumor. Cancer 25:564, 1970

22a. Hausman DH, Roitman HB: A malignant melanotic tumor of the uterus. Bull Ayer Clin Lab 4:79, 1962

23. Hewett P: Melanosis of the labium, and glands of the groin and pubes. Lancet 1:263, 1861

24. Jentys W, Sikorowa L, Mokrzanowski A: Primary melanoma of the vagina: Clinicopathologic study of 7 cases. Oncology 31:91, 1975

25. Jones HW III, Droegemueller W, Makowski EL: A primary melanocarcinoma of the cervix. Am J Obstet Gynecol 111:959, 1971

26. Karlen JR, Piver MS, Barlow JJ: Melanoma of the vulva. Obstet Gynecol 45:2, February 1975

27. Laufe LE, Bernstein ED: Primary malignant melanoma of the vagina. Obstet Gynecol 37:148, 1971

28. Leo S, Rorat E, Parekh M: Primary malignant melanoma in a dermoid cyst of the ovary. Obstet Gynecol 41:205, 1973

29. Long GC, Counseller VS, Dockerty MB: Primary melanoepithelioma of the female urethra. J Urol 55:520, 1946

30. Marcial-Rojas RA, de Arellano GAR: Malignant melanoma arising in a dermoid cyst of the ovary. Cancer 9:523, 1956

31. Masubuchi S Jr, Nagai I, Hirata M, et al.: Cytologic studies of malignant melanoma of the vagina. Acta Cytologica 19:6, 1975

32. Mino RA, Mino UH, Livingstone RG: Primary melanoma of the vagina with a review of the literature. Am J Obstet Gynecol 56:325, 1948

33. Mino RA, Livingstone RG, Hynes JF: Primary melanoma of the vagina. Ann West Med Surg 6:648, 1952

34. Morrow CP, DiSaia PJ: Malignant melanoma of the female genitalia: A clinical analysis. Obstet Gynecol Surv 31:4, 1976

35. Morrow CP, Rutledge FN: Melanoma of the vulva. Obstet Gynecol 39:745, 1972

36. Mullaney J: Primary melanoma of the vagina. J Pathol Bact 81:473, 1961

37. Nicholson GW: An epidermal heteromorphosis of the vaginal vault. J Pathol 43:209, 1936

38. Nigogosyan G, De La Pava S, Pickren JW: Melanoblasts in vaginal mucosa. Cancer 17:912, 1964

39. Norris HJ, Taylor HB: Melanomas of the vagina. Am J Clin Pathol 46:420, 1966

40. Novak ER, Woodruff D: Gynecologic and Obstetric Pathology, Ed 5, Philadelphia, WB Saunders Co., 1962

41. Otken LB: Primary melanotic sarcoma of the ovary. Am J Surg 55:160, 1942

42. Pack GT, Miller TR: The familial aspect of malignant melanoma. AMA Arch Dermatol 86:35, 1962

43. Pack GT, Oropeza R: A comparative study of melanomas and epidermoid carcinomas of the vulva: A review of 44 melanomas and 58 epidermoid carcinomas (1930–1965). Rev Surg (Philadelphia) 24:305, 1967

44. Park H, Kramer EE, Gray GF Jr: Primary malignant melanoma in an ovarian dermoid cyst. Am J Obstet Gynecol 106:942, 1970

45. Rabon NA: Malignant melanoma developing in a urethral caruncle. J Am Med Wom Assoc 19:855, 1964

46. Reed CAL: Melanosarcoma of the female urethra: Urethrectomy: Recovery. Am J Obstet Dis Wo Child 34:864, 1896

47. Schulz DM: A malignant melanotic neoplasm of the uterus resembling the "retinal anlage" tumors. Am J Clin Pathol 28:524, 1957

48. Simmons RJ: Melanoma of the vagina and cervix treated by radical surgery. Am J Obstet Gynecol 71:1137, 1956

49. Stegner HE: Uber melaninbildende pigmentzellen und pigmenttumoren der portio vaginalis uteri. Zentralbl Gynak 81:1686, 1959

50. Stewart JC: Benign melanosis: A supplementary report. JAMA 60:1358, 1913

51. Thiery M, Willighagen R: Melanoma of the female genital tract. Gynaecologia 161:466, 1966

52. Taylor CE, Tuttle HK: Melanocarcinoma of the cervix uteri and vaginal vault. Arch Pathol 38:60, 1944

53. Upton JR: Report of a malignant melanoma of the vestibule and external urethral meatus in a woman six months pregnant. West J Surg Obstet Gynecol 66:199, 1958

54. Wimhoffer H, Stoll P: Bericht uber ein malignes melanom der portio vaginalis uteri. Zentralbl Gynak 76:1840, 1954

CHAPTER TWENTY–NINE

MALIGNANT MELANOMA OF THE MALE GENITAL SYSTEM

IRVING M. ARIEL

The only organ of the male genitalia that harbors malignant melanoma is the penis, most frequently the cutaneous portion, and occasionally the mucous membrane of the urethra.

Although junction nevi, as well as other nevi, have been found frequently in the scrotum, no instances of malignant melanoma of the scrotal skin have been observed by us.

Only 40 cases of penile melanoma involving the skin, and only 12 patients with melanomas arising from the urethra have been recorded in the literature. The rarity of penile melanomas is emphasized by Das Gupta and Grabsted, who reported only two cases of penile melanoma seen at Memorial Hospital out of 1,200 patients with melanoma from various sites.[6] At the Columbia Presbyterian Hospital in New York, only one case of malignant melanoma was encountered among 83 patients with penile tumors, of which 64 were primary of the penis. The reason for its rarity is unknown, as it is far rarer than the amount of skin considered would indicate. It has been described in every race and in every continent including the United States, Europe, India, Malaya, and recently in Ireland. Four cases have been reported in Indians, one in a Malayan, one in a Thai, and one melanoma of the urethra was reported in a Chinese.

One melanoma of the terminal urethra was described by Girgis and colleagues in a Jewish male.[9] The only other cancer in their series involving penile melanoma in a Jewish male was a Kaposi sarcoma.

Melanomas are not generally observed in Negroes, but one malignant tumor of the penis which was treated by the author was considered by some pathologists to be a malignant melanoma of the penile skin. However, others considered it to be a squamous carcinoma (Fig. 29-1).

The first reported case has been credited to Murchison (according to Gross) in 1882.[12]

At the Pack Medical Group, only three malignant melanomas of the penis were observed. One presented with a large lesion with multiple sites of local spread (Fig. 29-2). This was treated by total penectomy and bilateral groin dissection, but the patient died of widespread metastases within one year. Another where the entire glans was involved was similarly treated without success. A third had a huge melanoma involving the glans with bilateral groin metastases. He was treated by surgery and preoperative and postoperative radium but died within three months from a "stroke" (metastases to brain) (Fig. 29-3).

AGE

The age of patients averaged from 30 years to 80 years, and the duration of symptoms varied from one month to three years. The old reports, such as those of Gould[11] and of Harrison,[15] describe symptoms whose duration varies from four to eight years, whereas in more recent reports such as those from Ellis and White[7] and Reid,[19] the symptoms lasted only from one to three months. This is probably the result of cancer education.

SYMPTOMS

Approximately half the patients described a dark brown lesion that had been present since childhood, remaining completely stationary in its biologic behavior until adulthood, when

507

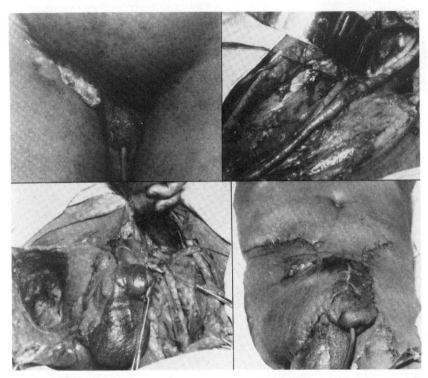

FIGURE 29–1.   Top left. Clinical appearance of extensive metastases to both inguinal regions in a 54-year-old Negro male whose penile melanoma had been treated elsewhere 1.5 years earlier by partial amputation of penis and x-ray therapy to inguinal regions. Note ligneous 10 cm size mass deeply infiltrating right inguinal region; fixity of the mass prohibited resection. A right hemipelvectomy was performed. Top right. Left radical groin dissection demonstrating the iliac and femoral vessels and the inguinal region stripped of the metastases to the lymph nodes. Bottom left. Left radical groin dissection and opened wound from previous right hemipelvectomy prepared for closure. Bottom right. Closure completed. Patient clinically free of evidence of melanoma six years after right hemipelvectomy and left radical groin dissection and was lost to follow-up.

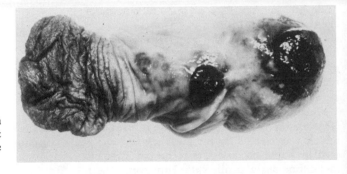

FIGURE 29–2.   Surgical   specimen after total penectomy for malignant melanoma of the penis with extensive local spread and satellitosis.

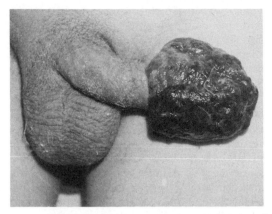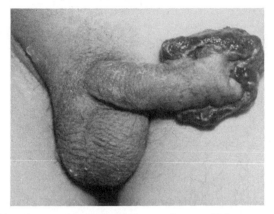

FIGURE 29-3.   The entire glans penis is invaded by a large exophytic malignant melanoma (right and left views).

the lesion increased in size, became more deeply pigmented, and slowly developed ulcerations with bleeding, and if it involved the prepuce, difficulty in withdrawing the prepuce.

In approximately half the patients, metastases will have occurred to the regional lymph nodes when the patient presents himself for treatment.

This history strongly suggests that the malignant melanoma developed in many instances upon a preexistent junction or compound nevus. As the disease progresses, patients complain of difficulty in micturition, fixation of the penis, making it immobile, and later, bleeding, especially on attempt to retract the prepuce. The glans penis is involved in most instances and more rarely the mucous membrane of the external urethral meatus. The coronal sulcus occasionally harbors malignant melanoma, but the shaft is usually spared from developing this form of neoplasm. Any pigmented lesion of the penis should be suspected of being malignant melanoma, as amelanotic melanomas have not been described for this organ.

Most melanomas vary in size from 2 to 4 cm, but a case reported by Roberts was 11 cm when the patient presented for treatment.[20]

Ocassionally, urethral fistulas may develop.

HISTOLOGY AND SPREAD

The histology is the same as that for malignant melanoma involving the skin anywhere. The question of origin of the melanocytes has been discussed at length, and the only questionable explanation is that of Batolo and D'Aquino who believe that the tumor may have arisen from cells of the nerve sheath. They are usually deeply infiltrating.

As the lesion progresses, it may spread by any one of the three usual routes: by local infiltration, which is a very common method, and microscopic deposits exist far beyond the confines that the surgeon thinks they do; by lymphatic spread, which is common; and by blood-borne metastases.

TREATMENT

The only treatment to date is surgical, and the best treatment is penectomy and bilateral radical groin dissection. Pack has advocated that if the lesion involves the glans or the external urethral meatus, a radical amputation together with bilateral groin dissection, which includes the inguinal, iliac, and obturator lymph nodes, should be performed with a permanent perineal urethrostomy. The metastasis may be to the deep iliac or obturator lymph nodes.

If the lesion involves the prepuce or the cutaneous envelope of the penis, a partial amputation of the penis with bilateral superficial groin dissection should suffice.

The most frequent error in treatment is to perform a partial amputation for melanoma of the glans or urethra, only to have signs of local spread to the penile stump present themselves at a later date. In a report from the University of Michigan, it is believed that inadequate partial amputation contributed to the eventual death of the patient.

However, Wheelock and Clark,[26] and Johnson and Ayala[16] report a ten- and a five-year cure, respectively, after only partial penectomy. Reid's 12-year survivor had only a local excision for multiple recurrences for the first 11 years before a groin dissection was done for inguinal metastases.[19]

There has been one report of endolymphatic isotope with ^{131}I lipiodol therapy, presented by Ellis and White, as a means of adjuvant therapy for metastases in the groin. (See Chapter 12.) Their patient remained well for over two years. Cascinelli[5] also reported a patient treated with ^{131}I ethadiol before performing the surgical procedure, but the patient died shortly thereafter of a heart attack, without evidence of melanoma.

PROGNOSIS

The prognosis is extremely poor, usually because the patient presents himself at a late stage, when local spread or metastases to regional lymph nodes or blood-borne metastases have occurred.

Two patients reported by Wheelock and Clark have survived for over ten years, and Reid reported one patient who survived over 12 years.

Orchiectomy and external irradiation have been tried without success.

Konigsberg and Gray have described an interesting case of benign melanosis of the glans, which involved practically all of the glans and which was originally misdiagnosed as malignant melanoma (Fig. 29–4). The patient has survived for 20 years after conservative therapy. A true penile melanoma seen by the same authors at the New York Hospital, New York, led to rapid death.

Melanomas arising from the urethra have been reported at different levels, including the meatus, fossa navicularis, and even the prostatic portion of the urethra. Posterior urethral melanomas warrant a pelvic node dissection along with a radical prostatectomy or prostatocystectomy, according to Konigsberg and Gray. No cures have been obtained as far as I can determine.

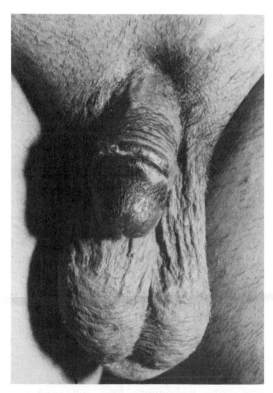

FIGURE 29–4. Benign melanosis of penile head originally considered a malignant melanoma. (Courtesy of Konigsberg HA, Gray GF: Benign melanosis and malignant melanoma of penis and male urethra. Urology 7(3):323, 1976. Published with permission of the author and The Williams & Wilkins Co., Baltimore.)

SUMMARY AND CONCLUSIONS

1. Malignant melanoma of the penis (skin or mucous membrane of the urethra) is very rare. Only about 65 cases have been reported.

2. It has been noted in all races and varying geographic regions. Only one questionable case has been observed in a Negro.

3. The treatment is surgical: Partial amputation and superficial groin dissection for melanomas of the prepuce; or radical penectomy with radical groin dissection for those of the glans and urethra.

4. The prognosis is bleak because the patient presents himself at a late stage, or because of surgical conservatism.

5. Improved oncologic education to the laity and a better understanding of the natural history by the surgeon may result in earlier diagnosis, more adequate treatment, and a better prognosis.

REFERENCES

1. Abeshouse BS: Primary and secondary melanoma of the genitourinary tract. South Med J 51:994, 1958
2. Banchieri FR, Gallizia G, Grandinetti C: Un cas de mélanome primitif de pénis. J Urol Nephrol 77:138, 1971
3. Batolo D, D'Aquino S: Melanoma del glande, Arch Ital Patol Clin Tumori 2:285, 1958
4. Bracken RB, Diokno AC: Melanoma of the penis and the urethra: 2 case reports and review of the literature. J Urol 111:198, 1974
5. Cascinelli N: Malignant melanoma of the penis. Tumori 55:313, 1969
6. Das Gupta T, Grabsted H: Melanoma of the genito-urinary tract. J Urol 93:607-614, 1965
7. Ellis H, White WF: Malignant melanoma of the penis. Endolymphatic therapy with ^{131}I Lipiodol. Br J Surg, 55:238-241, 1968
8. Fronstin MH, Hutcheson JB: Malignant melanoma of the penis. A report of two cases. Br J Urol 41:324-326, 1969
9. Girgis AS, Bergman H, Rosenthal H, Solomon L: Unusual penile malignancies in circumcised Jewish men. J Urol 110:696, 1973
10. Gojaseni P, Nitiyant P: Malignant melanoma of the penis. Br J Urol 44:143-146, 1972
11. Gould AP: A case of melanotic epithelioma of the penis. Amputation; Remarks. Lancet 1:438-439, 1880
12. Gross SD: A System of Surgery, ed 6, vol 2, Philadelphia, H. C. Lea, 1882, p 834
13. Guinn GA, Ayala AG: Male urethral cancer. J Urol 103:175, 1970
14. Gursel EO, Georgountzos C, Uson AC, et al.: Penile cancer. Urology 1:6, 1973
15. Harrison FG: Malignancies of the penis and urethra. Clinics 3:20, 1944
16. Johnson DE, Ayala AG: Primary melanoma of the penis. Urology 2:174, 1973
17. Konigsberg HA, Gray GF: Benign melanosis and malignant melanoma of penis and male urethra. Urology 7:3, 1976
18. Pack GT, Ariel IM: Treatment of Cancer and Allied Diseases. ed 2, vol 5. New York, Paul B Hoeber, 1962, pp 10-21
19. Reid JD: Melanocarcinoma of the penis: report of a case. Cancer 10:359, 1957
20. Roberts DI: Massive melanoma of the penis occurring in a Malayan. Br J Surg 39:561-568, 1952
21. Sampat MB, Sirsat MV: Malignant melanoma of the skin and mucous membranes in Indians. Indian J Cancer 3:4, 1966
22. Shanik GD, Jagoe SW: Case report: Malignant melanoma of the penis. Irish J Med Sci 145:6, 1976
23. Sirsat MV, Shrikande SS: Malignant melanoma of the penis in Indians: A report of two cases. Indian J Pathol Bacteriol 7:3, 1965
24. Talerman A: Malignant melanoma of the penis. Urol Int 27:66-80, 1972
25. Thomas JA, Fenn AS: Malignant melanoma of the penis: A report of a case and review of the literature. Indian J Pathol Bacteriol 10:372, 1969
26. Wheelock MC, Clark PJ: Sarcoma of the penis. J Urol 49:479, 1943

CHAPTER THIRTY

MALIGNANT MELANOMA INVOLVING THE CENTRAL NERVOUS SYSTEM

IRVING M. ARIEL

The central nervous system is involved by pigmented lesions, which can be divided into three categories: benign pigmentation (melanosis), primary malignant melanomas, and metastatic malanomas.

NEUROCUTANEOUS MELANOSIS SYNDROME

This is a nonfamilial disturbance characterized by giant pigmented nevi of the skin and melanosis of the leptomeninges. Malignant mclanomas may develop both in the cutaneous lesions and/or the central nervous system. Those that arise in the central nervous system are either pure melanomas or small-cell primitive neoplasms that usually show tumor cells with cytoplasmic melanin. Pigmented lesions of the skin are usually very extensive, producing the bathing trunk nevus or the garment nevus. They tend to spread over the posterior surface of the trunk and are frequently multiple. Benign leptomeningeal lesions show numerous melanocytes histologically, or clusters of small cells that resemble nevus cells. Perivascular collections of cells containing a great deal of pigment are often found, which resemble melanophores rather than melanocytes. The medulla is the most frequent part of the brain involved, but clusters of pigmented areas can be found elsewhere. Portions of the lesions may resemble a malignant schwannoma.

This disturbance often occurs in children, and unless a melanoma develops the pigmentation is usually harmless. Malignant mela-

nomas do occur in over half of these instances, and when they occur in the brain they are nearly always fatal.

Treatment, where possible, consists of attempted resection, but since the medulla is often involved, the resection is either impossible or unsuccessful.

PRIMARY MELANOMA OF THE CENTRAL NERVOUS SYSTEM

Primary melanomas of the brain are extremely rare and the treatment fraught with failure. Those arising within the spinal canal appear to be more frequent. Virchow[36] is credited with recording the first instance of a spinal cord melanoma in 1859. Kiel, Starr, and Hanson, in 1961, reviewed the world literature and cited 112 instances of melanoma of the central nervous system.[18] They recorded 41 examples of primary melanoma of the spinal cord, of which 22 were found at autopsy and 19 at operation. A report of Touraine in 1949 contains 66 cases of abnormal meningeal pigmentation, some of which were simple pigmentation and others were primary melanomas.[35] Lin and Cook[21] recorded two instances of primary melanoma of the spinal cord. They summarize the clinical features, and call attention to the long-term survival that may characterize primary melanomas of the spinal cord. They call attention to the fact that in order for the tumor to be labelled a primary melanoma of the spinal cord, evidence must exist to preclude it being metastatic. This is pertinent, because many of the patients do complain of various numbers and degrees of atypism in cutaneous lesions.

Primary tumors of the spinal cord seem to behave differently from melanomas of the skin or mucous membrane, in that there is usually a long survival period after removal of the lesion. Also, anaplasia is not a common finding on histologic examination. In fact, the tumors may have a benign appearance. There is no recorded case where a melanoma of the spinal cord produced a widespread dissemination. In approximately 120 recorded cases of primary meningeal melanomas of the spinal cord, males predominated in a ratio of 2:1. The melanomas were found in patients from 5 to 85 years, but were most common in the third and fourth decade. The only symptom that usually existed was that of increased cranial pressure, and the physical findings associated with this were those that presented themselves clinically. Increased protein in the cerebrospinal fluid could be noted, and a melanogen test of the spinal fluid was occasionally suggestive of the diagnosis as stressed by Nikonova and Usova.[27] The cells of origin are believed to be those arising from the neural crest. Rawles[28] has demonstrated in mice that only tissues containing neural crest elements can produce pigment. She demonstrated the migration of neural crest tissue to the epidermis, iris, and choroid of the eye and leptomeninges. Others believe that the meningeal sensory nerve endings, which are derived from the neural crest, are the pigmented cells that give rise to melanomas.

An interesting feature of leptomeningeal melanomas is the fact that two have been recorded in children (one by Touraine[35] and one by Spens et al.[34]) in which the histologic picture was truly malignant and the same as those seen in adult patients. They were not similar to the juvenile melanomas described by Spitz. This finding suggests that there may be some difference in response to hormonal stimulation between meningeal melanomas and those arising in the skin.

Meningeal melanomas are not infrequently associated with increased pigmentation or numerous lentigos or nevi. The prognosis is usually good, and patients who have had melanomas of the spinal cord removed have enjoyed good health for prolonged periods,

with a significant number surviving over ten years.

Lin and Cook[21] stress the need for total excision of the tumor without disruption and local dissemination of the tumor cells inasmuch as melanomas of the spinal cord, like melanomas elsewhere, do not have a strong cohesion between the melanoma cells. The cells are rather loosely packed and easily disrupted, and this permits local escape with resultant local recurrences.

Limas and Tio[19] reported a melanotic tumor of the leptomeninges with prolonged clinical course and benign histology. It was studied by light and electron microscopy. Similar tumors referred to as *pigmented* or *melanotic* meningiomas were also reviewed. They stress the fact that these tumors are characterized by the presence of numerous melanosomes and premelanosomes in their cytoplasm, and conclude that the term *meningeal melanocytoma* rather than *pigmented meningioma* is appropriate. They further stress that the benign histology and the favorable clinical course distinguish the meningeal melanocytoma from primary malignant melanomas of the leptomeninges. They call attention to the fact that the ultrastructure and behavior show similarities to melanocytic tumors of the dermis (the cellular blue nevus) and the uveal tract (spindle A melanomas). Although the tumors are cytologically and biologically benign, these tumors may cause neurologic disturbances through expanding growth, and early excision can be curative before a neurological complication becomes manifest.

The meningeal melanocytoma should be differentiated from melanotic meningeal lesions, which are the commonest, since melanomas comprise 12% to 16% of all tumors metastatic to the central nervous system.

Verma[35a] and colleagues reported a case of a meningeal melanocytoma in a 71-year-old woman treated by surgical excision. They believed that the surgery altered the blood-brain barrier and accordingly treated the patient with chemotherapy (dactinomycin and dacarbazine) supplemented by immunotherapy (intravenous *C. parvum*). After one year the patient was free of evidence of melanoma and all objective tests were negative. Treatment was discontinued. Three months later symptoms of recurrence developed.

It is problematic if continuation of the chemo/immunotherapy could have prevented the relapse.

METASTATIC MELANOMA TO THE BRAIN

The incidence of metastases to the brain in different series varies from practically one-third of autopsy cases to one-half of the patients who die of malignant melanoma. Das Gupta and Brasfield[8] recorded 39% of 105 autopsied patients who had metastases to their brain, and Einhorn et al.[9] recorded 54% of 85 autopsied.

At the Pack Medical Group, the incidence of metastases to the brain was 38% of 150 autopsied cases in which the brain was examined. Moseley, Nizze, and Morton,[26] from the University of California, Los Angeles Division, reviewed 712 patients seen since 1971. Twenty of these patients presented themselves with metastases to the brain and an additional 12 patients developed metastases to the brain simultaneously with other organ involvement (Fig. 30-1). Of those patients who developed dissemination, 2.8% developed brain metastases as a sole evidence of dissemination. Four of these patients (1.6% of all stage III patients) presented with a catastrophic event, such as a stroke or a seizure, with no antecedent symptoms. One of these patients presented with a seizure 19 years after excision of her primary tumor. In addition to the patients with brain metastases as the only evidence of tumor dissemination, 12 other patients (4.8%) had brain metastases diagnosed simultaneously with other organ involvement. Of the patients available for Clark's level of infiltration, three had level III melanoma, six had level IV, and one had level V. The symptoms of the patients, who presented without a catastrophic event, in decreasing order of frequency were: anorexia, nausea, vomiting, motor weakness, equilibrium disturbances, headache, parathesias,

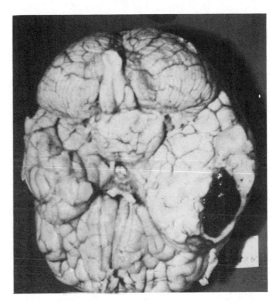

FIGURE 30-1. Example of metastatic melanoma to brain.

memory disturbances, visual disturbances, and pain.

The importance of metastases to the brain, presenting as a catastrophic event, is particularly significant as pertains to aircraft accidents. Bulcy[4] reported 17 cases of airline pilot incapacitation of which 16 of the 17 resulted from myocardial infarction. Harper et al.,[15] in the United Airlines study, in simulated incapacitation stated that the etiology, in decreasing order of frequency, was: reactive hypoglycemia, coronal cerebral atrophy, psychologic reactions, and early brain tumors. One case of a spontaneous subarachnoid hemorrhage from an unsuspected metastatic malignant tumor arising from the testis was recorded by Mason.[23]

A review of metastases of melanoma to the brain does not reveal any predominant site of harboring metastases.

The above focuses the need to consider a possible metastasis in any patient suffering from malignant melanoma or one who has previously been treated for melanoma who develops brain symptoms. This is emphasized by a study by Conrad et al.[7] from the Air Force Central Tumor Registry, who found that 7%

of patients with recurrent cancer, or 1.9% of their total series, presented with the first evidence of recurrent cancer in the central nervous system. They emphasized the fact that they were unable to document a single catastrophic event without prior symptoms suggestive of central nervous system involvement for days or even months prior to the development of seizure or stroke. They concluded that although metastases to the brain is a common site for cancer including malignant melanoma, the possibility of an occult metastasis causing a sudden catastrophe is extremely remote. They could not find a single case in the 640 patients of the Air Force Tumor Registry over a 20-year period.

TREATMENT OF METASTATIC MELANOMA TO THE BRAIN

The treatment of metastatic melanoma to the brain is usually unsuccessful. We have had good, but very temporary, results by immediately giving large doses of a diuretic and cortisone to reduce intracranial pressure and inflammation. One such patient, who was admitted unconscious, in six hours regained full consciousness and all sensory and motor activities, only to regress with no response from chemotherapy. Most of the chemotherapeutic agents used for treatment of metastatic cancer do not transgress the blood–brain barrier, and we have seen instances of temporary regression after a course of cancer chemotherapy in metastases to the skin, lymph nodes, and liver, only to have the metastases to the brain increase in size. A drug such as mithramycin, which does transgress the blood–brain barrier, may be used but it has not shown any outstanding effect upon malignant melanoma.

We have used intracarotid artery infusion of phenylalanine mustard and other chemotherapeutic agents with temporary but not significant response. Simon,[33] from Mount Sinai Hospital, has recorded the intracarotid artery injection of Yttrium-90 microspheres in the treatment of malignant tumors to the brain without any obvious hazard, and with slight benefit.

One of our patients who developed melanoma to the brain was treated by a resection of the melanoma, after which gelfoam soaked in radioactive chromic phosphate was inserted into the operative defect to give superficial irradiation to the neighboring tissue. The response was transient and the patient died within two months.

McGovern[25] has stated:

Metastases to the brain do not respond to immunotherapy and it also frequently happens that patients who have had metastatic disease in other sites which respond initially to immunotherapy, will come back in less than two years with cerebral metastases.

We have treated one patient who had a malignant melanoma develop upon a Hutchinson's freckle, which was treated by systemic DTIC and the local lesion treated by interstitial BCG. A good response was manifested by the lesion of the face, but huge metastases to regional lymph nodes developed with metastases to the brain, which killed the patient during the time that the initial lesion was regressing.

Clark[5] has reported 47 patients with metastases to the central nervous system. Of these, 26 received whole brain radiotherapy, and most received concomitant dexamethasone. An objective response was seen in eight of these patients and the median survival was five months.

Accordingly it may be stated that no adequate form of therapy is available to date for the treatment of metastatic melanoma to the brain, either as the only evidence of metastases or as one organ involved by bloodborne dissemination.

Gottlieb, Frei, and Luce,[12] reporting from the M.D. Anderson Hospital, recorded 41 patients with cerebral metastases of malignant melanoma. The patients were treated by radiotherapy, and some with combination chemotherapy and radiotherapy. The patients received a median tumor dose of 3,000 rads delivered to the entire brain over a two-week period. Twenty-four of the patients received concomitant chemotherapy and cortico-steroids, and 14 others received either chemotherapy or corticosteroids alone. The median and mean survival from completion of irradiation for all patients was 86.5 days and 103 days respectively, ranging from 4 to 436 days. Sixteen patients (39%) showed definite neurologic improvement and had a median survival of 131 days. The median survival of the 25 unresponding patients was only 17 days (p < .002). The median duration of improvement was 60 days (range 80–465 days). The most frequently seen response was return of limb function, disappearance of confusion, somnolence and coma, and cessation of headache, nausea, and vomiting. There was no statistical difference in the survival of patients receiving chemotherapy and/or cortico-steroids compared with those patients not receiving these agents.

Bremer, West, and Didolkar[3] reported on 32 patients from the Roswell Park Hospital in New York with metastatic malignant melanoma to the brain. Nineteen received craniotomy for removal of their tumor, and 13 were considered inoperable. Following intracranial surgery, neurologic defects were observed in 14 (74%) and the median survival was five to six months for the surgical group. The nonsurgical group with multiple metastases and multiple visceral involvement did not survive beyond a median of one month. Intratumor hemorrhage was present in seven (41%) of their 17 craniotomies, and intratumor hemorrhage was found at autopsy in 59% of the entire series. Two of these patients received chemotherapy after craniotomy and developed fatal intracranial hemorrhage. Their conclusion was that the patient with a single metastasis to the brain would benefit from surgical intervention. Six of their patients subjected to surgery (32%) survived from 8 to 15 months, and only one patient remains alive at the time of their writing (an average of 47 months[1] total survival time), and he is currently fully employed. They stress the early detection of metastases by the newer techniques of isotopic scanning and CAT scanning so that definitive surgery may be undertaken earlier than has been the custom in the past.

REFERENCES

1. Becker SM: Primary melanoma of the leptomeninges of the spinal cord. J Med Society of New Jersey 67:271–275, 1970.
2. Beresford HR: Melanoma of the nervous system: Treatment with cortico-steroids and radiation. Neurology 19:59–65, 1965
3. Bremer AM, West CR, Didolkar MS: An evaluation of the surgical management of melanoma of the brain. J Surg Oncol 10:211–219, 1978
4. Buley LE: Incidence, causes, and results of airline pilot incapacitation while on duty. Aerospace Med 40:64–69, 1969
5. Clark L: Melanomas: Basic properties and clinical behavior. V Reilly (ed): S Karger, vol 2, 1972, p 375
6. Cochran AJ: Malignant melanoma. A review of ten years experience in Glasgow, Scotland. Cancer 23:1190–1199, 1969
7. Conrad FG, Rossing RG, Allen MF, Bales HR: Hazard rate of recurrence in patients with malignant melanoma. Aerospace Med 42:1219–1225, 1971
8. Das Gupta T, Brasfield R: Metastatic melanoma: A clinicopathologic study. Cancer 17:1333–1339, 1964
9. Einhorn LH, Burgess MA, Vallejo CV, et al.: Prognostic correlations and response of treatment in advanced metastatic malignant melanoma. Cancer Res 34:1995–2004, 1974
10. Fox H, Emery J, Goodbody RA, Yates PO: Neurocutaneous Melanosis. Arch Dis Child 39:508–516, 1964
11. Gibson JB, Burrows D, Weir WP: Primary melanoma of the meninges. J Pathol Bacteriol 74:419–438, 1957
12. Gottlieb JA, Frei Emil III, Luce JK: An evaluation of the management of patients with cerebral metastases from malignant melanoma. Cancer 29:701–705, 1972
13. Grooms GA, Eilber FR, Morton DL: Failure of adjuvant immunotherapy to prevent central nervous system metastases in melanoma patients. J Surg Oncol 9:147–153, 1977
14. Harkin JC, Reed RJ: Tumors of the peripheral nervous system. fasc 3, 1968
15. Harper CR, Kidera GJ, Cullen JF: Study of simulated airline pilot incapacitation. Phase II. Subtle or partial loss of function. Aerospace Med 42:946–948, 1971
16. Hayward RD: Secondary malignant melanoma of the brain. Clin Oncol 2:227–232, 1976
17. Hilaris B, Raben M, Calabrese AS, Phillips RF,

Henschke UK: The value of radiation therapy for distant metastases from malignant melanoma. Cancer 16:765–773, 1963

18. Kiel FW, Starr LB, Hansen JL: Primary melanoma of the spinal cord. J Neurosurg 18: 616–629, 1961

19. Limas C, Tio FO: Meningeal melanocytoma (melanocytic meningioma). Cancer 30:1286–1294, 1972

20. Luse AS: Electron microscopic studies of brain tumors. Neurology 10:881–905, 1960

21. Lin TH, Cook AW: "Primary" melanoma within spinal canal. NY State J Med 1914–1916, July 15, 1966

22. Lerner AB: Melanin pigmentation. Am J Med 19:902, Dec 1955

23. Mason JK: Previous disease in aircrew killed in flying accidents. Aviat Space Environ Med 48:944–948, 1977

24. Masson P: Pigment cells in man. In Gordon M (ed): Biology of Melanomas, New York, NY Acad Sci, 1948, vol 4, p 15

25. McGovern WJ: Malignant melanoma of the skin and mucous membrane. In Milton CW (ed): Churchill Livingston, 1977, p 140

26. Moseley HS, Nizze A, Morton DL: Disseminated melanoma presenting as a catastrophic event. Aviat Space Environ Med 1342–1346, Nov 1978

27. Nikonova OS, Usova MK: Cerebral melanomas. Arch Nevropat Psikhiat 58:526, 1958 (Russian)

28. Rawles ME: Origin of melanophores and their role in development of color patterns in vertebrates. Physiol Rev 28:383, Oct 1948

29. Ray BS, Foot NC: Primary melanotic tumors of the meninges: resemblance to meningioma. Report of two cases in which operation was performed. Arch Neurol 44:104–117, 1940

30. Reed WB, Becker SW Jr, Nickel WR: Giant pigmented nevi, melanoma, and leptomeningeal melanocytosis. Arch Dermatol 91:100–107, 1965

31. Reyes D, Horrax: Metastatic melanoma of the brain. Report of a case with unusually long survival period following surgical removal. Ann Surg 131:237–242, 1971

32. Scott M: Spontaneous intracerebral hematoma caused by cerebral neoplasm. A report of 8 verified cases. J Neurosurg 42:338–345, 1975

33. Simon N: Intra-arterial irradiation. Bull NY Acad Med 45(4):358–372, 1969

34. Spens N, Parsons H, Begg CF: Primary melanoma of the meninges. NY State J Med Dec 1: 3777–3780, 1962

35. Touraine A: Les mélanoses neurocutanées. Ann Dermatol Syphil 9:489–524, 1949

35a. Verma DS, Spitzer G, Legha S, McCredie KB: Chemoimmunotherapy for meningeal melanocytoma of the thoracic spinal cord. JAMA 242(22):2435, 1979

36. Virchow R: Pigment und diffuse Melanose der Arachnoides. Arch Path Anat 16:180, 1859

37. Zimmerman LE: Melanocytes, melanocytic nevi and melanocytomas. Invest Ophthalmol 41:11–41, 1965

METASTATIC MALIGNANT MELANOMA TO THE LUNGS: PRINCIPLES OF SURGICAL TREATMENT AND RESULTS

IRVING M. ARIEL

The lungs represent a host organ for metastases from the vast majority of cancers including cutaneous melanomas. At Memorial Hospital, the lungs were involved in 70% of 125 autopsies. Einhorn et al.[21] record 87% of autopsies for melanoma revealed metastases to the lung. Patel et al.[31] record the lymph nodes and lungs to be involved in 75% of 216 autopsies. At the Pack Medical Foundation series of 300 autopsies, the lungs were found to be involved in 68% of patients dying from melanoma. Other series report 80% metastases to lungs.[19,28] Das Gupta found the lung to be the only site of metastases in 45 of 652 patients (7%) in patients with stage III melanoma.[19] No characteristic roentgenographic findings distinguish melanoma from other metastases or even certain primary neoplasms.

The notorious reputation for malignant melanoma with its previously low survival rate, the high incidence of metastases to the lungs, and the rarity of solitary metastases, has caused the average physician to consider any lesion of the lung in a patient previously treated for malignant melanoma to have metastases and accordingly to prognosticate a fatal outcome.

Patients with untreated metastases to lungs survive an average of 4.1 months.[27] Treatment by chemotherapy and/or immunotherapy in 39 patients with metastases exclusively to the lungs yield an average survival of ten months with no long-term survivors, as reported by Einhorn et al.

Great credit is owed to Dr. William G. Cahan[10] of Memorial Hospital, New York, for a thorough and critical investigation of the nature of solitary or multiple space-occupying lesions in the lung in patients with varying cancers. Instead of considering every tumor in the lung in a patient previously treated for melanoma as being metastases, four possibilities present themselves and warrant careful diagnostic attempts to determine the true nature of the lesion: (1) a benign lesion, (2) another primary cancer, (3) a primary melanoma, and (4) solitary metastatic melanoma. The following discussion leans heavily upon Cahan's reports.

With the maturation of thoracic surgery, greater attention has been placed upon the possibility of surgical intervention for solitary or even multiple metastases. The first melanoma metastatic to the lung removed at Memorial Hospital was in 1949; between 1949 and 1970, 29 patients have had resections performed for metastatic melanoma. There were 17 males and 12 females. Their ages varied from 24 to 68 years; the average age was 40 years. Nine patients had symptoms of cough, pneumonia, anorexia, weight loss, and chest pain, whereas 30 patients had no symptoms, but the diagnosis was suspected from roentgenograms, ten during a routine follow-up and ten had clinically retrogressed. All of the metastases were metachronous and appeared from 18 months to 16 years after treatment of the primary melanoma. Of the 13 patients with a solitary metastasis who were bronchoscoped, only one presented a positive diagnosis. In four patients with multiple metastases, biopsies in two patients showed melanoma, and one had cytologic evidence of melanoma. The surgical procedures performed consisted of eight wedge resections, eight segmental resections, nine lobectomies, and four pneumonectomies. Three radical pneumonectomies were performed for solitary metastases because of extensive involvement of the right upper lobe, the bronchus, involvement of the hilum, and a large mass in the right lower lobe that also invaded the right middle lobe. One radical pneumonectomy was performed for multiple metastases. Eighteen of their patients had a unilateral solitary metastasis, five had metastases that were unilateral but multiple, and six patients had bilateral multiple metastases, three of whom had synchronous metastases and two metachronous. Five of 18 patients with solitary metastases and four of 11 with multiple metastases had metastases to the pulmonary lymphatics.

Of the 29 patients treated, 19 died within two years after pulmonary excision (nine had solitary and ten had multiple metastases). Six patients survived from two to five years, one with multiple metastases. Of 12 patients who had their pulmonary excisions over five years ago, four are alive and free of evidence of melanoma.

This series emphasizes the situation in handling a suspect of metastases to the lung in a patient previously treated for melanoma. Arce[4] is credited with excising the first pulmonary metastases in 1936. In 1939, Ochsner and DeBakey,[29] and in 1942 Carlucci and Schleussner,[12] reported pneumonectomies. Each of their patients died postoperatively. Interesting features of that report were: (1) One case had had an eye enucleated 23 years before, but no metastases were encountered in the liver, the usual site for metastases from an eye melanoma; (2) the second case had no evidence of a primary tumor. This is not uncommon inasmuch as instances have been reported where the primary melanoma was either so cryptic, or had spontaneously regressed, that it no longer existed (see Chapter 7). The observation of no primary lesion has led to the report by Allen and Drash[3] of the existence of primary melanomas of the lung. Rosenberg, Polanco, and Blank[34] report an instance of multiple tracheal bronchial melanomas with a ten-year survival.

Cahan further reported that during an exploratory thoracotomy performed for presumed metastatic melanoma, nine patients were encountered who had suffered primary lung cancers. A higher incidence of other cancers in patients with malignant melanoma, or presumably cured malignant melanoma has been established.

McCormack and Martini[26a] updated the Memorial Hospital series in 1979. Of 448 patients operated upon with pulmonary metastases from various primary tumors, 40 were melanomas. There were four pneumonectomies, 20 lobectomies, and 20 wedge resections or segmentectomies. The overall five-year survival was 20% for the melanoma group but only those with solitary metastases survived the five-year period.

PRINCIPLES OF THE SURGICAL MANAGEMENT OF SUSPECTED METASTATIC MELANOMA TO THE LUNGS

The surgical management as described by Cahan is as follows: At exploratory thoracotomy, a solitary peripheral lesion that can be encompassed by a wedge or a segmental resection is initially excised for tissue diagnosis. If it proves to be a melanoma metastasis or a primary lung cancer, a radical lobectomy is completed. This is recommended because at least nine (31%) parenchymal melanoma deposits in his series showed no other metastasis to the regional lymphatics. For the same reason, should a metastasis (or a primary lung cancer) involve the main stem bronchus or extensively invade more than one of the major lobes, a radical pneumonectomy is recommended.

Two of his four five-year survivors had metastases in the hilar and mediastinal lymph nodes in the radical lobectomy specimens. Wedge and segmental resections were reserved for poor-risk patients.

Cahan noted no correlation between the time of the development of metastases and survival. Of the five-year survivors, four had metastases removed three, four, four and one-half, and 12 years after removal of the primary. In four other patients the fact that a shadow appeared as long as 11, 12, 15, and 16 years after the primary lesions did not seem to enhance survival, and these patients lived only three, 19, 25, and 28 months, respectively, following pulmonary surgery. Cahan believes that the reappearance of melanoma seems to signal a breakdown or resistance to the cancer and diffuse melanomatoses occurred thereafter. He calls attention to the fact that most patients who succumb to melanomas after pulmonary excision do so within two years, and the prospect is good for his two additional patients who survived 3 and 35 months after surgical resection.

The question of resecting multiple metastases is now being investigated by his group. Since beneficial results have been obtained with excising multiple metastases of osteogenic sarcoma, a similar program pertains. One of six patients with melanoma who had excisions for multiple unilateral metastases lived for more than two years. Six patients had bilateral pulmonary metastases: three synchronous, and three metachronous with each other. Four had unilateral excisions, two bilateral excisions, and died 11 and 25 months postoperatively.

Approximately 20 wedge resections or lobectomies have been performed at the Pack Medical Foundation for metastatic melanoma. The results have been discouraging. One patient with a small melanoma of her chest wall, Clark's level II, was treated by radical surgical resection. Two years later tiny metastases to the left lung necessitated a pneumonectomy. Six months later the patient suffered hemothorax with evidence of disseminated metastases and died within two months. No long survivors have been obtained.

Mathison, Flye, and Peabody[26] from the National Institutes of Health report:

Thirty-three patients over a 21-year period underwent thoracotomy for resection of suspected pulmonary metastases from malignant melanoma. Eleven patients were found to have nonmalignant disease (Group 1); 10 were found to have unresectable disease (Group 2); and 12 were rendered disease-free (Group 3). Of the patients found to have melanoma, 20 of 22 received postoperative chemotherapy. The median survival of the patients in Group 2 was 10.5 months (3 to 20 months); in Group 3 it was 12 months (3 to 35 months). There were no 5-year survivors. No factors distinguished the three groups preoperatively. Surgical resection still offers the greatest chance for long-term survival, based on reports of patients in the literature who have survived longer than 5 years following resection of pulmonary metastases from melanoma. Thoracotomy is especially useful for staging purposes in those patients found to have no metastatic disease.

They record 86 patients from the literature who underwent thoracotomy for melanoma with survival rate available in 71: ten patients (14%) survived less than one year, 32 patients (45%) survived one to two years, 14 patients (20%) survived two to five years, and 15 patients (21%) survived longer than five years. Two of the five-year survivors had two thoracotomies and two had multiple metastatic lesions. Of the 86 patients, 14 (16%) had positive hilar or mediastinal nodes.

Earlier diagnosis by CAT Scanning or isotope scanning (Gallium-61) may lead to earlier diagnosis and better results.

REFERENCES

1. Adkins PC, Wesselhoeft CW Jr, Newman W, et al.: Thoracotomy on the patient with previous malignancy: Metastasis or new primary. J Thorac Cardiovasc Surg 56:351, 1968
2. Alexander J, Haight C: Pulmonary resection for solitary metastatic sarcomas and carcinomas. Surg Gynecol Obstet 85:129, 1947
3. Allen MS Jr, Drash EC: Primary melanoma of the lung. Cancer 154, 1968
4. Arce MJ: Pneumonectomie totale (le tampon-drainage en chirugie endothoracique). Mem Acad Chir 62:1412, 1936
5. Beattie EJ Jr: Thoracotomy and pulmonary metastases (editorial). Ann Thorac Surg 27(4):294, Apr 1979
6. Borrie J: Secondary lung cancer treated surgically: A nine-year study. NZ Med J 69:71, 1969

7. Cahan WG: Excision of melanoma metastases to lung. Ann Surg 178:703, 1973
8. Cahan WG: Multiple primary cancers, one of which is lung. Surg Clin N Am 49(2):323, 1969
9. Cahan WG: Radical lobectomy. J Thorac Cardiovasc Surg 39(5):555, 1960
10. Cahan WG: The surgical management of melanoma metastatic to the lungs: Problems in diagnosis and managing, in Ariel IM (ed): Progress in Clinical Cancer. New York, Grune & Stratton, 1975, vol 6, pp 205–214
11. Cahan WG, Butler F, Watson WL, et al.: Multiple cancers: Primary in the lung and other sites. J Thorac Surg 20(3):355, 1950
12. Carlucci CA, Schleussner RC: Primary (?) melanoma of the lung. A case report. J Thorac Surg 11:643, 1942
13. Choksi L, Takita H, Vincent R: The surgical management of solitary pulmonary metastases. Surg Gynecol Obstet 134:479, 1972
14. Clerf LH: Melanoma of bronchus: Metastasis simulating bronchogenic neoplasm. Ann Otol Rhinol Laryngol 43:85, 1934
15. Cliffton E, Das Gupta T, Pool JL: Bilateral pulmonary resection for primary or metastatic lung cancer. Cancer 17:86, 1964
16. Cline R, Young WG: Long-term results following surgical treatment of metastatic pulmonary tumors. Am Surg 36:61, 1970
17. Creech O: Metastatic melanoma of the lung treated by pulmonary resection: (Report of a case). Med Rec Ann 45:426, 1951
18. Das Gupta T: Metastatic melanoma: A clinicopathologic study. Cancer 17:1325, 1964
19. Das Gupta T, Bowden L, Berg J: Malignant melanoma of unknown primary origin. Surg Gynecol Obstet 117:341, 1963
20. Edlich RF, Shea MA, Foker JE, et al.: A review of 26 years experience with pulmonary resection for metastatic cancer. Dis Chest 49:587, 1966
21. Einhorn LH, Burgess MA, et al.: Prognostic correlations and response to treatment to an advanced metastatic malignant melanoma. Cancer Res 34:1995–2004, 1974
22. Everson TC, Cole WH: Spontaneous regression of cancer: Preliminary report. Ann Surg 144:366, 1956
23. Fallon R: Operative treatment of metastatic pulmonary cancer. Ann Surg 166:263, 1967
24. Gliedman ML, Horowitz S, Lewis FJ: Lung resection for metastatic cancer. Surgery 42:521, 1957
25. Johnson R, Lindskog G: 100 cases of tumor metastatic to lung and mediastinum. JAMA 202:112, 1967
26. Mathisen DJ, Flye MW, Peabody J: The role of thoracotomy in the management of pulmonary metastases from malignant melanoma. Ann Thorac Surg 27(4):295, 1979
26a. McCormack PM, Martini N: The changing role of surgery for pulmonary metastases. Ann Thorac Surg 28(2):139–145, 1979
27. Minor G: A clinical and radiologic study of metastatic pulmonary neoplasms. J Thorac Surg 20:34, 1950
28. Nathanson L: Biologic aspects of human malignant melanoma. Cancer 20:650, 1967
29. Ochsner A, DeBakey M: Primary pulmonary malignancy. Surg Gynecol Obstet 68:435, 1939
30. Ochsner A, Rush V: Treatment of pulmonary metastatic disease. Surg Clin N Am 46:1469, 1966
31. Patel JK: Metastatic pattern of malignant melanoma: a study of 260 autopsied cases. Am J Surg 135:807–815, 1978
32. Polk J, Bailey A, Kalagayan H: Definitive surgery for metastatic lesions to the lung. Am J Surg 110:737, 1965
33. Ramsey HE, Cahan WG, Beattie J, et al.: The importance of radical lobectomy in lung cancer. J Thorac Cardiovasc Surg 58:225, 1969
34. Rosenberg LM, Polanco GB, Blank S: Multiple tracheobronchial melanomas with 10-year survival. JAMA 192:717–719, 1965
35. Turney S, Haight C: Pulmonary resection for metastatic neoplasms. J Thorac Cardiovasc Surg 61:784, 1971
36. Vidne B, Richter LM: Surgical treatment of solitary pulmonary metastasis. Cancer 38:2561, 1976

INDEX

Page numbers in *italics* indicate illustrations and tables.